Imaging Brain Diseases

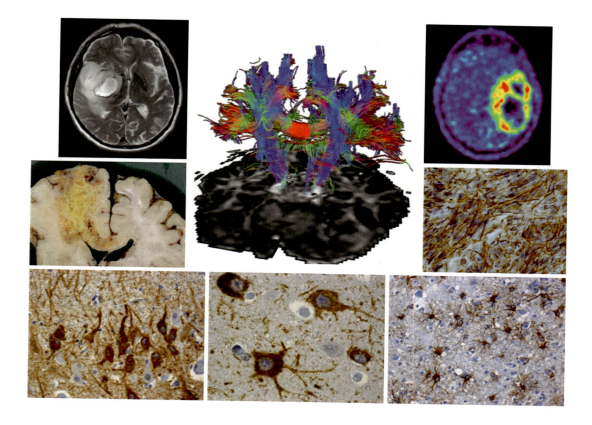

Serge Weis • Michael Sonnberger
Andreas Dunzinger • Eva Voglmayr
Martin Aichholzer • Raimund Kleiser
Peter Strasser

Imaging Brain Diseases

A Neuroradiology, Nuclear Medicine, Neurosurgery, Neuropathology and Molecular Biology-based Approach

Volume I

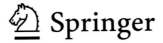

Serge Weis
Division of Neuropathology
Neuromed Campus
Kepler University Hospital
Johannes Kepler University
Linz
Austria

Michael Sonnberger
Department of Neuroradiology
Neuromed Campus
Kepler University Hospital
Johannes Kepler University
Linz
Austria

Andreas Dunzinger
Department of Neuro-Nuclear Medicine
Neuromed Campus
Kepler University Hospital
Johannes Kepler University
Linz
Austria

Eva Voglmayr
Department of Neuroradiology
Neuromed Campus
Kepler University Hospital
Johannes Kepler University
Linz
Austria

Martin Aichholzer
Department of Neurosurgery
Neuromed Campus
Kepler University Hospital
Johannes Kepler University
Linz
Austria

Raimund Kleiser
Department of Neuroradiology
Neuromed Campus
Kepler University Hospital
Johannes Kepler University
Linz
Austria

Peter Strasser
PMU University Institute for Medical &
Chemical Laboratory Diagnostics
Salzburg
Austria

ISBN 978-3-7091-1543-5   ISBN 978-3-7091-1544-2   (eBook)
https://doi.org/10.1007/978-3-7091-1544-2

© Springer-Verlag GmbH Austria, part of Springer Nature 2019

This work is subject to copyright. All rights are reserved by the Publisher, whether the whole or part of the material is concerned, specifically the rights of translation, reprinting, reuse of illustrations, recitation, broadcasting, reproduction on microfilms or in any other physical way, and transmission or information storage and retrieval, electronic adaptation, computer software, or by similar or dissimilar methodology now known or hereafter developed.

The use of general descriptive names, registered names, trademarks, service marks, etc. in this publication does not imply, even in the absence of a specific statement, that such names are exempt from the relevant protective laws and regulations and therefore free for general use.

The publisher, the authors, and the editors are safe to assume that the advice and information in this book are believed to be true and accurate at the date of publication. Neither the publisher nor the authors or the editors give a warranty, expressed or implied, with respect to the material contained herein or for any errors or omissions that may have been made. The publisher remains neutral with regard to jurisdictional claims in published maps and institutional affiliations.

This Springer imprint is published by the registered company Springer-Verlag GmbH, AT part of Springer Nature.
The registered company address is: Prinz-Eugen-Str. 8-10, 1040 Wien, Austria

*Dedicated
to my late mother Louise and my Aunt Marie-Antoinette
for their lifelong generous support and
to Denisa for our future adventures*
(Serge Weis)

to my brother Geri
(Michael Sonnberger)

*Dedicated
to my parents for their support and encouragement and
to my daughter Ella the sunshine of my life*
(Andreas Dunzinger)

*For my wife, my sons, and my daughter.
Thank you for being here with me, you make my life
worth living …*
(Peter Strasser)

Preface

The present book deals with picturing various diseases of the human nervous system using different imaging modalities. The appearances of the diseases are visualized on computerized tomography (CT) scans, magnetic resonance imaging (MRI) scans, nuclear medicine scans, surgical intraoperative pictures, gross anatomy, histology, and immunohistochemistry pictures. It is aimed at attracting the interest of neurologists, neuroradiologists, neurosurgeons, and neuropathologists as well as all allied neuroscientific disciplines. The information provided should facilitate the understanding of the disease processes in their daily routine work.

There exist many good and detailed books on the neuroradiologic aspects of brain diseases. Although these books contain hundreds of CT and MR scans, no histologic picture disclosing the microscopic features of the disorders dealt with is included. On the other hand, there exist excellent books describing the neuropathological features of brain disorders. Again, many light and electron microscopic pictures are included; however, the neuroradiologic scans are sparse or lacking. The correlative combination of nuclear medicine scans with either neuroradiologic scans or neuropathology images is nearly absent. The present book is, hence, an attempt to bridge the gap between neuro-clinicians, neuro-imagers, and neuropathologists.

It is our intention to present the brain disorders in a very systematic way allowing the reader to easily find the topics in which she or he is particularly interested. Although it might be considered monotonous, we feel that this approach is an effective didactic way in presenting data which can quickly be retrieved.

The book starts with a description of the various imaging modalities, i.e. computerized tomography and nuclear magnetic resonance imaging (Chap. 1). Here, the tremendous advances achieved during the last two decades are illustrated with the wealth of new imaging techniques available for daily routine diagnosis like spectroscopy, perfusion imaging, diffusion weighted imaging, and diffusion tensor imaging. Nuclear medicine imaging (Chap. 2) aims at representing the functional/metabolic state of the brain using different techniques (SPECT, PET) and applying various tracers like methionine, fluordeoxyglucose, fluorethyltyrosine, etc. in order to visualize various biochemical pathways (i.e., transmitter, amino acids, glucose). Chapter 3 describes the neuropathological approach for analyzing brain diseases. The cellular and tissue components of the normal nervous system are presented. The immunohistochemical typing of the various cells which make up the nervous system is presented in detail. A detailed description of the normal human brain and its vascular supply is provided in Chaps. 4–14 of Part II.

The subsequent chapters (Chaps. 15–83) of Part III to Part X deal with the various disorders involving the nervous system which can be grouped into the following disorders: hemodynamic (Chaps. 15 and 16), vascular (Chaps. 17–24), infectious (Chaps. 25–29), neurodegenerative (Chaps. 30–40), demyelination (Chaps. 41–43), epilepsy (Chaps. 44 and 45), trauma and intoxication (Chaps. 46–48), and the vast field of tumors (Chaps. 49–83).

The approach in presenting a brain disease entity is in the following order: brief definition of the entity, relative incidence, age incidence, sex incidence, predilection sites of the lesion, description of the characteristic CT findings with representative CT scans, description of the characteristic MRI findings with representative MRI scans, nuclear medicine findings, macroscopic features including intraoperative findings, microscopic features, ultrastructural features, immunohistochemical staining characteristics, spectrum of reactivities to proliferation markers, differential diagnosis, pathogenesis and molecular biological characteristics, treatment, and biologic behavior, prognosis, and prognostic factors.

Although molecular biology was and is undoubtedly the scientific trendsetter during the last decades and for the forthcoming years, however, some doubts about the promises made by medical molecular biologists are appropriate. In the future, people will see bands on blots, but they will not see anymore the cell, the tissue, and the organism and finally not anymore the patient. Okazaki in his *Fundamentals of Neuropathology* expressed the same opinion as follows: "Many residents are intelligent and well versed in the latest molecular biologic concepts or neurochemical advances, but they often have difficulties in recognizing actual brain lesions or interpreting histologic findings."

Furthermore, we want to impart to our young colleagues a sound and comprehensive knowledge on diseases involving the nervous system. Through this schematic, straightforward presentation, the aspiring clinical neuroscientist in training will hopefully not undergo the same frustrations that we experienced.

Special thanks are expressed to Johannes Trenkler, M.D. (Head, Department of Radiology); Robert Pichler, M.D., Ph.D. (Head, Department of Nuclear Medicine); and Prof. Andreas Gruber, M.D., Ph.D. (Head, Department of Neurosurgery), at the Neuromed Campus of the Kepler University Hospital (formerly Landes-Nervenklinik Wagner-Jauregg) for their fruitful collaboration. Dr. Weis thanks his medical team including Ognian Kalev, M.D. (senior consultant); Karoline Ornig, M.D. (trainee); and Dave Bandke, M.D., B.S.A. (trainee), for providing interesting cases. The help of Michaela Gnauer, clinical psychologist, for reviewing Chap. 14 is highly appreciated.

Finally, the authors acknowledge the skillful technical help of the following medical technologists (in alphabetical order):

- In neuropathology: Sabine Engstler, Susanne Fiedler, Gabriele Göberl, Christina Keuch, Anna Kroiss, Monika Lugmayr, and Christa Winter-Schwarz. Special thanks are necessary to appreciate the diligent work of Stefan Pirngruber as best mortuary technician and archivist of the histological blocks and sections. Birgit Kronfuss helped with secretarial work.
- In Neurosurgery: Hans-Peter Dahl, Franz Knogler, and Thomas Wimmer for registering the intraoperative images. Hans-Peter was very helpful with annotating some images.
- In neuroradiology: to the whole team of radiotechnologists (too many to name).
- In neuronuclear medicine: to the whole team of radiotechnologists (especially Silke Kern for her technical knowledge and her good memory of patients).

The authors thank Mag. Barbara Pfeiffer (Vienna), Claus-Dieter Bachem (Heidelberg), Andrea Ridolfi (Turin), Abha Krishnan, Jeyaraj Allwynkingsly, and Shanjini Rajasekaran (Chennai) from Springer-Verlag Wien, New York, for a smooth and perfect collaboration.

Linz, Austria	Serge Weis
Linz, Austria	Michael Sonnberger
Linz, Austria	Andreas Dunzinger
Linz, Austria	Eva Voglmayr
Linz, Austria	Martin Aichholzer
Linz, Austria	Raimund Kleiser
Salzburg, Austria	Peter Strasser

Contents

Volume I

Part I The Techniques

1 Imaging Modalities: Neuroradiology 3
   1.1   Introduction 3
   1.2   CT-Imaging 4
       1.2.1   Equipment 4
       1.2.2   Image Presentation. 5
       1.2.3   Characteristics of CT-Imaging. 6
       1.2.4   Contrast and Details Resolution. 6
       1.2.5   Artifacts 6
       1.2.6   Contrast Medium. 6
       1.2.7   Recent Developments and Trends 6
       1.2.8   CT-Angiography 7
       1.2.9   CT-Perfusion 7
   1.3   MR Imaging. 9
       1.3.1   Equipment 9
       1.3.2   Image Presentation. 9
       1.3.3   Characteristics of MR Imaging 11
       1.3.4   Contrast and Details Resolution. 13
       1.3.5   Imaging Protocols 13
       1.3.6   Artifacts 14
       1.3.7   Contrast Medium. 14
       1.3.8   Recent Developments and Trends 15
       1.3.9   MR Spectroscopy. 15
       1.3.10 MR Angiography 16
       1.3.11 MR-Perfusion Imaging 18
       1.3.12 MR Diffusion-Weighted Imaging (DWI). 19
       1.3.13 MR Diffusion Tensor Imaging (DTI). 19
       1.3.14 Functional MRI (fMRI). 20
       1.3.15 Neuronavigation and Intraoperative MRI 22
       1.3.16 Imaging Protocol Lists. 27
   Selected References 28

2 Imaging Modalities: Nuclear Medicine 29
2.1 Introduction 29
2.2 SPECT: Single Photon Emission Computed Tomography 39
2.3 PET—Positron Emission Tomography 42
2.4 FDG-PET 44
2.5 Amino Acid PET 48
2.6 123I-FP-CIT 49
2.7 D2 Receptor Ligands 50
2.8 Brain Perfusion SPECT 51
2.9 Amyloid Imaging 53
2.10 Indications for Nuclear Medicine Examinations 54
Selected References 55

3 Imaging Modalities: Neuropathology 57
3.1 Introduction 57
3.2 Removal, Fixation, and Cutting of the Brain and Spinal Cord 58
  3.2.1 Removal and Fixation of the Brain 58
  3.2.2 Removal and Fixation of the Spinal Cord 63
  3.2.3 Brain Cutting 65
  3.2.4 Gross Anatomical Examination of the Cut Brain 74
  3.2.5 Sampling of Brain Regions for Microscopic Examination 75
  3.2.6 Handling of Surgical Specimens 75
3.3 Fixation and Processing of Tissue 76
  3.3.1 Fixation of Sampled Tissue 76
  3.3.2 Processing of Tissue 78
3.4 Staining of Tissue 79
  3.4.1 Classical Stain 79
  3.4.2 Special Stains 83
  3.4.3 Special Neuro-stains 84
  3.4.4 Special Stains for Connective Tissue 87
  3.4.5 Other Special Stains 89
3.5 Immunohistochemistry 89
  3.5.1 General Principles 89
  3.5.2 Neuronal Markers 92
  3.5.3 Synaptic Markers 95
  3.5.4 Astroglial Markers 96
  3.5.5 Oligodendroglial Markers: Myelin Markers 97
  3.5.6 Microglial Markers 99
  3.5.7 Markers for Neurodegeneration 100
  3.5.8 Tumor Markers 102
  3.5.9 Vascular Markers 103
  3.5.10 Hematopoietic and Lymphatic Markers 105
  3.5.11 Proliferation Markers in Tumors 105
  3.5.12 Markers for Infectious Agents 107
  3.5.13 Immunohistochemical Panels 108

3.6	Other Techniques		108
	3.6.1	Electron Microscopy	108
	3.6.2	Fluorescence Microscopy	108
	3.6.3	Enzyme Histochemistry	108
	3.6.4	*In Situ* Hybridization (ISH)	111
	3.6.5	Molecular Biology	111
	3.6.6	Other Imaging Techniques	114
Selected References			114

Part II The Normal Human Brain

4 Subdivisions of the Nervous System 121
    4.1 Central Nervous System (CNS) and Peripheral
        Nervous System (PNS) 121
        4.1.1 Central Nervous System (CNS) 121
        4.1.2 Peripheral Nervous System (PNS) 122
    4.2 Cerebrospinal and Autonomic Nervous System 122
        4.2.1 Cerebrospinal Nervous System 122
        4.2.2 Autonomic Nervous System 123
    4.3 Cortical Areas 123
        4.3.1 Somatotopic Organization 123
        4.3.2 Primary Cortical Areas 123
        4.3.3 Secondary Cortical Areas 123
    4.4 Gray and White Matter 125
        4.4.1 Gray Matter 125
        4.4.2 White Matter 125
        4.4.3 Nuclei and Ganglia 125
        4.4.4 Tracts 125
        4.4.5 Neuropil 125
    Selected References 127

5 Gross Anatomy of the Nervous System 129
    5.1 Subdivisions of the Central Nervous System 129
    5.2 Telencephalon 129
        5.2.1 Superolateral Surface 131
        5.2.2 Medial Surface 135
        5.2.3 Inferior Surface 136
    5.3 Limbic System 137
    5.4 Hippocampal Formation 138
    5.5 Amygdala 142
    5.6 Basal Ganglia 143
        5.6.1 Caudate Nucleus 144
        5.6.2 Globus Pallidus 145
        5.6.3 Putamen 145
        5.6.4 Nucleus Accumbens 145
    5.7 White Matter 146
        5.7.1 Projection Fibers 147
        5.7.2 Association Fibers 147
        5.7.3 Commissural Fibers 148

	5.8	Diencephalon	150
		5.8.1 Thalamus	150
		5.8.2 Hypothalamus	153
		5.8.3 Subthalamus	155
		5.8.4 Epithalamus	155
	5.9	Mesencephalon	156
	5.10	Pons	156
	5.11	Medulla Oblongata	160
	5.12	Cerebellum	162
	5.13	Spinal Cord	163
	5.14	Pituitary Gland	164
	5.15	3D Reconstructions of the Brain and Cutplanes	166
		Selected References	168
6	**Ventricular System: Cerebrospinal Fluid (CSF)—Barriers**		169
	6.1	Introduction	169
	6.2	Ventricular System	169
		6.2.1 Lateral Ventricles	169
		6.2.2 Third Ventricle	174
		6.2.3 Fourth Ventricle	174
	6.3	Cerebrospinal Fluid (CSF)	174
	6.4	Choroid Plexus	176
	6.5	Barriers	176
		6.5.1 The Blood–Brain Barrier (BBB)	176
		6.5.2 The Brain–Liquor Barrier (BLB)	176
		6.5.3 The Blood–Liquor Barrier	176
		Selected References	177
7	**Meninges**		179
	7.1	Introduction	179
	7.2	Dura Mater	179
	7.3	Dural Sinuses	182
	7.4	Arachnoidea	186
	7.5	Pia Mater	186
	7.6	The Meningeal Spaces	188
	7.7	Arachnoidal Granulations	188
		Selected References	189
8	**Arterial Supply of the Brain**		191
	8.1	Introduction	191
	8.2	Carotid System	191
	8.3	Vertebro-Basilar System	199
	8.4	Clinical Vascular Syndromes	202
		8.4.1 Anterior Cerebral Artery Syndrome	202
		8.4.2 Middle Cerebral Artery Syndrome	208
		8.4.3 AICA Syndrome (Lateral Pontine Syndrome)	208
		8.4.4 Posterior Inferior Cerebellar Artery Syndrome (PICA Syndrome)	208
		8.4.5 Posterior Cerebral Artery Syndrome	209
		Selected References	209

9	**Venous Drainage of the Brain**	211
9.1	Introduction	211
9.2	Venous System	211
9.3	Dural Venous Sinuses	218
	Selected References	224

10	**Histological Constituents of the Nervous System**	225
10.1	Neuron	225
	10.1.1 Classification of Neurons	229
	10.1.2 Size of Neurons	231
	10.1.3 Types of Neuronal Connection	231
10.2	Synapse	232
	10.2.1 The Presynaptic Membrane	232
	10.2.2 The Postsynaptic Membrane	234
	10.2.3 The Synaptic Cleft	234
	10.2.4 Types of synapses	234
	10.2.5 Classification of synapses	235
10.3	Nerve Fibers and Peripheral Nerve	236
	10.3.1 Morphological Features of Nerve Fibers	236
	10.3.2 Classification of Nerve Fibers	238
	10.3.3 Structure of Peripheral Nerves	238
10.4	Glial Cells	239
10.5	Astroglia (Astrocytes)	240
10.6	Oligodendroglia (Oligodendrocytes)	245
10.7	Microglia	247
10.8	Ependymal Cells	249
10.9	Tanycytes	250
10.10	Molecular Composition of White Matter Myelin	250
	10.10.1 Lipids	250
	10.10.2 Myelin Basic Protein (MBP)	250
	10.10.3 Proteolipid Protein (PLP)	250
	10.10.4 Myelin-Associated Glycoprotein (MAG)	250
	10.10.5 Myelin Oligodendrocyte Glycoprotein (MOG)	251
	10.10.6 2′,3′-Cyclic Nucleotide 3′-Phosphodiesterase (CNP)	251
	10.10.7 Myelin Oligodendrocyte Basic Protein (MOBP)	251
	10.10.8 Other CNS Myelin Proteins	252
10.11	Meninges	252
	10.11.1 Dura mater	252
	10.11.2 Arachnoidea	252
	10.11.3 Pia Mater	252
	10.11.4 Sinuses	254
10.12	Choroid Plexus	254
10.13	Vessels	254
	10.13.1 Artery	255
	10.13.2 Arteriole	255
	10.13.3 Capillary	256
	10.13.4 Venule and Vein	258

		10.13.5	Endothelium	258
		10.13.6	Glymphatic System	259
	10.14	Neurovascular Unit		259
	Selected References			261

11 Microscopical Buildup of the Nervous System 267
    11.1 Cerebral Cortex 267
        11.1.1 Architectonics 269
        11.1.2 Layers and Networks of the Cerebral Cortex. 282
    11.2 Hippocampus. 294
        11.2.1 Cornu Ammonis (Hippocampus Proper) 295
        11.2.2 Gyrus Dentatus (Fascia Dentata, Gyrus Involutus). 299
        11.2.3 Entorhinal Cortex. 300
        11.2.4 Nucleus Basalis Meynert 300
    11.3 Amygdala. 300
    11.4 White Matter 301
    11.5 Basal Ganglia. 301
        11.5.1 Caudate Nucleus and Putamen. 301
        11.5.2 Globus Pallidus 304
    11.6 Diencephalon. 305
        11.6.1 Thalamus 305
        11.6.2 Hypothalamus 306
    11.7 Mesencephalon 306
        11.7.1 Substantia Nigra. 307
        11.7.2 Nucleus Ruber 308
    11.8 Pons 310
    11.9 Medulla Oblongata. 311
        11.9.1 Area Postrema 312
        11.9.2 Pyramis 312
        11.9.3 Inferior Olivary Complex. 313
    11.10 Cerebellum. 313
    11.11 Spinal Cord 318
    11.12 Ventricular System. 321
        11.12.1 Ventricular Lining 321
        11.12.2 Choroid Plexus. 321
    Selected References 323

12 Functional Systems 325
    12.1 Introduction 325
    12.2 Sensory System: Visual System. 325
    12.3 Motor System: Central Motor System. 333
        12.3.1 Corticospinal Tract. 333
    12.4 Motor System: Basal Ganglionic System 333
    12.5 Sensory System: Somatosensory System. 333
    12.6 Cerebral Cortex 341
    12.7 Limbic System. 342
    12.8 Hippocampal System. 345
        12.8.1 Polysynaptic Intrahippocampal Pathway. 345
        12.8.2 Direct Intrahippocampal Pathway 348
        12.8.3 Regulatory Circuits 348

	12.9 Amygdalar System.	349
	12.10 Cerebellum.	349
	12.11 Thalamic System	351
	12.12 Hypothalamus and Hypophyseal System.	351
	12.13 Two-stream Hypothesis	355
	12.13.1 Visual System: Two-Stream Hypothesis	355
	12.13.2 Ventral Stream	357
	12.13.3 Dorsal Stream.	360
	12.14 The Connectome	360
	12.15 Rich-Club Organization.	363
	Selected References	366
13	**Neurotransmitter Systems**	369
	13.1 Acetylcholine.	373
	13.2 Catecholamines Monoamines	376
	13.2.1 Dopamine.	376
	13.2.2 Noradrenaline.	381
	13.2.3 Monoamines: Adrenaline.	384
	13.2.4 Monoamines: Serotonin.	385
	13.3 Amino Acids	388
	13.3.1 γ-Aminobutyric Acid (GABA)	388
	13.3.2 Glutamic Acid (Glu)	391
	Selected References	395
14	**Localization of Brain Function**	401
	14.1 Frontal Cortex	403
	14.1.1 Primary Motor Cortex	403
	14.1.2 Supplementary Motor Area	403
	14.1.3 Premotor Cortex.	403
	14.1.4 Prefrontal Cortex (Frontal Association Cortex).	403
	14.1.5 Frontal Pole: Orbitofrontal Area	404
	14.1.6 Mesial Aspect: Cingulate Gyrus	404
	14.2 Parietal Cortex	404
	14.2.1 Primary Somatosensory Cortex	404
	14.2.2 Secondary Somatosensory Cortex	405
	14.2.3 Somatosensory Association Area.	405
	14.2.4 Postcentral Gyrus.	405
	14.2.5 Superior and Inferior Parietal Lobules.	405
	14.2.6 Supramarginal and Angular Gyri	405
	14.2.7 Angular Gyrus	406
	14.2.8 Mesial Aspect: Cuneus.	406
	14.3 Occipital Cortex.	406
	14.3.1 Primary Visual Cortex	406
	14.3.2 Visual Association Cortex	406
	14.3.3 Mesial Aspect.	406
	14.3.4 Lateral Aspect	407
	14.4 Temporal Cortex	408
	14.4.1 Primary Auditory Cortex	408
	14.4.2 Auditory Association Cortex	408

		14.4.3	Inferomedial Aspect (Amygdala and Hippocampus)	408

- 14.4.3 Inferomedial Aspect (Amygdala and Hippocampus) 408
- 14.4.4 Anterior Tip (Including Amygdala; Bilateral Lesions) 408
- 14.4.5 Latero-inferior Aspect 408
- 14.4.6 Latero-superior Aspect 408
- 14.4.7 Non-localizing 409
- 14.4.8 With Epileptogenic Lesions 409
- 14.5 Language Areas 409
- 14.6 Cortical Syndromes 412
- 14.7 Limbic System 413
  - 14.7.1 Hippocampus 413
  - 14.7.2 Amygdala 413
  - 14.7.3 Stria Terminalis 413
  - 14.7.4 Septal Nuclei 413
  - 14.7.5 Cingulate Cortex 413
- 14.8 Corpus Callosum 413
- 14.9 Basal Ganglia 415
- 14.10 Thalamus 416
- 14.11 Hypothalamus 417
- 14.12 Cerebellum 418
- 14.13 White Matter 419
- Selected References 422

Part III The Brain Diseases: Edema and Hydrocephalus

15 Brain Edema: Intracranial Pressure—Herniation 427
- 15.1 Definition 427
- 15.2 Epidemiology 427
- 15.3 Localization 428
- 15.4 General Imaging Findings 428
- 15.5 Neuropathology Findings 434
  - 15.5.1 Microscopic Features 439
  - 15.5.2 Ultrastructural Features 440
- 15.6 Molecular Neuropathology 440
- 15.7 Treatment and Prognosis 441
- Selected References 441

16 Hydrocephalus 443
- 16.1 Definition 443
- 16.2 Clinical Signs and Symptoms 443
- 16.3 Epidemiology 443
- 16.4 General Imaging Findings 444
- 16.5 Neuropathology Findings 449
- 16.6 Molecular Neuropathology 451
- 16.7 Treatment and Prognosis 451
- Selected References 451

Part IV The Brain Diseases: Vascular system

17 Vascular Disorders: Hypoxia 455
   17.1   Introduction 455
   17.2   Clinical Signs. 456
   17.3   Epidemiology. 456
   17.4   Neuroimaging Findings 456
   17.5   Neuropathology Findings. 463
   17.6   Molecular Neuropathology 466
   17.7   Treatment and Prognosis 470
   Selected References 470

18 Vascular Disorders: Ischemia–Infarction–Stroke 473
   18.1   Introduction 473
   18.2   Clinical Signs and Symptoms 473
   18.3   Epidemiology. 474
   18.4   Neuroimaging Findings 477
   18.5   Neuropathology Findings. 484
   18.6   Molecular Neuropathology 489
   18.7   Treatment and Prognosis 496
   Selected References 496

19 Vascular Disorders: Hemorrhage 499
   19.1   General Considerations 499
   19.2   Intracerebral Hemorrhage 500
         19.2.1   Clinical Signs and Symptoms 500
         19.2.2   Epidemiology. 500
         19.2.3   Neuroimaging Findings 500
         19.2.4   Neuropathology Findings. 501
         19.2.5   Molecular Neuropathology 501
         19.2.6   Treatment and Prognosis 503
   19.3   Subarachnoid Hemorrhage (SAH). 505
         19.3.1   Clinical Signs and Symptoms 505
         19.3.2   Epidemiology. 505
         19.3.3   Neuroimaging Findings 505
         19.3.4   Neuropathology Findings. 510
         19.3.5   Molecular Neuropathology 514
         19.3.6   Treatment and Prognosis 514
   19.4   Subdural Hemorrhage 520
         19.4.1   Clinical Signs and Symptoms 520
         19.4.2   Epidemiology. 520
         19.4.3   Neuroimaging Findings 520
         19.4.4   Neuropathology Findings. 521
         19.4.5   Molecular Neuropathology 522
         19.4.6   Treatment and Prognosis 524
   19.5   Epidural Hemorrhage (EDH). 529
         19.5.1   Clinical Signs and Symptoms 529
         19.5.2   Localization 529
         19.5.3   Neuroimaging Findings 529

		19.5.4	Neuropathology Findings.	530
		19.5.5	Molecular Neuropathology	530
		19.5.6	Treatment and Prognosis	533
	Selected References			533
20	**Vascular Disorders: Arteriosclerosis**			**537**
	20.1	Introduction		537
	20.2	Epidemiology		537
	20.3	Neuroimaging Findings		538
	20.4	Neuropathology Findings		538
	20.5	Molecular Neuropathology		540
	20.6	Treatment and Prognosis		542
	Selected References			548
21	**Vascular Disorders: Aneurysms**			**551**
	21.1	Definition		551
	21.2	Epidemiology		551
	21.3	Neuroimaging Findings		551
	21.4	Neuropathology Findings		552
	21.5	Molecular Neuropathology		558
	21.6	Treatment and Prognosis		570
	Selected References			576
22	**Vascular Disorders: Malformations**			**577**
	22.1	Introduction		577
	22.2	Arteriovenous Malformation (AVM)		577
		22.2.1	Epidemiology	577
		22.2.2	Neuroimaging Findings	577
		22.2.3	Neuropathology Findings	578
		22.2.4	Molecular Neuropathology	584
		22.2.5	Treatment and Prognosis	585
	22.3	Cavernous Hemangioma (Cavernoma)		585
		22.3.1	Epidemiology	585
		22.3.2	Neuroimaging Findings	585
		22.3.3	Neuropathology Findings	586
		22.3.4	Molecular Neuropathology	586
		22.3.5	Treatment and Prognosis	586
	22.4	Capillary Telangiectasia		593
		22.4.1	Epidemiology	593
		22.4.2	Neuroimaging Findings	596
		22.4.3	Neuropathology Findings	596
		22.4.4	Molecular Neuropathology	596
		22.4.5	Treatment and Prognosis	596
	22.5	Dural AV-Fistula		599
		22.5.1	Neuroimaging Findings	599
	Selected References			603
23	**Vascular Disorders: Angiopathies**			**605**
	23.1	Introduction		605
	23.2	Cerebral Amyloid Angiopathy		605
		23.2.1	Clinical Signs and Symptoms	605
		23.2.2	Epidemiology	606

		23.2.3	Neuroimaging Findings	606

			23.2.3	Neuroimaging Findings	606
			23.2.4	Neuropathology Findings	607
			23.2.5	Molecular Neuropathology	607
			23.2.6	Treatment and Prognosis	615
	23.3	Binswanger Disease			615
			23.3.1	Clincal Signs and Symptoms	615
			23.3.2	Epidemiology	616
			23.3.3	Neuroimaging Findings	616
			23.3.4	Neuropathology Findings	616
			23.3.5	Molecular Neuropathology	622
			23.3.6	Treatment and Prognosis	622
	23.4	Fahr Disease			622
			23.4.1	Clinical Signs and Symptoms	622
			23.4.2	Localisation	622
			23.4.3	Neuroimaging Findings	622
			23.4.4	Neuropathology Findings	622
			23.4.5	Molecular Neuropathology	626
			23.4.6	Treatment and Prognosis	626
	23.5	Cerebral Autosomal Dominant Arteriopathy (CADASIL)			626
			23.5.1	Clinical Signs and Symptoms	626
			23.5.2	Epidemiology	627
			23.5.3	Neuroimaging Findings	627
			23.5.4	Neuropathology Findings	628
			23.5.5	Molecular Neuropathology	632
			23.5.6	Treatment and Prognosis	632
	Selected References				633
24	**Vascular Disorders: Vasculitis**				635
	24.1	Definition			635
	24.2	Clinical Signs and Symptoms			636
	24.3	Epidemiology			637
	24.4	Neuroimaging Findings			637
	24.5	Neuropathology Findings			641
	24.6	Molecular Neuropathology			641
	24.7	Treatment and Prognosis			649
	Selected References				649

Part V   The Brain Diseases: Infections

25	**Infections: Bacteria**			653
	25.1	Clinical Signs and Symptoms		653
	25.2	Classification of Bacteria		653
	25.3	General Aspects		655
	25.4	Epidemiology		655
	25.5	Imaging Features		657
		25.5.1	Meningitis	657
		25.5.2	Encephalitis	661
		25.5.3	Brain Abscess	661
		25.5.4	Subdural Empyema	663

	25.6	Neuropathology Findings.	666
	25.7	Molecular Neuropathology	687
	25.8	Treatment and Prognosis	690
	Selected References		691

26 Infections: Viruses. 693

- 26.1 Clinical Signs and Symptoms 693
- 26.2 Classification of Viruses. 693
- 26.3 Epidemiology. 693
- 26.4 Neuroimaging Findings 696
- 26.5 Neuropathology Findings. 697
- 26.6 Molecular Neuropathology 698
- 26.7 Treatment and Prognosis 699
- 26.8 Unspecified Nodular Encephalitis 699
- 26.9 RNA Viruses: Human Immunodeficiency Virus (HIV)-1. 700
  - 26.9.1 HIV-1 Encephalitis (HIVE) 702
  - 26.9.2 HIV-1 Leukoencephalopathy (HIVL) 703
  - 26.9.3 Lymphocytic Meningitis (LM) and Perivascular Lymphocytic Infiltration (PLI) 703
  - 26.9.4 Vacuolar Myelopathy (VM) and Vacuolar Leukoencephalopathy (VL). 706
  - 26.9.5 Neuropathological Changes in Early Stages of HIV-1 Infection 706
  - 26.9.6 Neuropathological Changes in HIV-1-Infected Children 708
  - 26.9.7 Therapy: HAART Effects and Therapy-Induced Immune Restitution Inflammatory Syndrome (IRIS). 710
  - 26.9.8 The Sequalae of HIV-1 Infection of the Nervous System. 715
  - 26.9.9 Pathogenetic Mechanisms 717
- 26.10 DNA-Virus: Cytomegalovirus Infection (CMV) 720
  - 26.10.1 Neuroradiology Findings. 720
  - 26.10.2 Neuropathology Findings. 720
- 26.11 Progressive Multifocal Leukoencephalopathy (PML). 722
  - 26.11.1 Clinical Signs and Symptoms 722
  - 26.11.2 Neuroimaging Findings 725
  - 26.11.3 Neuropathology Findings. 725
  - 26.11.4 Molecular Nauropathology 730
- 26.12 Herpes Simplex Virus (HSV) Encephalitis 731
  - 26.12.1 Clinical Signs and Symptoms 731
  - 26.12.2 Neuroimaging Findings 731
  - 26.12.3 Neuropathology Findings. 736
  - 26.12.4 Molecular Neuropathology 736
  - 26.12.5 Treatment and Prognosis 736
- 26.13 Tick-Borne Encephalitis 736
  - 26.13.1 Clinical Signs and Symptoms 736
  - 26.13.2 Epidemiology. 737
  - 26.13.3 Neuroimaging Findings 737

		26.13.4	Neuropathology Findings.	739
		26.13.5	Molecular Neuropathology	741
		26.13.6	Treatment and Prognosis	742
	Selected References			742
27	**Infections: Parasites**			**749**
	27.1	Classification of Parasitic Agents.		749
	27.2	Clinical Signs and Symptoms		749
	27.3	*Toxoplasma gondii*		749
		27.3.1	Clinical Signs and Symptoms	749
		27.3.2	Epidemiology	751
		27.3.3	Neuroimaging Findings	752
		27.3.4	Neuropathology Findings.	752
		27.3.5	Molecular Neuropathology	752
		27.3.6	Treatment and Prognosis	756
	27.4	Taeniasis: Coenurosis/Cysticercosis		762
		27.4.1	Cysticercosis: Clinical Signs and Symptoms.	762
		27.4.2	Coenurosis: Clinical Signs and Symptoms	762
		27.4.3	Epidemiology	763
		27.4.4	Neuroimaging Findings	763
		27.4.5	Neuropathology Findings.	767
		27.4.6	Molecular Neuropathology	768
		27.4.7	Treatment and Prognosis	771
	Selected References			771
28	**Infections: Fungi**			**773**
	28.1	General Aspects		773
		28.1.1	Clinical Signs and Symptoms	773
		28.1.2	Epidemiology	773
		28.1.3	Classification of Fungi	773
		28.1.4	Neuroimaging Findings	775
		28.1.5	Neuropathology Stains	776
		28.1.6	Molecular Neuropathology	776
		28.1.7	Treatment	776
	28.2	*Aspergillus Fumigatus*		777
		28.2.1	Neuroimaging Findings	777
		28.2.2	Neuropathology Findings.	778
		28.2.3	Molecular Neuropathology	781
	28.3	*Cryptococcus Neoformans*		782
		28.3.1	Neuroimaging Findings	782
		28.3.2	Neuropathology Findings.	785
		28.3.3	Molecular Neuropathology	785
	28.4	*Candida Albicans*		787
		28.4.1	Neuropathology Findings.	787
		28.4.2	Molecular Pathology	787
	Selected References			793
29	**Prion Encephalopathies**			**797**
	29.1	General Aspects		797
		29.1.1	Clinical Signs and Symptoms	799
		29.1.2	Neuroimaging Findings	799
		29.1.3	Neuropathology Findings.	804

	29.1.4	Treatment and Prognosis	816
	29.1.5	Molecular Neuropathology	816
29.2	Creutzfeldt–Jakob Disease (CJD)		818
	29.2.1	Clinical Signs	818
	29.2.2	Macroscopic Features	819
	29.2.3	Microscopic Features	819
29.3	Variant CJD		820
	29.3.1	Clinical Signs and Symptoms	820
	29.3.2	Microscopic Features	821
	29.3.3	Molecular Neuropathology	821
29.4	Gerstmann–Sträussler–Scheinker Disease (GSS)		821
	29.4.1	Clinical signs	821
	29.4.2	Microscopic Features	821
29.5	Fatal Familial Insomnia (FFI)		822
	29.5.1	Clinical signs	822
	29.5.2	Microscopic Features	822
29.6	Kuru		822
	29.6.1	Clinical signs	822
	29.6.2	Macroscopical Features	822
	29.6.3	Microscopical Features	822
Selected References			823

Volume II

Part VI The Brain Diseases: Aging and Neurodegeneration

30 Neurodegeneration: General Aspects ... 827

30.1	Introduction		827
30.2	Clinical Signs and Symptoms		827
	30.2.1	Dementia	828
	30.2.2	Motor Disorders	830
30.3	Neuropathologic Changes		830
	30.3.1	Gross-anatomical Changes	830
	30.3.2	Microscopical Changes	830
	30.3.3	Amyloid Deposits	830
	30.3.4	Neurofibrillary Changes: Tauopathies	838
	30.3.5	Neuropil Threads	839
	30.3.6	Lewy Bodies	839
	30.3.7	Granulovacuolar Degeneration	840
	30.3.8	Ballooned Neurons	840
	30.3.9	Histological Visualization of Amyloid Deposits and Tangles	841
	30.3.10	Immunohistochemical Pattern in the Differential Diagnosis	844
	30.3.11	Frequencies of Neuropathology Diagnoses	844
30.4	Comparisons		844
30.5	Molecular Neuropathology		844
	30.5.1	Concepts of Neurodegenerative Diseases	844
	30.5.2	Relevant Proteins	846

		30.5.3	Amyloid and the Amyloid Cascade Hypothesis	847
		30.5.4	Tau	849
		30.5.5	Synuclein (α-Syn)	849
		30.5.6	TDP-43	851
		30.5.7	FUS	851
		30.5.8	Nucleotide Repeat Diseases	853

30.6 Biomarkers 853
30.7 Brief Sketch of the Differential Diagnoses 856
30.8 Differential Diagnoses: Lobar Atrophies 856
  30.8.1 Pick Disease 856
  30.8.2 Primary Progressive Aphasia (PPA) 856
  30.8.3 Motor Neuron Disease with Dementia 857
  30.8.4 Dementia Lacking Distinctive Histopathology (DLDH) . 857
30.9 Differential Diagnoses: Subcortical Dementias 857
  30.9.1 Progressive Subcortical Gliosis (PSG) 857
  30.9.2 Parkinson Disease with Dementia 857
30.10 Differential Diagnoses: Rare Cortical Dementias 857
  30.10.1 Chromosome 17-Associated Dementia 857
  30.10.2 Familial Presenile Dementia with Tangles (FPDT) ... 858
  30.10.3 Meso-Limbo-Cortical Dementia 858
30.11 Differential Diagnoses: Down Syndrome 858
30.12 Differential Diagnoses: Diffuse Neurofibrillary Tangles with Calcifications (DNTC) 859
30.13 Differential Diagnoses: Rare Neurodegenerative Disorders 859
  30.13.1 Thalamic Degeneration 859
  30.13.2 (Non) Hereditary Bilateral Striatal Necrosis 860
  30.13.3 Neuroacanthocytosis 860
  30.13.4 Pallidal Degenerations 860
  30.13.5 Dentato-Rubro-Pallido-Luysi an Degeneration 860
  30.13.6 Substantia Reticularis degeneration 861
30.14 Differential Diagnoses: Argyrophilic Grain Disease (AG) 861
30.15 Differential Diagnoses: Adult Polyglucosan Body Disease (APBD) 863
30.16 Differential Diagnoses: Normal Pressure Hydrocephalus (NPH) 863
30.17 Differential Diagnoses: Mitochondrial Encephalomyopathies 864
  30.17.1 Clinical Signs of Mitochondrial Encephalopathies .. 864
  30.17.2 Neuropathology Findings 864
30.18 Differential Diagnoses: Metabolic and Traumatic Disorders 866
  30.18.1 Hallervorden-Spatz Disease 866
  30.18.2 Leukodystrophies 866

		30.18.3	Wilson Disease: Hepato-Lenticular Degeneration	867
		30.18.4	Dementia Pugilistica	867
	Selected References			867

31 Normal Aging Brain ... 871

- 31.1 Introduction ... 871
  - 31.1.1 WHO Definition of Well-Being ... 871
- 31.2 Clinical Signs and Symptoms ... 872
- 31.3 Epidemiology ... 872
- 31.4 Neuroimaging Findings ... 872
- 31.5 Neuropathology Findings ... 874
- 31.6 Incidental White Matter Changes ... 877
- 31.7 Molecular Neuropathology ... 881
  - 31.7.1 Astrocytes ... 882
  - 31.7.2 Microglia ... 882
  - 31.7.3 Autophagy ... 883
  - 31.7.4 Unfolded Protein Response (UPR): Endoplasmic Reticulum Stress—Stress Response Pathways ... 883
  - 31.7.5 Mitochondria ... 884
  - 31.7.6 Advanced Glycation End-Product (AGE) ... 885
  - 31.7.7 cAMP Response Element Binding Protein (CREB) ... 885
  - 31.7.8 Ion Channels and ROS ... 885
  - 31.7.9 Sirtuins ... 885
  - 31.7.10 Translocator Protein (TSPO) ... 886
  - 31.7.11 Cathepsins ... 886
  - 31.7.12 Ghrelin ... 886
  - 31.7.13 Klotho ... 886
  - 31.7.14 Iron ... 886
  - 31.7.15 Insulin ... 887
  - 31.7.16 Signaling ... 887
- 31.8 Genetics of Successful Aging ... 887
- 31.9 Non-coding RNAs ... 888
- 31.10 DNA Damage ... 890
- 31.11 Treatment and Prognosis ... 890
- Selected References ... 892

32 Neurodegenerative Diseases: Alzheimer Disease (AD) ... 897

- 32.1 Clinical Signs and Symptoms ... 897
- 32.2 International Working Group (IWG) Clinical Criteria ... 897
- 32.3 Early-Onset AD Versus Late-Onset AD ... 900
- 32.4 Neuroimaging Findings ... 900
- 32.5 Neuropathology Findings ... 903
- 32.6 The Proposed Diagnostic Criteria ... 903
  - 32.6.1 Ball Criteria: The Hippocampal Criteria ... 903
  - 32.6.2 Newcastle Criteria (Tomlinson, Roth, Blessed) ... 915
  - 32.6.3 NIH Criteria (Khachaturian) ... 915

		32.6.4	NINCDS-ADRA	916
		32.6.5	CERAD Criteria.........................	917
		32.6.6	NIH/Reagan............................	918
	32.7	Staging of Neurofibrillary Tangle Development		919
	32.8	Phases of Aß-deposition by Thal et al. (2002)...........		923
	32.9	Molecular Neuropathology		923
		32.9.1	Genetics...............................	923
		32.9.2	Aberrations in Mitochondrial DNA (mtDNA)...........................	926
		32.9.3	Epigenetics.............................	927
	32.10	Treatment and Prognosis		928
	Selected References			928
33	**Neurodegenerative Diseases: Lewy Body Dementia**			933
	33.1	Clinical Signs and Symptoms		933
	33.2	Epidemiology.....................................		933
	33.3	Neuroimaging Findings............................		935
	33.4	Neuropathology Findings...........................		939
	33.5	Molecular Neuropathology		939
	33.6	Treatment and Prognosis		939
	Selected References			943
34	**Neurodegenerative Diseases: Fronto-temporal Lobar Degeneration**			945
	34.1	Clinical Signs and Symptoms		945
	34.2	Epidemiology.....................................		945
	34.3	Neuroimaging Findings............................		945
	34.4	Neuropathology Subgroups		953
	34.5	Types of FTLD....................................		954
		34.5.1	Fronto-temporal Lobar Degeneration with TDP-43 Proteinopathy.................	954
		34.5.2	Fronto-temporal Lobar Degeneration with Motor Neuron Disease Type Inclusions.....	956
		34.5.3	Fronto-temporal Lobar Degeneration with *GRN* Mutation	958
		34.5.4	Fronto-temporal Lobar Degeneration with *VCP* Mutation	959
		34.5.5	Fronto-temporal Lobar Degeneration with *C9ORF* Mutation.....................	959
		34.5.6	Fronto-temporal Lobar Degeneration with Ubiquitin-Positive Inclusions (FTLD/UPS)	960
		34.5.7	Fronto-temporal Lobar Degeneration with Tauopathy..........................	960
		34.5.8	Pick Disease............................	960
		34.5.9	Cortico-basal Degeneration	962
		34.5.10	Progressive Supranuclear Palsy	962
		34.5.11	Argyrophilic Grain Disease	962
		34.5.12	Sporadic Multiple System Tauopathy with Dementia	962

		34.5.13	White Matter Tauopathy with Globular Glial Inclusions	964

        34.5.13 White Matter Tauopathy with Globular
                 Glial Inclusions 964
        34.5.14 Tangle-Only Dementia...................... 964
        34.5.15 Fronto-temporal Lobar Degeneration
                 with *MAPT* Mutation...................... 965
        34.5.16 Fronto-temporal Lobar Degeneration
                 with FUS Proteinopathy.................... 965
        34.5.17 Neuronal Intermediate Filament Inclusion
                 Disease (NIFID)........................... 966
        34.5.18 Basophilic Inclusion Body Disease (BIBD)..... 966
        34.5.19 Atypical Fronto-temporal Lobar
                 Degeneration with Ubiquitin-Positive
                 Inclusions (FTLD-U)....................... 967
        34.5.20 Fronto-temporal Lobar Degeneration
                 with No Inclusions........................ 967
   34.6 Molecular Neuropathology 968
   34.7 Treatment and Prognosis 968
   Selected References 968

35 Neurodegenerative Diseases: Progressive Supranuclear Palsy (PSP)–Cortico-Basal Degeneration (CBD) 973
   35.1 Introduction 973
   35.2 Progressive Supranuclear Palsy (PSP).................. 973
        35.2.1 Clinical Signs................................ 973
        35.2.2 Epidemiology................................ 973
        35.2.3 Neuroimaging Findings 974
        35.2.4 Neuropathology Findings.................... 976
        35.2.5 Molecular Neuropathology 978
        35.2.6 Treatment and Prognosis 978
   35.3 Cortico-Basal Degeneration (CBD)................... 978
        35.3.1 Clinical Signs................................ 978
        35.3.2 Neuroimaging Findings 978
        35.3.3 Neuropathology Findings.................... 981
        35.3.4 Molecular Neuropathology 984
        35.3.5 Treatment and Prognosis 984
   Selected References 984

36 Neurodegenerative Diseases: Vascular Dementia 987
   36.1   Introduction 987
   36.2   Clinical Signs and Symptoms 988
   36.3   Diagnostic Criteria................................ 989
   36.4   Epidemiology..................................... 989
   36.5   Neuroimaging Findings 989
   36.6   Neuropathology Findings.......................... 991
   36.7   Leuko-araiosis 995
   36.8   Morbus Binswanger................................ 995
   36.9   Cerebral Amyloid Angiopathy...................... 995
   36.10 CADASIL 995
   36.11 Molecular Neuropathology 995
   36.12 Treatment and Prognosis 995
   Selected References 1000

37	**Neurodegenerative Diseases: Parkinson Disease**	1001
37.1	Clinical Signs and Symptoms	1001
37.2	Epidemiology	1003
37.3	Neuroimaging Findings	1003
37.4	Neuropathology Findings	1007
37.5	Molecular Neuropathology	1012
	37.5.1 Pathogenesis	1012
	37.5.2 Genetics	1013
	37.5.3 Epigenetics	1017
37.6	Treatment and Prognosis	1018
	Selected References	1019
38	**Neurodegenerative Diseases: Multiple System Atrophy (MSA)**	1021
38.1	Introduction	1021
38.2	Clinical Signs and Symptoms	1021
38.3	Epidemiology	1022
38.4	Neuroimaging Findings	1022
38.5	Neuropathology Findings	1027
38.6	Molecular Neuropathology	1034
38.7	Treatment and Prognosis	1034
	Selected References	1035
39	**Neurodegenerative Diseases: Motor Neuron Diseases**	1037
39.1	Introduction	1037
39.2	Clinical Signs and Symptoms	1037
39.3	Diagnostic Criteria	1037
39.4	Epidemiology	1039
39.5	Neuroimaging Findings	1039
39.6	Neuropathology Findings	1042
39.7	Molecular Neuropathology	1045
	39.7.1 Pathogenetic Mechanisms	1045
	39.7.2 Genes	1050
39.8	Treatment and Prognosis	1055
	Selected References	1056
40	**Neurodegenerative Diseases: Huntington Disease**	1059
40.1	Introduction	1059
40.2	Clinical Signs and Symptoms	1059
40.3	Epidemiology	1059
40.4	Neuroimaging Findings	1059
40.5	Neuropathology Findings	1063
40.6	Molecular Neuropathology	1065
	40.6.1 Genetics	1067
	40.6.2 Epigenetics	1067
40.7	Treatment and Prognosis	1067
	Selected References	1067

Part VII The Brain Diseases: Myelin Disorders

41 Demyelinating Diseases: Multiple Sclerosis 1071
- 41.1 Introduction 1071
- 41.2 Clinical Signs and Symptoms 1071
- 41.3 Epidemiology.................................... 1073
- 41.4 Neuroimaging Findings 1073
- 41.5 Neuropathology Findings......................... 1077
- 41.6 Molecular Neuropathology 1087
- 41.7 Treatment and Prognosis 1092
- Selected References 1093

42 Demyelinating Diseases: Neuromyelitis Optica Spectrum Disorder 1097
- 42.1 Clinical Signs and Symptoms 1097
- 42.2 Epidemiology.................................... 1098
- 42.3 Neuroimaging Findings 1098
- 42.4 Neuropathology Findings......................... 1101
- 42.5 Molecular Neuropathology 1101
- 42.6 Treatment and Prognosis 1103
- Selected References 1103

43 Demyelinating Diseases: Acute Demyelinating Encephalomyelitis (ADEM) 1105
- 43.1 Introduction 1105
- 43.2 Clinical Signs and Symptoms 1105
- 43.3 Epidemiology.................................... 1105
- 43.4 Neuroimaging Findings 1105
- 43.5 Neuropathology Findings......................... 1106
- 43.6 Molecular Neuropathology 1115
- 43.7 Treatment and Prognosis 1115
- Selected References 1115

Part VIII The Brain Diseases: The Epilepsies

44 Epilepsies: General Aspects 1119
- 44.1 Introduction 1119
- 44.2 Definitions 1119
- 44.3 Classification of the Epilepsies 1121
  - 44.3.1 International League Against Epilepsy (ILEA) Classification-1981 1121
  - 44.3.2 International League Against Epilepsy (ILEA) Classification-1989 1121
  - 44.3.3 International League Against Epilepsy (ILEA) Classification-2010 1122
  - 44.3.4 International League Against Epilepsy (ILAE) Classification-2017 1122
  - 44.3.5 International Classification of Diseases Classification (ICD)-2012 1123
  - 44.3.6 Electroclinical Syndromes................... 1123

	44.4	Neuroimaging Findings 1124
		44.4.1 Transient Seizure Related Imaging Features 1124
	44.5	Etiological Classification of Epilepsies 1129
	44.6	Neuropathological Lesions Associated with the Epilepsies 1129
	44.7	Molecular Neuropathology 1132
	44.8	Malformations Due to Genetic Changes 1135
	44.9	Treatment 1138
	Selected References 1139
45	**Epilepsies: Temporal Lobe Epilepsy** 1143
	45.1	Introduction 1143
	45.2	Clinical Signs. 1143
	45.3	Neuroimaging Findings 1143
	45.4	Neuropathology Findings. 1147
	45.5	Molecular Neuropathology 1153
	45.6	Treatment and Prognosis 1154
	Selected References 1154
46	**Epilepsies: Malformations of Cortical Development—Focal Cortical Dysplasia (FCD)**. 1157
	46.1	Introduction 1157
	46.2	Neuroimaging Findings 1157
	46.3	Neuropathology Findings. 1158
	46.4	Historical Classification. 1165
	46.5	Molecular Neuropathology 1168
	Selected References 1168
47	**Epilepsies: Malformations of Cortical Development—Heterotopia** 1171
	47.1	Definition 1171
	47.2	Neuroimaging Findings 1171
	47.3	Neuropathology Findings. 1171
		47.3.1 White Matter Heterotopia 1171
		47.3.2 Nodular Heterotopia. 1175
		47.3.3 Periventricular Nodular Heterotopia 1176
		47.3.4 Subcortical Laminar Heterotopias 1178
	47.4	Molecular Neuropathology 1179
	Selected References 1179

Part IX   The Brain Diseases: Trauma and Intoxication

48	**Trauma**. 1185
	48.1	Definition 1185
	48.2	Epidemiology. 1185
	48.3	Clinical Signs and Symptoms 1185
	48.4	Classification of TBI 1186
	48.5	Neuroimaging Findings 1192
		48.5.1 Cerebral Contusions. 1192
		48.5.2 Chronic Traumatic Brain Injury. 1192

48.6   Focal Injuries 1196
   48.7   Diffuse Injuries 1207
   48.8   Chronic Traumatic Encephalopathy. 1212
   48.9   Molecular Neuropathology 1214
   48.10 Treatment and Prognosis 1218
   Selected References 1220

49 Intoxication: Alcohol. 1223
   49.1   Introduction 1223
   49.2   Ethanol: Acute and Chronic Alcoholism 1223
          49.2.1   Clinical Signs and Symptoms 1223
          49.2.2   Epidemiology. 1223
          49.2.3   Neuroimaging Findings 1224
          49.2.4   Neuropathology Findings. 1224
   49.3   Wernicke–Korsakoff Encephalopathy 1228
          49.3.1   Clinical Signs. 1228
          49.3.2   Neuroimaging Findings 1228
          49.3.3   Neuropathology Findings. 1230
          49.3.4   Molecular Neuropathology 1230
   49.4   Cerebellar Degeneration 1230
          49.4.1   Clinical Signs. 1230
          49.4.2   Neuropathology Findings. 1230
   49.5   Central Pontine Myelinolysis. 1233
          49.5.1   Clinical Signs. 1233
          49.5.2   Neuroimaging Findings 1233
          49.5.3   Neuropathology Findings. 1233
          49.5.4   Molecular Neuropathology 1233
   49.6   Marchiafava–Bignami Disease 1235
          49.6.1   Clinical Signs. 1235
          49.6.2   Neuroimaging Findings 1235
          49.6.3   Neuropathology Findings. 1238
   49.7   Fetal Alcohol Spectrum Disorders (FASD) 1238
          49.7.1   Clinical Signs. 1238
          49.7.2   Neuropathology Findings. 1239
          49.7.3   Molecular Neuropathology 1240
   Selected References 1240

50 Intoxication: Street Drugs 1243
   50.1   Introduction 1243
          50.1.1   General Aspects 1243
          50.1.2   Clinical Signs and Symptoms 1243
          50.1.3   Neuroimaging Findings 1244
   50.2   Opiates 1244
          50.2.1   Neuroimaging Findings 1244
          50.2.2   Neuropathology Findings. 1245
          50.2.3   Molecular Neuropathology 1247
   50.3   Cocaine 1253
          50.3.1   Clinical Signs and Symptoms 1253
          50.3.2   Neuroimaging Findings 1254

		50.3.3	Neuropathology Findings.	1254

- 50.3.3 Neuropathology Findings. 1254
- 50.3.4 Molecular Neuropathology 1254
- 50.4 Cannabis. 1255
  - 50.4.1 CNS Complications of Cannabis 1255
  - 50.4.2 Neuroimaging Findings 1256
  - 50.4.3 Neuropathology Findings. 1256
  - 50.4.4 Molecular Neuropathology 1256
- 50.5 Amphetamine and Methamphetamine. 1257
  - 50.5.1 Clinical Signs and Symptoms 1257
  - 50.5.2 Neuroimaging Findings 1257
  - 50.5.3 Neuropathology Findings. 1257
  - 50.5.4 Molecular Neuropathology 1257
- 50.6 Designer Drugs 1258
  - 50.6.1 Substances 1258
  - 50.6.2 Modes of Action. 1258
  - 50.6.3 Molecular Neuropathology 1259
  - 50.6.4 Outcome. 1259
- Selected References 1259

Volume III

Part X The Brain Diseases: Tumors

51 Tumors of the Nervous System: General Considerations 1263
- 51.1 Clinical Signs and Symptoms 1263
- 51.2 Definitions 1264
  - 51.2.1 Neuro-oncology. 1264
  - 51.2.2 Tumor. 1264
  - 51.2.3 Neoplasia 1264
  - 51.2.4 Brain Tumor. 1264
  - 51.2.5 Malignant Versus Benign. 1264
  - 51.2.6 Seeding and Metastases 1264
  - 51.2.7 Various Modalities of Therapy. 1265
  - 51.2.8 Endpoints on Clinical Trials 1265
- 51.3 Histologic Tumor Characteristics 1266
  - 51.3.1 Cellularity 1266
  - 51.3.2 Anaplasia 1266
  - 51.3.3 Metaplasia 1266
  - 51.3.4 Pleomorphism 1266
  - 51.3.5 Mitoses. 1266
  - 51.3.6 Reactive Versus Neoplastic 1267
  - 51.3.7 Endothelial Proliferation and Neovascularity ... 1268
  - 51.3.8 Necrosis. 1268
  - 51.3.9 Encapsulation and Invasion 1269
  - 51.3.10 Rosettes 1269
  - 51.3.11 Palisades and Pseudopalisades. 1270
  - 51.3.12 Desmoplasia. 1270
  - 51.3.13 Reactive Astrogliosis 1271
  - 51.3.14 Microglial Activation. 1271

		51.3.15 Perivascular Lymphocytic Cuffing 1271
	51.4	WHO Classification of Tumors of the Central Nervous System 1271
	51.5	Grading Systems for Brain Tumors 1273
		51.5.1 WHO Grading System 1273
		51.5.2 Kernohan et al. (1949) 1273
		51.5.3 Ringertz (1950) 1273
		51.5.4 St. Anne/Mayo 1274
		51.5.5 Smith Grading for Oligodendroglioma 1274
	51.6	Frequencies of Brain Tumors 1275
	51.7	Molecular Neuropathology: The Hallmarks of Cancer 1275
	51.8	Molecular Neuropathology: Cell Cycle 1277
		51.8.1 The Cell Cycle in Normal Cells 1277
		51.8.2 The Cell Cycle in Cancer Cells 1280
	51.9	Molecular Neuropathology: DNA Damage Response 1281
		51.9.1 Mechanisms of DNA Damage Recognition 1281
		51.9.2 Mechanisms of DNA Damage Repair 1282
	51.10	Molecular Neuro-oncology: Oncogenes 1285
	51.11	Molecular Neuropathology: Tumor Suppressors 1286
	51.12	Molecular Neuropathology: Cell Death 1289
		51.12.1 Apoptosis 1289
		51.12.2 Autophagy 1293
		51.12.3 Necroptosis 1296
		51.12.4 Ferroptosis 1296
		51.12.5 Pyroptosis 1296
		51.12.6 Parthanatos 1297
		51.12.7 NETosis 1297
		51.12.8 Caspase-Independent Cell Death 1297
	51.13	Molecular Neuropathology: Genomic Instability 1300
	51.14	Molecular Neuropathology: Signal Transduction Pathways 1302
		51.14.1 PKC 1305
	51.15	Molecular Neuropathology: Epigenetic Changes 1305
	51.16	Molecular Neuropathology: Telomeres and Telomerase ... 1306
	51.17	Molecular Neuropathology: Angiogenesis 1306
		51.17.1 Features of Tumor Endothelial Cells 1307
	51.18	Molecular Neuro-oncology: Glioma Invasion and Microenvironment 1310
	51.19	Molecular Neuro-oncology: MicroRNAs 1315
	51.20	Molecular Neuro-oncology: Stem Cell Hypothesis 1315
	51.21	Carcinogenic Agents 1317
	51.22	Common Molecular Changes in Brain Tumors 1318
	51.23	Treatment for Brain Tumors 1325
	Selected References 1327
52	**Diffuse Astrocytoma WHO Grade II** **1333**
	52.1	Epidemiology 1333
	52.2	Neuroimaging Findings 1334
	52.3	Neuropathology Findings 1334

	52.4	Molecular Neuropathology 1344
		52.4.1 Pathogenesis............................. 1344
		52.4.2 Genetics 1344
		52.4.3 Epigenetics............................... 1344
		52.4.4 Gene Expression 1345
	52.5	Treatment and Prognosis 1345
	Selected References 1345

53 Anaplastic Astrocytoma WHO Grade III 1347
    53.1 Epidemiology...................................... 1348
    53.2 Neuroimaging Findings 1348
    53.3 Neuropathology Findings........................... 1352
    53.4 Molecular Neuropathology 1358
    53.5 Treatment and Prognosis 1358
    Selected References 1359

54 Glioblastoma 1361
    54.1 Epidemiology...................................... 1362
    54.2 Neuroimaging Findings 1362
    54.3 Neuropathology Findings........................... 1374
    54.4 Molecular Neuropathology 1389
        54.4.1 Pathogenesis............................. 1389
        54.4.2 Genetics 1390
        54.4.3 Epigenetics............................... 1395
        54.4.4 Gene Expression 1395
    54.5 Treatment and Prognosis 1398
        54.5.1 Treatment: State of the Art................. 1398
        54.5.2 Treatment: Historical Aspects 1399
    Selected References 1400

55 Gliosarcoma WHO Grade IV-Giant Cell Glioblastoma WHO Grade IV 1403
    55.1 Gliosarcoma WHO Grade IV........................ 1403
        55.1.1 Epidemiology............................. 1403
        55.1.2 Neuroimaging Findings 1403
        55.1.3 Neuropathology Findings................... 1406
        55.1.4 Molecular Neuropathology 1406
        55.1.5 Treatment and Prognosis 1410
    55.2 Giant Cell Glioblastoma WHO Grade IV 1410
        55.2.1 Epidemiology............................. 1411
        55.2.2 Neuroimaging Findings 1411
        55.2.3 Neuropathology Findings................... 1411
        55.2.4 Molecular Neuropathology 1414
        55.2.5 Treatment and Prognosis 1414
    Selected References 1414

56 Gliomatosis Cerebri 1417
    56.1 Epidemiology...................................... 1417
    56.2 Neuroimaging Findings 1418
    56.3 Neuropathology Findings........................... 1421

	56.4	Molecular Neuropathology 1421
	56.5	Treatment and Prognosis 1421
	Selected References 1423

57 Pilocytic Astrocytoma WHO Grade I 1425
    57.1   Epidemiology.. 1425
    57.2   Neuroimaging Findings 1426
    57.3   Neuropathology Findings........................... 1426
    57.4   Molecular Neuropathology 1435
            57.4.1   Pathogenesis.............................. 1435
            57.4.2   Genetics................................. 1435
            57.4.3   Epigenetics............................... 1436
    57.5   Treatment and Prognosis 1436
    Selected References 1437

58 Oligodendroglioma WHO Grade II-Anaplastic Oligodendroglioma WHO Grade III....................... 1439
    58.1   Oligodendroglioma WHO Grade II 1439
            58.1.1   Epidemiology............................. 1439
            58.1.2   Neuroimaging Findings 1440
            58.1.3   Neuropathology Findings................... 1440
            58.1.4   Molecular Neuropathology 1446
            58.1.5   Treatment and Prognosis 1450
    58.2   Anaplastic Oligodendroglioma WHO Grade III 1450
            58.2.1   Epidemiology............................. 1451
            58.2.2   Neuroimaging Findings 1451
            58.2.3   Neuropathology Findings................... 1454
            58.2.4   Molecular Neuropathology 1454
            58.2.5   Treatment and Prognosis 1458
    Selected References 1458

59 Oligo-astrocytoma WHO Grade II-Anaplastic Oligo-astrocytoma WHO Grade III 1461
    59.1   Oligo-astrocytoma WHO Grade II................... 1461
            59.1.1   Epidemiology............................. 1461
            59.1.2   Neuroimaging Findings 1461
            59.1.3   Neuropathology Findings................... 1464
            59.1.4   Molecular Neuropathology 1468
            59.1.5   Treatment and Prognosis 1468
    59.2   Anaplastic Oligo-astrocytoma WHO Grade III 1468
            59.2.1   Epidemiology............................. 1469
            59.2.2   Neuroimaging Findings 1469
            59.2.3   Neuropathology Findings................... 1469
            59.2.4   Molecular Neuropathology 1478
            59.2.5   Treatment and Prognosis 1478
    Selected References 1478

60 Ependymal Tumors.................................... 1481
    60.1   General Aspects 1481
            60.1.1   Clinical Signs and Symptoms 1481
            60.1.2   Nuclear Medicine Imaging Findings 1481

		60.1.3	Molecular Neuropathology	1481
	60.2	Ependymoma WHO Grade II		1483
		60.2.1	Epidemiology	1484
		60.2.2	Neuroimaging Findings	1484
		60.2.3	Neuropathology Findings	1486
		60.2.4	Treatment and Prognosis	1491
	60.3	Anaplastic Ependymoma WHO Grade III		1491
		60.3.1	Epidemiology	1492
		60.3.2	Neuroimaging Findings	1492
		60.3.3	Neuropathology Findings	1492
		60.3.4	Treatment and Prognosis	1497
	60.4	Myxopapillary Ependymoma (WHO Grade I)		1497
		60.4.1	Epidemiology	1498
		60.4.2	Neuroimaging Findings	1498
		60.4.3	Neuropathology Findings	1498
		60.4.4	Treatment and Prognosis	1499
	60.5	Subependymoma (WHO Grade I)		1502
		60.5.1	Epidemiology	1503
		60.5.2	Neuroimaging Findings	1503
		60.5.3	Neuropathology Findings	1503
		60.5.4	Treatment and Prognosis	1510
	Selected References			1510
61	**Choroid Plexus Tumors**			**1513**
	61.1	General Aspects		1513
		61.1.1	Epidemiology	1513
		61.1.2	Nuclear Medicine Imaging Findings	1513
		61.1.3	Differential Diagnosis	1514
		61.1.4	Molecular Neuropathology	1514
		61.1.5	Treatment and Prognosis	1514
	61.2	Choroid Plexus Papilloma WHO Grade I		1514
		61.2.1	Neuroimaging Findings	1515
		61.2.2	Neuropathology Findings	1515
	61.3	Atypical Choroid Plexus Papilloma (WHO Grade II)		1521
		61.3.1	Neuroimaging Findings	1522
		61.3.2	Neuropathology Findings	1522
	61.4	Choroid Plexus Carcinoma WHO Grade III		1522
		61.4.1	Neuroimaging Findings	1526
		61.4.2	Neuropathology Findings	1526
		61.4.3	Molecular Neuropathology	1526
	Selected References			1531
62	**Dysembryoplastic Neuroepithelial Tumor (DNT)**			**1533**
	62.1	Epidemiology		1533
	62.2	Neuroimaging Findings		1534
	62.3	Neuropathology Findings		1534
	62.4	Molecular Neuropathology		1537
	62.5	Treatment and Prognosis		1542

Selected References 1542

63 Desmoplastic (Infantile) Astrocytoma/Ganglioglioma (DIA/DIG) 1545
    63.1 Epidemiology 1545
    63.2 Neuroimaging Findings 1546
    63.3 Neuropathology Findings 1546
    63.4 Molecular Neuropathology 1549
    63.5 Treatment and Prognosis 1551
    Selected References 1551

64 Ganglioglioma/Gangliocytoma 1553
    64.1 Ganglioglioma 1553
        64.1.1 Epidemiology 1554
        64.1.2 Neuroimaging Findings 1554
        64.1.3 Neuropathology Findings 1556
        64.1.4 Molecular Neuropathology 1558
        64.1.5 Treatment and Prognosis 1563
    64.2 Anaplastic Ganglioglioma 1563
        64.2.1 Epidemiology 1563
        64.2.2 Neuroimaging Findings 1564
        64.2.3 Neuropathology Findings 1564
        64.2.4 Molecular Neuropathology 1564
        64.2.5 Treatment and Prognosis 1565
    Selected References 1565

65 Neurocytoma: Central—Extraventricular 1567
    65.1 Epidemiology 1567
    65.2 Neuroimaging Findings 1568
    65.3 Neuropathology Findings 1570
    65.4 Molecular Neuropathology 1572
    65.5 Treatment and Prognosis 1574
    Selected References 1574

66 Rosette-Forming Glioneuronal Tumor (RGNT) 1575
    66.1 Epidemiology 1575
    66.2 Neuroimaging Findings 1575
    66.3 Neuropathology Findings 1579
    66.4 Molecular Neuropathology 1583
    66.5 Treatment and Prognosis 1583
    Selected References 1584

67 Pineal Parenchymal Tumors 1587
    67.1 General Aspects 1587
        67.1.1 Epidemiology 1587
        67.1.2 Nuclear Medicine Imaging Findings 1587
        67.1.3 Differential Diagnosis 1587
        67.1.4 Molecular Neuropathology 1587
    67.2 Pineocytoma 1588
        67.2.1 Neuroimaging Findings 1588

		67.2.2	Neuropathology Findings.	1591

- 67.3 Pineal Parenchymal Tumor of Intermediate
  Differentiation 1595
  - 67.3.1 Neuropathology Findings. 1595
  - 67.3.2 Treatment and Prognosis 1597
- 67.4 Pineoblastoma 1597
  - 67.4.1 Neuroimaging Findings 1597
  - 67.4.2 Neuropathology Findings. 1599
  - 67.4.3 Treatment and Prognosis 1599
- Selected References 1601

68 Medulloblastoma. 1605
- 68.1 Epidemiology. 1606
- 68.2 Neuroimaging Findings 1606
- 68.3 Neuropathology Findings. 1609
- 68.4 Molecular Neuropathology 1621
  - 68.4.1 Pathogenesis. 1621
  - 68.4.2 Molecular Classification of Medulloblastomas . . . 1621
  - 68.4.3 Epigenetics. 1623
- 68.5 Treatment and Prognosis 1623
- Selected References 1626

69 Embryonal Tumors: Other CNS Embryonal Tumors 1629
- 69.1 General Aspects 1629
- 69.2 CNS Embryonal Tumor, NOS 1630
  - 69.2.1 Epidemiology. 1631
  - 69.2.2 Neuroimaging Findings 1631
  - 69.2.3 Neuropathology Findings. 1631
  - 69.2.4 Molecular Neuropathology 1636
  - 69.2.5 Treatment and Prognosis 1636
- 69.3 Embryonal Tumors with Multilayered Rosettes,
  C19MC-Altered. 1636
  - 69.3.1 Epidemiology. 1636
  - 69.3.2 Neuropathology Findings. 1636
  - 69.3.3 Molecular Neuropathology 1638
  - 69.3.4 Treatment and Prognosis 1639
- 69.4 Medulloepithelioma. 1639
  - 69.4.1 Epidemiology. 1639
  - 69.4.2 Neuropathology Findings. 1639
  - 69.4.3 Molecular Neuropathology 1640
  - 69.4.4 Treatment and Prognosis 1640
- Selected References 1640

70 Embryonal Tumors: Atypical Teratoid/Rhabdoid
Tumor (ATRT). 1643
- 70.1 Epidemiology. 1643
- 70.2 Neuroimaging Findings 1643

	70.3	Neuropathology Findings. 1645
	70.4	Molecular Neuropathology 1648
	70.5	Treatment and Prognosis. 1649
	Selected References 1649

71 Tumors of the Peripheral Nervous System 1651
- 71.1 General Aspects 1651
  - 71.1.1 Clinical Signs and Symptoms 1651
  - 71.1.2 Classification of Tumors of the Peripheral Nervous System. 1651
  - 71.1.3 Nuclear Medicine Imaging Findings 1652
- 71.2 Schwannoma 1654
  - 71.2.1 Epidemiology. 1654
  - 71.2.2 Neuroimaging Findings 1654
  - 71.2.3 Neuropathology Findings. 1657
  - 71.2.4 Molecular Neuropathology 1665
  - 71.2.5 Treatment and Prognosis 1665
- 71.3 Neurofibroma. 1665
  - 71.3.1 Epidemiology. 1665
  - 71.3.2 Neuroimaging Findings 1666
  - 71.3.3 Neuropathology Findings. 1666
  - 71.3.4 Molecular Neuropathology 1668
  - 71.3.5 Treatment and Prognosis 1670
- 71.4 Perineurioma 1670
  - 71.4.1 Epidemiology. 1672
  - 71.4.2 Neuroimaging Findings 1672
  - 71.4.3 Neuropathology Findings. 1674
  - 71.4.4 Molecular Neuropathology 1674
  - 71.4.5 Treatment and Prognosis 1674
- 71.5 Hybrid Nerve Sheath Tumors 1675
  - 71.5.1 Neuropathology Findings. 1675
- 71.6 Malignant Peripheral Nerve Sheath Tumor (MPNST) 1675
  - 71.6.1 Epidemiology. 1678
  - 71.6.2 Neuroimaging Findings 1678
  - 71.6.3 Neuropathology Findings. 1679
  - 71.6.4 Molecular Neuropathology 1681
  - 71.6.5 Treatment and Prognosis 1682
- 71.7 Neurofibromatosis Type 1 (NF1). 1682
  - 71.7.1 Incidence and Diagnostic Criteria 1682
  - 71.7.2 Neuroimaging Findings 1683
  - 71.7.3 Neuropathology Findings. 1683
  - 71.7.4 Molecular Neuropathology 1683
- 71.8 Neurofibromatosis Type 2 (NF2). 1683
  - 71.8.1 Incidence and Diagnostic Criteria 1686
  - 71.8.2 Neuroimaging Findings 1688
- 71.9 Schwannomatosis. 1688
  - 71.9.1 Incidence and Diagnostic Criteria 1688
- 71.10 Molecular Neuropathology 1688

Contents

	71.10.1 Neurofibromatosis Type 1 (NF1)	1689
	71.10.2 Neurofibromatosis Type 2 (NF2)	1689
	71.10.3 Schwannomatosis	1690
	71.10.4 Malignant Peripheral Nerve Sheath Tumor (MPNST)	1691
	71.10.5 Epigenetics	1692
Selected References		1692

72 Tumors of Meningothelial Cells: Meningiomas 1695
- 72.1 Introduction 1695
- 72.2 General Aspects 1695
  - 72.2.1 Clinical Signs and Symptoms 1695
  - 72.2.2 Epidemiology 1695
  - 72.2.3 Neuroimaging Features 1696
- 72.3 Meningioma 1705
  - 72.3.1 Neuropathology Findings 1707
- 72.4 Atypical Meningioma 1727
  - 72.4.1 Neuropathology Findings 1727
- 72.5 Anaplastic (Malignant) Meningioma 1729
  - 72.5.1 Microscopic Features 1729
- 72.6 Common Neuropathology Aspects 1729
- 72.7 Molecular Neuropathology 1733
  - 72.7.1 Pathogenesis 1733
  - 72.7.2 Genetics 1733
  - 72.7.3 Signaling Pathways 1733
  - 72.7.4 Hh (Hedgehog) Pathway 1733
  - 72.7.5 Wnt (Wingless) Pathway 1734
  - 72.7.6 Chromosomal Aberrations and Mutations 1734
  - 72.7.7 Epigenetics 1735
  - 72.7.8 Gene Expression 1736
- 72.8 Treatment and Prognosis 1736
- Selected References 1738

73 Tumors of the Sellar Region 1741
- 73.1 Classification of Tumors of the Sellar Region 1741
- 73.2 Craniopharyngioma 1741
  - 73.2.1 Clinical Signs and Symptoms 1742
  - 73.2.2 Epidemiology 1742
  - 73.2.3 Neuroimaging Findings 1742
  - 73.2.4 Neuropathology Findings 1743
  - 73.2.5 Molecular Neuropathology 1752
  - 73.2.6 Treatment and Prognosis 1753
- 73.3 Pituicytoma 1753
  - 73.3.1 Epidemiology 1753
  - 73.3.2 Neuroimaging Findings 1753
  - 73.3.3 Neuropathology Findings 1754
  - 73.3.4 Molecular Neuropathology 1755
  - 73.3.5 Treatment and Prognosis 1755

	73.4	Granular Cell Tumor of the Sellar Region............. 1757
		73.4.1 Epidemiology............................. 1758
		73.4.2 Neuroimaging Findings..................... 1758
		73.4.3 Neuropathology Findings................... 1758
		73.4.4 Molecular Neuropathology.................. 1762
		73.4.5 Treatment and Prognosis................... 1762
	73.5	Spindle Cell Oncocytoma........................... 1763
		73.5.1 Epidemiology............................. 1763
		73.5.2 Neuroimaging Findings..................... 1763
		73.5.3 Neuropathology Findings................... 1763
		73.5.4 Molecular Neuropathology.................. 1764
		73.5.5 Treatment and Prognosis................... 1764
	Selected References.................................... 1764

74 Tumors of the Pituitary Gland........................... 1767
- 74.1 Epidemiology...................................... 1767
- 74.2 Classification of Pituitary Tumors..................... 1767
  - 74.2.1 Clinical Classification of Pituitary Tumors...... 1768
  - 74.2.2 Radiologic Classification of Pituitary Tumors.... 1768
- 74.3 Radiological Features of Pituitary Tumors............. 1769
  - 74.3.1 Microadenoma............................ 1769
  - 74.3.2 Macroadenoma........................... 1770
- 74.4 Neuropathology Classification of Pituitary Tumors...... 1774
  - 74.4.1 Historical Histological Classification of Pituitary Tumors...................... 1774
  - 74.4.2 Immunohistochemical Classification of Pituitary Tumors...................... 1774
- 74.5 Molecular Neuropathology........................... 1774
- 74.6 Treatment... 1780
- 74.7 Prognostic Clinicopathological Classification of Pituitary Tumors................................ 1781
- 74.8 Pituitary Adenomas................................. 1781
  - 74.8.1 Somatotroph Adenoma..................... 1781
  - 74.8.2 Lactotroph Adenoma...................... 1785
  - 74.8.3 Thyrotroph Adenoma...................... 1787
  - 74.8.4 Corticotroph Adenoma.................... 1789
  - 74.8.5 Gonadotroph Adenoma.................... 1790
  - 74.8.6 Null Cell Adenoma........................ 1792
  - 74.8.7 Plurihormonal and Double Adenoma......... 1794
- 74.9 Atypical Pituitary Adenoma.......................... 1796
- 74.10 Pituitary Carcinoma................................ 1798
  - 74.10.1 Clinical Signs and Symptoms............... 1798
  - 74.10.2 Epidemiology............................ 1798
  - 74.10.3 Neuroimaging Findings.................... 1798
  - 74.10.4 Neuropathology Findings.................. 1798
  - 74.10.5 Molecular Neuropathology................. 1800
  - 74.10.6 Prognosis................................ 1800
- 74.11 Pituitary Blastoma................................. 1800

		74.11.1	Clinical Signs and Symptoms	1801
		74.11.2	Epidemiology	1801
		74.11.3	Neuropathology Findings	1801
		74.11.4	Molecular Neuropathology	1801
		74.11.5	Prognosis	1801
	74.12	Apoplexia of the Pituitary		1802
		74.12.1	Clinical Signs and Symptoms	1802
		74.12.2	Epidemiology	1802
		74.12.3	Neuroimaging Findings	1802
		74.12.4	Neuropathology Findings	1802
		74.12.5	Molecular Neuropathology	1802
		74.12.6	Treatment and Prognosis	1805
	Selected References			1808
75	**Cystic Lesions**			**1811**
	75.1	Introduction		1811
	75.2	General Aspects		1811
	75.3	Epidermoid Cyst		1811
		75.3.1	Epidemiology	1811
		75.3.2	Neuroimaging Findings	1812
		75.3.3	Neuropathology Findings	1812
		75.3.4	Molecular Neuropathology	1817
		75.3.5	Treatment and Prognosis	1817
	75.4	Dermoid Cyst		1817
		75.4.1	Epidemiology	1819
		75.4.2	Neuroimaging Findings	1821
		75.4.3	Neuropathology Findings	1821
		75.4.4	Molecular Neuropathology	1825
		75.4.5	Treatment and Prognosis	1825
	75.5	Rathke's Cleft Cyst		1825
		75.5.1	Epidemiology	1825
		75.5.2	Neuroimaging Findings	1829
		75.5.3	Neuropathology Findings	1829
		75.5.4	Molecular Neuropathology	1833
		75.5.5	Treatment and Prognosis	1833
	75.6	Colloid Cyst of the Third Ventricle		1833
		75.6.1	Epidemiology	1834
		75.6.2	Neuroimaging Findings	1834
		75.6.3	Neuropatholog Findings	1834
		75.6.4	Molecular Neuropathology	1838
		75.6.5	Treatment and Prognosis	1838
	75.7	Enterogeneous cyst		1841
		75.7.1	Epidemiology	1841
		75.7.2	Neuroimaging Findings	1841
		75.7.3	Neuropathology Findings	1841
		75.7.4	Molecular Neuropathology	1844
		75.7.5	Treatment and Prognosis	1844
	75.8	Arachnoidal Cyst		1845

		75.8.1	Epidemiology........................... 1845

- 75.8.1 Epidemiology.......................... 1845
- 75.8.2 Neuroimaging Findings.................. 1845
- 75.8.3 Neuropathology Findings................ 1845
- 75.8.4 Molecular Neuropathology.............. 1849
- 75.8.5 Treatment and Prognosis............... 1849
- Selected References... 1851

76 Germ Cell Tumors... 1855
- 76.1 General Aspects.. 1855
  - 76.1.1 Epidemiology.................................... 1855
  - 76.1.2 Nuclear Medicine Imaging Findings........... 1856
  - 76.1.3 Immunophenotype............................... 1856
  - 76.1.4 Differential Diagnosis.......................... 1857
  - 76.1.5 Molecular Neuropathology..................... 1857
  - 76.1.6 Treatment and Prognosis....................... 1857
- 76.2 Germinoma.. 1858
  - 76.2.1 Neuroimaging Findings......................... 1858
  - 76.2.2 Neuropathology Findings....................... 1858
- 76.3 Yolk Sac tumor... 1861
  - 76.3.1 Neuropathology Findings....................... 1863
- 76.4 Embryonal Carcinoma................................. 1865
  - 76.4.1 Neuroimaging Findings......................... 1865
  - 76.4.2 Neuropathology Findings....................... 1865
- 76.5 Choriocarcinoma....................................... 1869
  - 76.5.1 Neuroimaging Findings......................... 1870
  - 76.5.2 Neuropathology Findings....................... 1870
- 76.6 Teratoma.. 1870
  - 76.6.1 Neuroimaging Findings......................... 1872
  - 76.6.2 Neuropathology Findings....................... 1874
- Selected References... 1878

77 Lymphomas... 1881
- 77.1 Introduction.. 1881
- 77.2 Primary CNS Lymphoma:............................. 1884
  - 77.2.1 Clinical Symptoms and Signs.................. 1884
  - 77.2.2 Epidemiology.................................... 1884
  - 77.2.3 Neuroimaging Findings......................... 1884
  - 77.2.4 Neuropathology Findings....................... 1885
  - 77.2.5 Molecular Neuropathology..................... 1894
  - 77.2.6 Treatment and Prognosis....................... 1903
- 77.3 Intravascular Lymphoma.............................. 1904
  - 77.3.1 Clinical Signs and Symptoms.................. 1904
  - 77.3.2 Epidemiology.................................... 1904
  - 77.3.3 Neuroimaging Findings......................... 1904
  - 77.3.4 Neuropathology Findings....................... 1904
  - 77.3.5 Molecular Neuropathology..................... 1908
  - 77.3.6 Treatment and Prognosis....................... 1908
- 77.4 Post-Transplant Lymphoproliferative Disorder (PTLD)... 1909
  - 77.4.1 Epidemiology.................................... 1909

		77.4.2	Neuroimaging Findings	1909
		77.4.3	Neuropathology Findings	1910
		77.4.4	Molecular Neuropathology	1910
		77.4.5	Treatment and Prognosis	1910
	77.5	Plasmacytoma	1914
		77.5.1	Epidemiology	1914
		77.5.2	Neuroimaging Findings	1915
		77.5.3	Neuropathology Findings	1915
		77.5.4	Molecular Neuropathology	1920
		77.5.5	Treatment and Prognosis	1920
	Selected References	1920

78 Histiocytic Tumors 1923

	78.1	General Considerations	1923
		78.1.1	Definitions	1923
		78.1.2	Epidemiology	1923
		78.1.3	Nuclear Medicine Imaging Findings	1924
	78.2	Langerhans Cell Histiocytosis (LCH)	1924
		78.2.1	Clinical Signs and Symptoms	1924
		78.2.2	Epidemiology	1924
		78.2.3	Neuroimaging Findings	1925
		78.2.4	Neuropathology Findings	1927
		78.2.5	Molecular Neuropathology	1930
		78.2.6	Treatment and Prognosis	1930
	78.3	Non-Langerhans Cell Histiocytoses	1930
		78.3.1	Epidemiology	1930
		78.3.2	Neuroimaging Findings	1931
		78.3.3	Neuropathology Findings	1931
		78.3.4	Molecular Neuropathology	1934
		78.3.5	Treatment and Prognosis	1934
	Selected References	1941

79 Soft Tissue Tumors: Mesenchymal, Non-meningothelial Tumors 1943

	79.1	General Aspects	1943
		79.1.1	Classification of Soft tissue tumors	1943
		79.1.2	Grading of Soft Tissue Tumors	1943
		79.1.3	Incidence	1944
		79.1.4	Pathogenesis	1944
	79.2	Solitary Fibrous Tumor/Hemangiopericytoma	1944
		79.2.1	Epidemiology	1945
		79.2.2	Neuroimaging Findings	1945
		79.2.3	Neuropathology Findings	1948
		79.2.4	Molecular Pathology	1952
		79.2.5	Treatment and Prognosis	1952
	79.3	Hemangioblastoma	1956
		79.3.1	Epidemiology	1956
		79.3.2	Neuroimaging Findings	1956
		79.3.3	Neuropathology Findings	1959

	79.3.4	Molecular Pathology 1960
	79.3.5	Treatment and Prognosis 1961
79.4	Lipoma.. 1961	
	79.4.1	Definition 1961
	79.4.2	Neuroimaging Findings 1962
	79.4.3	Neuropathology Findings............. 1962
79.5	Undifferentiated High-Grade Pleomorphic Sarcoma: Malignant Fibrous Histiocytoma (MFH)............... 1967	
	79.5.1	Neuropathology Findings............. 1967
79.6	Other Mesenchymal Tumors 1967	
	79.6.1	Hemangioma 1967
	79.6.2	Epithelioid Hemangioendothelioma 1967
	79.6.3	Angiosarcoma 1970
	79.6.4	Kaposi Sarcoma....................... 1970
	79.6.5	Ewing Sarcoma/Peripheral Primitive Neuroectodermal Tumor 1970
	79.6.6	Angiolipoma 1972
	79.6.7	Hibernoma 1972
	79.6.8	Liposarcoma........................... 1972
	79.6.9	Desmoid-Type Fibromatosis 1972
	79.6.10	Myofibroblastoma 1972
	79.6.11	Inflammatory Myofibroblastic Tumor 1973
	79.6.12	Benign Fibrous Histiocytoma 1973
	79.6.13	Fibrosarcoma 1973
	79.6.14	Undifferentiated Pleomorphic Sarcoma/Malignant Fibrous Histiocytoma 1973
	79.6.15	Leiomyoma 1973
	79.6.16	Leiomyosarcoma 1973
	79.6.17	Rhabdomyoma......................... 1974
	79.6.18	Rhabdomyosarcoma................. 1974
Selected References 1974		

80 Bone Tumors 1977
- 80.1 General Aspects of Bone Tumors 1977
  - 80.1.1 Classification of Bone tumors 1977
  - 80.1.2 Incidence 1977
  - 80.1.3 Nuclear Medicine Imaging Findings 1977
  - 80.1.4 Molecular Pathogenesis...................... 1977
  - 80.1.5 Treatment and Prognosis 1984
- 80.2 Osteoma.. 1985
  - 80.2.1 Localization 1985
  - 80.2.2 Neuroimaging Findings 1985
  - 80.2.3 Pathology Findings 1985
- 80.3 Osteoid Osteoma 1986
  - 80.3.1 Localization 1986
  - 80.3.2 Neuroimaging Findings 1986
  - 80.3.3 Pathology Findings 1987
- 80.4 Osteoblastoma 1992

		80.4.1	Localization 1992
		80.4.2	Pathology Findings 1992
	80.5	Osteosarcoma................................ 1992	
		80.5.1	Localization 1992
		80.5.2	Imaging Findings......................... 1992
		80.5.3	Pathology Findings 1994
	80.6	Chondroma................................... 1996	
		80.6.1	Localization 1996
		80.6.2	Pathology Findings 1996
	80.7	Chondrosarcoma 1998	
		80.7.1	Localization 1998
		80.7.2	Imaging Findings......................... 1998
		80.7.3	Pathology Findings 2000
	80.8	Fibrous Dysplasia............................. 2005	
		80.8.1	Localization 2005
		80.8.2	Imaging Findings......................... 2005
		80.8.3	Pathology Findings 2005
	80.9	Chordoma................................... 2005	
		80.9.1	Localization 2010
		80.9.2	Imaging Findings......................... 2010
		80.9.3	Pathology Findings 2010
	80.10	Giant Cell Tumor............................. 2010	
		80.10.1	Localization 2010
		80.10.2	Imaging Findings......................... 2014
		80.10.3	Pathology Findings 2014
	80.11	Aneurysmal Bone Cyst 2016	
		80.11.1	Localization 2017
		80.11.2	Imaging Findings......................... 2017
		80.11.3	Pathology Findings 2018
	Selected References 2020		
81	**Metastatic Tumors** 2025		
	81.1	General Aspects.............................. 2025	
		81.1.1	Epidemiology............................ 2025
		81.1.2	Neuroimaging Findings 2025
		81.1.3	Neuropathology Findings................... 2038
		81.1.4	Histologic Features 2038
		81.1.5	Molecular Neuropathology 2041
		81.1.6	Treatment and Prognosis 2041
		81.1.7	Immunohistochemical Approach 2045
	81.2	Lung Tumors 2051	
		81.2.1	General Aspects.......................... 2051
		81.2.2	Neuropathology Findings................... 2051
		81.2.3	Immunophenotype........................ 2051
	81.3	Breast Tumors 2051	
		81.3.1	General Aspects.......................... 2051
		81.3.2	Neuropathology Findings................... 2051
		81.3.3	Immunophenotype........................ 2061

- 81.4 Skin Tumors: Melanoma 2061
  - 81.4.1 General Aspects 2064
  - 81.4.2 Neuropathology Findings. 2064
  - 81.4.3 Immunophenotype 2070
- 81.5 Renal Tumors. 2073
  - 81.5.1 General Aspects 2073
  - 81.5.2 Neuropathology Findings. 2073
  - 81.5.3 Immunophenotype 2073
- 81.6 Urinary Tract Tumors. 2073
  - 81.6.1 General Aspects 2073
  - 81.6.2 Neuroimaging Findings 2073
  - 81.6.3 Immunophenotype 2073
- 81.7 Prostate Tumors 2076
  - 81.7.1 General Aspects 2076
  - 81.7.2 Neuropathology Findings. 2076
  - 81.7.3 Immunophenotype 2082
- 81.8 Testicular Tumors. 2082
  - 81.8.1 General Aspects 2082
  - 81.8.2 Neuropathology Findings. 2082
  - 81.8.3 Immunophenotype 2084
- 81.9 Gastro-Intestinal Tumors 2084
  - 81.9.1 General Aspects 2084
- 81.10 Colon Carcinoma. 2085
  - 81.10.1 Neuropathology Findings. 2085
  - 81.10.2 Immunophenotype 2085
- 81.11 Esophageal Carcinoma. 2085
  - 81.11.1 Neuropathology Findings. 2085
- 81.12 Gastric Carcinoma 2085
  - 81.12.1 Neuropathology Findings. 2085
  - 81.12.2 Immunophenotype 2085
- 81.13 Liver Carcinoma 2085
  - 81.13.1 Neuropathology Findings. 2085
  - 81.13.2 Immunophenotype 2085
- 81.14 Pancreas. 2093
  - 81.14.1 Neuropathology Findings. 2093
  - 81.14.2 Immunophenotype 2093
- 81.15 Female Genital Tract 2093
  - 81.15.1 General Aspects 2093
- 81.16 Ovarian Carcinoma 2093
  - 81.16.1 Neuropathology Findings. 2095
  - 81.16.2 Immunophenotype 2099
- 81.17 Carcinoma of the Vagina and Cervix 2099
  - 81.17.1 Neuropathology Findings. 2099
  - 81.17.2 Immunophenotype 2101
- 81.18 Uterine Carcinoma. 2101
  - 81.18.1 Neuropathology Findings. 2101
  - 81.18.2 Immunophenotype 2101

Selected References 2104

82	**Therapy-Induced Lesions**		2107
	82.1	Introduction	2107
	82.2	General Imaging Findings	2107
	82.3	Radiation Necrosis	2107
		82.3.1 Epidemiology	2108
		82.3.2 Neuroimaging Findings	2108
		82.3.3 Neuropathology Findings	2108
		82.3.4 Molecular Neuropathology	2114
		82.3.5 Treatment and Prognosis	2116
	82.4	Therapy-Induced Leukoencephalopathy	2116
		82.4.1 Clinical Signs	2116
		82.4.2 Neuroimaging Findings	2116
		82.4.3 Neuropathology Findings	2116
		82.4.4 Molecular Neuropathology	2117
	82.5	Therapy-Induced Secondary Neoplasms	2117
		82.5.1 Molecular Neuropathology	2117
	Selected References		2117
83	**Tumor Progression– Pseudoprogression**		2119
	83.1	Introduction	2119
	83.2	Neuroimaging Findings	2119
	83.3	Neuroimaging Criteria for Therapeutic Outcome	2122
		83.3.1 RANO Response Criteria for *Low-Grade Glioma*	2122
		83.3.2 The Immunotherapy Response Assessment in Neuro-Oncology (iRANO) Criteria	2125
	83.4	Nuclear Medicine Findings	2125
	83.5	Molecular Neuropathology	2125
	Selected References		2137
84	**Autoimmune Encephalitis: Paraneoplastic Syndromes**		2139
	84.1	Definitions	2139
	84.2	Epidemiology	2139
	84.3	Clinical Signs	2139
	84.4	Autoimmune Encephalitides	2142
		84.4.1 Limbic Encephalitis (LE)	2142
		84.4.2 Paraneoplastic Limbic Encephalitis (PLE)	2142
		84.4.3 NMDA-R Encephalitis	2142
		84.4.4 Voltage-Gated Potassium Antibody Syndromes	2143
		84.4.5 Morvan Syndrome	2145
		84.4.6 AMPAR (GluR1, GluR2) Antibody Syndrome	2145
		84.4.7 Glycine Receptor Antibody Syndrome	2146
		84.4.8 Dopamine 2 Receptor Antibody Syndrome (D2RA)	2146
		84.4.9 GABA Receptor Ab Syndrome	2146
		84.4.10 Metabotropic Glutamate Receptor Antibody Syndrome	2147
		84.4.11 IgLON5 Ab Syndrome	2147

	84.5	Neuroimaging Findings............................ 2148
		84.5.1 General Imaging Findings................... 2148
	84.6	Neuropathology Findings........................... 2148
	84.7	Molecular Neuropathology 2151
		84.7.1 Predisposition to Autoimmunity 2153
	84.8	Treatment and Prognosis........................... 2155
	Selected References 2164

Appendix A: WHO Classification of Tumors of the Central Nervous System................................. 2167

Appendix B: WHO Classification of Tumors................... 2181

References 2209

Index... 2215

About the Authors

Serge Weis is the head of the Division of Neuropathology at the Neuromed Campus of the Kepler University Hospital, Johannes Kepler University, Linz, Austria. He is a native of Luxembourg and studied medicine at the University of Vienna (Austria). He was trained in neuropathology at the Ludwig Maximilians University, Munich, Germany. He was deputy director at the Department of Neuropathology, Otto von Guericke University Magdeburg, (Germany) and director of neuropathology at the Stanley Medical Research Institute, Bethesda, MD, USA. His scientific interests are focused on brain tumors, neurodegeneration, and biological psychiatry. He edited the largest book in German-speaking countries on Alzheimer disease and wrote a book, published in 1993, on 3D reconstruction of the brain (serge.weis@kepleruniklinikum.at).

Michael Sonnberger is a senior consultant in neuroradiology at the Department of Neuroradiology of the Neuromed Campus of the Kepler University Hospital, Johannes Kepler University, Linz, Austria. He studied medicine at the University of Innsbruck (Austria) and was trained in radiology/neuroradiology at the University of Regensburg (Germany) and at the State Neuropsychiatric Hospital Wagner-Jauregg, Linz, Austria. His fields of expertise are interventional neuroradiology and stroke (michael.sonnberger@kepleruniklinikum.at).

Andreas Dunzinger is a senior consultant in nuclear medicine at the Department of Nuclear Medicine of the Neuromed Campus of the Kepler University Hospital, Johannes Kepler University, Linz, Austria. He studied medicine at the University of Vienna (Austria). He was trained as a general physician at the Hospital of the Sisters of Mercy, Linz, Austria, and in nuclear medicine at the Medical University of Graz and at the State Neuropsychiatric Hospital Wagner-Jauregg, Linz, Austria. His field of expertise is neuronuclear medicine and neuroendocrinology (andreas.dunzinger@kepleruniklinikum.at).

Eva Voglmayr is a trainee in radiology and neuroradiology at the Department of Neuroradiology of the Neuromed Campus of the Kepler University Hospital, Johannes Kepler University, Linz, Austria. She studied medicine at the University of Vienna. Her field of interest is neurodegeneration (eva.voglmayr@kepleruniklinikum.at).

Martin Aichholzer is deputy head of the Department of Neurosurgery at the Neuromed Campus of the Kepler University Hospital, Johannes Kepler University, Linz, Austria. He studied medicine at the University of Vienna and was trained at the Department of Neurosurgery of the Medical University of Vienna (Austria). His field of expertise is skull base surgery (martin.aichholzer@krpleruniklinikum.at).

Raimund Kleiser is a medical physicist and is the head of the imaging center at the Institute of Neuroradiology at the Kepler University Hospital in Linz. He studied physics in Freiburg im Breisgau (Germany) and supplemented his training with the specialization in medical physics. His focus is on functional imaging, for which he established fMRT measuring equipment in prestigious institutions in Germany, Switzerland, and Austria (Raimund.kleiser@kepleruniklinikum.at).

Peter Strasser is molecular biologist at the PMU University Institute for Medical & Chemical Laboratory Diagnostics of the Paracelsus Medical University in Salzburg, Austria. He studied general biology at the University of Salzburg and specialized in biochemistry and molecular genetics. Dr. Strasser's current focus of interest lies in the genetic background of neurological diseases (p.strasser@salk.at).

Part I
The Techniques

Imaging Modalities: Neuroradiology

1.1 Introduction

Neuroradiology is a subspecialization of radiology which evaluates the brain and spine as well as the face, the neck, and the brachial plexus.

Neuroradiologic techniques include:

- Plain radiographs/X-rays
- CT
- MRI
- Fluoroscopy
- Ultrasonography

The fields of neuroradiology are characterized in Table 1.1 while the applications of the various neuroradiology techniques are shown in Table 1.2.

It is not the aim of this chapter to describe the fundamental physical principles of different imaging techniques in depth. Several comprehensive books already exist on this topic. Details of these physical techniques are beyond the scope of this chapter. The aim is rather to illustrate the physiological-physical context as well as to describe the source of the measurable signal, and the different physiological components around the signal which can be measured with the respective method. In the following, the two main neuroradiological diagnostic methods, i.e., computer tomography

Table 1.1 The various fields of neuroradiology

Diagnostic neuroradiology		• Interpretation of images • Plain radiographs/X-rays • CT • MRI • Fluoroscopy • Ultrasonography
Interventional neuroradiology	Vascular—Diagnostic	• Four-vessel angiogram • Six-vessel angiogram • Spinal angiogram • Arterial and venous sampling
	Vascular—Interventional	• Aneurysm • Arteriovascular malformation • Venous malformation • Stenting • Clot retrieval • T-PA and vasodilation
	Non-vascular—Diagnostic	• Biopsies • Discogram
	Non-vascular—Interventional	• Vertebroplasty • Kyphoplasty • Epidural injection • MILD surgery • Rhizotomies

Table 1.2 Applications of the neuroradiologic techniques

Plain radiographs	• Trauma in primary care facilities • Shunts, e.g., ventriculoperitoneal shunts, ventriculopleural shunts • Foreign bodies, i.e., metallic foreign bodies in the orbital and face • Sinusitis
Computed tomography	• Trauma • Stroke (hemorrhagic vs non-hemorrhagic stroke) • Preoperative planning • Reconstruction procedures • Rule out metallic foreign body • In patients with contraindications to MRI study
Magnetic resonance imaging	• Stroke (first 3–24 h) • Preoperative planning and postoperative follow-up in neoplasms • Non-neoplastic conditions • Arterial and venous structures • Subtle hemorrhage • Physiologic examinations • Fetal MRI studies
Angiography and fluoroscopy	• Diagnostic vascular imaging • Diagnostic non-vascular imaging • Interventional vascular procedures • Interventional non-vascular procedures

(CT) and magnetic resonance tomography (MRT), with their wide scope of applications are described.

1.2 CT-Imaging

In conventional projection radiography, an X-ray image shows for each pixel of the image the sum of the attenuation of the ray intensity along its projection. Computed tomography follows the principles of conventional radiography: a region section of the body, i.e., a slice, is penetrated by the X-ray beam. After the passage of the ray through the slice, the resulting profile of the ray intensity is measured. In contrast to conventional radiography, in computed tomography the attenuation of the ray intensity by the body is not directly displayed on plain film, but is registered with scintillation detectors. The principle of computed tomography was developed by Hounsfield in 1968.

In computed tomography, the scintillation detectors are very sensitive and, thus, enable the use of lower doses of radiation than in conventional radiology. The attenuation of the X-ray intensity depends on the density and the size of the object. The higher the density, the larger the size of the object, i.e., the longer the distance of projection of the X-ray, the smaller is the registered ray intensity.

The projections are described by equations that contain several variables. For other projections of the same slice, new equations will result, but the number of variables will remain constant. These variables are called linear attenuation coefficients and can only be calculated when the number of equations exceeds the number of variables. This implicates that a larger number of projections is necessary for a greater number of voxel (resolution). The reiterative solution of the equations is very protracted. Therefore, in most CT scanners, an algorithm, known as filtered back-projection, is applied. To reconstruct the image, the linear attenuation coefficients of every pixel are calculated. These attenuation coefficients are converted into gray values and displayed on a screen or a film.

1.2.1 Equipment

The mechanism of scanning has been developed very fast. Originally, for every projection, the object was scanned with a pencil beam and a single detector (scanners of the first generation). To complete a projection, a set of parallel shots was necessary. Subsequently, the X-ray tube and the detector were rotated a few degrees to perform the next projection. The scanners of the second generation are very similar to those of the first generation. In contrast, not a pencil beam but a fan beam is employed and is detected by a detector array. Currently, only

1.2 CT-Imaging

scanners of the third or fourth generation are used, particularly to reduce scan time. In both types of these scanners, a wide fan beam is used, which covers the whole extent of a slice. In CT scanners of the third generation, the X-ray tube and the opposite detector array are rotating for every projection. In scanners of the fourth generation, only the X-ray tube is rotating, while the X-ray fan is registered by a stationary detector array.

1.2.2 Image Presentation

Per definition, water has a CT density of 0 HU (Hounsfield Units). The CT density of the other structures can be calculated as follows:

$$\text{HU} = \frac{\mu}{\mu_w} - 1 * 1000$$

μ: linear attenuation coefficient of the voxel
μ_w linear attenuation coefficient of water

Thus, air typically has CT densities of -1000 HU. The density of soft tissues ranges between 10 and 80 HU. CT densities of more than 150 HU are characteristic for bone or metallic materials. Usually, not the entire spectrum of CT densities is shown, but only a part of it. For example, the imaging of the brain is performed in a window between -10 and 80 HU. Structures with a CT density less than -10 HU appear black, whereas structures with a density of more than 80 HU appear white. Thus, only the values between -10 HU and 80 HU are encoded by gray values. The advantage of the window setting is to improve the contrast between the structures of interest. The disadvantage is that structures with CT values out of the chosen window range cannot be differentiated since they are shown uniformly black or white. If bone or bony structures are of interest, a wide window is necessary (ranging from -1000 to $+1000$ HU). In this case, brain structures like the basal ganglia cannot be differentiated.

Because computed tomography measures the linear attenuation coefficient of X-rays, it is particularly well suited for the imaging of bony structures. However, the attenuation coefficients of different brain structures differ very little and, as compared to magnetic resonance imaging, only a small contrast for these structures can be achieved (Fig. 1.1).

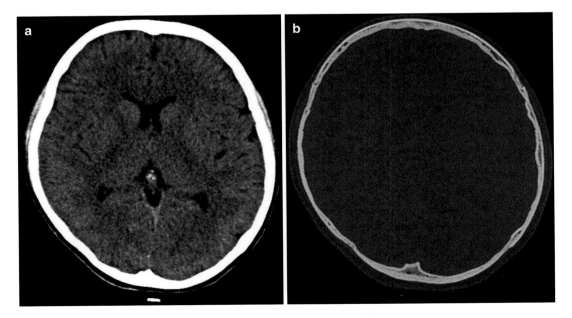

Fig. 1.1 CT image without contrast (**a**) and bone window CT (**b**) of the head

1.2.3 Characteristics of CT-Imaging

In computed tomography, the linear attenuation coefficient of each voxel of the slice is measured. If structures with different densities are located within one voxel (e.g., CSF and gray matter), a mean value proportional to the structure densities results after imaging. This can simulate pathologic findings resembling infarcts or epidural hematoma. This effect is called *partial volume effect*. It has to be considered when examining the borders of different structures in order to avoid diagnostic errors. If an automatic segmentation by thresholding is performed, then partial volume can cause problems by over- or underestimating the segmented structure.

1.2.4 Contrast and Details Resolution

The resolution of a CT image depends on different parameters. The spatial resolution is dependent on the size of a voxel and the slice thickness. Also, the algorithm for reconstruction of the image (kernel) influences the spatial resolution. The thinner the slice and the smaller the voxel slice, the greater is the spatial resolution. By minimizing the voxel size, the signal-to-noise ratio will decrease, and subsequently, an increase of the radiation dose is necessary to compensate for this effect. An increase of the signal-to-noise ratio by the factor 2 implies an increase of the radiation dose by the factor 4.

Contrast resolution depends on the slice thickness. By increasing the slice thickness, the signal-to-noise ratio and, therefore, the contrast resolution will increase. On the other hand, the contrast resolution depends on the object size. The bigger an object, the smaller are the differences in intensity, which can be differentiated. Conversely, a high difference in density is needed to differentiate small objects from the environment.

1.2.5 Artifacts

One source of artifacts is the patient himself. In contrast to conventional radiology, the scan time takes a few seconds. Movements of restless patients during the scanning process lead to miscalculation in the reconstructed image. These artifacts appear as bright, often curved streaks.

Another cause of artifacts is the algorithm of filtered back-projection. At the border of structures with great differences in density, streaky artifacts occur, for example, around metallic materials. Another typical artifact appearing at the skull base is a streak of low density between both petrous temporal bones, which is caused by the bone/air-borders of the mastoid.

1.2.6 Contrast Medium

The contrast medium used in computed tomography does not differ from that used in conventional radiology. A nonionic iodinated contrast medium is usually applied intravenously. A contrast enhancement is observed in vascular or highly vascularized structures, like angioma or the choroid plexus, or in structures with a disturbed blood–brain barrier, for example, in abscess or glioblastoma. The intrathecal use of contrast medium is also possible, and is usually performed for myelography with postmyelographic CT. Rarely, the contrast medium is applied intrathecally to perform a cisternography. An indication for this is the imaging of posttraumatic fistulas.

1.2.7 Recent Developments and Trends

1.2.7.1 High-Resolution-CT

A special algorithm and filter function (kernel) is used for edge enhancement. Application on thin slices (1–2 mm) allows a detailed imaging, particularly of the bone structure. This type of computed tomography is used in the imaging of the petrous temporal bone and inner ear.

1.2.7.2 Spiral-CT

In this type of computed tomography, the table positioning is not only performed during the delay between the scans, but the table is moved continuously. Thus, the X-ray tube describes a helical movement around the patient rather than a circle. The major advantage is that in a minimum of time a maximum of data can be acquired. The data represents the entire volume (not only a set of slices), of which the interesting slices can be calculated. If contrast medium is injected during the scanning process, a homogenous contrast enhancement results. Subsequently, 3D images of the vessels can be performed.

1.2.8 CT-Angiography

Computed tomography angiography (CTA) uses an injection of iodine-rich contrast material and CT-scanning to help diagnose and evaluate blood vessel disease or related conditions, such as aneurysms or blockages.

Angiographic images are acquired through contrast injection of the vessel of interest (Fig. 1.2). Like most arterial angiographic procedures, intra-arterial access is obtained by placement of a catheter (a hollow plastic tube), most often, into the superficial femoral artery. It is an ideal vessel for access, since it is large, superficial, compressible, and not responsible for supply of a vital organ. From the SFA, the catheter is navigated, under X-ray guidance, into the descending aorta, and from there into the great vessels. A variety of catheters and wires are available for safe catheterization of appropriate vessels. Needless to say, angiographic safety and diagnostic yield are extremely operator dependent. It is usually not necessary to place the catheter into the brain vessels themselves; rather, the catheter is maintained within a vessel in the neck. An X-ray dye, usually a nonionic, near-isosmolar X-ray contrast agent, is then injected through the catheter and carried by blood flow into the vessels of the brain. As the X-ray dye (the same dye as used for CT-angiography) passes through the arteries, capillaries, and veins of the brain, a series of X-ray images are made, usually by two cameras located at the front and on the side of the patient's head. The frequency of image acquisition can be varied, as directed by necessity to obtain dynamic information while minimizing radiation exposure. Typical cerebral angiography involves catheterization of both carotid arteries and at least one vertebral artery though exact protocol depends on the indication. Diagnostic angiography is usually performed awake or under mild sedation (the inside of blood vessels has no nerve endings, and therefore the patient does not, for most part, feel the catheter once it is inside the body). Local anesthesia (typically lidocaine) is administered at the groin prior to cannulation of the SFA. For most patients, this is all that is required. The advantage of performing angiography in awake state is that the patient may be given instructions in anticipation of particular diagnostic maneuvers and is better able to hold still during injections, which produces higher quality images. The actual injection of contrast is not painful, but rather perceived by most people as a warm sensation in the distribution of the selected vessel. Other sensations, such as flashes of lights behind one or both eyes, intermittent dizziness, or taste changes, may be experienced depending on the vessel of interest. Most diagnostic angiograms last less than 1 h of actual catheter time, but may vary widely based on indication, vascular health, and other considerations. At conclusion of the study, the catheter is removed from the groin and hemostasis achieved by direct manual compression or deployment of a vascular closure device. Subsequent recovery depends primarily on the particular method of closing the groin puncture site.

1.2.9 CT-Perfusion

Perfusion computed tomography allows rapid qualitative and quantitative evaluation of cerebral perfusion by generating maps of cerebral blood flow (CBF), cerebral blood volume (CBV), and mean transit time (MTT). The technique is based on the central volume principle (CBF = CBV/MTT) and requires the use of commercially available software employing complex deconvolution algorithms to produce the perfusion maps. Some controversies exist regarding this technique, including which artery to use as input vessel, the accuracy of quantitative results, and the reproducibility of results. Despite these controversies, perfusion CT has been found to be useful for noninvasive diagnosis of cerebral ischemia

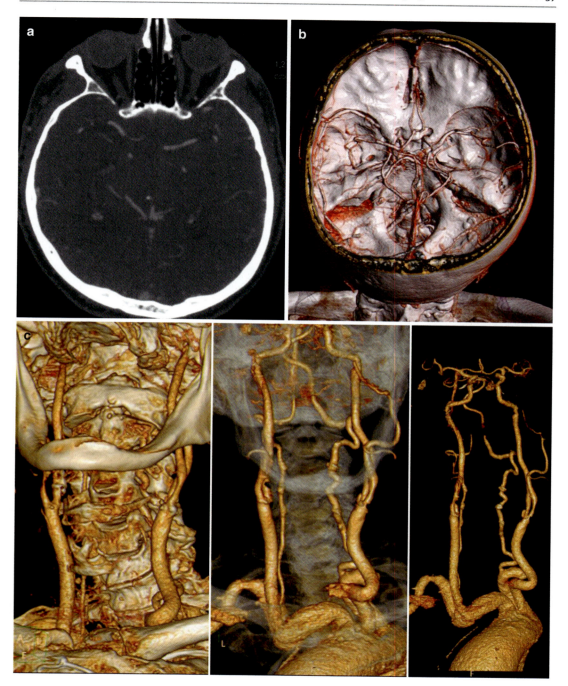

Fig. 1.2 CT-Angiography with contrast axial (**a**) and volume rendering (**b**). Bone substraction of an extracranial CT-Angiography (**c**)

and infarction and for evaluation of vasospasm after subarachnoid hemorrhage. Perfusion CT has also been used for assessment of cerebrovascular reserve by using acetazolamide challenge in patients with intracranial vascular stenoses who are potential candidates for bypass surgery or neuroendovascular treatment, for the evaluation of patients undergoing temporary balloon occlusion to assess collateral flow and cerebrovascular reserve, and for the assessment of microvascular permeability in patients with intracranial neoplasms.

1.3 MR Imaging

Besides CT, magnetic resonance imaging (MRI) is used for in vivo examination of the human brain. Magnetic resonance is a dynamic and flexible technology that allows one to adapt the imaging study to the anatomic part of interest and to the disease process being investigated. As compared to CT, MRI presents a lot of advantages:

- good delineation of anatomic structures, i.e., differentiation between gray and white matter, basal ganglia, and thalamus
- no limitations in orientation of the cutplanes; every direction is possible (e.g., sagittal cuts)
- acquisition of other parameters, i.e., T1, T2, spin density
- no exposure of the patient to ionizing radiation

For a basic understanding of MRI imaging, the physical principles will shortly be explained. The principles of MRI are quite complex, but in the following steps they are described with some simplifications.

1.3.1 Equipment

An MR system consists of the following components:

- a strong magnet to generate the static magnetic field
- shim coils to make the magnetic field as homogeneous as possible
- gradient coils to provide spatial localization of the signals
- a radiofrequency (RF) coil to transmit a radio signal into the body part being imaged—the protons interact with the radio frequency pulse and after switch off the stimulated nuclei return to equilibrium and send a radio frequency signal
- the emitted signal is registered by radio frequency receiver coils
- a computer to reconstruct the radio signals into the final image, whereas the calculation and reconstruction of the image is done after a series of radio frequency pulses

1.3.2 Image Presentation

Protons and neutrons possess a spin, i.e., they rotate around an axis through their midpoint. Nuclei with an odd number of protons or neutrons induce a weak magnetic field. The rotation of the electric charge is causing this induction. In magnetic resonance tomography, the following nuclei can be registered: ^1H, ^{31}P, ^{13}C, ^{23}Na.

Only ^1H, which consists of one proton, will be considered here because this nucleus is usually registered in MRI. If an external magnetic field is applied, the protons are oriented parallel or antiparallel to the external field. Then, they spin around the axis of the external field like a spinning top on the ground. This spinning is also called precession. The precession frequency is proportional to the strength of the external magnetic field and can be calculated following the Larmor equation:

$$\omega = \gamma * B_0$$

ω: precessional frequency
γ: gyro magnetic constant—nuclei-specific constant
B_0: strength of the external magnetic field

The difference in energy between the antiparallel and the parallel state is very small. Thus, only a small excess of the nuclei exists in the energetically favorable parallel state. Applying a magnetic field strength of 1.5 Tesla (T) (for comparison the magnetic field strength of the earth is about 30 µT), the ratio of the parallel to antiparallel oriented spins amounts around 1,000,007/1,000,000 and is a little bit dependent on the temperature. The resulting net magnetization along the axis of the external field is very weak, even considering the large number of ^{1}H in the human body. After the protons are aligned parallel and antiparallel, a radio frequency pulse is applied. The applied pulse corresponds to the precession frequency and provokes two modifications of the proton alignment:

- Some protons interact with the radio frequency pulse and change into the higher energetic antiparallel state, which leads to a change of the net magnetization. The longitudinal magnetization (M_z) along the external magnetic field (z-axis) decreases. A radio frequency pulse, called 90° pulse, causes a rotation of 90° into the xy-plane. Accordingly, a 180° pulse produces a rotation by 180° opposite to the direction of the magnetic field. This is not only a simple rotation from the z-axis to the xy-plane, but rather a helical movement of the net magnetization along the surface of a sphere. For a better comprehension, this fact is described with respect to a rotating system of coordinates (i.e., rotation around the z-axis with precession frequency), and the helical movement corresponds to a simple shift.
- The precession of the protons is synchronized, i.e., the protons are rotating in phase. Previously, the vectors perpendicular to the z-axis did neutralize themselves, but after synchronization, they sum up which results in a transversal net magnetization.

After ending the radio frequency pulse, the protons return to equilibrium. Thereby, they emit energy in the form of a radio frequency signal. Due to the rotation of the transversal magnetization (xy-plane), the emitted radio frequency is a sinusoidal signal, oscillating with the precession frequency. This signal is measured by radio frequency coils and is called free induction decay (FID).

T1 and T2 relaxation processes influence the FID. After ending the radio frequency pulse, the stimulated protons return to the equilibrium state, which means that the original longitudinal net magnetization recovers. Mathematically, this can be described by the following equation:

$$M_z = M_{z0} * \left(1 - e^{-\left(\frac{t}{T1}\right)}\right)$$

M_z: longitudinal magnetization at the time t after a 90° pulse
M_{z0}: longitudinal magnetization before the 90° pulse
T1: spin-lattice relaxation

The T1 constant (spin-lattice relaxation) corresponds to the time t till 63% of the original longitudinal net magnetization M_{z0} has recovered.

Following a 90° pulse, a progressive dephasing of the synchronized transversal magnetization occurs. The following two factors produce this dephasing process:

- inhomogeneity of the micromagnetic environment
- inhomogeneity of the external magnetic field.

Temporal and spatial alterations of the micromagnetic environment of protons, for example, inhomogeneities caused by intramolecular movements or diffusion, lead to a progressive desynchronization. The dephasing of the protons results in an increasing loss of transversal magnetization. The constant T2 (spin-spin relaxation) corresponds to the time t till the transversal magnetization reaches 37% of the original transversal magnetization M_{xy0}.

The loss of transversal magnetization is expressed by the following relation:

1.3 MR Imaging

$$M_{xy} = M_{xy0} * e^{-\left(\frac{t}{T2}\right)}$$

M_{xy}: transversal magnetization at the time t after a 90° pulse
M_{xy0}: transversal magnetization before the 90° pulse
T2: spin-spin relaxation constant

In addition to the inhomogeneity of the micromagnetic environment described above, inhomogeneities of the applied external magnetic field can be observed, which also cause a progressive dephasing. Thus, the loss of transversal magnetization occurs quicker than expected. The time constant of this faster decrease of the transversal magnetization is called T2*.

With its dependence on the more biologically variable parameters of proton density, longitudinal relaxation time (T1) and transverse relaxation time (T2), variable image contrast can be achieved by using different pulse sequences and by changing the imaging parameters. Signal intensities on T1, T2, and proton density-weighted images relate to specific tissue characteristics. For example, the changing chemistry and physical structure of hematomas over time directly affects the signal intensity on MR images, providing information about the age of the hemorrhage. Moreover, with MR's multiplanar capability, the imaging plane can be optimized for the anatomic area being studied, and the relationship between lesions and eloquent areas of the brain can be defined more accurately. Flow-sensitive pulse sequences and MR angiography yield data about blood flow as well as displaying the vascular anatomy. Even brain function can be investigated by having a subject perform specific mental tasks and registering changes in regional cerebral blood flow and oxygenation. Finally, MR spectroscopy has enormous potential for providing information about the biochemistry and metabolism of tissues. As an imaging technology, MR has advanced considerably over the past 10 years, but it continues to evolve and new capabilities will likely be developed.

1.3.3 Characteristics of MR Imaging

The signal intensity on the MR image is determined by four basic parameters: (1) T1 relaxation time, (2) T2 relaxation time, (3) proton density, and (4) flow. The T1 and T2 relaxation times define the way that the protons revert back to their resting states after the initial RF pulse. Proton density is the concentration of protons in the tissue in the form of water and macromolecules (proteins, fat, etc.). The most common effect of flow is loss of signal from rapidly flowing arterial blood.

The contrast on the MR image can be influenced by changing the pulse sequence parameters. A pulse sequence sets the specific number, strength, and timing of the RF and gradient pulses. The two most important parameters are the repetition time (TR) and the echo time (TE). The TR is the time between consecutive 90° RF pulses. The TE is the time between the initial 90° RF pulse and the echo.

The most common pulse sequences are the T1-weighted and T2-weighted spin-echo sequences (Table 1.3) (Fig. 1.3). The T1-weighted sequence uses a short TR and short TE. The T2-weighted sequence uses a long TR and long TE. The T2-weighted sequence can be employed as a dual echo sequence.

The first or shorter echo (TE < 30 ms) is proton density (PD) weighted or a mixture of T1 and T2. This image is very helpful for evaluating periventricular pathology, such as multiple sclerosis, as the hyperintense plaques are contrasted against the lower signal of the cerebrospinal fluid (CSF). More recently, the Fluid-Attenuated Inversion Recovery (FLAIR) sequence has replaced the PD image. FLAIR images are T2-weighted with the CSF signal suppressed.

The TR, matrix size, and NEX (number of excitations) are the only parameters that affect scanning time. Increasing any one of these param-

Table 1.3 Comparisons between TR and TE in T1 and T2 imaging

	TR	TE
T1-weighted	TR < 1000 ms	TE < 30 ms
T2-weighted	TR > 2000 ms	TE > 80 ms

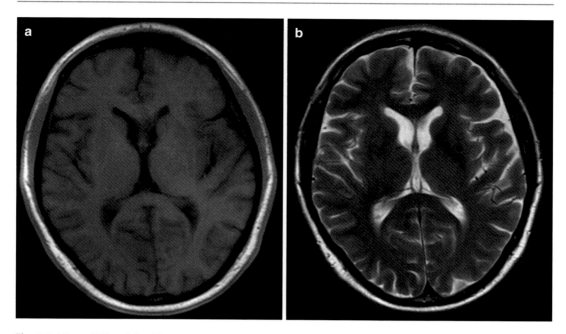

Fig. 1.3 T1- and T2-weighted images: (**a**) In T1, the ventricles appear dark, whereas they are bright in T2 (**b**)

eters increases the minimum scan time. Spatial resolution is determined by matrix size, FOV, and slice thickness. Increasing matrix size or decreasing FOV and slice thickness increases spatial resolution, but at the expense of either decreased signal-to-noise or increased scan time. To obtain images of high resolution with high signal-to-noise requires longer scan times. All of the scan parameters affect signal-to-noise. The signal within an image can be improved by increasing TR, FOV, slice thickness, and NEX or by decreasing TE and matrix size. The most direct way to increase signal is by increasing NEX, but one must keep in mind that increasing NEX from two to four, for example, doubles the scan time, but increases the signal by only the square root of two. Finally, TE does not affect scanning time; however, it does determine the maximum number of slices in the multislice mode. Increasing the TE or shortening TR decreases the number of slices that can be obtained with one pulse sequence.

Specialized techniques for reducing motion and other artifacts on the images also have applications for brain imaging. Gradient moment rephasing or flow compensation techniques effectively reduce ghost artifacts resulting from CSF flow. They should be used for T2-weighted spin-echo and gradient-echo acquisitions, but not with T1-weighted imaging because they increase the signal from CSF. Flow compensation techniques do not contribute to SAR (a measure of power deposition), but the extra gradient pulses lengthen the minimum TE, and gradient heating may limit the number of slices, the minimum FOV, and slice thickness. Cardiac gating also reduces artifacts from CSF pulsations, resulting in superior object contrast and resolving power in the temporal lobes, basal ganglia, and brain stem.

Saturation (SAT) techniques use extra RF pulses to eliminate artifacts from moving tissues outside the imaging volume, such as swallowing or respiratory artifacts, and from unsaturated protons that enter the imaging volume through vascular channels. SAT should be used for T1-weighted imaging of the sella, internal auditory canals, and the spine. The extra RF pulses increases SAR and time, lengthening the minimum TR or decreasing the maximum number of slices in a multislice mode.

Methods for eliminating wrap-around or aliasing should be requested when imaging small anatomic areas, such as the sella and internal auditory canals, with smaller FORs. The "no phase wrap" option is most effective in the anterior-posterior

1.3 MR Imaging

direction for sagittal and axial scans. On newer MR systems, many of these specialized techniques are automatically added to the appropriate sequences.

1.3.4 Contrast and Details Resolution

When studying an MR image, the easiest way to determine which pulse sequence was used, or the "weighting" of the image, is to look at the CSF spaces (i.e., ventricular system). If the CSF is bright (high signal), then it is a T2-weighted image. If the CSF is dark, it is a T1-weighted image.

On MR images of the brain, the primary determinants of signal intensity and contrast are the T1 and T2 relaxation times (Table 1.4). The contrast is distinctly different on T1 and T2-weighted images. In T1-weighted imaging tissues with high fat content (e.g., white matter) appear bright and compartments filled with water (e.g., CSF) appear dark. In T2-weighted imaging compartments filled with water (e.g., CSF compartments) appear bright and tissues with high fat content (e.g., white matter) appear dark. This is good for demonstrating pathology since most (not all) lesions are associated with an increase in water content. PD-weighted imaging is used to differentiate anatomical structures based on their proton density, i.e., the scanning parameters are set (long TR/short TE) to minimize T1 and T2 relaxation effects (Table 1.4). Brain pathologies have some common signal characteristics. Thus, pathologic lesions can be divided into five major groups by their specific signal characteristics on the three basic images: T1-weighted, T2-weighted, and proton density-weighted PD.

Table 1.4 The five major groups of lesions

	T1-weighted	T2-weighted	PD
Solid mass	Dark	Bright	Bright
Cyst	Dark	Bright	Dark
Subacute blood	Bright	Bright	Bright
Acute and chronic blood	Gray	Dark	Dark
Fat	Bright	Dark	Bright

1.3.5 Imaging Protocols

Since studies have shown that T2-weighted images are most sensitive for detecting brain pathology, patients with suspected intracranial lesions should be screened with T2-weighted spin-echo and FLAIR images. The axial plane is commonly used because of our familiarity with the anatomy from CT. The other scan parameters include a 256 × 256 matrix, 1 NEX, 22 cm FOR, and 5 mm slice thickness for a scan time of less than 4 min and a voxel size of 5 × 0.86 × 0.86 mm. A 1–2 mm interslice gap prevents RF interference between slices.

If an abnormality is found, additional modalities help characterize the lesion. Non-contrast T1-weighted images are needed only if the preliminary scans suggest hemorrhage, lipoma, or dermoid. Otherwise, contrast-enhanced scans are recommended. Gadolinium-based contrast agents for MR are paramagnetic and have demonstrated excellent biologic tolerance. No significant complications or side effects have been reported. It is injected intravenously at a dose rate of 0.1 mmol/kg. The gadolinium contrast agents do not cross the intact blood–brain barrier. If the blood–brain barrier is disrupted by a disease process, the contrast agent diffuses into the interstitial space and shortens the T1 relaxation time of the tissue, resulting in increased signal intensity on T1-weighted images. The scans should be acquired between 3 and 30 min post-injection for optimal results.

Contrast enhancement is especially helpful for extra-axial tumors because they tend to be isointense to brain on plain scans. It also identifies areas of blood–brain barrier breakdown associated with intra-axial lesions. Gadolinium enhancement is essential for detecting leptomeningeal inflammatory and neoplastic processes. Contrast scans are obtained routinely in patients with symptoms of pituitary adenoma (elevated prolactin, growth hormone, and so forth) or acoustic schwannoma (sensorineural hearing loss). To screen for brain metastases in patients with a known primary, contrast-enhanced T1-weighted scans alone are probably sufficient.

Gadolinium does not enhance rapidly flowing blood. If vascular structures are not adequately seen on plain scans, the positive contrast provided by gradient-echo techniques or MR angiography may be helpful to confirm or disprove a suspected carotid occlusion or cerebral aneurysm, to evaluate the integrity of the venous sinuses, and to assess the vascularization of lesions. Gradient-echo imaging also enhances the magnetic susceptibility effects of acute and chronic hemorrhage, making them easily observable, even on low- and mid-field MR systems.

Although the axial plane is the primary plane for imaging the brain, the multiplanar capability of MR allows selecting the optimal plane to visualize the anatomy of interest. Coronal views are good for parasagittal lesions near the vertex and lesions immediately above or below the lateral ventricles (corpus callosum or thalamus), temporal lobes, sella turcica, and internal auditory canals. The coronal plane can be used as the primary plane of imaging in patients with temporal lobe seizures. Sagittal views are useful for midline lesions (sella, third ventricle, corpus callosum, pineal region) and for the brain stem and cerebellar vermis.

Scan techniques are slightly different for the sella and cerebellopontine angle. For the sella, the plain and contrast-enhanced scans are obtained in the coronal and sagittal planes using a smaller FOR and thin (3 mm or less) contiguous or overlapping sections. For patients with a sensorineural hearing loss or suspected acoustic schwannoma, contrast-enhanced scans with T1-weighting are obtained through the internal auditory canals, using thin overlapping sections.

1.3.6 Artifacts

As in CT, movements of the patient provoke artifacts, which are visible as blurred images. Pulsating vessels also provoke these artifacts, resulting in a multiple representation of the vessel along the phase encoding gradient.

Another cause of artifacts is given by differences in susceptibility. This is particularly evident for the border between air and tissue in gradient-echo pulse sequences. These differences in susceptibility cause local inhomogeneities of the magnetic field and produce a shortening of $T2*$. In extreme cases, a loss of signal is visible.

In different chemical metabolites, protons show different frequencies of the resonance signal. This effect is known as chemical shift and can produce artifacts since the frequency is also used for spatial localization. Therefore, along the frequency encoding gradient, a local shift of tissues containing a large amount of different metabolites, like fat as compared to CSF, is visible.

1.3.7 Contrast Medium

In magnetic resonance imaging, paramagnetic and superparamagnetic substances are used.

1.3.7.1 Paramagnetic Contrast Medium

The external magnetic field induces a weak magnetic field in the substance. This produces a local increment of the magnetic field. The best known paramagnetic contrast medium is gadolinium complexed with diethylenetriaminepentaacetate (DTPA). The resulting Gd-DTPA-dimeglumine solution is applied in a concentration of 0.1–0.2 mmol/kg body weight. Gd-DTPA does not pass the blood–brain barrier. Similar substances are Gd-DOTA and Gd-DO3A.

1.3.7.2 Superparamagnetic Contrast Medium

This contrast medium shows a similar behavior as the paramagnetic substances, which means they can be magnetized by an external field. In contrast to paramagnetic substances, this effect can be produced by a weak magnetic field. Magnetizers, like ferrite particles, are superparamagnetic substances and are particularly used in the imaging of the reticuloendothelial system. They are not applied in the imaging of the brain.

Supplementary diamagnetic substances show a negative susceptibility, which means, they cause a decrease of the local magnetic field. This is the reason, why they are not used as contrast medium. The contrast medium causes a shortening of the T1 and T2 values, which results in an increase of the signal in T1-weighted images and a decrease in T2-weighted images.

1.3.8 Recent Developments and Trends

The development of magnetic resonance imaging is not yet at its end. Particularly, the following techniques could be integrated in clinical imaging:

Many improvements in MR hardware and software components lead to improved spatial and temporal resolutions. Here the developments to higher magnetic fields up to 7 T play an important role.

Increased interest in molecular imaging using MRI is increasing the number of processes that can be imaged in the brain. Combined PET/MR allows using the high sensitivity of PET-imaging to depict molecular, metabolic, and functional processes in conjunction with the excellent soft tissue contrast and the functional imaging capabilities of MR.

MRI is a more versatile imaging technique than CT since it measures a number of physiological and metabolic characteristics of human tissue. Whereas MRI is used to produce structural images of subjects' brain, the following described functional components allow an in vivo measurement of brain activity.

1.3.9 MR Spectroscopy

MR spectroscopy allows tissue to be interrogated for the presence and concentration of various metabolites. The basic principle is the electron cloud around an atom that shields the nucleus from the magnetic field to a lesser or greater degree. The electron cloud around different chemical compounds shields the resonant atoms to varying degrees depending on the specific compound. This results in slightly different resonant frequencies, what induces a slightly different MR signal.

In radiology practice, the investigated spectra are usually of protons although other nuclei can also be targeted to examine different components. Therefore, different coils are available:

- ^{1}H MRS
- ^{13}C (carbon)
- ^{23}Na (sodium)
- ^{17}O (oxygen)
- ^{31}P (phosphorus)
- ^{39}K (potassium)

If a raw signal of H-MR spectroscopy was processed, then the spectra would be dominated by water, which would make all other spectra invisible. Water suppression is therefore part of any MR spectroscopy sequence; either via inversion recovery or chemical shift selective (CHESS). Additional water suppression is also part of the offline analysis. If water suppression is not successful a general slope to the baseline can be revealed, changing the relative heights and integrals of the peaks.

Many sequences used for MR imaging can also be used for spectroscopy (Fig. 1.4). The simplest sequence consists of a 90° RF pulse without any gradients with reception of the signal by the RF coil immediately after the signal RF pulse. The essential difference between an imaging and a spectroscopy sequence is that for spectroscopy a read out gradient is not used during the time the RF coils are receiving the signal. Instead of using the frequency information to provide spatial information, it is used to identify different chemical compounds (Table 1.5).

Various relationships of metabolites allow improved differential diagnosis (Table 1.6).

MRS can be performed by two methods—single-voxel spectroscopy (SVS), where a single sample volume is selected and a spectrum

Fig. 1.4 ¹H-MRS: Glioblastoma with high choline peak and low NAA peak

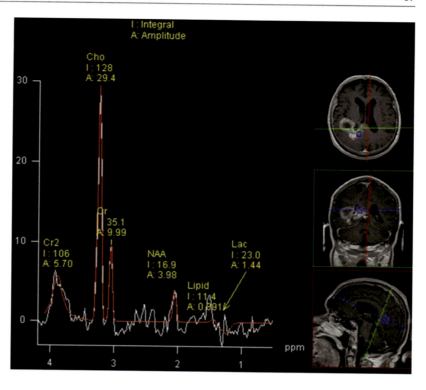

obtained from it, or multi-voxel spectroscopy where spectra are obtained from multiple voxels in a single slab of tissue. SVS gives a better signal-to-noise ratio and is a more robust technique. The disadvantage is that only a single spectrum is obtained. The placement of the volume of interest (VOI) becomes critical and may lead to errors of interpretation if not done correctly. With multi-voxel MRS, a much larger area can be covered, eliminating the sampling error to an extent. This however is done at the expense of a significant weakening in the signal-to-noise ratio and a longer scan time. Both SVS and multi-voxel imaging utilize specialized MR pulse sequences. The two most widely used are the Point Resolved Excitation Spin-echo Sequence (PRESS) and the STimulated Echo Acquisition Mode (STEAM) technique.

1.3.10 MR Angiography

MR angiography is a noninvasive method in which the application of contrast agent is not needed. This is possible because fresh blood shows a high signal in T1-weighted and T2-weighted images. MR angiography is based on assessing the differences in the contrast between blood and the surrounding tissue. To enhance this contrast, the following two methods are applied.

1.3.10.1 Phase Contrast MR Angiography

The differences in phase due to the movement of blood are registered. This method is particularly suitable for imaging a slow blood flow. A relatively high spatial resolution is typical, showing also small vessels. However, phase contrast MRA is often disturbed by subject's movement artifacts.

Table 1.5 List of the resonance peaks for the most important metabolites

Metabolite	Resonance (ppm)	Marker
Myoinositol	3.5	• Concerning about inositol phosphates in intracellular signal processing • More concentrated in glial cells than neurons
Choline	3.2	• Marker for cellular membrane turnover
Creatine	3.0	• Present in metabolically active tissue • Maintained at a relatively constant level • Is predominantly used as a convenient internal standard and allows for ratio calculations
N-acetylaspartate (NAA)	2.0	• Marker of neuronal viability
Lipids	1.3	• Markers of severe tissue damage with liberation of membrane lipids
Lactate	1.3	• Marker of anaerobic metabolism with no peak seen in normal spectra • With a characteristic double peak at long TEs • It is however superimposed on the lipid band, and using an intermediate TE (e.g., 144 ms) will invert only lactate allowing it to be distinguished

Table 1.6 Selection of important pathologies with tendencies of metabolite changes

	Myoinositol	Choline	Creatine	NAA	Lipids	Lactate
Glioma[a]	–	↑	↓	↓	↑	↑
Non-glial tumor				↓		
Ischemia	–	–	–	–	–	↑
Infarction	–	–	–	–	–	↑
Infection				↓		
PML	↑	–	–	–	–	–
Mitochondrial	–	↑	–	↓	–	(↑)

[a]To a higher grade

1.3.10.2 Time-of-Flight MR Angiography

The surrounding tissue in every slice is saturated. The non-stimulated protons entering with the blood flow into the slice give a high signal. The maximum of contrast is achieved, when the slice is positioned perpendicular to the vessel. Usually, this method is applied to image rapid blood flow.

A transversal 3D-gradient-echo pulse sequence (usually FISP-3D) is applied for MR angiography of intracranial vessels. This allows the imaging of the circle of Willis and its branches (Fig. 1.5). In contrast, phase contrast MR angiography is used to image the dural sinus.

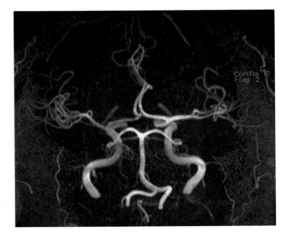

Fig. 1.5 MR angiography

1.3.11 MR-Perfusion Imaging

Perfusion is a fundamental biological function that refers to the delivery of oxygen and nutrients to tissue by means of blood flow. Perfusion MRI is sensitive to microvasculature and has been applied in a wide variety of clinical applications, including the classification of tumors, identification of stroke regions, and characterization of other diseases (Fig. 1.6). Perfusion MRI techniques are classified with or without using an exogenous contrast agent. Bolus methods, with injections of a contrast agent, provide better sensitivity with higher spatial resolution, and are therefore more widely used in clinical applications.

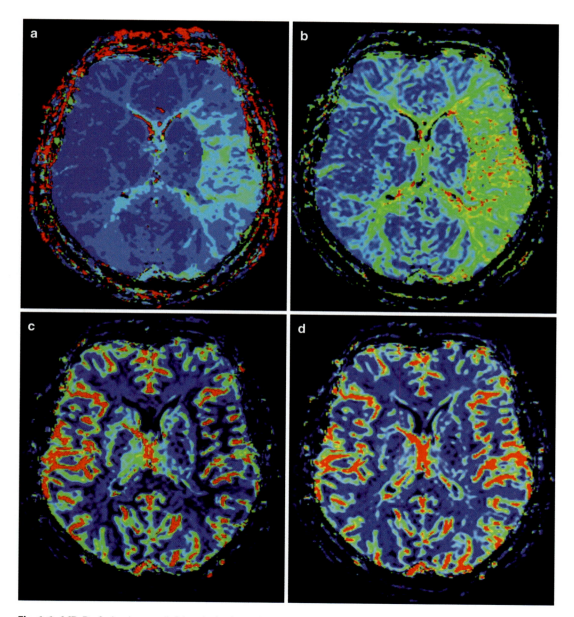

Fig. 1.6 MR-Perfusion in acute left hemispheric stroke TTP (**a**), MTT (**b**), CBF (**c**) and CBV (**d**), and in a glioblastoma WHO grade IV (**e**)

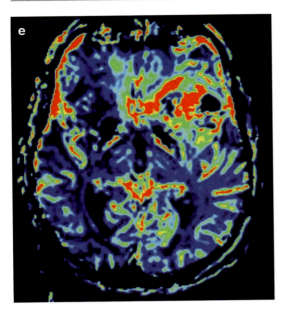

Fig. 1.6 (continued)

However, arterial spin labeling methods provide a unique opportunity to measure cerebral blood flow without requiring an exogenous contrast agent and have better accuracy for quantification. Importantly, MRI-based perfusion measurements are minimally invasive overall and do not use any radiation and radioisotopes. In this review, we describe the principles and techniques of perfusion MRI. This review summarizes comprehensive updated knowledge on the physical principles and techniques of perfusion MRI.

1.3.12 MR Diffusion-Weighted Imaging (DWI)

Diffusion-weighted imaging (DWI) is a form of MR imaging based upon measuring the random Brownian motion of water molecules within a voxel of tissue. The relationship between histology and diffusion is complex; however, in general, highly cellular tissues or those with cellular swelling exhibit lower diffusion coefficients, and thus diffusion is particularly useful in tumor characterization and cerebral ischemia.

As opposed to free diffusion of water kept inside a container, diffusion of water inside a voxel of brain tissue, for example, is hindered primarily by cell membrane boundaries, and thus represents the combined water diffusion in a number of compartments:

- diffusion within the intracellular fluid
    - within the cytoplasm generally
    - within organelles
- diffusion within extracellular fluid
    - interstitial fluid
    - intravascular
    - lymphatic
    - various biological cavities, e.g., ventricles of the brain
- diffusion between intra- and extracellular compartments

The contribution of each one of these will depend on the tissue and pathology. For example, in acute cerebral infarction it is believed that the decrease in ADC values is the result of a combination of water moving into the intracellular compartment (where its diffusion is more impeded by organelles than it is in the extracellular space) and the resulting cellular swelling narrowing the extracellular space 6. Similar mechanisms result in low ADC values in highly cellular tumors (e.g., small round blue cell tumors (e.g., lymphoma/PNET) and high-grade gliomas (GBM)).

1.3.13 MR Diffusion Tensor Imaging (DTI)

DTI is a promising MRI method for studying noninvasively the anatomical organization of major white matter fiber systems (Fig. 1.7). White matter bundles carry functional information between brain regions. The diffusion of water molecules is hindered across the axes of these bundles such that measurements of water diffusion can reveal information regarding the location of large white matter pathways.

A key problem for accurate reconstruction of neuronal fibers is the selection of a suitable tracking algorithm. In certain areas of the white matter, such as the corona radiata or the occipi-

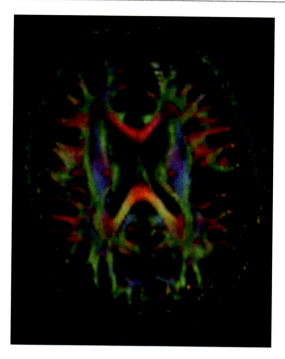

Fig. 1.7 Diffusion tensor imaging (DTI). The direction in which fiber tracts run are color-coded. Red: commissural fibers, Green: association fibers, Blue: projection fibers

tal white matter where an abundant crossing and/or merging of different fiber systems takes place, the main diffusion intravoxel direction does not necessarily correspond to the main fiber direction. This is due to the tensor's voxel averaged quantity and the limited resolution of available DTI acquisitions. Consequently, simple tracking algorithms, which incorporate only the main diffusion direction for determining the propagation pathway (or track) are not adequate in such anatomically complex areas, and the reconstructed trajectories are often compromised by the wrong directional. More complex tracking algorithms have been developed to overcome these limitations, particularly to ameliorate tracking results in crossing and branching situations. This problem can be addressed by using a tracking algorithm called "advanced Fast Marching" (aFM), which has been specifically developed in order to improve reconstruction of white matter trajectories in anatomically complex areas.

1.3.14 Functional MRI (fMRI)

One of the most exciting methodologies in the clinical neurosciences evolving towards the end of the twentieth century was functional magnetic resonance imaging (fMRI) (Fig. 1.8). fMRI has provided new insights into human cognitive functions. fMRI is a type of specialized MRI scan and based on the supposition that there is a relationship between brain function and cerebral blood dynamics. When a neural event occurs in a region of the brain, there is a subsequent increase in local blood flow that changes the ratio of oxyhemoglobin to deoxyhemoglobin in the local microvasculature of the activated region. This change leads to an increase in fMRI signal that has been called the blood oxygenated level-dependent (BOLD) response. Thus, fMRI is an *indirect* measure of neural activity. There is a possible mismatch between the location of the BOLD signal and the actual site of neural activity that can be reduced to a maximum error of 3–6 mm with dedicated MR imaging and postprocessing techniques. The BOLD signal reflects the total amount of deoxyhemoglobin ($dHBO_2$) and is thus a complex function of cerebral blood flow (CBF), the cerebral rate of oxygen metabolism

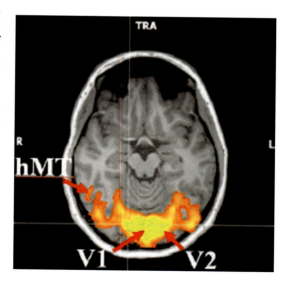

Fig. 1.8 Functional MRI: Activation of the primary visual cortex after visual stimulation

($CMRO_2$), cerebral blood volume (CBV), and the magnetic field strength. Furthermore, the interpretation of changes in the BOLD signal can be complicated by variations in these physiological quantities due to factors such as age, disease, or the presence of vasoactive agents.

1.3.14.1 Task Design and Image Analysis Methods

The choice of the cerebral activation paradigm is perhaps one of the most difficult issues because not enough is known regarding how exactly brain functions are organized. The choice of a paradigm depends on the objective of a study and it deserves careful consideration. What stimuli are presented depends firstly on what functions one wants to measure, and secondly on how closely comparison stimuli can be matched. For an fMRI experiment, one has to devise a task which contains at least two different conditions in order to create a meaningful activation paradigm. During an investigation based on the block design, the patient performs a task of usually 20–30 s, in which specific brain functions are invoked and alternated with periods of a control task. Calculated and compared to a rest condition with nearly no specific brain activation, the whole brain activation related to the performed task is shown. To identify a particular function, the control task should invoke all the functions that are involved in the experimental stimuli, except for the function of interest. Although regions involved in both tasks remain undetected, cognitive processes involved in processing stimuli are generally complex, and can differ considerably between subjects. Accordingly, there are various cognitive functions that require more than one type of control stimulus due to complicated interactions between brain systems. One way of dealing with this is to devise multiple tasks, each of which contains the function of interest plus several functions that need to be filtered out. This is referred to as "conjunction design" and is used for instance in language studies, e.g., in order to isolate "language comprehension."

Temporal resolution of fMRI is generally low, as the BOLD response lags behind the neural response by several seconds and lasts for a single event up to 10–20 s. Methods to increase temporal resolution have received considerable attention, and it is referred to as the event-related design. This term is, however, generally used to indicate the type of data analysis that is applied, in that the hemodynamic BOLD response is an important factor in building the factors for image analysis.

A task may involve presentation of a series of experimental stimuli with an interval of 2 or 3 s, alternating with a series of comparison stimuli. The data can be analyzed with a boxcar function with on and off periods, but alternatively each stimulus can be modeled as a task-related brief event. This impulse function can be transformed to a series of BOLD response curves. Extractions of the BOLD response from the data require a special scheme of varying stimulus onset times and/or inter-stimulus intervals and can be achieved without any comparison stimuli.

Characteristics of the brain processes that are invoked by a stimulus determine whether a block design or an event-related design should be used. For instance, perception of simple visual stimuli involves predictable rapid and brief instances of neuronal activity and can be modeled adequately. Memory tasks, however, cannot be modeled very well in time, making it difficult to construct an adequate impulse function. In this case, a block design may be better suited. Even more complicated is the situation with patients, when, for example, strategies to perform a task are changed. Small differences in the instruction or comprehension can induce major differences in activated brain regions. Therefore, it is necessary that all confounds (e.g., functions one is not interested in) are controlled.

Many of the currently available fMRI data analysis programs make use of multiple regression algorithms based on the General Linear Model. This type of analysis essentially determines whether the fMRI signal time series in each voxel correlates with the task, showing the events that take place when the task is performed, as well as factors that contribute to noise in the dataset. Once an fMRI protocol has been composed, which includes data acquisition method (pulse sequence), task design (paradigm), and image analysis (preprocessing and statistical algorithms)—in which all of them can affect the quality—an fMRI experiment can be tested. Interpretation of results of fMRI experiments is rarely straightforward, and it is important to test the results on the basis of validity, sensitivity, and reliability. Performance is a valuable measure in fMRI because it can indicate not only whether a function is invoked, but also the demand imposed by the task on the underlying brain system. In addition, the quantification of different performance parameters can be used for a parametric statistical analysis and can contribute to a more specific view.

Most MR imaging units today have software for real-time automatic analysis and display results during imaging. The corresponding performance is not a trivial issue and in neuropsychology, performance is generally the readout variable and is used to describe a persons' cognitive abilities. In fMRI, task performance can give rise to problems in image interpretation. Poor performance may be associated with abnormal task solving strategies. For example, the strategy determines how much the working memory system is taxed, and this affects the levels of brain activity as measured with fMRI. In addition, the level of difficulty may also be adjusted for each individual subject, based on a practice session before scanning. An alternative solution is to adjust the statistical analysis to performance by separating scans acquired during correct responses from scans acquired during incorrect responses.

Abnormal fMR imaging activation can, of course, be truly false-positive resulting from movement artifacts or low statistical threshold, but it can also represent variations in normal anatomy and physiology or reflect brain plasticity. On the other hand, failure to detect activity can be caused by several factors; some of them are difficult or impossible to control. Furthermore, a tumor can distort the brain or cause blood flow abnormalities that may alter or diminish the BOLD signal. Absence does not necessarily imply absence of relevant neural activity. Even activity inside the tumor can be detected and may be functionally relevant.

1.3.14.2 Arterial Spin Labeling

BOLD is the most widely used functional MR imaging method, but others such as perfusion fMRI based upon arterial spin labeling (ASL) methods offers another useful complement to BOLD fMRI. In contrast to BOLD, it can provide quantitative measures of both baseline and functional changes in CBF that can aid in the interpretation of the BOLD signal change. Changes in CBF are thought to be more directly linked to neuronal activity than BOLD, so that perfusion fMRI also has the potential to offer more accurate measures of the spatial location and magnitude of neural function. The CBV fMRI is expected to show only microvascular activation regions, which are localized in the brain parenchyma. However, different types of ASL sequences are still under development and have some restrictions especially with regard to number of the acquired image volume and spatial resolution compared to BOLD fMRI. Nevertheless, CBV fMRI can be combined with other fMRI methods to study different aspects of the hemodynamic responses during functional activation and/or physiological challenges. The spatial and temporal characteristics of these multimodal fMRI responses can provide us with a tool for quantitative evaluation of brain physiology, and it can be investigated how the brain regulates its blood supply and maintains homeostasis during normal state and in pathology.

1.3.15 Neuronavigation and Intraoperative MRI

Neuronavigation was developed within the last 20 years in order to improve the safety of brain surgery and to improve functional outcome of the patients' suffering from different kinds of intracranial lesions. In its infancy, the purpose of stereotactic and neuronavigationally guided technologies was to create a mathematical model describing a coordinate system for the space within the closed structure of the skull. The history of neuronavigation, thus, is quite short, but full of highly promising achievements. The advent of neuronavigation, however, would have been impossible without the development of modern imaging technology, electronics, and space technology.

1.3 MR Imaging

The examinations done by highly sophisticated neuroimaging technologies are related to the actual patient's brain during surgery. Computer-graphic modeling and accelerated manipulation of data through complex mathematical algorithms with recent computer technologies facilitate the real-time quantitative spatial depiction of images of a patient's brain creating an individual "fiducial coordinate system." This fiducial spatial system uses fiduciary or natural landmarks as a reference to describe with high accuracy the position of specific structures within a defined space.

1.3.15.1 Neuronavigation Procedure

A diagnostic CT and/or MRI scan image of the patient's anatomy usually taken the day before surgery is loaded into the neuronavigation computer workstation (Fig. 1.9). Similar to navigating in a city on the basis of landmarks, a surgeon uses landmarks in the image scan. The surface of the

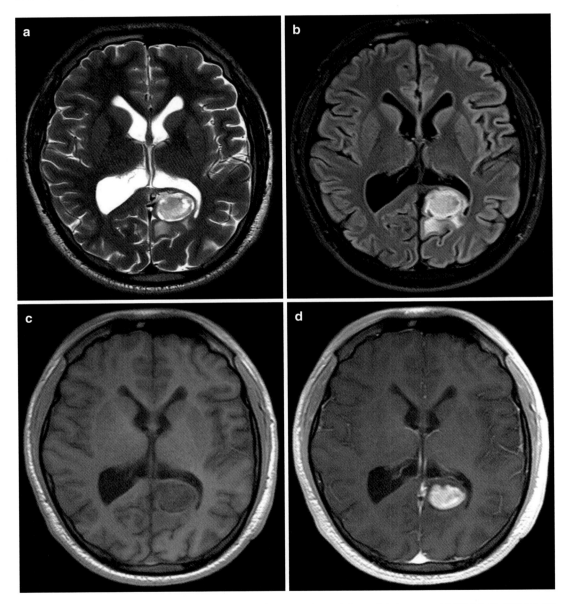

Fig. 1.9 Neuronavigation—part 1: Preoperative MR demonstrating a right occipital tumor with T2 (**a**), FLAIR (**b**), T1 (**c**), T1 contrast (**d**) and intraoperative after Resection T2 (**e**), FLAIR (**f**), T1 (**g**), T1 contrast (**h**)

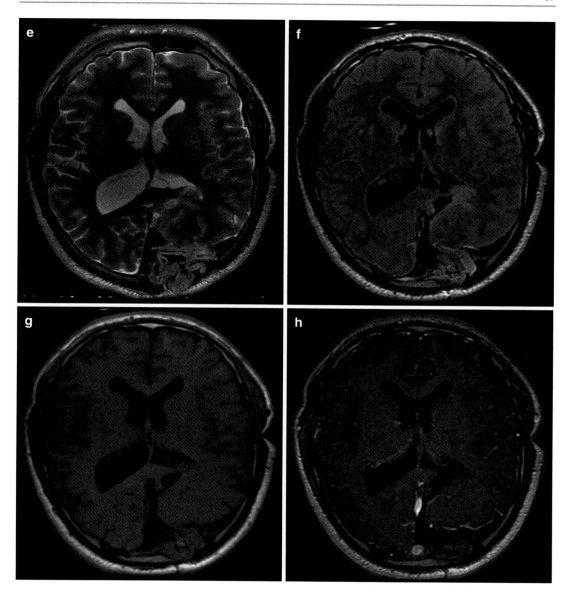

Fig. 1.9 (continued)

head, however, often needs artificial markers because the head is relatively featureless, except for facial features. Therefore, mostly artificial landmarks on the patient's head are used to serve as markers. As alternative, natural landmarks of the head (tip of the nose, bridge of the nose, the inner angel of the eye, etc.) can be used as natural fiducials and superimposed on the 3D images.

The scan is then used to create a 3D model of the patient's brain anatomy. Thus, the patient's unique anatomy can be viewed on the computer monitor of the neuronavigation workstation. Then, entry point, target points, risk zones, targeted resection borders, and vessels are built and displayed in a 3D-manner. Eventually, surgical trajectories and the targeted boarder of the resection area are defined on the computed image and can be anticipated even during the planning period.

These data are then transferred to the computer in the operating room. After anesthesia is administered, before the start of surgery, the surgeon maps the patient's anatomy to the 3D model of the scanned information, using an image-guided probe of the patient's anatomy; this process is known as registration process (also called reference process). As the registration process begins, the neurosurgeon touches the center of the fiducials that have been placed on the patient's head or touches natural landmarks with an image-guided instrument (image-guided pointer or probe). Then the neurosurgeon touches that point on the screen with the instrument. Point by point, on the patient's head in the operation room and then on the monitor, the neurosurgeon builds a correlation between the head and the screen image. By matching the scan with the real anatomy of the individual patient during surgery, the neurosurgeon can accurately "see" the location of the instrument tip in the brain; registration thus means matching a patient's physical anatomy with the 3D computer scan information (Fig. 1.10).

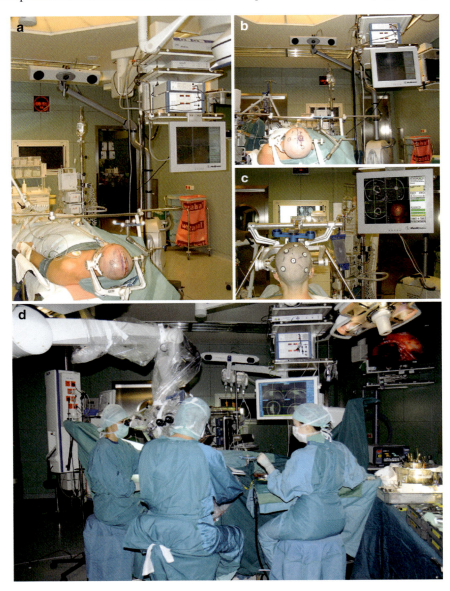

Fig. 1.10 Neuronavigation—part 2: The head of the patient is fixed (**a**); the positions for the reference markers are drawn on the head (**b**); the reference markers are fixed to the skin (**c**); the surgical team views the MRI images with the target (**d**); example of the images with the target provided to the neurosurgeon (**e**, **f**); the region of the tumor is projected onto the bony skull (**g**); the region of the tumor to be targeted is projected onto the cerebral surface (**h**)

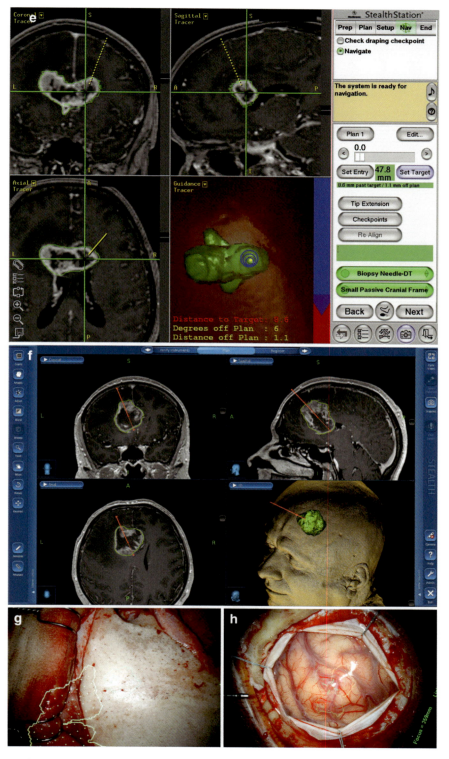

Fig. 1.10 (continued)

As the surgeon moves an instrument in the brain, its position is precisely calculated. The neurosurgeon now can track instrumentation as it proceeds into the operative field as well as view its relative position and trajectory to the operative field allowing the visualization of exact placement and direction of the moving instrument or the microscope. During surgery, the tip of surgical instruments or the focus of the surgical microscope will be displayed dynamically as cross-hairs in all three orthogonal anatomical views on the monitor. This also enables the neurosurgeon to visualize the proximity of the instruments to critical anatomic structures, such as eloquent brain regions, cerebral arteries, venous structures, and cranial nerves. Ultimately, neuronavigation helps the surgeon to accurately detect where he or she is working in the patient's brain at every moment during surgery.

1.3.15.2 Intraoperative MR

Intraoperative MR imaging (iMRI) is a procedure to create and thereby update MR images of the brain during surgery. Neurosurgeons trust on iMRI technology to create accurate pictures of the brain that guide them in removing brain tumors and other abnormalities during operations. Already during opening of the skull but also during surgery it can lead to strong brain shifts, which makes presurgical imaging no longer exactly precise. Intraoperative MRI locates abnormalities if the brain has shifted. MR imaging during the operation gives surgeons the most accurate information. Furthermore, it can be difficult to distinguish the edges of a brain tumor and separate normal tissue from abnormal tissue. Imaging with iMRI during surgery helps to confirm successful removal of the entire brain tumor and to achieve a more complete removal of some brain tumors. For this reason, iMRI has become the standard of care for operations to remove certain brain tumors.

1.3.16 Imaging Protocol Lists

Typical imaging protocols used in diagnostic neuroradiology are shown in Table 1.7.

Table 1.7 Typical imaging protocols used in neuroradiology

Brain routine protocol	• T1_tra_4mm • T2_tra_4mm • flair_tra_4mm • diffusion_tra_4mm • *contrast agent* • T1_mpr_sag • T1_tra_4mm
Tumor protocol	• T2_tse_tra_4mm • flair_tra_4mm • T1_se_tra_4mm • T2_ge_hemo_tra_4mm • DTI_30/30 directions • perfusion *(with contrast agent)* • T1_mpr_sag • T1_se_tra__4mm
Stroke protocol	• diffusion_tra_4mm • swi_tra_4mm • tof_3d_tra_4mm • perfusion *(with contrast agent)* • ge_3d_cor.dyn.carotis • flair_tra_4mm • T1_se_tra_4mm
Epilepsy protocol	• T1_mpr_sag • T2_tse_tra_4mm • flair_tra_4mm • T2_tse_cor_2mm (hippocampus) • T2_tse_tra_2mm (hippocampus) • flair_space_sag • *or* • t2_space_sag • diffusion_tra_4mm • *contrast agent* • T1_mpr_sag • T1_tra_4mm
Neurodegeneration protocol	• *same as Brain routine protocol* • T2*_tra_4mm

Selected References

Bottomley PA, Griffiths JR (eds) (2016) Handbook of magnetic resonance spectroscopy in vivo: MRS theory, practice and applications. Wiley

Brown RW, Cheng YCN, Haacke EM (2014) Magnetic resonance imaging: physical principles and sequence design, 2nd edn. Wiley-Blackwell

Bushong SC (2014) Magnetic resonance imaging: physical and biological principles, 4th edn. Mosby

Buxton RB (2009) Introduction to functional magnetic resonance imaging: principles and techniques, 2nd edn. Cambridge University Press

Constantinides C (2014) Magnetic resonance imaging. Routledge

Huettel SA, Song AW, McCarthy G (2014) Functional magnetic resonance imaging, 3rd edn. Sinauer

Jackson A (ed) (2015) Magnetic resonance spectroscopy. MI Books International

Johansen-Berg H, Behrens TEJ (eds) (2013) Diffusion MRI. From quantitative measurement to in vivo neuroanatomy, 2nd edn. Elsevier-Academic Press

Leite C, Castillo M (eds) (2015) Diffusion weighted and diffusion tensor imaging: a clinical guide. Thieme

Mettler FA (2013) Essentials of radiology. Elsevier

Mori S, Tournier JD (2013) Introduction to diffusion tensor imaging, 2nd edn. Elsevier

Newton HB, Jolesz FA (eds) (2008) Handbook of neuro-oncology neuroimaging. Elsevier-Academic Press

Rinck PA (ed) (2018) Magnetic resonance in medicine: a critical introduction. Books on Demand

Osborn AG, Blaser SI, Salzman KL, Katzman GL, Provenzale J, Castillo M, Hedlund GL, Illner A, Harnsberger HR, Cooper JA, KOnes BV, Hamilton BE (2007) Diagnostic imaging: brain. Amirsys

Stagg C (2014) Magnetic resonance spectroscopy: tools for neuroscience research and emerging clinical applications. Elsevier

Stieltjes B, Brunner RM, Fritzsche K, Laun P (2012) Diffusion tensor imaging: introduction and atlas. Springer

van Hecke W, Emsell L, Sunaert S (eds) (2016) Diffusion tensor imaging: a practical handbook. Springer

Wang Y (2012) Principles of magnetic resonance imaging: physics concepts, pulse sequences, & biomedical applications. CreateSpace Independent Publishing Platform

Weishaupt D, Kochli VD, Marincek B (2008) How does MRI work? An introduction to the physics and function of magnetic resonance imaging, 2nd edn. Springer

Imaging Modalities: Nuclear Medicine

2.1 Introduction

Nuclear medicine is a medical discipline which uses molecular imaging by labeling a pharmaceutical molecule with a radioactive compound in order to visualize the metabolism of the labeled molecule in the human body.

It provides noninvasive quantification of

- metabolism
- receptor binding
- assessment of regional blood flow

Nuclear medicine is used for

- diagnosis
- treatment planning
- outcome prediction
- control of the effectiveness of therapy

It has a widespread use in oncology, neurology, cardiology, and internal medicine.

Radiation used in nuclear medicine originates from the nucleus of the atom (as the name suggests); in contrast, X-rays arise from the atomic shell. The molecules used are able to bind with certain receptors or are incorporated into cells by specific uptake mechanisms and thereby display the metabolic state of the cells. The spatial resolution of nuclear medicine images is lower than those in radiology. Visualizing the metabolism of living cells not only provides valuable information about the normal functioning of the brain but also gives insight into the nature of the pathological processes at work and the alterations of neurochemical pathways. This molecular approach provides the opportunity to visualize and quantify the state of living cells even if only minor structural changes are present. Thus, different pathological structures or even benign processes can be differentiated by nuclear medicine. This information enables one to make significant changes in the therapeutic regimens for the patient indispensable.

The first step is to know which structure should be visualized. Specific tracers have to be chosen to investigate the desired target and thereby identifying the normal brain function or its dysfunction. Then, the suitable pharmaceutical for this purpose has to be chosen and will be labeled with the appropriate radioactive compound. Although this approach sounds simple, it represents the main challenge in nuclear medicine. For example, a pharmaceutical which accumulates too much in other human tissues than that of interest would not be suitable, especially when it concentrates in neighboring structures. It thereby would influence the image quality and cause useless radiation burden to the patient. The labeling of the pharmaceutical can be tricky as well; specialized radio-pharmacists have to fulfill this task. One has to keep in mind, that, although we measure the radioactivity of the radioisotope, the interpretation of these results (as they are transformed into images) requires a lot of experience, whereby several influencing parameters have to be taken into account as described below.

Information about the patient's medical history has to be obtained. The history of diseases includes mandatory information about trauma, the current neurological and/or psychiatric status, past surgical interventions and radiation.

The nuclear medical techniques can be used in vitro and in vivo, but here we concentrate on its use in vivo. A special case represents the diagnosis of brain death: because of brain edema there is no uptake of a brain perfusion tracer and the skull appears empty.

Among the nuclear medical techniques, one can distinguish between

- **SPECT** (Single Photon Emission Computed Tomography) tracers emitting gamma rays
- **PET** (Positron Emission Tomography) tracers emitting positrons (positively charged electrons—antimatter) which collide with electrons and thereby emit annihilation radiation.

These different techniques are described in the following two subchapters.

Changes in the distribution of the radiotracer during the time of image collection have to be taken into account as well as the natural decay of the radiotracer. Thus, too long acquisition times should be avoided (patients in poor health condition would not tolerate long motionlessness). On the other hand, appropriate count statistics have to be obtained (which can be achieved by longer recording times or higher administered doses).

Half-life time plays an important role in nuclear medicine. It is defined as the time in which half of the amount, and thereby the activity, of the radiotracer has declined to half of that in the beginning. This is of importance, as it is mandatory to use a radioisotope with the appropriate half-life for the examination; thus, it is meaningless to use a radioisotope with a very short half-life when we want to observe a slow metabolism and vice versa. Half-life plays also a role in the choice of a radiotracer with regard to its delivery to the hospital: a very short half-life radiotracer would have decayed before it reaches the clinician. For example, carbon-11 can only be used by specialized PET centers (these are facilities which have a cyclotron on site) because of its short half-life of 20 min. A longer half-life gives us the opportunity to perform scans for a longer time period and thereby to acquire dynamic scans. The radioisotope fluoride-18 has an easy to handle half-life of 110 min. On the other hand, fluoride chemistry can be difficult. The labeling with fluoride can also change the biological behavior of the tracer; it is thus necessary to test whether there is a significant change in activity. Half-life does not mean only physical half-life but also biological half-life because the human body is decomposing or excreting the radiopharmaceuticals through various mechanisms or along various organ systems (first of all by urinary excretion). In theory, radioisotopes with a short half-life can be administered several times a day; thus, different examinations before and after an intervention or examinations of different structures can be performed on the same day. In practice, this is of little importance but could be of interest for the future when more structures should be observed simultaneously.

The **energy of emission** is also important as it influences the modality of detection. First, the energy should be so high that it can penetrate the human body and reach the detector. For example, FDG the most commonly used PET tracer has an energy of 511 keV; the most commonly used isotope for SPECT examinations is 99mTc and its energy peaks at about 140 keV. In SPECT, different collimators are used for different radioisotopes whereby the detection window can be adjusted to the used radioisotope. When the energy, on the one hand, is too high, it can trouble the imaging device; on the other hand, the energy of emission plays a major role in the therapeutic approach. When the energy of the emitted particle is higher, more of the surrounding tissue is treated. For example, in

2.1 Introduction

the treatment of larger lesions in neuroendocrine tumors Yttrium-90 is used rather than Lutetium-177 because of its higher energy and consequently higher penetration in tumor tissue.

The **type of radiation** generated in an atomic nucleus is also of importance because the use of a radionuclide depends on it. One can distinguish the following types of radiation (Fig. 2.1):

- gamma radiation consisting of photons
- beta radiation consisting of electrons
- alpha radiation consisting of two protons and two neutrons (the nucleus of helium)

On the one hand, particle emitters are easier to shield (e.g., alpha particles by a sheet of paper); on the other hand, radionuclide emitting particles (beta or even alpha particles) would cause potentially more damage to the patient because of its higher interaction with human tissue (especially if it is incorporated). Because of this interaction, the use of such would not contribute to an adequate image quality (in some cases as with Yttrium-90 Bremsstrahlung images can be obtained, but are of low quality compared to imaging radionuclides). Particle emitters are already used as therapeutic tools and more of these are still under development. Often one tries to label diagnostic pharmaceuticals with alpha or beta emitters, when they have a very good tumor-to-background ratio, in order to use the same pharmaceutical for both diagnostic and therapeutic purposes. In some cases (e.g., Iodine-131), they can be used without a pharmaceutical as they are absorbed through the physiological pathways of the targeted tissue (e.g., thyroid gland).

Tracer kinetics is of importance because they differ for each tracer or examination. It is mandatory to know how fast a tracer reaches the target and is absorbed by it. Furthermore, a tracer can be released or metabolized by the target so that after a while the activity in the target is reduced. In addition, it is also important to know when the background activity is as low as possible, in order to achieve the best target-to-background ratio. Tracer kinetics and half-life are related to each other for

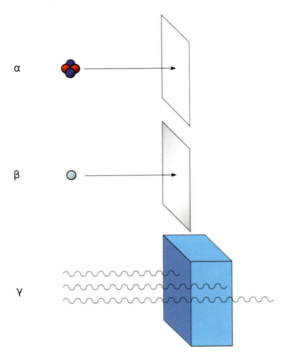

Fig. 2.1 Alpha (nucleus of helium), beta (electron), and gamma radiation (photons) and scheme of needed shielding (source: https://de.wikipedia.org/wiki/Datei:Alfa_beta_gamma_radiation.svg)

the following reason: if the uptake phase lasts longer the background activity may be reduced; however, there might also be a significant reduction of the radioisotope in the target because of its natural decline. Because of these facts, the uptake time has to be defined and kept constant, especially when the same patient is examined two times or more often, particularly if a quantification of the tracer uptake has to be done.

Appropriate **patient preparation** and **standardized acquisition protocols** are prerequisites for an optimal result. Especially for brain studies, the influence of medication and food intake has to be taken into account; on the one hand, they could alter brain metabolism and, on the other hand, interfere with the radiopharmaceutical agent given to the patient. It is mandatory to understand the physiological function of the brain, the pathophysiology of disease processes, and the effects of medication.

Patients have to be positioned properly in the scanner. Usually, the patient is in supine position and the head is fixed with the help of foamed plastic to provide a stable position of the patient throughout the whole examination. Often the orbitomeatal line is used for standardization of patient positioning. Patients are instructed to avoid movements of the head and should also void the bladder for maximum comfort and to minimize radiation burden when the tracer is excreted by the urinary system. In some cases (i.e., FDG-PET and CBF-scans), patients should be positioned comfortably in a quiet, dark room prior to and after tracer injection. For tracer injection, a cannula which is rinsed with a sodium chloride solution has to be used to avoid paravenous tracer injection (the tracer would not harm the patient, but would influence the image quality or leads to lack for image acquisition and make thereby the correct assessment of the image impossible).

Because of differences in uptake kinetics, standardized acquisition protocols with a fixed uptake time and acquisition parameters are recommended, in order to make scans from different patients and repeated scans from the same patient comparable.

During the study, patients have to be under **continuous supervision**. Especially if sedation is necessary, patients have to be monitored adequately; an emergency backup and an antidote is mandatory.

Data analysis can be performed in different ways. Most commonly, a visual interpretation of the images is done, but automated analysis is available for different purposes. The challenge of these automated programs is to compare the patient's metabolism with a "normalized" metabolism, which is reconstructed by signal averaging of healthy control subjects. On the one hand, these databases can differ for age, gender, or even continents. On the other hand, it could be a valuable tool to exclude subjective bias of the investigator. Due to these circumstances, it would be best to create own databases for the different study protocols. In PET, semi-quantitative analysis is available by calculating the standardized uptake value (SUV).

In order to avoid pitfalls and to interpret the functional images accurately, the past clinical history of the patient, its present neurological and/or psychiatric status, the results from past examinations (SPECT, PET, CT, MRI, EEG, etc.), and the actual intake of medication (i.e., psychotropic medication and the last intake) have to be known by the physician.

The most common pitfalls include: patient movement during the study, contamination with the radiotracer (e.g., with urine), dysfunction of the cannula, former therapies (i.e., surgery, radiation, chemotherapy), influence of medication on the metabolism of the radiotracer (e.g., sedatives), food intake (i.e., FDG and amino acid PET), other diseases, processing failures, age-dependency.

The images can be viewed in the three axes parallel to the body planes (Fig. 2.2):

- transversal: at right angles to the long axis of the body
- sagittal: from the back to the front, like the sagittal suture
- coronal: from the left to the right, like the coronal suture
- three-dimensional mode

Three-dimensional display may be particular helpful for a more accurate topographic orientation in some clinical questions (but always in combination with the standardized plane slices to avoid pitfalls by artifacts) (Fig. 2.3).

It is mandatory to check the images for movements of the patient between the CT- and PET-scan because this would cause artifacts by the attenuation correction (Fig. 2.4).

Attenuation correction is part of the data analysis. This means that the radiation which originates in the body is attenuated by the surrounding human tissue. Several possibilities for correction can be used. Transmission imaging with a 68Ge source, CT scans, MRI, and

2.1 Introduction

mathematical models are available. If there is patient movement between the transmission and emission scan, attenuation correction leads to misleading interpretation.

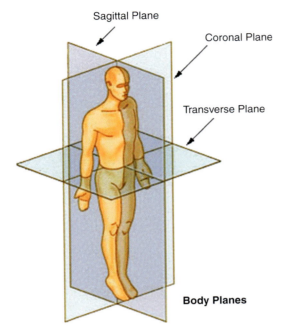

Fig. 2.2 Body planes (source: https://de.wikipedia.org/wiki/Datei:BodyPlanes.jpg)

Data analysis also means applying filtering methods (most commonly used filters include the Hanning and Shepp-Logan filters in PET systems and low-pass filters like Butterworth in SPECT systems), iterative reconstruction methods and reorientation procedures of the images (the intercommissural line is the most commonly used method). Quantification can be done by calculating the SUV or, especially in SPECT systems, comparing the uptake behavior with that of a region with disease-independent constant uptake. If possible, data should be compared with age-matched normal controls.

For the visual assessment of the images, many different scales can be used. It has to be taken into account that the selection of the scale can markedly influence the display. The scale should not only show different shades of color but should also allow the discrimination of structures at the same time (Fig. 2.5). A threshold has to be chosen appropriately to allow the correct interpretation of the image by visualizing all shades of the scale. Images should be read on the computer screen rather than from hard copies to allow the variation of the color scale and thresholding (Fig. 2.6). For comparison, age-matched databases are preferably used especially those databases which are

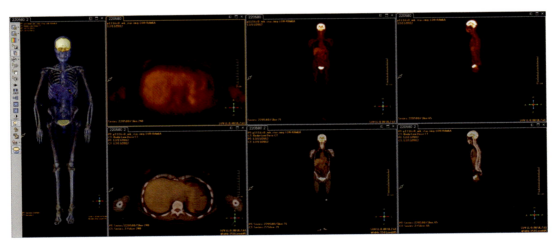

Fig. 2.3 Example of a whole body examination (from left: 3D fused PET/CT, transversal plane, coronal plane, sagittal plane)

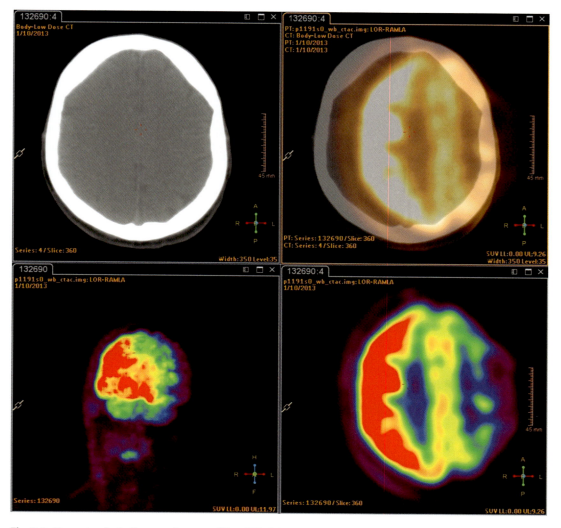

Fig. 2.4 Example of misalignment between CT and FDG-PET acquisition

acquired on the same type of camera and with the same processing conditions (reconstruction, filtering, and attenuation correction) as the study.

For quantification, ROI (region of interest) techniques are used in SPECT as well as in PET systems. With this technique the specific structure can be chosen and the tracer accumulation measured and compared to a reference region with usually low specific tracer binding. In PET systems, the SUV (standardized uptake value) can be calculated for the ROIs (even for three-dimensional ROIs). For the interpretation of nuclear medicine studies, morphological changes revealed by CT or MRI have to be taken into consideration.

Reporting has to be adequate. It should include all pertinent information like name of the patient, birth date, relevant patient's medical history, reasons for the examination, potential pit-

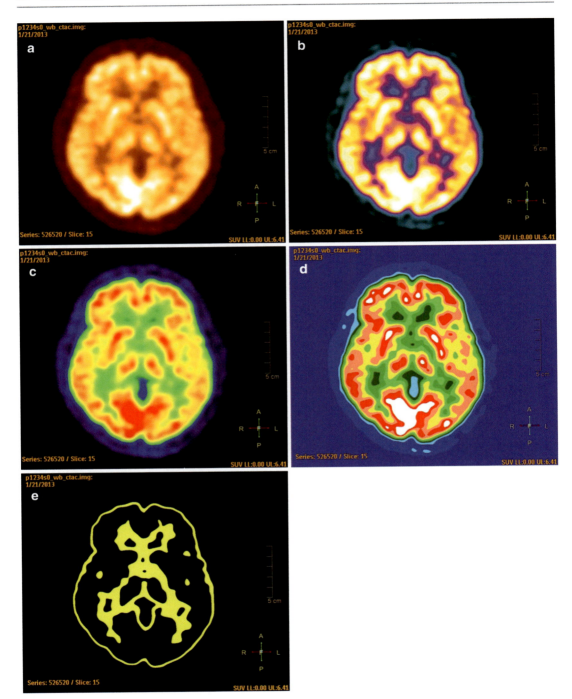

Fig. 2.5 (**a–e**) Examples of different color scales and their influence on the impression of the image (the threshold is kept the same for all images)

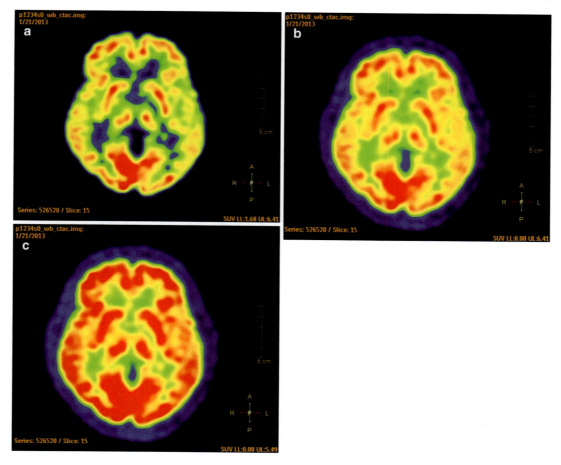

Fig. 2.6 Influence of thresholding on the impression of the image with the same color scale. (**a**) High lower threshold, (**b**) mean lower and upper threshold, (**c**) high upper threshold

falls (i.e., interfering medication, hyperglycemia), type of examination, date of examination, radiopharmaceutical, administered activity, used acquisition protocol, sedation, findings (physiological and pathologic) with a description of the localization and intensity (i.e., semi-quantitative and quantitative) of the uptake, limitations (i.e., patient's movement, small lesions, localization of the lesion near a physiologically high uptake), answer on clinical issues and comparative data (previous studies, CT and MRI). At the end of the report, the interpretation and conclusion should state the most probable diagnosis based on generally accepted disease patterns (subjective interpretation of the images has to be stated), differential diagnoses (if appropriate), and additional or follow-up studies should be recommended, if appropriate.

Contraindications for nuclear medicine studies have to be mentioned. In general, pregnancy and breast feeding are (relative) contraindications because of the radiation burden. Due to the absence of adverse reactions against radiopharmaceuticals, they are generally tolerated well. In some cases, there could be a contraindication in circumstances with an additional stimulation (e.g., for Diamox) or in certain patient condition (e.g., humpback, hyperglycemia). Furthermore, lack of cooperation is a relative contraindication (if sedation is not applicable).

For the **production of radionuclides** a generator, a nuclear reactor or a cyclotron can be used (Figs. 2.7, 2.8, and 2.9) (Tables 2.1, 2.2, and 2.3). Most PET tracers are produced in a cyclotron, so a short explanation of the function of such a facility should not be lacking. Charged particles are accelerated in a vacuum by an electromagnetic field on their helical path. This beam of charged particles is directed on a (stable) target when it reaches the desired velocity and thereby energy. On the target, they produce an altered nucleus which is unstable. The target material has to be pure in order to avoid other radioisotopes than the desired. The cyclotron has to be shielded well to prevent the staff from maximal radiation burden.

Quality Assurance

For both, SPECT and PET systems quality controls are essential to provide the best performance of the system and thereby the best image quality. These control tests contain spatial resolution, energy resolution, spatial distortion, non-uniformity, count rate characteristics, sensitivity, center of rotation, tomographic resolution, tomographic uniformity, and pixel size calibration.

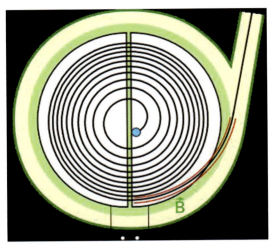

Fig. 2.7 Working principle of a cyclotron (source: https://de.wikipedia.org/wiki/Datei:Zyklotron_Prinzipskizze02.svg)

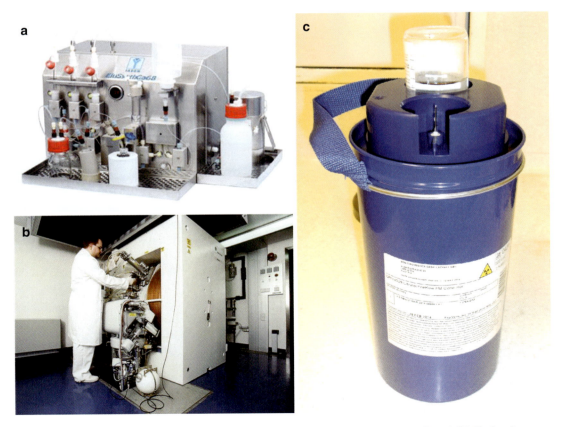

Fig. 2.8 Example of a germanium/gallium generator (Iason) (**a**), example of a cyclotron (Iason) (**b**), Technetium generator (**c**)

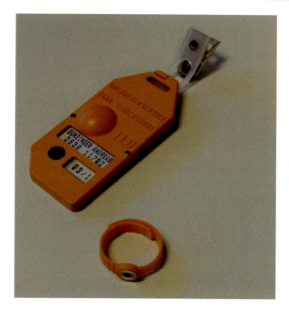

Fig. 2.9 Dosimeter for whole body measurement (above) and ring dosimeter for measurement of hand exposure

Table 2.1 Some examples of radionuclides used for gamma camera systems

Radionuclide	Production	Half-life
99mTc	Generator	6 h
123I	Cyclotron	13 h
131I	Reactor	8 days
111In	Cyclotron	2.8 days
201Tl	Cyclotron	73 h
67Ga	Cyclotron	78 h

Table 2.2 Some examples of radionuclides used for PET systems

Radionuclide	Production	Half-life
18F	Cyclotron	110 min
11C	Cyclotron	20 min
15O	Cyclotron	2 min
68Ga	Generator	68 min
124I	Cyclotron	4.2 days

Table 2.3 Some examples of radionuclides used for therapy

Radionuclide	Production	Half-life
131I	Reactor	8 days
177Lu	Reactor	6.6 days
90Y	Generator	2.7 days
89Sr	Reactor	50 days
153Sm	Reactor	1.9 days

Table 2.4 Deterministic effects of ionizing radiation

Threshold dose 0.25 Sv	• Short-lasting changes in blood count
Temporary radiation syndrome 1 Sv	• Illness • Blood count changes • Loss of hair after 2 weeks • Gastrointestinal problems
Mean lethal dose 4 Sv	• 50% of the people die
Lethal dose 6 Sv	• Nausea and vomiting after 1 h • Diarrhea • Fever • Cachexia • 100% of the people die

Radiation Protection

Ionizing radiation has the potential to interfere with human tissue by causing serious and long-lasting damage, like cell death and chromosomal aberrations, thereby leading to long-term effects. Radiation protection includes the protection of the patient, his family, the general population, and the nuclear medicine staff. There are explicit laws in each country concerning these fields.

It has to be mentioned that different human tissues have different radiosensitivities. Bone marrow is relatively sensitive so that already at lower doses changes in blood count can be observed. In contrast, skin is relatively insensitive.

For the calculation of the effective dose, one has to consider the biological effect of radiation depending on the type of radiation (alpha, beta, gamma) and the sensitivity of the human tissue. The unit used to characterize the effective dose is called Sievert (Sv) and in practice we talk about milli-Sievert (mSv).

One can differentiate between **deterministic effects** (Table 2.4), which are well defined and take place at a certain dose, and **stochastic effects** (e.g., mutagenesis and carcinogenesis). For stochastic effects, only doses above a relatively high dose of 100 mSv is a linear dose–effect relationship defined. Below this level, one can only assume what takes place. For example, *hormesis theory* says that a small amount of radiation would increase the repair systems and thereby minimize the potential harmful effect of radiation. Most of the physicians believe there is a linear dose–effect relationship also at lower doses.

Some factors contribute to the dose:

- the activity (the higher the administered activity is, the higher the dose—here the ALARA principle should be mentioned which is the abbreviation for As Low As Reasonable Achievable and means that the administered dose should be high enough to get usable images but not higher)
- the time (the longer the time a person is near the source of radiation, the higher would be the dose)
- the distance (doubling the distance to the source of radiation would quarter the dose)
- the shielding (it depends on the kind of radiation (higher energy of radiation needs better shielding), but in general the better the shielding, the lower the dose).

The unit of activity of a radioactive tracer is Bequerel (1 Bq is one decay per second) and in practice, we have to handle with Megabequerel (MBq). The patient is asked to drink enough to flush the urinary system and void the bladder frequently to reduce radiation burden. For radiation, protection only defined amounts of radioactivity are administered to the patient.

Nuclear medicine staff wears personal dosimeters (mostly thermo-luminescence-dosimeters TLD) for monitoring. Special finger dosimeters are available to detect the obtained finger radiation dose. Furthermore, radiation detectors to measure contamination of the hands, feet, and clothes are available at a Department of Nuclear Medicine. In case of contamination, decontamination facilities are necessary. When leaving the nuclear medicine department, the clothes and shoes have to be changed to prevent staff from carrying radioactivity with them. Eating and drinking in the department is prohibited to avoid ingestion of radioactivity.

For the protection of the population, only patients with a radiation dose under a defined limit are allowed to leave the nuclear medicine department. In general, the administered amount of radioactivity for diagnostic purposes is so low

Table 2.5 Examples for radiation burden in nuclear medicine examinations

99m-TC ECD (brain perfusion SPECT)	550 MBq	2.7 mSv
111-In DTPA (liquor SPECT)	25 MBq	0.53 mSv
123-I FP-CIT (dopamine receptor SPECT)	185 MBq	4.35 mSv
18-F FDG (glucose-PET)	200 MBq	3.8 mSv
11-C MET (amino acid PET)	400 MBq	2.08 mSv
68-Ga DOTATOC (somatostatin receptor PET)	100 MBq	3.45 mSv
18-F FET (amino acid PET)	200 MBq	3 mSv

to cause no problem (Table 2.5). Only in therapeutic cases, could it be necessary to keep the patient in the department for a defined time. Especially for children, dosage cards (i.e., from the European Association of Nuclear Medicine) are available and dose reduction has to be conducted.

2.2 SPECT: Single Photon Emission Computed Tomography

SPECT has the advantage over planar imaging to produce 3D pictures. Planar imaging shows a two-dimensional image of a three-dimensional tracer distribution, thus overlaying or subjacent structures can influence the targeted formation. Most of the systems are dual-headed; for brain imaging, three-headed systems or dedicated brain imaging devices are of advantage because of better count statistics. SPECT is used in investigating the brain, the myocardium, the lung, or used even in tumor imaging or skeletal imaging as an additional technique.

For SPECT acquisition, planar images are recorded 360° around the patient. Therefore, a step and shoot technique (moving the camera head to the next position and record an image) in which different numbers of images can be chosen, Furthermore, the recording time of the single image can be modified to get a better count statistic, or a faster examination can be chosen. Alternatively, a continuous mode can be selected (the camera head rotates slowly around the patient and records images continuously during the rotation period). The images can be viewed transversally, sagittally, and coronally. The continuous mode may provide shorter acquisition times and reduce mechanical wear to the imaging device.

For the sake of simplicity: the photon leaves the targeted structure, passes human tissue, and leaves the body. The gamma camera (Fig. 2.10) has lead collimators (different collimators are available for the different purposes, resolutions, and radionuclides with their corresponding different energies of emission) which separate the photons so that they can impact on the scintillating crystal. There they cause a short flash of light which is increased by a photomultiplier (Figs. 2.11 and 2.12) and then counted by the computer system. The counts have to be filtered and analyzed.

Attenuation correction is available, but not needed in general (it can be obtained by a long living radioisotope which is implemented in the camera or nowadays by CT or MRI). Especially for images of the brain, arithmetical attenuation correction is possible due to the homogeneity of the brain tissue and the skull. Jewelry or other metallic things have to be removed from the patient, as far as it is possible, because of the attenuation caused by them. For the analysis of the images, filtered back-projection and iterative reconstructions are available. The camera can be set on the peak of emission energy of the used

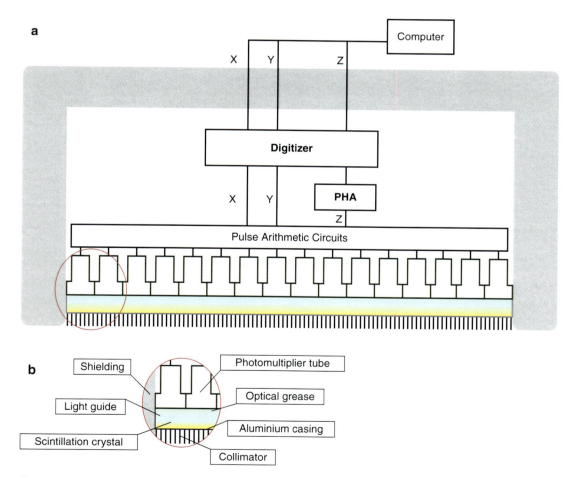

Fig. 2.10 Scheme of a gamma camera detection device (source: (**a**) https://commons.wikimedia.org/wiki/File:Gamma_camera_cross_section.PNG (**b**) https://de.wikipedia.org/wiki/Datei:Gamma_Camera_Cross_Section_detail.png)

2.2 SPECT: Single Photon Emission Computed Tomography

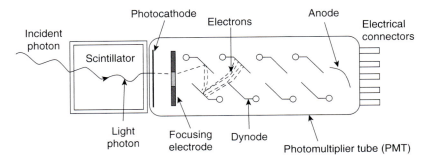

Fig. 2.11 Scheme of a photomultiplier (source: https://de.wikipedia.org/wiki/Datei:Photomultipliertube.png)

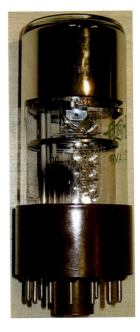

Fig. 2.12 Photomultiplier (source: https://de.wikipedia.org/wiki/Datei:Pmside.jpg)

radioisotope (with a defined window), so scattered photons or photons of other origin can be excluded.

Gamma cameras can be used for PET-imaging when they are designed for coincidence detection. These systems have a relatively poor spatial resolution and a lower sensitivity compared to PET systems. The crystals used in gamma cameras (NaI) are not the same as in PET cameras (BGO, LSO, GSO), and the thickness of these crystals plays a major role too. Furthermore, PET systems are designed as a ring of crystals, while gamma cameras have one, two, or three heads.

The number of camera heads is important for the image acquisition, as more heads allow to acquire a better count statistic and therefore results in more impressive images with a better target-to-background ratio which provides a more accurate diagnosis.

The distance of the gamma camera head to the patient is important too, as the nearer the camera head is to the patient, the better is the spatial resolution of the image. In this regard, compromises have sometimes to be made because of the constitution of the patient (e.g., patients with a humpback or patients with claustrophobia). The patient has to be fixed properly, so that there is no (or nearly no) movement during the image recording, which can last up to 20 or 30 min. Patient movement would result in blurred images or even suggest different diagnoses (e.g., two pathological focuses resulting from one, which is moved to another localization).

In order to get a better count statistic, dedicated brain imaging systems have been developed, but are not commonly used, because the newer SPECT systems with camera heads are nearly equal and can also be used in other studies (e.g., skeletal system, heart kidney, lung) as well. Another development consists in the development of hybrid SPECT/CT systems. In these systems, SPECT and CT can be performed in a "one-stop-shop" examination. The question whether the combination of CT with SPECT is helpful, has to be answered by each physician himself. The invention and subsequent use of PET/CT in brain imaging seems to be of limited benefit for neurological patients.

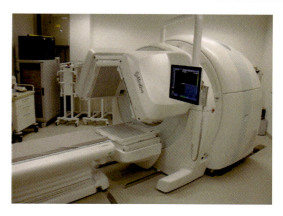

Fig. 2.13 Example of a three-headed gamma camera

Attenuation correction can be performed by calculation (according to Chang), by transmission scan or, nowadays, by CT in SPECT/CT systems (Fig. 2.13).

2.3 PET—Positron Emission Tomography

PET is based on the use of an unstable isotope which emits positively charged electrons, called positrons. They have to travel a very short distance in human tissue before colliding with electrons and thereby emitting annihilation radiation from two photons with an energy of 511 keV emitted in opposite directions (nearly 180°). They are scattered and attenuated by human tissue and find their way to the photosensitive crystals. The crystals in PET systems are circularly arranged to collect the annihilation radiation. The photons are only accepted when they arrive simultaneously at 180° (coincident events) (in contrast to SPECT which is characterized by a single photon).

PET can be used in a two-dimensional mode with barriers between the crystals or in a three-dimensional mode without these barriers. In the 3D mode, all coincidences are counted (including the oblique planes). Thus, the 3D mode allows a much better count statistic, but needs more computing capacity (which is not a problem with the new systems). The newest PET/CT systems acquire only 3D mode images and thereby enhance the image quality and sensitivity of the examination. 3D mode PET/CT also allows shorter acquisition times. The flashes are collected, intensified, filtered, and analyzed (with an attenuation correction using a transmission scan for example with Ge68). PET systems nowadays are always offered as a hybrid system PET/CT (or PET/MR), hence this correction can be obtained by the anatomical information (Figs. 2.14 and 2.15).

PET/MR systems are on the march; however, they face some problems with this attenuation correction and are more expensive. First comparative studies showed that the diagnostic accuracy (e.g., in glioma patients) is not lesser than in PET/CT; the question remains whether there is a future for this modality in the clinical routine, or if it should be used only in research or specialized centers. PET/MR is propagated particularly in neurological investigations; experience showed that a co-registration of PET with MR in separated systems is no problem (the brain is not moving in the skull between two examinations and the computer capacity is high enough to fuse the two images properly). The benefit in daily routine for a patient consists in a "one-stop-shop" exploration, like it is nowadays possible in hybrid PET/CT devices. Especially for PET/MR systems, it would be helpful to use the newest designed systems (like time-of-flight systems and 3 T MR) because of shorter examination time. When using contrast media for CT, we have to consider the effect on attenuation correction especially for oral contrast media.

Computing capacity has to be relatively high for PET systems; beside true coincidences, there can be an accidental coincidence (the two photons arriving in a coincidence having origins from different sources), scatter (one photon has undergone Compton scattering before detection), or multiple coincidences (more than two photons arrive in coincidence). Coincidence in the case of PET includes a short time difference of some nanoseconds due to physical and technical reasons.

PET studies can be performed as a dynamic scanning (the data collection at multiple time points) or as a static study. Dynamic scanning can be used for the absolute quantification of glucose

2.3 PET—Positron Emission Tomography

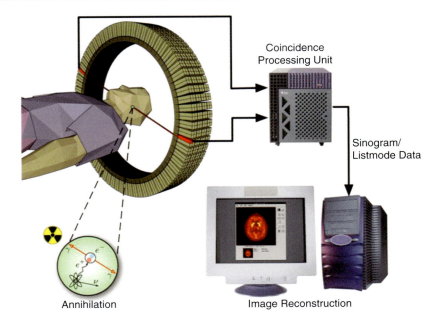

Fig. 2.14 Scheme of a PET system (source: Wikipedia14: https://de.wikipedia.org/wiki/Datei:PET-schema.png)

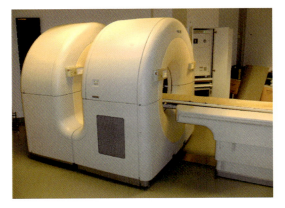

Fig. 2.15 Example of a PET/CT system with the CT element in the front, the PET element in the rear

metabolism or to monitor the changes in uptake behavior of the selected target over time. Dynamic scanning can be useful in agitated patients. The sinograms of the different images can be checked and thereby eliminating image frames with patient's movement. In most clinical settings, static image acquisition is used by most centers.

One of the advantages of PET is the possibility of quantifying the tracer uptake with the so-called SUV (standardized uptake value), which is corrected for the administered dose, the decay, and the body weight or the body surface, respectively. Unfortunately, the different PET systems do not produce comparable SUV values. Massive efforts to standardize and harmonize this SUV calculation are needed in order to make different PET systems comparable. The newest computing systems allow the calculation not only of the SUV in one layer but also SUV calculation in the three-dimensional mode combined with the assessment of the included volume (i.e., the gross tumor volume in glioma patients). For SUV calculation, standardized uptake times are necessary because of tracer-kinetics to make scans of different patients and repeated scans of the same patient comparable. In addition to SUV calculation, a calibration factor is needed. Another advantage is that the spatial resolution of PET is better than in SPECT systems (about 5 mm).

Two facts limit the potential of better spatial resolution. First, the positron travels a short distance in human tissue before being annihilated. Second, the positron still has some energy when it meets an electron. This energy is the cause for the angle of the annihilation radiation to be $180° \pm 6°$. Thus, the combined effect of these factors limits the potential resolution of the system to 2–3 mm.

2.4 FDG-PET

FDG [fluorine-18 fluoro-2-deoxyglucose] was introduced in 1976 and behaves as an analog to glucose. It is transported into the cells by the glucose transporter Glut-1. In the cell, FDG is phosphorylated to 18FDG-6-PO4 which is trapped into the cell and only metabolized very slowly. In contrast to glucose, FDG is excreted by the urinary system at normal blood glucose levels. FDG-PET scans of the brain are most commonly performed 30 min after injection. The administered dose is 125–300 MBq in the 3D mode in adults.

In the brain, glucose provides about 95% of the ATP production required for brain function. Glucose and, thereby, FDG uptake is closely related to neuronal activity, and changes in neuronal activity can be observed by FDG-PET before structural changes occur.

The most common indications for cerebral FDG-PET are: dementia, epilepsy, movement disorders, and neuro-oncology.

Before injection, the patient should fast for at least 4 h to allow an optimal cerebral FDG uptake which is not influenced by food intake or elevated blood glucose levels. The blood glucose level should be under 160 mg/dL, since at higher levels there is an increased competition between the blood glucose and FDG at the Glut-1 and thereby resulting in lower FDG uptake leading to a lower diagnostic accuracy. The patients with diabetes should be at stable blood glucose levels because the acute correction of hyperglycemia with insulin improves only partly the image quality. The patient should avoid excessive stimulants, alcohol, and any drug affecting brain activity.

Patient preparation includes the positioning of the patient in a quiet, dark room some minutes before and at least 20 min after injection of FDG. A cannula for the intravenous injection should be placed beforehand. Furthermore, it is recommended that the patient should void the bladder before and after scanning to minimize radiation burden (FDG is excreted by the urinary system). The history of neurological and/or psychiatric diseases and status, the results from former examinations (SPECT, PET, CT, MRI, EEG, etc.), and the medication (i.e., psychotropic medication and the last intake) have to be known by the physician.

If sedation is necessary, it should be performed as late as possible because of its influence on FDG uptake. Short-acting medication is preferred for sedation and the patient has to be monitored with pulse oximetry. An emergency backup (i.e., an antidote) has to be available.

The patient should be positioned comfortably, the head should be fixed, and the patient should be advised to avoid voluntary movement to prevent artifacts. The position of the patient should be standardized. Attenuation correction has to be done by transmission scan or nowadays by CT or MRI.

Emission scan acquisition usually starts 30 min after FDG injection. For tumor imaging, the uptake phase could be longer to achieve a better delineation of the tumor from the healthy tissue (for this indication amino acid PET is usually performed today). Standardized acquisition protocols with a fixed uptake time and acquisition parameters are recommended to make scans from different patients and repeated scans from the same patient comparable, due to tracer-kinetics.

Especially for quantification purposes, SUV calculation is used. Standardized uptake and acquisition times are mandatory. In general, data acquisition needs about 15 min and a minimum of 10 min is recommended to get an appropriate count statistic. In agitated patients, shorter acquisition times can be helpful; however, an inferior image quality and thereby diagnostic accuracy has to be accepted. Normally 50–200 million coincidental events are collected. Transmission scans are being performed with CT nowadays.

2.4 FDG-PET

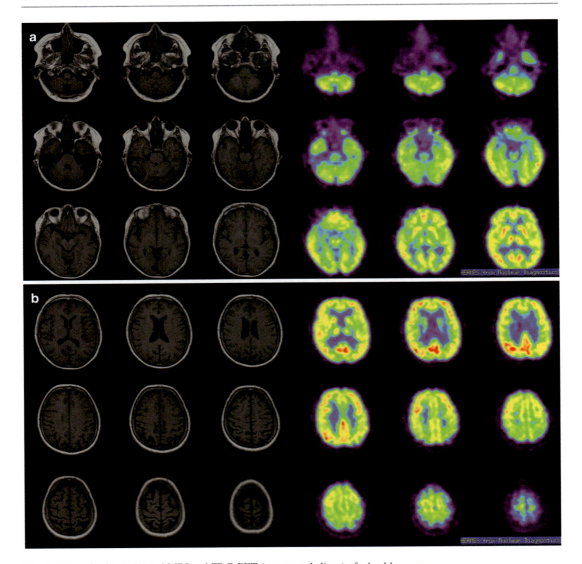

Fig. 2.16 (**a**, **b**) Co-registered MRI and FDG-PET (transversal slices) of a healthy person

Reformatting to standardize plane orientation can be performed, if necessary.

Analysis includes a visual interpretation and can be based on a semi-quantitative analysis by the comparison with a "normalized" data base. The images have to be matched with morphology obtained by CT and MRI (Figs. 2.16, 2.17, and 2.18).

The most common pitfalls are: patient movement, cerebral activation (i.e., the visual and motor cortex), elevated blood glucose and medication (especially sedation and psychotropic drugs).

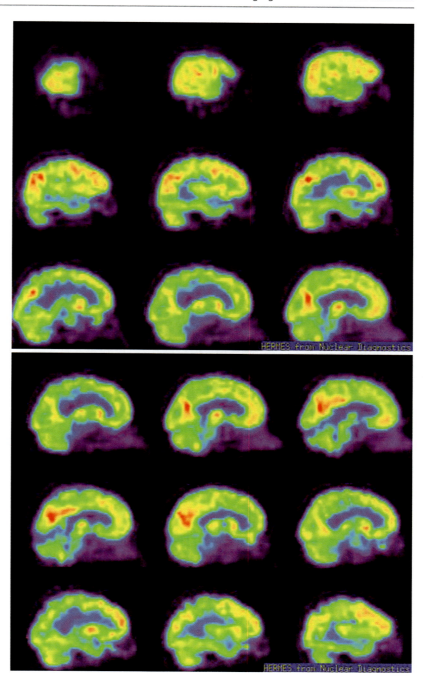

Fig. 2.17 Sagittal slices of an FDG-PET

2.4 FDG-PET

Fig. 2.18 Coronal slices of an FDG-PET

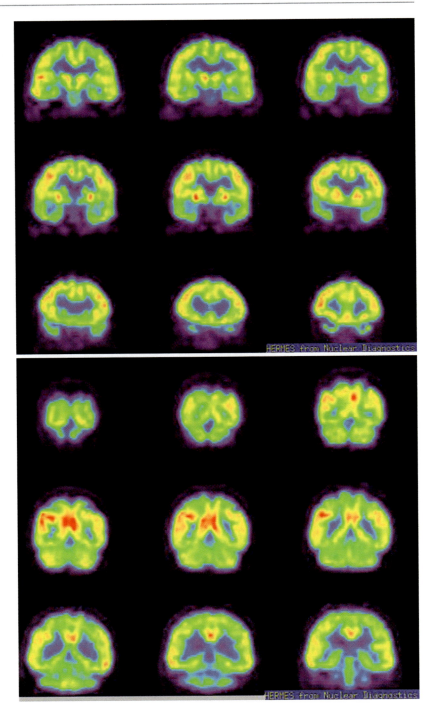

2.5 Amino Acid PET

Amino acid uptake in brain tumor cells results from overexpression of the transporter system and cell proliferation. The tumor-to-background ratio is much better than in FDG-PET or in conventional anatomical imaging, as there is nearly no amino acid uptake in healthy brain tissue due to the lack of proliferation. Furthermore, amino acids are more tumor specific because of lesser uptake in inflammation.

[Methyl-11C]-L-methionine (MET) is frequently used, but has the disadvantage of a short half-life of about 20 min; thus, it is only applicable in PET centers with a cyclotron on site. O-(2-[18F]fluoroethyl)-L-tyrosine (FET) is one of the tracers which were developed to overcome the disadvantages of MET. It uses the same transporter system, i.e., L-system, but is not incorporated into proteins and has a longer half-life of 110 min due to the use of 18fluorine. FET has a fast uptake kinetic, a high in vivo stability and can, in contrast, easily be synthesized. Results of MET and FET-PET are similar although FET is preferred in many institutions because of the advantages described above.

The common indications are:

- Detection of viable tumor tissue (differentiation of viable tumor from non-neoplastic changes, i.e., radiation necrosis)
- tumor delineation (estimation of the gross tumor volume—FET-PET is superior to CT and MRI and has a much better tumor-to-background ratio than FDG, which is taken up in normal cortex and basal ganglia)
- selection of the biopsy site (identification of the part of the tumor with the highest grade of malignancy for stereotactic biopsy to prevent sampling error due to the heterogeneity of gliomas)
- noninvasive tumor grading (at the moment the discussion about the value of amino acid PET is ongoing—FDG seems to be better suited for this purpose)
- prognostic marker (the uptake activity in low-grade gliomas seems to be a marker of cell proliferation and thereby the biological activity of the tumor—higher uptake is correlated with a poorer prognosis)
- radiation therapy planning (in combination with anatomical imaging amino acid, PET can be used to define the gross tumor volume to include all active proliferating areas which might be missed by CT or MRI)
- tumor response (the change of amino acid uptake can predict the response to radiotherapy and chemotherapy)
- tumor recurrence (possible early detection of residual or recurring tumor after surgery)

Patients should be fasting for a minimum of 4 h prior to amino acid PET to assure stable metabolic conditions. Some studies showed a higher uptake in patients pre-loaded with amino acids although there is a competition between the labeled and unlabeled amino acids. It seems that transport outside of the unlabeled amino acids in exchange for the labeled ones takes place. In contrast to FDG-PET, sedation is not a problem in amino acid PET due to the very low uptake in healthy brain tissue and the independence of amino acid uptake in brain tumors to neuronal activity. The patient should empty the bladder before scanning, to prevent maximum discomfort and to minimize radiation burden, as in FDG-PET. The patient's head should be fixed; the patient should be positioned comfortably and advised to avoid voluntary movements. The positioning of the patient should be standardized. As in FDG-PET, the patient's medical history has to be known (especially previous surgical interventions, chemotherapy and radiation as well as former nuclear medicine examinations). The typically administered dose is 200–250 MBq in adults.

Images can be performed as static (i.e., 30 min p.i.) or dynamic images (20–40 min p.i.). The patients should be positioned properly to avoid movement artifacts. Attenuation correction and image processing has to be done as described above. Reformatting, to standardize plane orientation, can be performed if necessary.

Image interpretation can be done visually or by quantification. It is necessary to use the same interpretation method for each patient and for repeated studies. The optimal way is to gather information from the own patients and create a database on which cut offs are defined. There are several possibilities: quantification by SUV alone or by using a contralateral reference region. The images have to be matched with morphology obtained by CT and MRI.

Pitfalls include: artifacts, insufficient attenuation correction, physiologic MET uptake, inappropriate reference region, brain hematoma, close to surgery or radiotherapy, brain abscess, acute ischemic lesions resulting in postischemic hyperperfusion, false-negative results in low-grade gliomas (20%) (but indicating a better prognosis in these patients), false-negative results due to Bevacizumab therapy and false-negative results in gliomatosis cerebri.

2.6 123I-FP-CIT

Various cocaine analogs labeled with 123I are suitable for the assessment of the DAT (dopamine transporter) system in the presynaptic neurons which are responsible for the reuptake of dopamine from the synaptic cleft. The presynaptic terminals of neurons projecting from the substantia nigra connect to the postsynaptic nerves by using dopamine as neurotransmitter. The most commonly used tracers are [123I]β-CIT and [123I]FP-CIT.

The indications for imaging include parkinsonism and dementia with Lewy bodies. The tracers can differentiate between parkinsonian syndromes related to Parkinson disease, multiple system atrophy, and progressive supranuclear palsy on the one hand and from essential tremor or side effects from neuroleptic drugs on the other hand. The tracer cannot differentiate between PD, multiple system atrophy, and progressive supranuclear palsy.

Patient preparation in these investigations is discussed frequently. The patients should avoid taking any medication which could significantly influence the analysis (i.e., amphetamines, CNS stimulants, Modafinil, antidepressants, adrenergic agonists, anticholinergic drugs, opioids, anesthetics). It is understood that the withdrawal can only be done if the patient can tolerate it, whereby the omission of the medication should be started at least five times the drug's biological half-life time before the date of the examination. Antiparkinsonian drugs do not affect DAT binding significantly and therefore they don't have to be withdrawn. Smoking may interfere but does not have a significant effect on DAT binding.

Prior to injection, the thyroid gland has to be blocked (e.g., with sodium perchlorate) to prevent free radioactive iodine from accumulating in the thyroid. The history of neurological and/or psychiatric diseases and status, the results from former examinations (SPECT, PET, CT, MRI, EEG, etc.), and the medication (i.e., psychotropic medication and the last intake) have to be known by the physician. Contraindications have to be taken into account (pregnancy, breast feeding, and inability to cooperate).

The typically administered dose is 150–250 MBq (most commonly 185 MBq) in adults. In children, there are no established clinical indications. If necessary, the recommendations of a pediatric task group have to be adopted. Data acquisition is started 3–6 h after injection for FP-CIT and 18–24 h after injection for β-CIT. As described above, a fixed interval between injection and image acquisition is recommended to make the investigations comparable between patients and for intra-individual follow-up studies. The patient should void the bladder before and after the scan to minimize radiation burden. The patient should be informed about the acquisition time and about the necessity of avoiding voluntary movements of the head. Sedation can be used in uncooperative patients, if necessary. The head should be fixed comfortably to avoid movements.

As in all brain imaging studies, triple or dual head SPECT cameras should be used (or even specific brain imaging devices) due to the better count rate and thereby the better image quality and validity (for FP-CIT more than three million detected events and for β-CIT at least one million detected events are requested). The scanning time is usually around 30 min (single head camera systems would need a longer acquisition time and higher administered doses of the radiotracer).

The data have to be reconstructed (filtered back-projection or iterative reconstruction) and filtered (usually with a low-pass filter); attenuation correction has to be done (calculated according to Chang or measured with a transmission or CT scan). The slices have to be reformatted in the three orthogonal planes (standardized), and semi-quantitative evaluation with ROIs (striatum, caudate nucleus, putamen, and reference regions like occipital cortex or cerebellum) has to be applied.

The image interpretation is done by visual assessment and semi-quantitatively with a ROI (region of interest) technique. For ROI definition, morphology as obtained by CT or MRI can be used. For semi-quantitative analysis, usually transverse/oblique slices are selected and the slices with the striatal binding are added together. The following features have to be described: the shape of tracer accumulation, asymmetries in tracer accumulation, differences between caudate nucleus and putamen, and tracer binding in contrast to reference regions with low tracer uptake (e.g., cerebellum, occipital cortex, and frontal cortex). Ideally, data from age-matched normal controls are available for comparison.

Some pitfalls have to be considered, which include: medication (as described above), technical artifacts, and age dependency of DAT reduction.

Reporting should include a precise diagnosis based on standardized criteria or on the recommendation of further investigations, like D2 receptor imaging of FDG-PET.

2.7 D2 Receptor Ligands

For the assessment of D2 receptors, the following radiotracers are available:

- For SPECT: 123I-IBZM and 123I-epidepride
- for PET: 11C-raclopride, 18F-fallypride, and 18F-desmethoxyfallypride(DMFP)

For the dopaminergic system, D1, D2, D3, D4, and D5 receptors are described and are divided into D1-like receptors (D1 and D5) and D2-like receptors (D2, D3, and D4). The radiotracers bind also to D3 receptors, but the vast majority of D2-like receptors in the striatum are D2 receptors. Thus, the clinical assessment of the D2 status is possible and we can refer to the radiotracers as D2 receptor ligands. These radiotracers are dopamine receptor antagonists. The affinity and selectivity differs between the tracers, making it mandatory that these differences have to be taken into account by calculating specific binding ratios and the optimal time point for acquisition.

The most common indication for the use of D2 receptor ligands is the differentiation of Parkinson disease from other neurodegenerative parkinsonian syndromes, like multiple system atrophy and progressive supranuclear palsy. They can also be used in the assessment of Wilson disease (to show the degree of neuronal damage), Huntington disease (for this purpose, FDG is widely available), assessment of D2 receptor blockade with neuroleptic drugs, and the assessment of the dopamine receptor status in pituitary adenoma. The common contraindications have to be taken into consideration (pregnancy, breast feeding, and inability to cooperate).

If 123Iodine ligands are used, the thyroid has to be blocked (e.g., sodium perchlorate 200 mg) before tracer injection. The patient's history and current status (i.e., neurological and psychiatric), medication (i.e., dopamine agonists, neuroleptics, metoclopramide, amphetamine), and results of morphological and prior nuclear medicine imaging studies have to be known by the physician. The withdrawal of medication, especially neuroleptics and dopamine agonists, is discussed controversially because the time of withdrawal depends on the biological half-life of the drug, which can mean it would have to be withdrawn for months. Furthermore, in some cases, the patient needs the medication and it is not appropriate to withdraw it. Nevertheless, if possible the medication should be stopped and images should be acquired at OFF conditions.

Injection should be given via a tested cannula as a slow intravenous bolus. The administered activity in adults is 150–250 MBq (typically 185 MBq) of 123I-IBZM, 123I-epidepride, 18F-fallypride, and 18F-DMFP. Due to the short half-life of 11C, 220–370 MBq of 11C-raclopride should be administered. If an administration to a child is necessary, the dosage has to be adapted based on valid guidelines.

For the different radiotracers, specific uptake times are established:

- 1.5–3 h for 123I-IBZM
- 2–3 h for 123I-epidepride
- 1–1.5 h for 18F-DMFP
- 2.5–3 h for 18F-fallypride
- 30–60 min for 11C-raclopride (with a dynamic PET acquisition of 50–60 min can be performed).

A fixed uptake time and constant acquisition parameters make the study comparable to prior or later studies of the same patient and to studies of other patients.

The patient should void the bladder before and after the image acquisition to ensure maximum comfort and reduce radiation burden. The patient should be positioned comfortably and be instructed to avoid any voluntary movement. Sedation can be used in uncooperative patients if necessary. The head should be fixed comfortably to avoid movements.

For SPECT acquisition, dual or triple head cameras are recommended (single head cameras would need a much longer acquisition time and higher administered doses of the radiotracer). Usually, more than three million detected events are necessary. The scanning time varies depending on the camera system. Attenuation is done by calculation (Chang), transmission, or CT.

For PET scans, usually 3D acquisitions are performed. Static or dynamic imaging is possible and attenuation correction by transmission, CT or MRI has to be done. The acquired data have to be filtered (usually low-pass filters in SPECT systems and Hanning or Shepp-Logan in PET systems) and reconstructed according to the specifications of the camera system. Reformatting has to be performed to standardize plane orientation.

Image interpretation is mainly based on semi-quantitative evaluation with a ROI (region of interest) technique assisted by visual interpretation. For ROI definition, morphology obtained by CT or MRI can be used. Usually, transverse/oblique slices are selected and added together. ROIs can be defined in different ways. Standardized ROIs with the same shape and dimensions have the advantage of reproducibility but the disadvantage that they don't fit properly in every patient. ROIs drawn with an isocontour function have the advantage of covering the metabolic active parts of the striatum but the disadvantage of low comparability between different patients. ROIs drawn with anatomical landmarks from CT or MRI have the advantage of covering the anatomical structure of the patients correctly but the disadvantage of greater technical requirements.

The shape of tracer accumulation has to be described, also asymmetries, differences between caudate nucleus and putamen and the tracer binding in contrast to reference regions with low tracer uptake (e.g., cerebellum, occipital cortex, frontal cortex). Especially, the ROIs of the reference regions have to be standardized in a department to make the studies of different patients comparable. Ideally, data from age-matched normal controls should be available for comparison.

The most common pitfalls include: age dependency, patient movement, thresholding, technical artifacts, and medication.

Reporting should include a precise diagnosis based on standardized criteria or on the recommendation of further investigations or follow-up studies.

2.8 Brain Perfusion SPECT

Two different radiopharmaceuticals are commonly used for the assessment of brain perfusion:

- ECD (ethyl cysteine dimer)
- HMPAO (hexamethyl propylene amine oxime)

Both are labeled with 99mTc. At the moment, only HMPAO is commercially available. Other brain perfusion tracers like 123I-IMP, 123I-HIPDM, 133Xe, and 127Xe have some disadvantages, i.e., unfavorable dosimetry and lower energy.

Due to its lipophilic structure, the compound enters the brain cells rapidly and is trapped there as a result of its conversion into a hydrophilic structure, consequently making redistribution impossible. The images reflect the regional cerebral blood flow (rCBF) at a short time window after tracer injection and are independent of later variations in rCBF. The peak brain activity is at 2 min after injection; the brain uptake is 2–3% for HMPAO and 4–7% for ECD; the gray-to-white-matter ratio is 2–3:1 for HMPAO and 4:1 for ECD. The images do not provide absolute quantitative flow values but allow the estimation of relative regional blood flow differences.

The most common indications for imaging are: cerebrovascular disease, presurgical localization of epileptogenic foci (ictal and interictal studies), dementia (for this indication nowadays FDG is often used), inflammation, and brain death. Some studies indicate the usefulness in depression. The common contraindications have to be taken into account which include: pregnancy, breast feeding, uncooperative patient.

The patient should avoid excessive stimulants, alcohol and drugs, affecting the cerebral blood flow. The withdrawal of drugs has to be discussed with the clinician. A cannula should be inserted, the patient should be placed in a quiet, dark room and positioned comfortably. The patient should close the eyes and relax without any movement for a minimum of 5 min before and 5 min after the injection. If sedation is necessary, it should be administered shortly before data acquisition and the patient has to be monitored appropriately with pulse oximetry. The history of neurological and/or psychiatric diseases and status, the results from former examinations (SPECT, PET, CT, MRI, EEG, etc.), and the medication (i.e., psychotropic medication and the last intake) have to be known by the physician.

The time interval for injection is 30 min for unstabilized 99mTc-HMPAO, 4 h for stabilized 99mTc-HMPAO, and 6 h for 99mTc-ECD. The administered activity is 555–1110 MBq (usually 740 MBq) in adults. In children, dose adoption is necessary. Data acquisition starts 30–60 min after tracer injection to allow the wash-out of unspecific uptake. The patient should void the bladder before and after the image acquisition to ensure maximum comfort and reduce radiation burden. The patient should be positioned comfortably and be instructed to avoid any voluntary movement. Sedation can be used in uncooperative patients if necessary. The head should be fixed comfortably to avoid movements.

For SPECT acquisition, dual or triple head cameras are recommended (single head cameras would need a much longer acquisition time and higher administered doses of the radiotracer). Usually, more than five million detected events are necessary. The scanning time varies depending on the camera system. Attenuation is done by calculation (Chang), transmission, or CT.

A vasodilatory challenge can be performed with acetazolamide (this is a carboanhydrase inhibitor and leads to an increase of rCBF in normal cerebral vessels). It is used for the evaluation of the cerebrovascular reserve. Contraindications include allergy, acute stroke (within 3 days), migraine, and renal or hepatic insufficiency (relative contraindications).

Usually, the dose is 1000 mg in adults and 14 mg/kg in children. It has a diuretic effect and can lead to mild vertigo, tinnitus, nausea, perioral paresthesia, and hypotension. It has to be mentioned that the diagnostic use of acetazolamide is not mentioned in the information sheet of the drug. The tracer should be injected 15–20 min after acetazolamide. A second study without acetazolamide has to be performed in order to compare the images and estimate the effect.

For the assessment of focal epilepsy, ictal (tracer injection as soon as possible after seizure onset with the patient being under video-EEG monitoring) and interictal studies have to be performed and compared, in order to localize the origin of the seizure. In interictal studies, EEG monitoring is also of value to avoid the possibility of a seizure occurs before or after injection and thereby affects the image.

The data have to be reconstructed (filtered back-projection or iterative reconstruction) and filtered (usually with a low-pass filter). Attenuation correction has to be done (calculated according to Chang or measured with a transmission or CT scan), the slices have to be reformatted in the three orthogonal planes (standardized). Reformatting has to be performed to standardize plane orientation (e.g., AC-PC line).

Image interpretation can be done visually using semi-quantitative analysis with ROI techniques, and with automated image analysis methods like SISCOM (subtraction ictal SPECT co-registered to MRI). For this technique, an ictal SPECT is subtracted from an interictal one of the same patient. SPM (statistical parametric mapping) means spatial normalization based on normal databases and voxel-based analysis. For the interpretation of the study, morphological changes revealed by CT or MRI have to be considered and if possible data should be compared with age-matched normal controls.

The most common pitfalls include: patient movement, medication, unintended cerebral activation, thresholding, technical artifacts.

Reporting should include a precise diagnosis based on standardized criteria or on the recommendations of further investigations or follow-up studies.

2.9 Amyloid Imaging

Several compounds for amyloid imaging are available or tested in clinical phase III trials. The most commonly known radiotracer is the 11C-Pittsburgh-Compound-B (11C-PIB) which is used in clinical studies since about 10 years. Some fluorine-18 labeled tracers like florbetapir, florbetaben, and flutemetamol are either in clinical trial studies or have recently gained approval. Some studies have been performed to compare fluorine-18 labeled tracers with PIB and these studies found a very good correlation of the results. Histopathological correlation between PIB and postmortem assessment of amyloid-β has been shown.

Despite some unsolved questions, the Society of Nuclear Medicine and Molecular Imaging (SNMMI) and the Alzheimer Association (AA) have jointly developed criteria to assist the use of amyloid imaging radiotracers. They defined the following three criteria for appropriate use: (1) patients with persistent or progressive unexplained mild cognitive impairment (MCI), (2) patients fulfilling core clinical criteria for possible AD, because of unclear clinical presentation, either an atypical clinical course or an etiologically mixed presentation, (3) patients with progressive dementia and atypically early-onset of symptoms (usually defined as 65 years or younger in age).

One of the ongoing discussions is the problem on how to handle amyloid-β positive people without clinical signs of dementia (positive amyloid PET rates are less than 5% between 50 and 60 years of age, 10% between 60 and 70 years of age, 25% between 70 and 80 years of age, and more than 50% between 80 and 90 years of age) (Moghbel et al. 2012; Villemagne et al. 2012).

Usually, 370 MBq of the fluorine-18 radiotracer is injected and acquisition is performed at 30 min after injection. 11C-PIB is administered at a dose of 300–555 MBq with a time window of data acquisition of 50–70 min.

The patient should void the bladder before and after the image acquisition to ensure maximum comfort and reduce radiation burden. The patient should be positioned comfortably and be instructed to avoid any voluntary movement. Sedation can be used in uncooperative patients if necessary. The head should be fixed comfortably to avoid movements.

The data have to be reconstructed (filtered back-projection or iterative reconstruction) and filtered (usually with a low-pass filter). Attenuation correction has to be done (calculated according to Chang or measured with a transmission or CT scan) and the slices have to be reformatted in the three orthogonal planes (standardized). Reformatting has to be performed to standardize plane orientation (e.g., AC-PC line).

Some circumstances have to be considered, for example, amyloid PET is frequently positive in dementia with Lewy bodies and in patients with cerebral amyloid angiopathy. Because of these findings and the age-dependent amyloid deposition in healthy people, amyloid PET has to be seen in the context of the clinical findings, like neurological and psychiatric status, and other imaging results like MRI and FDG-PET.

At present image interpretation criteria, the clinical significance of positive and negative amyloid PET and technical aspects are evolving. Interpretation is done mainly visually, i.e., interpreting a scan as amyloid positive (amyloid-β is found) and negative (amyloid-β is absent). Indeterminate results have to be reported and the reasons have to be discussed. Automated image interpretation systems are under development but their clinical usefulness has to be proven.

2.10 Indications for Nuclear Medicine Examinations

SPECT tracers are listed in Table 2.6 while PET tracers are given in Table 2.7.

Table 2.6 SPECT tracers

Tracer	Radionuclide	Main indications	Target
ECD	m99Tc	• Epilepsy • Dementia • Cerebrovascular disease • Brain death • Encephalitis	rCBF
HMPAO	m99Tc	• Epilepsy • Dementia • Cerebrovascular disease • Brain death • Encephalitis	rCBF
FP-CIT	123I	• Parkinsonism	Dopamine transporter
β-CIT	123I	• Parkinsonism	Dopamine transporter
IBZM	123I	• Atypical parkinsonism	D2 receptor
Tectrotyd	m99Tc	• Meningioma	SSR
Octreotide	111In	• Meningioma	SSR
201TlCl	201Tl	• Tumor	Na-K-ATPase
Sestamibi	M99Tc	• Tumor	Mitochondria

Table 2.7 PET tracers

Tracer	Radionuclide	Main indications	Target
FDG	18F	• Dementia • Tumor • Carcinoma of unknown primary • Huntington disease	Glut-1/ glucose-6-phosphatase
FET	18F	• Gliomas • Head and neck tumors	L-system
FLT	18F	• Gliomas	DNA synthesis
MET	11C	• Gliomas	L-system
DOPA	18F	• Parkinsonism • Neuroendocrine tumor	Dopamine decarboxylase
DOTATOC/-NOC	68Ga	• Neuroendocrine tumor • Meningioma	Somatostatin receptor
Fallypride	18F	• Atypical parkinsonism	D2 receptor
Raclopride	11C	• Atypical parkinsonism	D2 receptor
Mefway	18F	• Depression	5HT1A receptor
Flumazenil	18F	• Epilepsy • Dementia	GABA A receptor
H2O	15O	• Cerebrovascular disease	Cerebral blood flow
Pittsburgh compound B	11C	• Dementia	Amyloid deposition
Flutemetamol	18F	• Dementia	Amyloid deposition

Selected References

Akdemir UO, Atay Kapucu LO (2016) Nuclear medicine imaging in pediatric neurology. Mol Imaging Radionucl Ther 25(1):1–10. https://doi.org/10.4274/mirt.49389

Alexiou GA, Tsiouris S, Voulgaris S, Kyritsis AP, Fotopoulos AD (2012) Glioblastoma multiforme imaging: the role of nuclear medicine. Curr Radiopharm 5(4):308–313

Balon HR, Brown TL, Goldsmith SJ, Silberstein EB, Krenning EP, Lang O, Dillehay G, Tarrance J, Johnson M, Stabin MG (2011) The SNM practice guideline for somatostatin receptor scintigraphy 2.0. J Nucl Med Technol 39(4):317–324. https://doi.org/10.2967/jnmt.111.098277

Bennett P, Oza UD (2015) Diagnostic imaging: nuclear medicine, 2nd edn. Elsevier, Amsterdam

Bernier DR, Christian PE, Langan JK (2003) Nuclear medicine: technology and techniques, 4th edn. Mosby, St. Louis

Beyer T, Antoch G, Muller S, Egelhof T, Freudenberg LS, Debatin J, Bockisch A (2004) Acquisition protocol considerations for combined PET/CT imaging. J Nucl Med 45(Suppl 1):25s–35s

Bombardieri E, Weber W (2012) Diagnosis of brain tumors and nuclear medicine imaging. Q J Nucl Med Mol Imaging 56(2):101–102

Bombardieri E, Giammarile F, Aktolun C, Baum RP, Bischof Delaloye A, Maffioli L, Moncayo R, Mortelmans L, Pepe G, Reske SN, Castellani MR, Chiti A (2010) 131I/123I-metaiodobenzylguanidine (mIBG) scintigraphy: procedure guidelines for tumour imaging. Eur J Nucl Med Mol Imaging 37(12):2436–2446. https://doi.org/10.1007/s00259-010-1545-7

Busemann Sokole E, Plachcinska A, Britten A (2010a) Acceptance testing for nuclear medicine instrumentation. Eur J Nucl Med Mol Imaging 37(3):672–681. https://doi.org/10.1007/s00259-009-1348-x

Busemann Sokole E, Plachcinska A, Britten A, Lyra Georgosopoulou M, Tindale W, Klett R (2010b) Routine quality control recommendations for nuclear medicine instrumentation. Eur J Nucl Med Mol Imaging 37(3):662–671. https://doi.org/10.1007/s00259-009-1347-y

Chang LT (1978) A method for attenuation correction in radionuclide computed tomography. IEEE Trans Nucl Sci 25:638–643

Czernin J, Auerbach MA (2005) Clinical PET/CT imaging: promises and misconceptions. Nuklearmedizin 44(Suppl 1):S18–S23

Czernin J, Phelps ME (2002) Positron emission tomography scanning: current and future applications. Annu Rev Med 53:89–112. https://doi.org/10.1146/annurev.med.53.082901.104028

Czernin J, Schelbert HR (2007) PET/CT in cancer patient management. Introduction. J Nucl Med 48(Suppl 1):2s–3s

Darcourt J, Booij J, Tatsch K, Varrone A, Vander Borght T, Kapucu OL, Nagren K, Nobili F, Walker Z, Van Laere K (2010) EANM procedure guidelines for brain neurotransmission SPECT using (123)I-labelled dopamine transporter ligands, version 2. Eur J Nucl Med Mol Imaging 37(2):443–450. https://doi.org/10.1007/s00259-009-1267-x

Del Sole A, Moncayo R, Tafuni G, Lucignani G (2004) Position of nuclear medicine techniques in the diagnostic work-up of brain tumors. Q J Nucl Med Mol Imaging 48(2):76–81

Donohoe KJ, Agrawal G, Frey KA, Gerbaudo VH, Mariani G, Nagel JS, Shulkin BL, Stabin MG, Stokes MK (2012) SNM practice guideline for brain death scintigraphy 2.0. J Nucl Med Technol 40(3):198–203. https://doi.org/10.2967/jnmt.112.105130

Elgazzar AH (2014) The pathophysiologic basis of nuclear medicine. Springer, Berlin

Ell PJ, Gambhir SS (2004) Nuclear medicine in clinical diagnosis and treatment. Churchill Livingstone, 3rd edn

Giussani A, Hoeschen C (2013) Imaging in nuclear medicine. Springer, Berlin

Goethals I, Dierckx R, Van Laere K, Van De Wiele C, Signore A (2002) The role of nuclear medicine imaging in routine assessment of infectious brain pathology. Nucl Med Commun 23(9):819–826

Gregoire V, Chiti A (2010) PET in radiotherapy planning: particularly exquisite test or pending and experimental tool? Radiother Oncol 96(3):275–276. https://doi.org/10.1016/j.radonc.2010.07.015

Ito K, Inui Y, Kizawa T, Kimura Y, Kato T (2017) Current and future prospects of nuclear medicine in dementia. Rinsho Shinkeigaku 57(9):479–484. https://doi.org/10.5692/clinicalneurol.cn-001016

Johnson KA, Minoshima S, Bohnen NI, Donohoe KJ, Foster NL, Herscovitch P, Karlawish JH, Rowe CC, Hedrick S, Pappas V, Carrillo MC, Hartley DM (2013) Update on appropriate use criteria for amyloid PET imaging: dementia experts, mild cognitive impairment, and education. Amyloid Imaging Task Force of the Alzheimer's Association and Society for Nuclear Medicine and Molecular Imaging. Alzheimers Dement 9(4):e106–e109. https://doi.org/10.1016/j.jalz.2013.06.001

Kapucu OL, Nobili F, Varrone A, Booij J, Vander Borght T, Nagren K, Darcourt J, Tatsch K, Van Laere KJ (2009) EANM procedure guideline for brain perfusion SPECT using 99mTc-labelled radiopharmaceuticals, version 2. Eur J Nucl Med Mol Imaging 36(12):2093–2102. https://doi.org/10.1007/s00259-009-1266-y

Lassmann M, Chiesa C, Flux G, Bardies M (2011) EANM Dosimetry Committee guidance document: good practice of clinical dosimetry reporting. Eur J Nucl Med Mol Imaging 38(1):192–200. https://doi.org/10.1007/s00259-010-1549-3

Mascalchi M, Vella A (2012) Magnetic resonance and nuclear medicine imaging in ataxias. Handb Clin Neurol 103:85–110. https://doi.org/10.1016/b978-0-444-51892-7.00004-8

Mettler FA, Guiberteau MJ (2012) Essentials of nuclear medicine imaging, 6th edn. Elsevier, Philadelphia

Minoshima S, Drzezga AE, Barthel H, Bohnen N, Djekidel M, Lewis DH, Mathis CA, McConathy J, Nordberg A, Sabri O, Seibyl JP, Stokes MK, Van Laere K (2016) SNMMI procedure standard/EANM practice guideline for amyloid PET imaging of the brain 1.0. J Nucl Med 57(8):1316–1322. https://doi.org/10.2967/jnumed.116.174615

Moghbel MC, Saboury B, Basu S, Metzler SD, Torigian DA, Langstrom B, Alavi A (2012) Amyloid-beta imaging with PET in Alzheimer's disease: is it feasible with current radiotracers and technologies? Eur J Nucl Med Mol Imaging 39(2):202–208. https://doi.org/10.1007/s00259-011-1960-4

Muehllehner G (1985) Effect of resolution improvement on required count density in ECT imaging: a computer simulation. Phys Med Biol 30(2):163–173

Patil S, Biassoni L, Borgwardt L (2007) Nuclear medicine in pediatric neurology and neurosurgery: epilepsy and brain tumors. Semin Nucl Med 37(5):357–381. https://doi.org/10.1053/j.semnuclmed.2007.04.002

Phelps ME, Huang SC, Hoffman EJ, Selin C, Sokoloff L, Kuhl DE (1979) Tomographic measurement of local cerebral glucose metabolic rate in humans with (F-18)2-fluoro-2-deoxy-D-glucose: validation of method. Ann Neurol 6(5):371–388. https://doi.org/10.1002/ana.410060502

Pichler R, Dunzinger A, Wurm G, Pichler J, Weis S, Nussbaumer K, Topakian R, Aigner RM (2010a) Is there a place for FET PET in the initial evaluation of brain lesions with unknown significance? Eur J Nucl Med Mol Imaging 37(8):1521–1528. https://doi.org/10.1007/s00259-010-1457-6

Pichler R, Wurm G, Nussbaumer K, Kalev O, Silye R, Weis S (2010b) Sarcoidois and radiation-induced astrogliosis causes pitfalls in neuro-oncologic positron emission tomography imaging by O-(2-[18F]fluoroethyl)-L-tyrosine. J Clin Oncol 28(36):e753–e755. https://doi.org/10.1200/jco.2010.30.5763

Sathekge M, McFarren A, Dadachova E (2014) Role of nuclear medicine in neuroHIV: PET, SPECT, and beyond. Nucl Med Commun 35(8):792–796. https://doi.org/10.1097/mnm.0000000000000139

Sharp PF, Gemmell HG, Murray AD (2005) Practical nuclear medicine. Springer, London

Silverman DH (2008) Evaluating pathology in the brain with nuclear medicine. Semin Nucl Med 38(4):225–226. https://doi.org/10.1053/j.semnuclmed.2008.03.002

Tatsch K, Asenbaum S, Bartenstein P, Catafau A, Halldin C, Pilowsky LS, Pupi A (2002a) European Association of Nuclear Medicine procedure guidelines for brain neurotransmission SPET using (123)I-labelled dopamine D(2) receptor ligands. Eur J Nucl Med Mol Imaging 29(10):Bp23–Bp29

Tatsch K, Asenbaum S, Bartenstein P, Catafau A, Halldin C, Pilowsky LS, Pupi A (2002b) European Association of Nuclear Medicine procedure guidelines for brain neurotransmission SPET using (123)I-labelled dopamine D(2) transporter ligands. Eur J Nucl Med Mol Imaging 29(10):Bp30–Bp35

Tatsch K, Asenbaum S, Bartenstein P, Catafau A, Halldin C, Pilowsky LS, Pupi A (2002c) European Association of Nuclear Medicine procedure guidelines for brain perfusion SPET using (99m)Tc-labelled radiopharmaceuticals. Eur J Nucl Med Mol Imaging 29(10):Bp36–Bp42

Townsend DW, Carney JP, Yap JT, Hall NC (2004) PET/CT today and tomorrow. J Nucl Med 45(Suppl 1):4s–14s

Van Laere K, Varrone A, Booij J, Vander Borght T, Nobili F, Kapucu OL, Walker Z, Nagren K, Tatsch K, Darcourt J (2010) EANM procedure guidelines for brain neurotransmission SPECT/PET using dopamine D2 receptor ligands, version 2. Eur J Nucl Med Mol Imaging 37(2):434–442. https://doi.org/10.1007/s00259-009-1265-z

Vander Borght T, Asenbaum S, Bartenstein P, Halldin C, Kapucu O, Van Laere K, Varrone A, Tatsch K (2006) EANM procedure guidelines for brain tumour imaging using labelled amino acid analogues. Eur J Nucl Med Mol Imaging 33(11):1374–1380. https://doi.org/10.1007/s00259-006-0206-3

Varrone A, Asenbaum S, Vander Borght T, Booij J, Nobili F, Nagren K, Darcourt J, Kapucu OL, Tatsch K, Bartenstein P, Van Laere K (2009) EANM procedure guidelines for PET brain imaging using [18F]FDG, version 2. Eur J Nucl Med Mol Imaging 36(12):2103–2110. https://doi.org/10.1007/s00259-009-1264-0

Villemagne VL, Klunk WE, Mathis CA, Rowe CC, Brooks DJ, Hyman BT, Ikonomovic MD, Ishii K, Jack CR, Jagust WJ, Johnson KA, Koeppe RA, Lowe VJ, Masters CL, Montine TJ, Morris JC, Nordberg A, Petersen RC, Reiman EM, Selkoe DJ, Sperling RA, Van Laere K, Weiner MW, Drzezga A (2012) Abeta Imaging: feasible, pertinent, and vital to progress in Alzheimer's disease. Eur J Nucl Med Mol Imaging 39(2):209–219. https://doi.org/10.1007/s00259-011-2045-0

Virgolini I, Ambrosini V, Bomanji JB, Baum RP, Fanti S, Gabriel M, Papathanasiou ND, Pepe G, Oyen W, De Cristoforo C, Chiti A (2010) Procedure guidelines for PET/CT tumour imaging with 68Ga-DOTA-conjugated peptides: 68Ga-DOTA-TOC, 68Ga-DOTA-NOC, 68Ga-DOTA-TATE. Eur J Nucl Med Mol Imaging 37(10):2004–2010. https://doi.org/10.1007/s00259-010-1512-3

Weih M, Degirmenci U, Kreil S, Suttner G, Schmidt D, Kornhuber J, Lewczuk P, Kuwert T (2011) Nuclear medicine diagnostic techniques in the era of pathophysiology-based CSF biomarkers for Alzheimer's disease. J Alzheimers Dis 26(Suppl 3):97–103. https://doi.org/10.3233/jad-2011-0020

Ziessman HA, O'Malley JP, Thrall JH (2013) Nuclear medicine: the requisites, 4th edn. Elsevier, Philadelphia

Imaging Modalities: Neuropathology

3.1 Introduction

Neuropathology is the medical discipline concerned with the study of diseases affecting the central and peripheral nervous system as well as muscle. Its aim is to describe the structural, biochemical, molecular, and functional changes in the various cells which make up the nervous system. Using morphologic, immunologic, and molecular biological techniques, neuropathology tries to explain the signs and symptoms of patients. Delivering a clear-cut diagnosis provides the rational basis for patient care and therapy.

The following four aspects are at the core of the neuropathology endeavor:

- Morphologic and molecular changes, i.e., structural and biochemical changes occurring in affected cells
- Clinical manifestations, i.e., the functional consequences of the structural and biochemical changes in the cells
- Etiology, i.e., the cause of the disease
- Pathogenesis, i.e., mechanisms leading to disease

Neuropathology is the bridge between the

- Basic neurosciences
  - Molecular biology
  - Neurochemistry
  - Neuroimmunology
- Clinical neuromedicine
  - Neurology
  - Neurosurgery
  - Neuropediatrics
  - Psychiatry
  - Neuroradiology
  - Neuronuclear medicine

Specimens are analyzed at the following levels:

- Gross anatomy
- Light microscopy
- Electron microscopy (ultrastructural)

Specimens are derived from:

- Brain
- Spinal cord
- Meninges
- Peripheral nerves
- Muscle
- Bone and soft tissues surrounding the brain and spinal cord
- Cerebrospinal fluid

Specimens are obtained through:

- Autopsy (brain, spinal cord, meninges)
- Open brain surgery
- Biopsy (stereotactic or navigated biopsy, muscle and nerve biopsy)
- Lumbar puncture

In the next chapters, the general procedures for removal of brain and spinal cord, tissue fixation, tissue processing, and tissue staining are described.

3.2 Removal, Fixation, and Cutting of the Brain and Spinal Cord

3.2.1 Removal and Fixation of the Brain

Before removing the brain, a thorough examination of the head should take place (Fig. 3.1):

- ears (bleeding as a sign of trauma)
- nose (bleeding as a sign of trauma)
- eyes (hemorrhage as a sign of trauma, intraretinal bleeding)
- wounds (sutured or non-sutured, entry or exit of bullets or strangulation marks in case of suicide)
- surgically placed drainage tubes or shunts

The skull is opened in the following way (Fig. 3.2):

- The hair is parted with a comb at an imaginary line connecting both ears.
- The frontal part of the hair is combed towards the front while the posterior part is combed backwards.
- The scalp is cut by an incision with a knife at an imaginary line connecting both ears.
- The anterior scalp segment is gently moved anteriorly by dislocating the skin from the skull by use of the scalpel or blunt dissection.
- The posterior scalp segment is reflected in the same way.
- The temporalis muscle of both sides is incised by a knife.
- The calvarium is cut open with an electric saw describing a horizontal line.
  - starting 1 cm above the supra-orbital ridge
  - running backwards until reaching approximately 1 cm above the ear pinna
  - extending posteriorly until the occipital protuberance
- The calvarium is gently loosened and then removed with a T-piece avoiding lacerations or ruptures of the dura mater.
- The intact dura mater is inspected for pathological findings (e.g., epidural hemorrhages).
- The superior sagittal sinus should **not** be opened with scissors, as one would dislocate and move mechanically a possible thrombus.
- The dura is cut with scissors, removed, and subsequently fixed.
- If present, a subdural hemorrhage should be described with regard to color, consistency, dimensions, and weight.
- The exposed surface of the brain is inspected for pathological findings (e.g., subarachnoidal hemorrhage, signs of brain atrophy of the frontal lobe, fibrosis of the leptomeninges, yellowish-greenish meningeal discoloration in case of meningitis).

The brain is removed in the following way (Fig. 3.3):

- The frontal lobes are lifted by placing the fingers of the left hand under the frontal poles which are gently retracted.
- The optic chiasm and the optic nerves become visible. The optic nerves are incised with the scalpel at the level of the optic foramina.
- The pituitary stalk and the internal carotid arteries become visible. They are transected with the scalpel.
- The tentorium cerebelli is transsected gently while cutting with the scalpel along the ridge of the petrous temporal bone.
- The brain is supported posteriorly with the left hand. The more advanced the previous incisions are the more the brain is falling backwards.

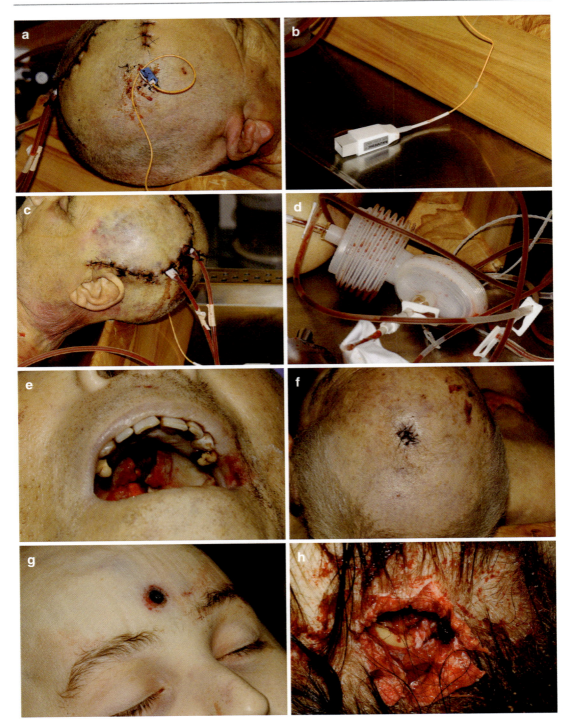

Fig. 3.1 Careful examination of the head reveals the presence of wounds as signs of trauma and surgical interventions (**a**). Cable of the device for measuring brain pressure (**a**), connection for the registration device (**b**), drainage tubes for hemorrhages (**c**), collection device for drainage unit (**d**), entry of bullet with destruction of the palate in case of suicidal gunshot (**e**), exit of the bullet (**f**), entry of bullet in suicidal gunshot (**g**), exit wound (**h**), small entry wound of bullet (**i**) with galeal hemorrhage (**j**), hemorrhage of the eyeball (**k**), severe hemorrhage and protrusion of the eyeball (**l**)

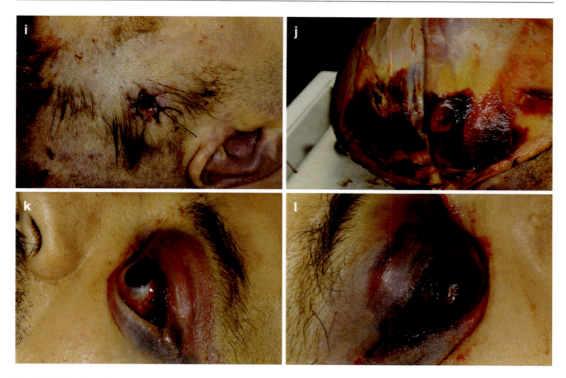

Fig. 3.1 (continued)

- The exposed cranial nerves are cut with the scalpel as close as possible to the bone.
- The brain stem and its transition into the spinal cord at the level of the foramen magnum can be inspected.
- The upper part of the spinal cord is dissected by placing a thin long scalpel as deep as possible into the vertebral canal and transsecting the spinal cord as well as the vertebral arteries.
- The brain can now be removed.
- The weight of the fresh brain is taken after letting the remaining blood and cerebrospinal fluid drain off.
- In case of a ruptured aneurysm:
  - The brain is placed in a plastic mold, thus, avoiding distortion while removing the aneurysm.
  - The unaffected blood vessels are exposed and freed of any debris by blunt dissection.
  - In case of an aneurysm of the basilar artery, the blood clot can be bluntly removed by using the handle of the scalpel.
  - In case of an aneurysm of the middle cerebral artery, the temporal pole is dislocated or even removed. The origin of the middle cerebral artery from the internal carotid artery is identified; its course is followed laterally until abutting on the blood clot. The blood clot is gently removed by blunt dissection until the bifurcation of the artery becomes visible. Now, the remaining blood clot is gently removed until the aneurysm becomes visible. While gently scraping off the blood one might feel when the scalpel is touching the coil or the metallic clip.
  - In case of an aneurysm of the anterior communicating branch, both hemispheres should be loosened from each other by separating them bluntly with the handle of the scalpel holder. The origin of the anterior cerebral artery from the internal carotid artery is identified, its course followed, the lower parts of the frontal lobe slightly dislocated in order to expose the anterior communicating branch.

3.2 Removal, Fixation, and Cutting of the Brain and Spinal Cord

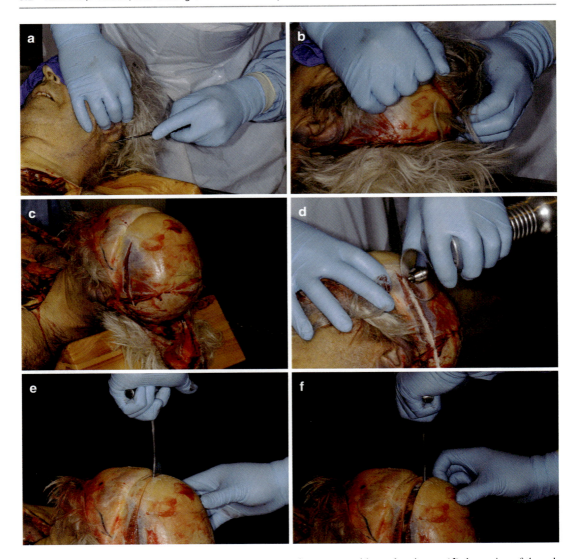

Fig. 3.2 Opening of the skull: The scalp is incised with a knife at an imaginary line connecting both ears (**a**); gentle removal of the anterior scalp segment blunt dissection (**b**), reflection of the posterior scalp segment (**c**), the calvarium is cut open with an electric saw (**d**), loosening of the calvarium with a T-piece (**e**), and removal of the calvarium with a T-piece (**f**)

The brain is fixed in the following way (Fig. 3.4):

- In case that the whole brain is fixed:
  - A thread is passed under the basilar artery; a forceps can be used to first pass under the basilar artery, cover the thread, and move it under the basilar artery.
  - The brain is then suspended in a plastic bucket with 4% formalin.
  - Both ends of the thread are then fixed at the sides of the bucket in order to avoid that the brain sinks to the bottom of the bucket and thus causing distortion.
- In case that one hemisphere is frozen:
  - Both hemispheres are separated by a cut using a knife which is introduced in the interhemispheric fissure; the hemispheres are torn away by using the hand; the corpus callosum is transsected; the hemispheres

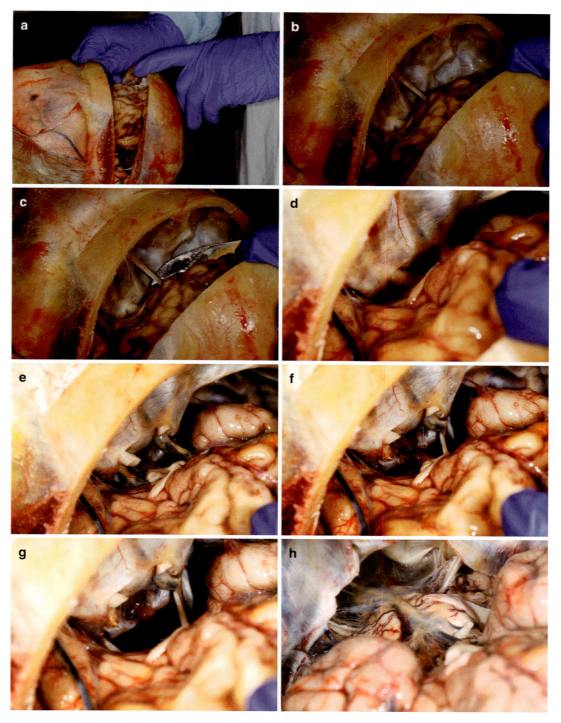

Fig. 3.3 Removal of the brain: Retraction of the frontal poles (**a**); the olfactory nerve becomes visible (**b**); transection of the olfactory nerve (**c**); the optic nerves become visible (**d**); after transection of the optic nerves, the internal carotid arteries become visible (**e**); after transection of the internal carotid arteries, the pituitary stalk becomes visible (**f**); transection of the pituitary stalk (**g**); inspection of the basilar artery and transection the vertebral arteries (**h**); after sectioning the cerebellar tentorium, the cerebellum is removed from the posterior fossa (**i**); inspection of the cerebellar tonsils (**j**); the whole brain is removed from the skull (**k**); inspection of the surface of the brain. A reddish-discolored area is seen in the central area (**l**, **m**)

3.2 Removal, Fixation, and Cutting of the Brain and Spinal Cord

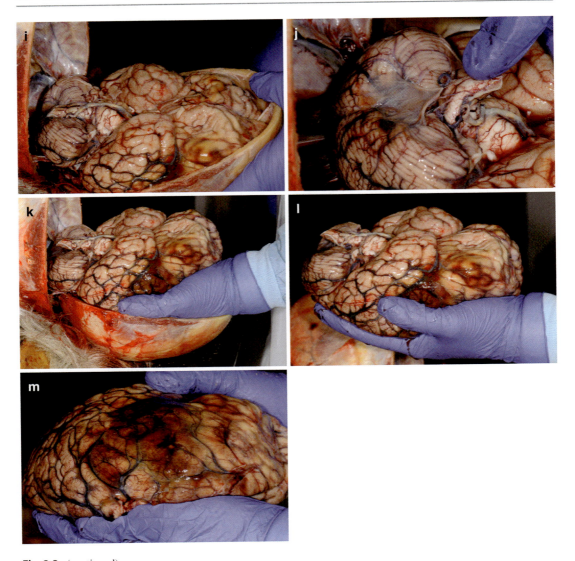

Fig. 3.3 (continued)

are separated from each other with the hand; finally, the brain stem is transsected in its midline with the knife.
- One hemisphere is placed in a bucket with formalin for fixation resting on its medial surface.
- The other hemisphere is freshly cut into a series of 1 cm thick slices, which are placed on a hard paper support covered by a sheet of plastic. The slices are then frozen in a −80° Celsius freezer.

3.2.2 Removal and Fixation of the Spinal Cord

The spinal cord can be removed by:

- Anterior approach
- Posterior approach

The *anterior approach* is performed in the following steps:

- Finishing the body autopsy.

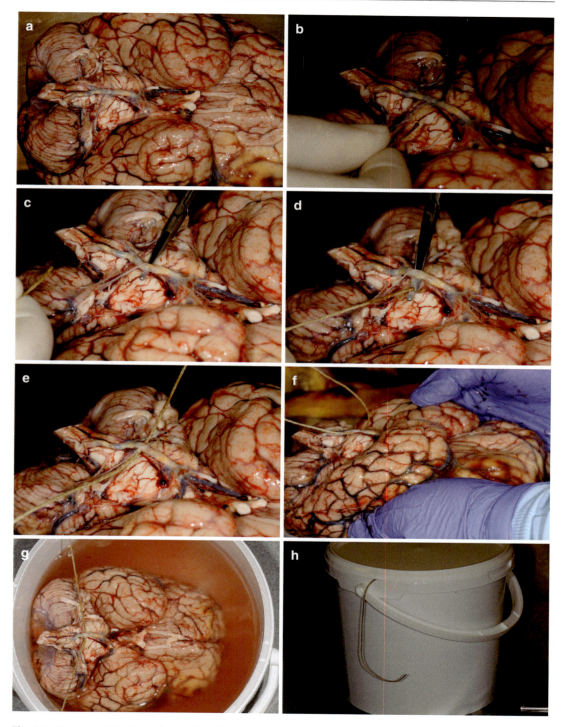

Fig. 3.4 Fixation of the brain: Inspection of the basilar artery (**a**); positioning of a thread under the basilar artery (**b**–**f**); the brain is placed in a bucket filled with formaldehyde (**g**) while the thread is placed at the borders of the bucket and fixed with its cover (**h**)

3.2 Removal, Fixation, and Cutting of the Brain and Spinal Cord

- Evisceration of all the organs.
- Exposure of the vertebral column by removal of the remaining paravertebral soft tissue.
- Cutting up the pedicles of the vertebrae behind the vertebral body by use of either a special chisel or an electric vibrating saw.
- After cutting through the vertebral disc at level L4, the lumbar segment can be worked free with a T-piece.
- After the loosened piece of column is lifted smoothly while any connections of soft tissue are cut with the scalpel, it can be removed completely.
- The lumbar dural sac is lifted gently with a surgical forceps and the cauda equina is cut.
- Holding the spinal cord wrapped into the dura up in the air all connections, i.e., the roots are cut using the scalpel while being careful to leave some root tissue as well as spinal ganglia attached to the specimen.

The *posterior approach* is performed (Fig. 3.5):

- By an incision of the skin along the vertebral spines.
- The paravertebral muscles are then moved laterally.
- By use of either a special chisel or an electric vibrating saw, the pedicles of the vertebrae behind the vertebral body are cut up.
- After cutting through the vertebral disc at level L4, the lumbar segment can be worked free with a T-piece.
- After the loosened piece of column is lifted smoothly while any connections of soft tissue are cut with the scalpel, it can be removed completely.
- The lumbar dural sac is lifted gently with a surgical forceps and the cauda equina is cut.
- Holding the spinal cord wrapped into the dura up in the air all connections, i.e., the roots are cut using the scalpel while being careful to leave some root tissue as well as spinal ganglia attached to the specimen.

The spinal cord should be fixed in a long glass container by passing a thread on each side through the dura mater; both ends of the thread are then fixed at the sides of the glass container allowing the free-floating spinal cord to fix. Alternatively, the spinal cord wrapped by the dura mater can be placed in a large-sized plastic container, by spreading it out along the container's sides, thus, avoiding kinking.

3.2.3 Brain Cutting

In the routine diagnostic neuropathology workflow, the brain is fixed for a minimum duration of 1 week. Before cutting the brain, it should be placed in running water for at least 2 h, thus, avoiding irritation of the eyes and nose.

The weight of the fixed brain is measured.

The brain cutting is done in the following ways (Fig. 3.6):

- External *visual* examination of the brain by describing:
  - the opacity/lucency of the leptomeninges (subarachnoidal hemorrhage, signs of meningitis)
  - the topographical orientation of the gyri and sulci (gyrification abnormalities)
  - the status of the vasculature (arteriosclerotic plaques, aneurysms)
  - discoloration of brain tissue (brownish discoloration in case of ischemia)
  - tissue damage and brownish discoloration (in case of trauma)
- External *tactile* examination of the brain by describing:
  - softening of brain tissue of the cerebral and cerebellar hemispheres (in case of ischemia and hemorrhage)
- The brain is laid on the dissection table with its basal surface facing upwards.
- The lower brain stem (i.e., pons and medulla oblongata) and cerebellum are removed by a

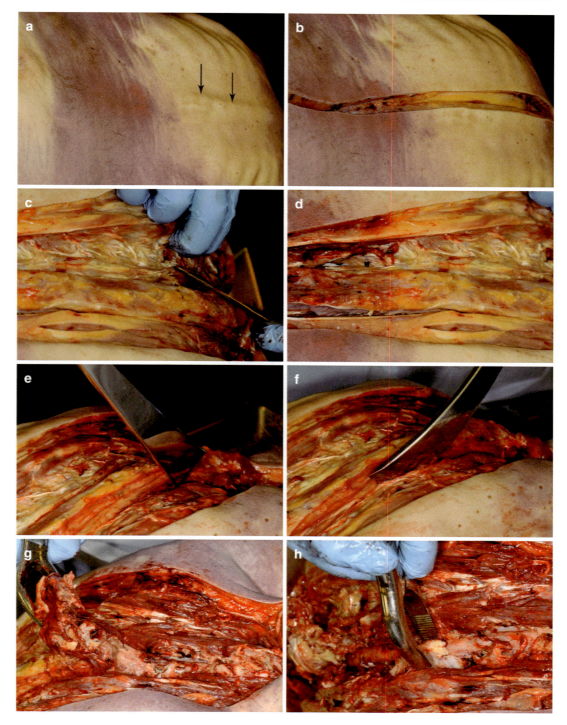

Fig. 3.5 Posterior approach for the removal of the spinal cord: Localization of the vertebral spines (→) (**a**), cutting the skin (**b**), removal of the paravertebral muscles (**c**), exposing the vertebral spine (**d**), cutting the pedicles of the vertebrae by a special chisel (**e**, **f**), loosening the column (**g**, **h**), exposing the spinal cord (**i**, **j**), gentle removal of the spinal cord (**k**, **l**), lining the spinal cord for length measurement (**m**, **n**)

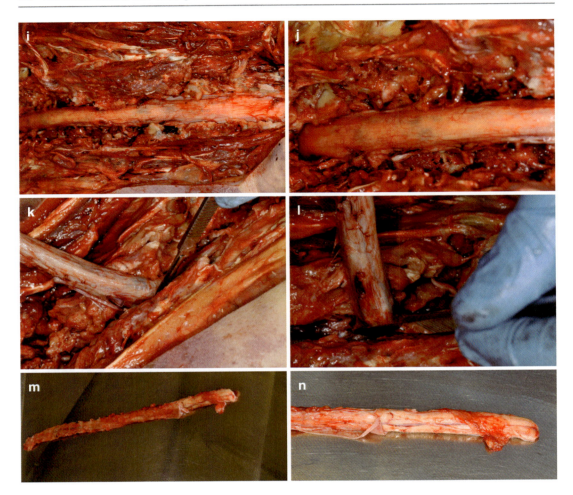

Fig. 3.5 (continued)

horizontal cut at the border between the upper pons and lower mesencephalon.
- The scalpel is placed in the interpeduncular fossa and through a horizontal cut the mesencephalon is transsected, thus, resulting in a section displaying the substantia nigra and the red nucleus.
- The frontal lobes are separated from the brain by placing the knife apposed to the temporal poles. This ensures that the subsequent sections through the remaining brain can be cut perpendicular to the midline.
- The frontal lobes are placed with the cut surface on the dissection table. Horizontal 1 cm thick cuts are now performed.
- Coronal 1 cm thick serial cuts are performed through the remaining brain. Attention should be drawn in order to perform cuts through
  – 1 cm behind the temporal pole
  – rostral edge of the optic chiasm

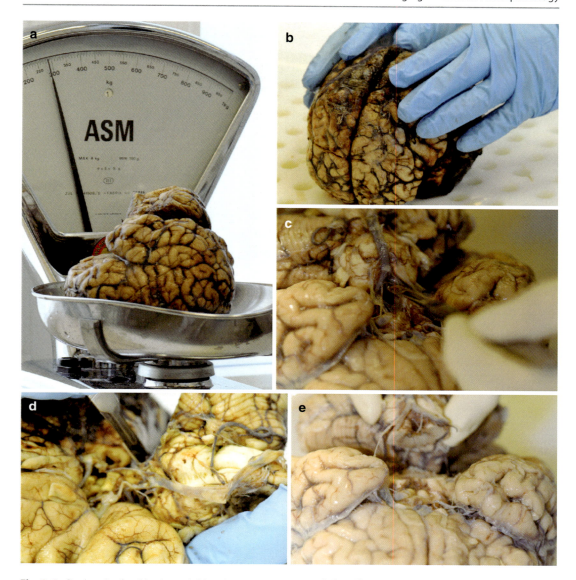

Fig. 3.6 Cutting the fixed brain: weighing the brain (**a**), visual and tactile examination (**b**), removal of the lower brain stem (i.e., pons and medulla oblongata) and cerebellum by a horizontal cut at the border between the upper pons and lower mesencephalon (**c–e**), removal of the mesencephalon (**f**), cutting the leptomeninges in order to inspect the middle cerebral artery (**g, f**), generating frontal sections (**i–r**) by either cutting the brain free hand (**i–l**) or using devices (**m–r**), positioning the cut brain slices for examination (**s, t**)

3.2 Removal, Fixation, and Cutting of the Brain and Spinal Cord

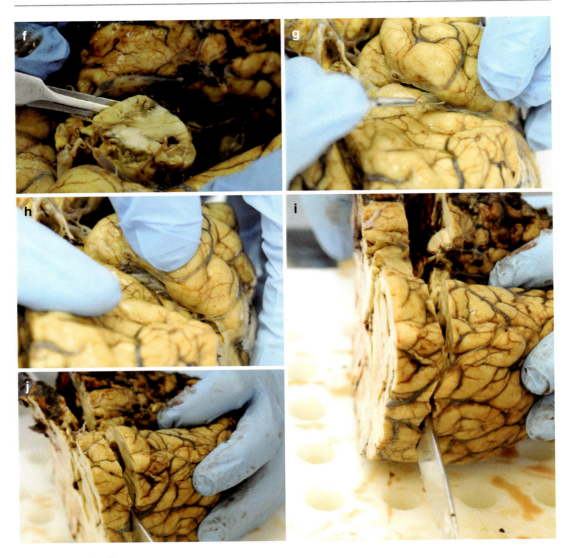

Fig. 3.6 (continued)

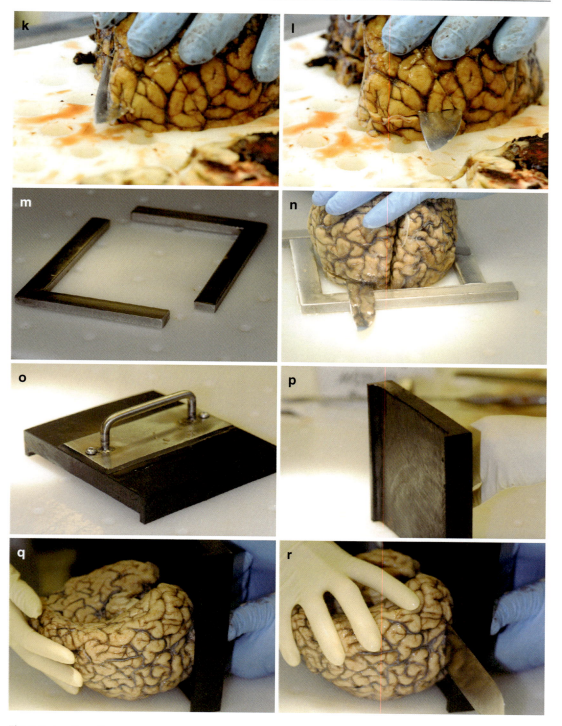

Fig. 3.6 (continued)

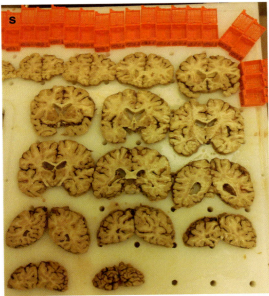
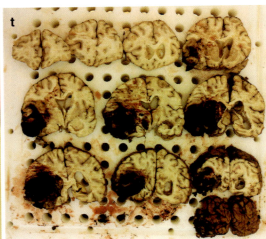

Fig. 3.6 (continued)

- infundibulum of the pituitary gland
- mammillary bodies
- red nucleus
- through the cerebral aqueduct
- posterior part of the mesencephalon
- occipital lobe
• The slices are laid out on the dissection table starting from the first frontal slice up to the last occipital slice. The slices are laid in such a way that the examiner looks at the slice from backwards, i.e., the left hemisphere is displayed at the left side of the examiner.

There are two ways of cutting the brain stem and the cerebellum (Fig. 3.7):

• The brain stem and cerebellum are not separated from each other
  – To be used if hemorrhagic ventricular tamponade is suspected.
  – The unseparated brain stem and cerebellum is heod in the left hand in such a way that the upper cerebellar hemispheres are touching the inner of the palm.
  – Sections are generated through the specimen perpendicular to the rostro-caudal axis of the brain stem.
  – The slices are laid out on the dissection table starting with the most rostral slice.
• The brain stem and cerebellum are separated from each other
  – To be used in all other situations.
  – The cerebellum can be separated from the brain stem in the following two ways:
    ○ Sectioning through the superior, middle, and inferior cerebellar peduncles on each side.
    ○ Sectioning the vermis, extending both cerebellar hemispheres from each other, inspecting the floor of the fourth ventricle, and the sectioning through the superior, middle, and inferior cerebellar peduncles on each side.

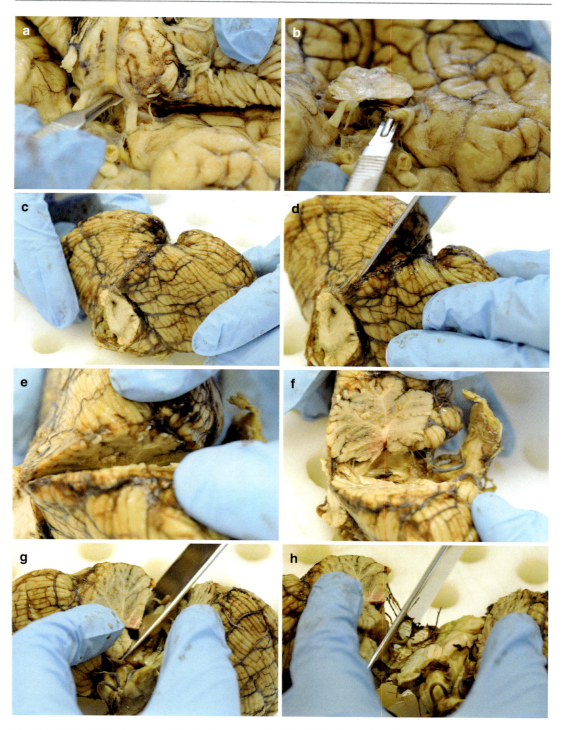

Fig. 3.7 Cutting the brain stem and cerebellum: removal of the brain stem and cerebellum by a cut at the border between the Mesencephalon and pons (**a**, **b**), removal of the cerebellum from the brain stem by sectioning the vermis (**c**, **d**), extending both cerebellar hemispheres from each other (**e**, **f**), inspecting the floor of the fourth ventricle, and the sectioning through the superior, middle, and inferior cerebellar peduncles on each side (**g**, **h**); the left cerebellar hemisphere is sectioned into 5 mm thick slices parallel to the vermis (**i**, **j**); the right cerebellar hemisphere is placed with the vermis on the dissection table (**k**, **l**), sections are generated at an angle of 45° through the hemisphere (**m**), in the resulting slices, the dentate nucleus can be seen at its largest extension (**n**); the sections through the brain stem are generated perpendicular to its superior-inferior axis (**o**); positioning the cut brain slices for examination (**p–r**)

3.2 Removal, Fixation, and Cutting of the Brain and Spinal Cord

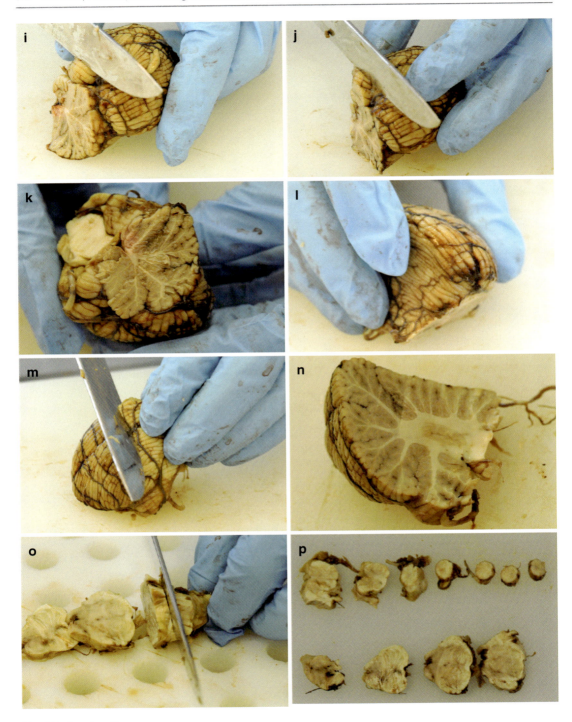

Fig. 3.7 (continued)

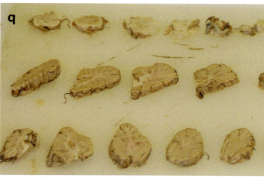
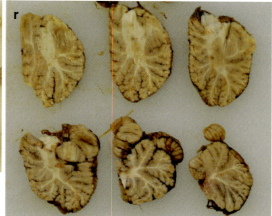

Fig. 3.7 (continued)

- The brain stem is cut into 5 mm thick slices at the following anatomical landmarks:
  - superior colliculi
  - inferior colliculi
  - pontomesencephalic junction
  - root of the fifth cranial nerve (mid-pons)
  - medullo-pontine junction (sixth, seventh, eighth cranial nerves)
  - mid-olivary level
  - caudal end of olives
  - pyramidal decussation
- The left cerebellar hemisphere is sectioned into 5 mm thick slices parallel to the vermis.
- The right cerebellar hemisphere is placed with the vermis on the dissection table. Sections are generated at an angle of 45° through the hemisphere. In the resulting slices, the dentate nucleus can be seen at its largest extension.

- *Visual* examination of the slice by describing:
  - the border between gray and white matter
  - size of gyri (atrophy, polymicrogyria)
  - the size of the ventricular system
  - discoloration of brain tissue (brownish discoloration in case of ischemia with reperfusion bleeding)
  - tissue damage and brownish discoloration (in case of trauma)
  - tissue damage and dark reddish to blackish discoloration (in case of hemorrhage)
  - tissue discoloration with glassy appearance (in case of multiple sclerosis)
- *Tactile* examination of the slices by describing:
  - softening of brain tissue of the cerebral and cerebellar hemispheres (in case of ischemia and hemorrhage)

Examples of typical brain lesions are given in Fig. 3.8.

3.2.4 Gross Anatomical Examination of the Cut Brain

Each brain slice is examined as follows:

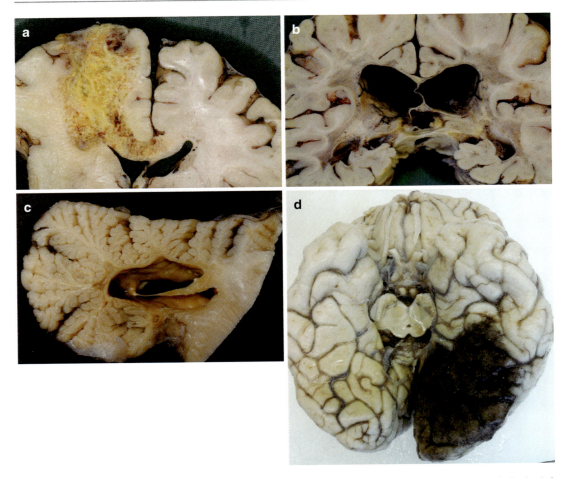

Fig. 3.8 Examples of gross anatomically visible lesions: brain tumor (glioblastoma WHO grade IV) (**a**), large areas of demyelination (**b**), old ischemic necrosis in the cerebellum (**c**), acute ischemic hemorrhagic necrosis in the left occipital lobe (**d**)

3.2.5 Sampling of Brain Regions for Microscopic Examination

Depending on the diagnostic/scientific question, several sampling schemes are applied and can be grouped as follows:

- No brain involvement in the course of the disease
- Neurodegenerative disorder
- Brain trauma
- Infant brain
- Epilepsy brain

Defined brain regions (Table 3.1) and all abnormally appearing brain regions have to be sampled (Fig. 3.9).

3.2.6 Handling of Surgical Specimens

The surgical specimen is characterized by:

- Taking its weight
- Measuring its size
- Describing its color
- Judging its firmness/softness

Table 3.1 The various parts of the brain are sampled in the following ways

Frontal lobe	Frontal superior including the superior frontal gyrus and the frontal medial gyrus (suited to examine watershed ischemia)
	Middle frontal gyrus as part of the superolateral prefrontal cortex (biological psychiatry)
	Frontal orbital including the straight gyrus
Temporal lobe	Hippocampal formation with the entorhinal region
	Superior and middle temporal gyri
	Amygdala
Parietal lobe	Superior parietal lobule
Occipital lobe	Primary visual cortex (Brodman area 17) and adjacent occipital cortex (Brodman areas 18, 19)
Cingulate gyrus	Anterior part above the genu corporis callosi
Basal ganglia	Anterior level including the caudate nucleus, putamen, and accumbens nucleus
	Middle level including the caudate nucleus, putamen, and globus pallidus
	Posterior level including the putamen and globus pallidus as well as part of the thalamus (latero-posterior putamen in multi-system atrophy)
Diencephalon	Thalamus
Cerebellum	Vermis (upper vermis atrophy in alcoholism, autism)
	Cerebellar cortex including gray and white matter as well as the dentate nucleus
Brain stem	Substantia nigra and red nucleus
	Pons
	Medulla oblongata with pyramid and inferior olivary nucleus

The tumor sample is sectioned by cutting the specimen in a series of equidistant 0.5 cm thick sections. All sections are processed for histological examination (Fig. 3.10).

3.3 Fixation and Processing of Tissue

A detailed description of tissue fixation and processing is given by Spencer et al. (2012), Rhodes (2012), and Usman and Asim (2005).

3.3.1 Fixation of Sampled Tissue

The aim of fixation is to:

- Harden tissue
- Preserve tissue
- Prevent loss of specific molecules due to catabolic enzymatic activity
- Prevent tissue destruction by microorganisms during storage

Fixation almost always leads to shrinkage, swelling, hardening of tissues, and color variations in various histochemical stains.

The mechanisms of fixation are manyfold and include:

- Covalent addition of reactive groups and of cross-links between proteins, individual protein moieties, within nucleic acids, and between nucleic acids and proteins
- Dehydration
- Effects of acids, salt formation, and heat
- Combinations of the above

The various types of fixation include:

- Physical methods (usually not applied or applied in conjunction with a chemical method):
  – Heat fixation
  – Microwave fixation
  – Freeze-drying and freeze substitution
- Chemical methods

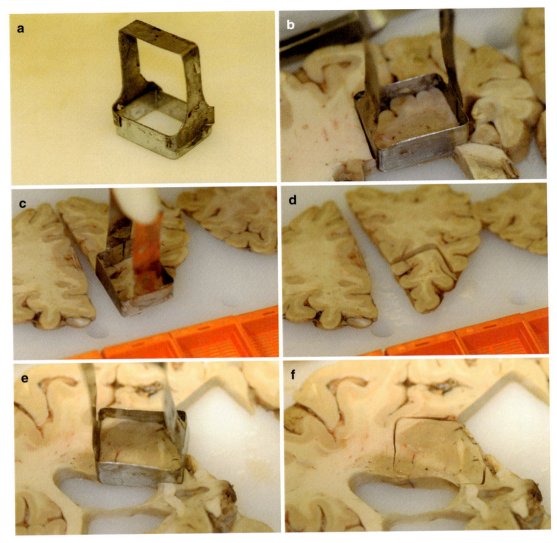

Fig. 3.9 Sampling brain regions. Use of a special device for sampling brain regions (**a, b**); generating a sample from the superior frontal gyrus (**c, d**) and basal ganglia with accumbens and anterior commissure (**e, f**) for histological examination

- Coagulant fixatives (coagulate proteins making them insoluble)
- Dehydrant coagulant fixatives (e.g., alcohol, ethanol, methanol, acetone)
- Non-coagulant cross-linking fixatives
    - Formaldehyde (4% neutral buffered formaldehyde)
    - Glutaraldehyde (used in electron microscopy)
    - Osmium tetroxide fixation (used in electron microscopy)

Factors that influence the quality of fixation include buffer, pH, duration of fixation, size of the specimen, temperature of fixation, concen-

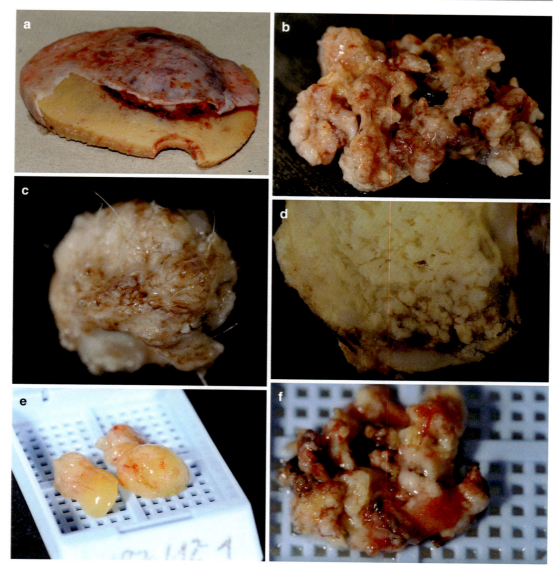

Fig. 3.10 Surgical specimens: Samples for histological examination from a metastasis growing through the skull bone (**a**), glioblastoma WHO grade IV (**b**), dermoid cyst (**c**), and metastasis from breast cancer (**d**); the specimens are placed in plastic cassettes for further tissue processing (**e**, **f**)

tration of fixative, osmolality of fixatives, ionic composition of fixatives, and additives to fixatives.

A universal or ideal fixative has not yet been identified. Thus, the choice of a fixative is always a compromise balancing between beneficial and detrimental effects.

3.3.2 Processing of Tissue

Tissue processing is aimed at:

- Removing all extractable water from tissue
- Replacing it with a support medium in order to

- Provide sufficient rigidity
- Enable the sectioning of tissue without damage or distortion

Tissue processing takes place in the following steps:

- Dehydration:
  - removal of unbound water and aqueous fixative from the tissue
  - is done slowly
  - in a graded alcohol series starting with 70% ethanol, followed by 95%, and terminated in 100%
  - excessive dehydration leads to hard, brittle, and shrunken tissue
- Clearing:
  - removal of dehydrating solutions
  - making the tissue components receptive to the infiltrating medium
  - clearing agents are aromatic hydrocarbons or short-chain aliphatic hydrocarbons (CAVE: environmental issue), i.e., xylene, chloroform
- Infiltrating:
  - permeation of the tissue with a support medium, i.e., paraffin
  - paraffin forms a matrix which prevents tissue distortion during microtomy
- Embedding:
  - correct orientation of the properly processed tissue in a support medium, i.e., paraffin filling all the spaces within the tissue and allowing it to solidify.
  - done with the use of an embedding center which consists of a paraffin dispenser, a cold plate, and a heated storage area for molds and tissue cassettes.

Factors which influence the rate of processing include:

- Agitation
- Heat
- Viscosity
- Vacuum

A self-contained vacuum tissue processor is usually used in routine work (Fig. 3.11a–f):

- Tissues in their cassettes are placed in a retort chamber.
- Reagents used for dehydration and clearing as well as the melted paraffin are moved into and out of the retort chamber using vacuum and pressure.
- Each step of the procedure can be individually programmed by adjusting temperature, time, or vacuum/pressure.

Subsequently, the processed tissue blocks are embedded in paraffin (Fig. 3.11g) and from the formalin-fixed, paraffin-embedded (FFPE) tissue blocks 5 μm thick sections are cut using a microtome (Fig. 3.11h–j). Additional equipment of a neuropathology laboratory includes staining machine for routine or special stains (Fig. 3.11k), slide cover slipping machine (Fig. 3.11l), automated immunohistochemistry strainers (Fig. 3.11m–p), and cryostat for the generation of frozen sections (Fig. 3.11q). The formalin-fixed, paraffin-embedded (FFPE) tissue blocks are archived and stored for 20 years (legal requirement) (Fig. 3.11r).

3.4 Staining of Tissue

3.4.1 Classical Stain

Hematoxylin and Eosin Stain (H&E) (Fig. 3.12)
- The classical universally applied stain
- Used to study the general morphology of the tissue
- Stain results:
  - Nuclei—blue
  - Other tissue components—pink
- Indications in neuropathology:
  - cytoarchitectonical buildup of the cerebral and cerebellar cortex
  - neuronal loss, neuronal swelling
  - glial changes

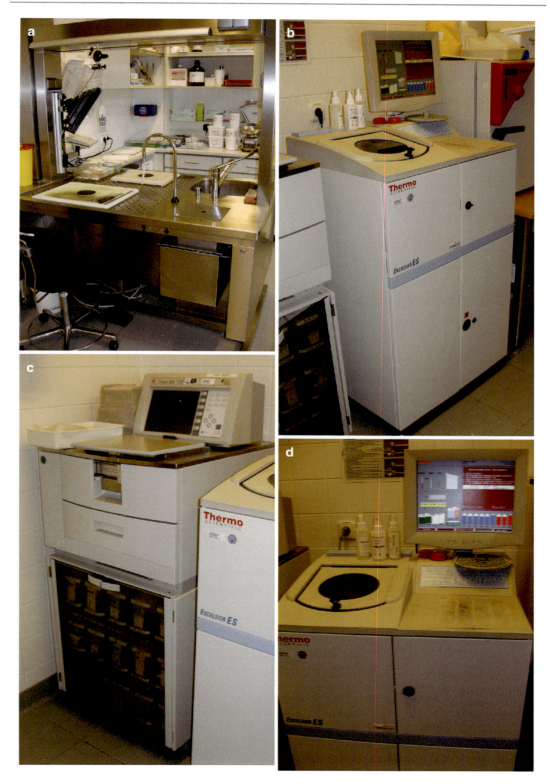

Fig. 3.11 Processing tissues: table for sectioning and sampling the received tissue (**a**), tissue processor (**b–f**), paraffin embedding processor (**g**), microtome (**h**), water bath (**i**), heating plate (**j**), device for routine staining (**k**), glass slide covering (**l**), immunohistochemical staining machine (**m–p**), cryostat (**q**), archiving the paraffin blocks (**r**)

3.4 Staining of Tissue

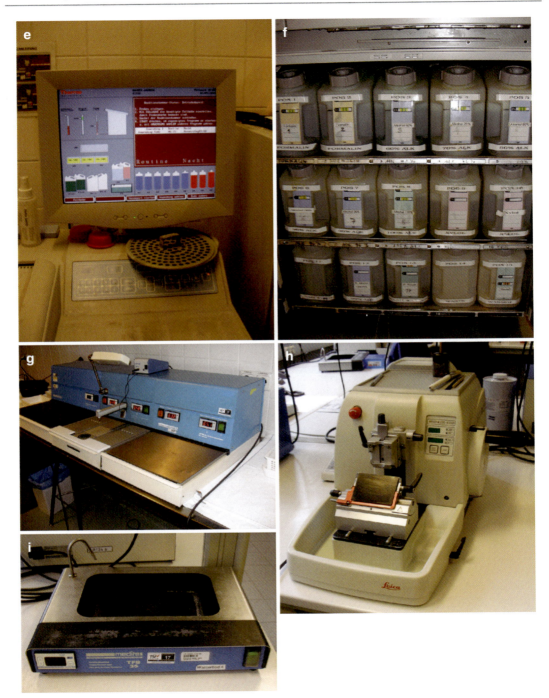

Fig. 3.11 (continued)

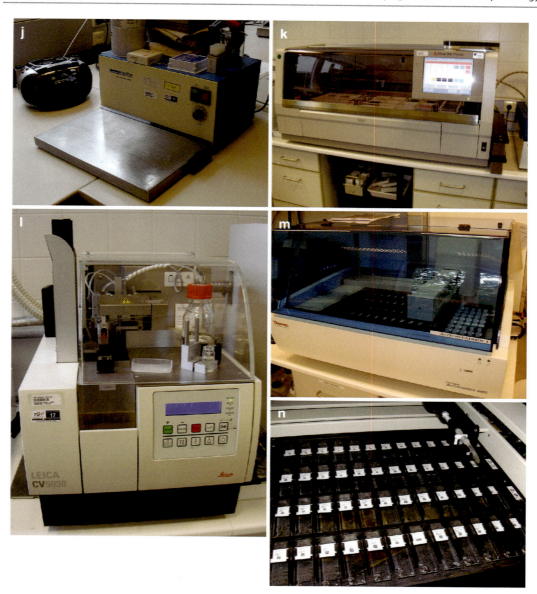

Fig. 3.11 (continued)

3.4 Staining of Tissue

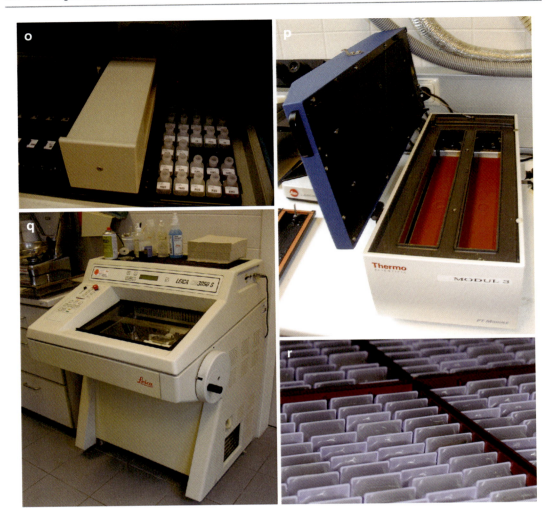

Fig. 3.11 (continued)

- vascular changes
- hemorrhagic tissue damage
- ischemic tissue destruction
- tumor growth
- evidence of inflammatory cells (lymphocytes, granulocytes, macrophages)

3.4.2 Special Stains

Periodic Acid-Schiff (PAS) (Fig. 3.13a)
- Used to show carbohydrate moieties, glycogen in muscle, mucin in adenocarcinoma
- Stain results:
  - PAS-positive material—magenta
  - Nuclei—blue
  - Background—pale pink
- Indications in neuropathology:
  - Fungal pathogens
  - Corpora amylacea
  - Lipofuscin
  - Basement membranes (better demonstrated with immunohistochemistry for collagen type IV)
  - Glycogen in muscle tissue
  - Mucin in metastatic adenocarcinoma

Diastase-Sensitive PAS or PAS with Diastase Digestion
- Depolymerization of glycogen into smaller sugar units by diastase and amylase; the later

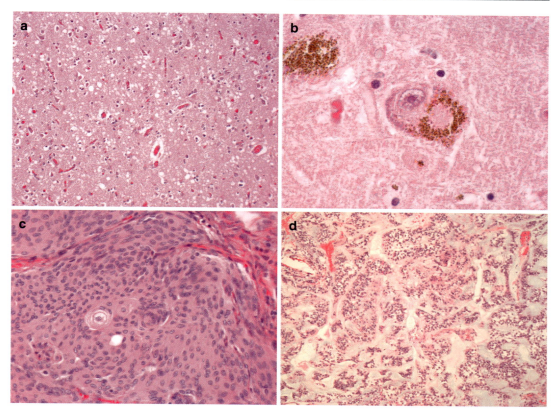

Fig. 3.12 Hematoxylin and Eosin stained tissues/structures: spongiform changes in the cerebral cortex of a case with Creutzfeldt–Jakob disease (**a**), neuron of the substantia nigra with Lewy body in Parkinson disease (**b**), meningioma (**c**), ependymoma (**d**)

are washed out retaining other substances attached to sugars (i.e., mucopolysaccharides)
- Stain results:
  - Glycogen is bright/magenta in the untreated stain
  - Glycogen should be absent in the diastase-treated slide
- Indications in neuropathology:
  - Glycogenosis

Alcian Blue (Fig. 3.13b, c)
- Used to show mucins
- Stain results:
  - Acid mucin—blue
  - Proteoglycans and hyaluronic acid—blue
  - Nuclei—red
- Indications in neuropathology:
  - Mucinous background in ependymomas

3.4.3 Special Neuro-stains

Special stains used in neuropathology to demonstrate various components of the normal and diseased nervous system are listed in Table 3.2.

Some of these special neuro-stains will be briefly mentioned. Although some of them are routinely used in diagnostic neuropathology (i.e., cresyl violet, Luxol fast blue, modified Bielschowsky, and Gallyas stain), it has to be stated that for each of the above-mentioned cells/structures there exist today reliable markers for immunohistochemical staining (see Sect. 3.3).

Cresyl Violet (Nissl Stain) (Fig. 3.14a–d)
- Nissl substance, abundant in the neuronal cytoplasm is stained with the cresyl violet

3.4 Staining of Tissue

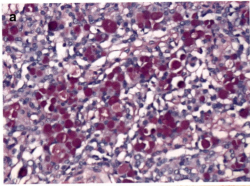
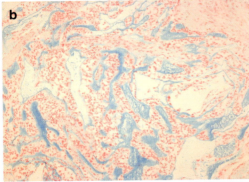
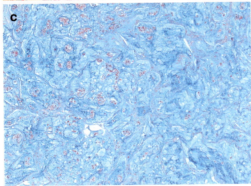

Fig. 3.13 Special stains: Alcian blue-positive structures in a papillary ependymoma (WHO grade I) (**b**), metastasis of a mucoid adenocarcinoma of the lung (**c**)

- Stain results:
  - Nissl substance—dark purple/blue
  - Nuclei—purple/blue
  - Background—colorless
- Indications in neuropathology:
  - Demonstration of neurons (e.g., in tumors)
  - Evaluation of the correct cytoarchitectonic buildup of the cortex (cortical dysplasia causing epilepsy)
  - Morphometric evaluation of brain tissue

Table 3.2 The special neurohistological stains can be grouped following the cells/structures they stain

Cell/structure	Stain
Neurons	• Cresyl violet (Nissl stain) • Golgi Cox silver impregnation
Axons and neuronal processes	• Bielschowsky • Palmgren • Marsland, Glees, and Erikson • Holmes
Myelin	• Luxol fast blue (LFB) • Loyez iron aluminum • Marchi method for degenerated myelin • Wölke iron hematoxylin • Holmes
Glial cells	• Phosphotungstic acid hematoxylin (PTAH) (astrocytes) • Holzer (astrocytes) • Hortega silver carbonate (microglia) • Penfield silver nitrate (oligodendrocytes) • Cajal gold chloride (astrocytes)
Neurodegeneration	• Modified Bielschowsky • Methenamine silver • Haga • Garvey uranyl-silver nitrate • Gallyas • Cross's modified Palmgren stain • Bodian • Thioflavin S

Luxol Fast Blue (LFB) (Fig. 3.14e, f)
- Used to demonstrate myelin
- Stain results:
  - Myelin—blue
  - Red blood cells—blue
  - Nuclei—purple
  - Nissl substance—purple
- Indications in neuropathology:
  - Determination of myelin pallor, loss, demyelination

Phosphotungstic Acid Hematoxylin (PTAH)
- Used to stain for astrocytes and glial fibers
- Stain results:
  - Glia and glial fibers—blue
  - Neurons—pink
  - Nuclei—blue
  - Myelin—purple-blue

- Indications in neuropathology:
  - Usefulness limited to gray matter, areas of demyelination, reactive astrocytes

Modified Bielschowsky (Fig. 3.14g, h)
- Used to stain axons, senile plaques, neuritic plaques, and neurofibrillary tangles

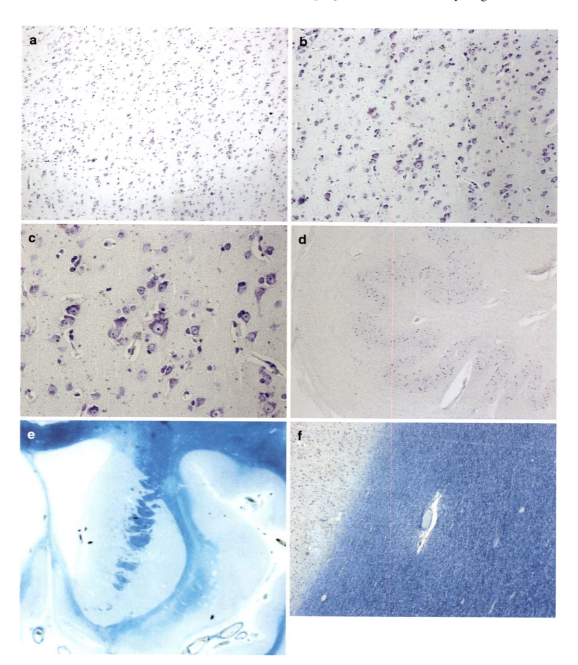

Fig. 3.14 Special Neuro-stains: Cresyl violet (**a–d**) showing neurons in the cerebral cortex (**a–c**) and in the inferior olivary nucleus of the medulla oblongata (**d**), Luxol fast blue (**e, f**) showing white matter (in blue) (**e**: basal ganglia) and cerebral cortex with the border between gray and white matter (**f**), Bielschowsky stain (**g, h**) demonstrating nerve fibers in the cerebral cortex (**g**) and white matter (**h**); Gallyas stain (**i, j**) of the hippocampal formation showing white matter (in dark) (**i**) and neurofibrillary tangles (**j**)

3.4 Staining of Tissue

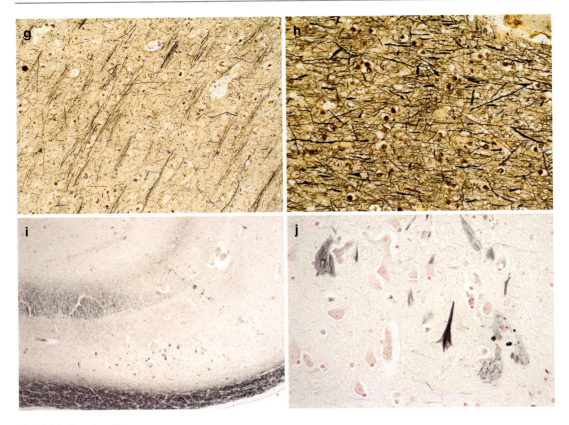

Fig. 3.14 (continued)

- Stain results:
  - Senile plaques, neuritic plaques—black
  - Neurofibrillary tangles—black
  - Axons—black
  - Background—pink
- Indications in neuropathology:
  - Neurodegenerative diseases, e.g., Alzheimer disease

Gallyas (Fig. 3.14i, j)
- Used to stain neurofibrillary tangles
- Stain results:
  - Neurofibrillary tangles—black
  - Senile plaques—black
  - Nuclei—red to pink
  - Background—red to pink
- Indications in neuropathology:
  - Neurodegenerative diseases, e.g., Alzheimer disease
  - Oligodendroglial inclusions (Papp and Lantos inclusions) in multi-system atrophy
  - Neuropil threads
  - Argyrophilic grains in argyrophylic grain disease

3.4.4 Special Stains for Connective Tissue

Trichrome (Masson)
- Used for the demonstration of collagen
- Stain results:
  - Collagen—blue
  - Fibrin—red
  - Nuclei—blue/black
- Indications in neuropathology:
  - Vascular changes
  - Fibrosis or desmoplasia in tumors

Elastica van Gieson (Fig. 3.15a–d)
- Used for the demonstration of elastic fibers
- Stain results:

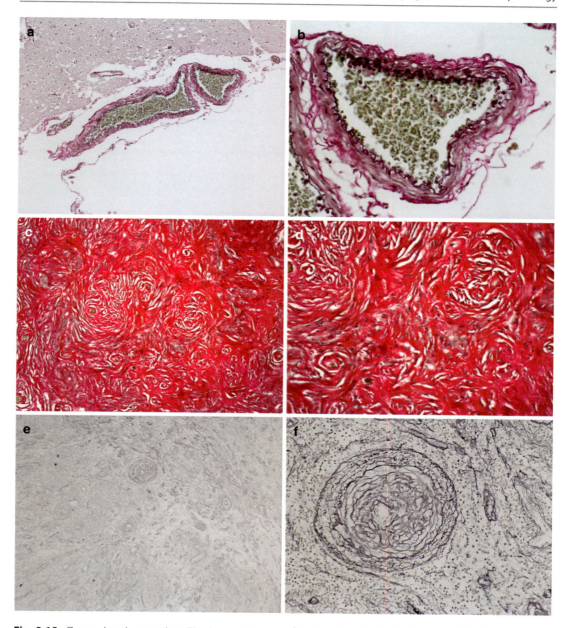

Fig. 3.15 Connective tissue stains: Elastic van Gieson stain (**a–d**) displaying the arterial wall (**a, b**) and connective tissue in a fibroblastic meningioma (WHO grade I) (**c,** **d**). Reticulin stain (**e, f**) shows reticulin fibers in case of lymphoma

- Elastic fibers—blue/black
- Collagen—red
- Other tissues—yellow
• Indications in neuropathology:
  - Assessment of vessel walls, aneurysmatic sac

Reticulin (Fig. 3.15e, f)
• Used for the demonstration of reticulin fibers
• Stain results:
  - Reticulin fibers—black
  - Collagen—pink/gray
  - Nuclei—pink

3.5 Immunohistochemistry

- Indications in neuropathology:
  - Growth pattern of tumors, i.e., glioblastoma vs gliosarcoma
  - Abnormal structural changes in lymphoma

3.4.5 Other Special Stains

Besides special neuro-stains, other stains are used to visualize normal or abnormal material in the nervous system (Table 3.3) (Fig. 3.16).

Table 3.3 Other special stains used in diagnostic neuropathology

Visualized product	Method	Stain results
Hemosiderin (Fig. 3.16a, b)	Perl's Prussian blue	• Hemosiderin—blue • Ferric salts—blue • Nuclei—pink
Amyloid (Fig. 3.16c, d)	Congo red (polarized light)	• Amyloid—red/pink on unpolarized light, apple-green with polarized light • Nuclei—blue
	Thioflavin S (fluorescence light)	• Amyloid—yellow-green
Lipofuscin	Schmorl	• Lipofuscin—dark blue • Melanin—blue • Nuclei—pink
Lipids	Oil red O (frozen sections only)	• Neutral lipids—red • Nuclei—blue
	Sudan black B (frozen sections only)	• Lipids—blue/black • Nuclei—pink
Calcium	Von Kossa	• Calcium deposits—black
Ferrous iron	Turnball blue	• Blue
Ferric iron	Prussian blue	• Blue
Glycogen	Best carmine	• Bright red
Carbohydrate	Periodic acid-Schiff (PAS) with and without diastase	• Bright rose red

Table 3.3 (continued)

Visualized product	Method	Stain results
Bacteria	Gram stain	• Gram-positive bacteria—blue/black • Gram-negative bacteria—red • Nuclei—pink
	Gomori methenamine silver (GMS)	• Gram-positive bacteria-black
Mycobacterium tuberculosis	Ziehl-Neelsen	• Mycobacteria—red • Nuclei—pale blue
Spirochaetes	Warthin Starry	• Spirochaetes—black • Background—yellow
Fungi (Fig. 3.16e, f)	Grocott	• Fungi—black • Basement membranes—black • Background—green
	Gomori methenamine silver (GMS)	• Fungi—black

3.5 Immunohistochemistry

A detailed description about immunohistochemistry is given by Jackson and Blythe (2012)

3.5.1 General Principles

Immunohistochemistry aims at identifying cellular or tissue constituents by means of an antigen-antibody interaction, whereby the cellular or tissue component is considered to be the antigen. The site of the antigen-antibody reaction, i.e., antibody binding is visualized either by direct labeling or by use of a secondary labeling method.

Primary antibodies might be:

- Polyclonal antibodies
- Monoclonal antibodies
- Lectins

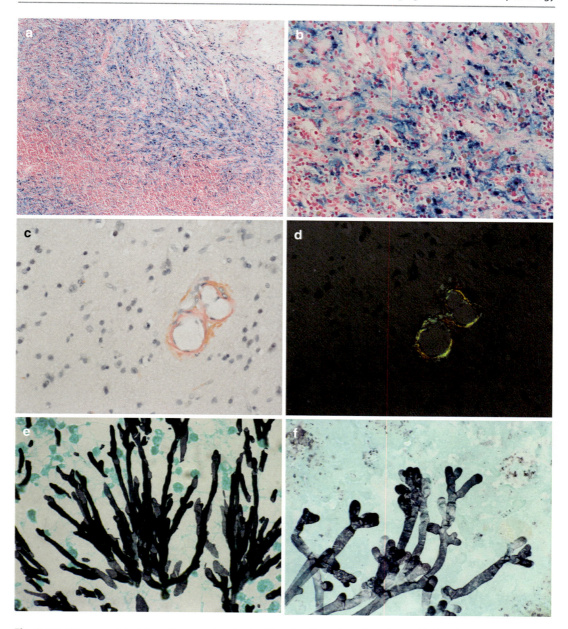

Fig. 3.16 Other special stains: Congo red stain (**a**, **b**) viewed under unpolarized light (**a**) and under polarized light (**b**) used to show amyloid deposition; Prussian blue (**c**, **d**) used to show hemosiderin; Grocott stain used to demonstrate fungi (in these pictures aspergillus) (**e**, **f**)

The used labels fall into the following categories:

- Enzyme labels
- Colloidal metal labels
- Fluorescent labels
- Radiolabels

The used immunohistochemical methods are:

- Direct method (one-step staining method)
- Indirect, two-step method
  - Polymer chain two-step indirect technique
  - Unlabeled antibody-enzyme complex techniques (PAP and APAP)

3.5 Immunohistochemistry

- Immunogold silver staining (IGSS)
- (Strept)avidin-biotin techniques
- Hapten labeling technique
- Mirror image complementary antibody labeling technique (MICA)

A variety of factors might influence the results of immunohistochemical staining procedures (Table 3.4).

The rationale for the application of immunohistochemistry is given as:

- Diagnosis of tumors
  - Classification of poorly differentiated neoplasms
  - Diagnosis of carcinoma of unknown primary
  - Diagnosis of invasion
- Assessment of markers reflecting prognosis
  - Ki67/MIB1 (see later)
  - P53
- Assessment of markers reflecting a therapeutic response
  - HER2 (herceptin for breast cancer)
  - ER/PR (tamoxifen for breast cancer)
  - Braf (melanoma)
  - IDH1 (gliomas)
- Detection of microinvasion
- Identification of infectious agents (see Sect. 3.4.12)
  - Viruses
  - Other organisms (Toxoplasma)

The correct interpretation of immunohistochemistry is the evaluation of the location of the targeted antigen:

- Nuclear reactivity
  - Transcription factors
  - Steroid hormone receptors
  - Proliferation markers (Ki67)
- Cytoplasmic reaction
  - Intermediate filaments (GFAP)
  - Contractile proteins (actin)
  - Secretory products (pituitary hormones)
  - Functional proteins

Table 3.4 Issues influencing the outcome of immunohistochemical staining, modified after (Alafuzoff et al. 2015)

Agonal state	• Premortem condition (infectious disease, malignancy treated with cytostatics)
Mode of death	• Rapid death • Prolonged death with poor circulation
Postmortem delay	• None to hours • Even months
Fixative	• Paraformaldehyde, glutaraldehyde, formaldehyde, ethanol, and others • Percentage of fixative • Buffered or unbuffered fixative
Fixation time	• Hours • Days • Months • Years
Paraffin	• Melting point of the embedding medium (wax, paraffin, paraplast, others)
Storage time and storage temperature of blocks	• Days to years • Room temperature • 4 °C
Storage time and storage temperature of sections	• Days to months • Room temperature • 4 °C
Pretreatment strategy	• No pretreatment • Enzymes • Heat • Acids
Antibody applied	• Various clones for one protein • Made in-house or commercial • Polyclonal or monoclonal
Incubation time and temperature	• Minutes to overnight • 37–4 °C

Detection systems	• Amplification of signal based on
	  – avidin-biotin complex
	  – labeled streptavidin-biotin
	  – polymers
	• Variability in the polymers produced by different companies
	• Sensitivity based on first-, second-, and third-generation systems
	• Various chromogens

Mode of staining	• Automatic • Manual • In-house protocols

Table 3.5 Cellular localization of various antigens

Immunoreactivity	
Nuclear	• Transcription factors • Steroid hormone receptors • Proliferation markers (Ki67)
Cytoplasmic	• Intermediate filaments (GFAP) • Contractile proteins (actin) • Secretory products (pituitary hormones) • Functional proteins
Cytoplasmic granular	• Napsin
Cytoplasmic dot-like	• Hodgkin lymphoma (CD30, CD15) • Neuroendocrine tumors (cytokeratins)
Membranous	• Cluster of differentiation (CD)-markers (CD3, CD20) • Surface receptors (EGFR, HER2) • Adhesion molecules (E-cadherin)
Nuclear and cytoplasmic	• S100 • Calretinin • ß-catenin
Negative	• True negative • False negative

Table 3.6 Biomarkers associated with central neural cell types

Cell type	Biomarker
Multipotential neural stem cells	• Nestin • GFAP • LewisX glycosphingolipid3-fucosyl-N-acetyl-lactosamine (LeX/CD15) • Musashi homolog (MSI) 1&2 • Hes 1&5 • PDGFRα • Prominin-1 (CD33/PROM1) • Sex determining region Y-box 2 (SOX2) • Minichromosome maintenance complex component 2 (MCM2) • Oligodendrocyte lineage transcription factor 2 (OLIG2)
Transit amplifying cells	• LeX/CD15 • OLIG2 • Distal-less homeobox 2 (DLX2) • Epithelial growth factor receptor (EGFR) • Chondroitin sulfate proteoglycan (NG2)
Neuroblasts/neuronal progenitors	• PSA-NCAM • Doublecortin (DCX) • ß-III tubulin • Microtubulie-associated protein (MAP2)
Mature neurons	• NeuN • Neurofilament protein (NFP) • Neuron-specific enolase (NSE)

- Cytoplasmic granular reactivity
  - Napsin
- Cytoplasmic dot-like reactivity
  - Hodgkin lymphoma (CD30, CD15)
  - Neuroendocrine tumors (cytokeratins)
- Membranous reactivity
  - CD-markers (CD3, CD20)
  - Surface receptors (EGFR, HER2)
  - Adhesion molecules (E-cadherin)
- Nuclear and cytoplasmic reactivity
  - S100
  - Calretinin
  - ß-catenin
- Negative immunoreactivity
  - True negative
  - False negative

The knowledge about the localization of various antigens corresponding to specific cellular sites (i.e., nuclear, cytoplasmic, and membranous) is of utmost importance (Table 3.5).

3.5.2 Neuronal Markers

Immunohistochemical biomarkers for neuronal lineage cells and neurons are listed in Table 3.6.

- Neuron-specific enolase (NSE)
  - Reacts with neurons and neuroendocrine cells
  - Highly nonspecific
  - Sensitive
- NeuN (Neuronal Nuclei) (Mullen et al. 1992) (Fig. 3.17a–f)
  - Reacts with neuronal nuclei
  - Expression in most neuronal cell types throughout the nervous system

3.5 Immunohistochemistry

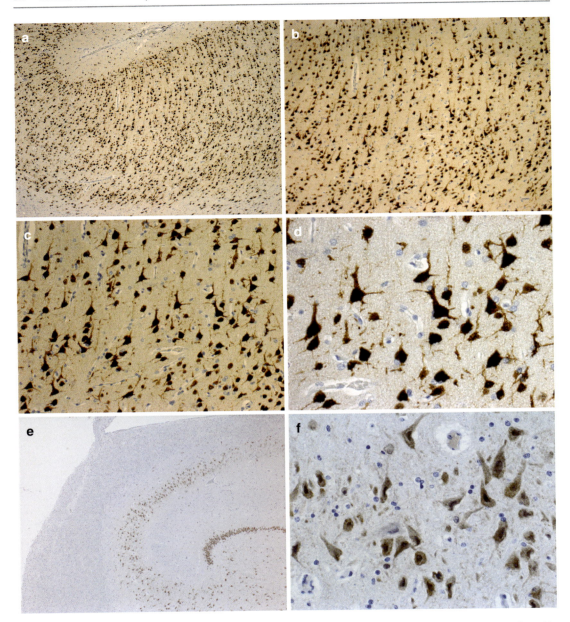

Fig. 3.17 Neuronal markers: Immunohistochemistry for NeuN (**a–f**) show neurons in the cerebral cortex (**a–d**) and in the hippocampal formation (**e, f**)

- Lack of immunoreactivity in cerebellar Purkinje cells, olfactory bulb mitral cells, and retinal photoreceptor cells
- Microtubule-associated protein (MAP2) (Dehmelt and Halpain 2005; Friedrich and Aszodi 1991; Sanchez et al. 2000) (Fig. 3.18c, d)
  - Selectively located in the somatodendritic compartment of neurons
  - Predominantly expressed in dendrites
  - Regulates neuronal plasticity and dendritic extension
  - Promotes structure modulation and morphological stabilization in neurons
  - Stabilize microtubules against depolymerization
  - Stiffening effect on microtubules
- SMI-31 (Johnstone et al. 1997; Shea and Beermann 1993)

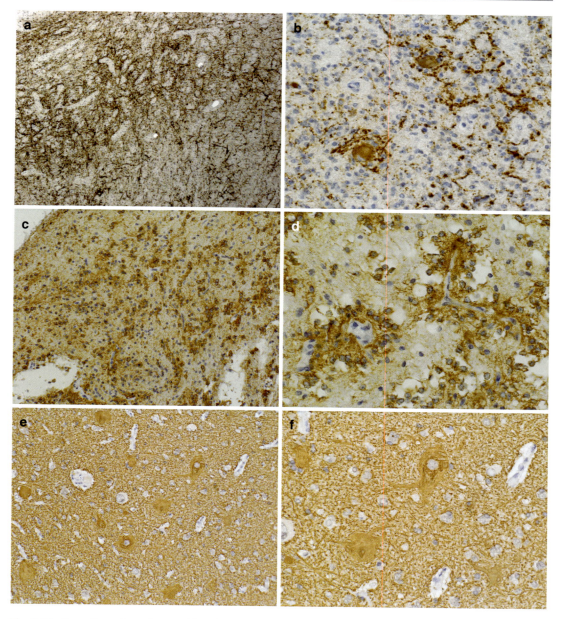

Fig. 3.18 Synaptic markers: Immunohistochemistry for synaptophysin (**a**, **b**) in focal cortical dysplasia (**a**) and ganglioglioma (**b**), for microtubule-associated protein (MAP2) (**c**, **d**) in rosette-forming glioneuronal tumor, for neurofilament (**e**, **f**)

- SMI-31 reacts with a phosphorylated epitope in extensively phosphorylated neurofilament H.
- Reacts with axons.
- Some dendrites such as basket cell dendrites, but not Purkinje cell dendrites are positive.
- Nerve cell bodies are generally unreactive.

• SMI-32 (Gottron et al. 1995; Voelker et al. 2004; Morel et al. 2002)
  - Reacts with a nonphosphorylated epitope in neurofilament H of most mammalian species.
  - Stains neuronal cell bodies.
  - Stains dendrites and some thick axons in

the central and peripheral nervous systems, but thin axons are not marked.
  – Labels a neuronal population with enhanced vulnerability to kainate toxicity most of which are GABA-ergic and reveal kainate-activated Ca^{2+} uptake.
- Nestin
  – type IV intermediate filament
  – widely expressed in neural stem cells

The cellular localization of neuronal markers is given in Table 3.7.

Markers for interneurons include among others:

- Calbindin (Buffa et al. 1990; Schwaller et al. 2002; Schmidt 2012)
  – calcium-binding protein
  – marker for double-bouquet, Martinotti cells
  – interneurons in layer II and to a lesser extent in layer III-IV
- Parvalbumin (Hof et al. 1999; DeFelipe 1997; Hu et al. 2014)
  – calcium-binding protein
  – marker for GABA-ergic interneurons
- Calretinin (Cauli et al. 2014; Barinka and Druga 2010; Camp and Wijesinghe 2009; Rogers et al. 1990)
  – Synonym: 29 kDa calbindin
  – Vitamin D-dependent calcium-binding protein
  – Involved in calcium signaling
  – Role in diverse cellular functions, including message targeting and intracellular calcium buffering
  – Modulator of neuronal excitability
  – Expressed in neurons
- Somatostatin (Barnett 2003; Epelbaum et al. 1994; Kawaguchi and Kondo 2002; Schindler et al. 1996; Tallent 2007)
  – Peptide
  – Acts as hormone
  – Affects neurotransmission and cell proliferation via interaction with G-protein-coupled somatostatin receptors

Table 3.7 Cellular localization of neuronal markers

Antibody	Reactivity
Neuron-specific enolase	Cytoplasm
NeuN	Neuronal nuclei
MAP2	Dendrites
SMI-31	Axons
SMI-32	Cell body
SMI-311	Pan-neurofilaments

- Cholecystokinine
  – Peptide
  – Functions as hormone
- Neuropeptide Y (Benarroch 2009; Heilig and Widerlov 1995; Protas et al. 2003; Sperk et al. 2007)
  – 36-Amino acid neuropeptide
  – Acts as a neurotransmitter in the brain and in the autonomic nervous system of humans
  – Produced in the hypothalamus

Layer-specific markers were recently identified and used sparsely in research (Fauser et al. 2013):

- ER81
  – Transcription factor of the ETS family
  – Layer 5 projection neurons
- RORß
  – Layer IV
  – Internal granule cell layer neurons
- SMI32
  – Nonphosphorylated neurofilament H
  – Corticospinal projection neurons in Layers III and V
- TLE4
  – Transcriptional activator
  – Localized in nuclei of layer V/VI neurons

3.5.3 Synaptic Markers

- Synaptophysin (Thiel 1993; Wiedenmann 1991) (Fig. 3.18a, b)
  – transmembrane glycoprotein
  – reacts with synaptic vesicles
  – cell membranes and cytoplasm is stained

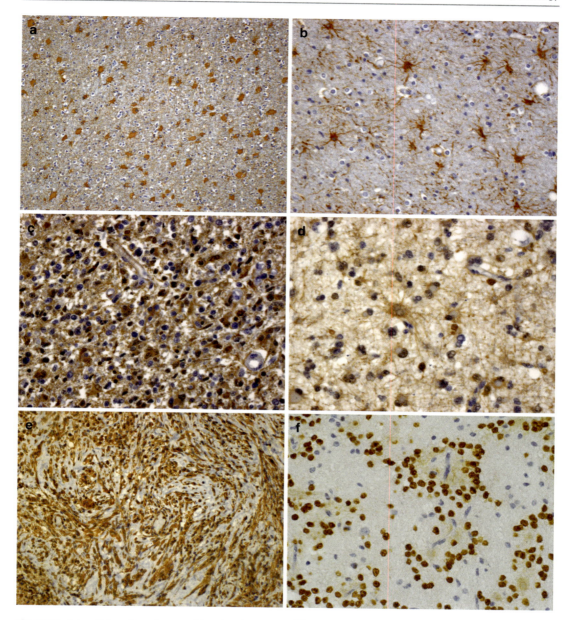

Fig. 3.19 Astroglial markers: Immunohistochemistry for GFAP (glial fibrillary acidic protein) (**a**, **b**) in a case of Creutzfeldt–Jakob disease, S100 (**c**, **d**) in glioblastoma (WHO grade IV) (**c**) and anaplastic astrocytoma (WHO grade III) (**d**); Vimentin in glioblastoma (WHO grade IV) (**e**); Olig2 in rosette-forming glioneuronal tumor (**f**)

- Chromogranin (Hendy et al. 1995; Lloyd 1987; Loh et al. 2012; O'Connor et al. 2000; Willis et al. 2011)
  - acidic glycoprotein located in neurosecretory granules
  - reacts with synaptic vesicles
  - positive in neuroendocrine tumors

3.5.4 Astroglial Markers

- GFAP (Eng 1985; Eng and Ghirnikar 1994; Eng et al. 2000; Middeldorp and Hol 2011) (Fig. 3.19a, b)
  - Cytoplasmic intermediate filament
  - 50 KDa molecular weight

- The major component of glial fibrils
- Marker of astrocytic differentiation
- S100 (family) (Donato et al. 2013; Heizmann 1999; Heizmann et al. 2002; Kligman and Hilt 1988; Nash et al. 2008; Zimmer et al. 1995) (Fig. 3.19c, d)
  - Soluble in 100% ammonium sulfate
  - S100 gene family is the largest subfamily of acidic, dimeric, calcium-binding proteins of EF-hand type
  - At least 25 distinct members of this subgroup have been described
  - 22 of these genes are clustered at chromosome locus 1q21
  - Functions include: regulation of calcium homeostasis, cell proliferation, apoptosis, cell invasion and motility, cytoskeleton interactions, protein phosphorylation, regulation of transcriptional factors, autoimmunity, chemotaxis, inflammation, and pluripotency
  - Most sensitive melanocytic marker
  - Low specificity; reacts with nerve sheath tumors, gliomas, chordomas, granular cell tumors
- Vimentin (Clarke and Allan 2002; Evans 1998; Minin and Moldaver 2008; Pekny 2001) (Fig. 3.19e)
  - Cytoplasmic 57 kDA type III intermediate filament protein
  - Characteristic of cells of mesenchymal nature (endothelial cells, fibroblasts, and vascular smooth muscle cells)
  - Expressed early in astrogliogenesis
  - Stains mainly the perinuclear region
  - Tendency to be expressed more consistently in higher grade astrocytomas
- Glt1 (Morel et al. 2013; Schmitt et al. 1996; Yang et al. 2009, 2010)
  - Astrocyte glutamate transporter
  - Responsible for the vast majority of functional uptake of extracellular glutamate in the CNS
- GLAST1 (Rauen and Wiessner 2000; Stoffel et al. 2004)
  - High affinity, Na(+)-dependent, electrogenic glial L-glutamate transporter
- Aldh1
  - Aldehyde dehydrogenase 1
  - It is a cytosolic detoxifying enzyme responsible for the oxidation of intracellular aldehydes

3.5.5 Oligodendroglial Markers: Myelin Markers

- Carbonic anhydrase II (Cammer and Brion 2000; Giacobini 1987)
  - a zinc-containing enzyme that catalyzes the reversible hydration of carbon dioxide
- Galactocerebroside (GC) (Jessen et al. 1985; Rostami et al. 1984; Uchida et al. 1981)
  - is a major glycolipid of myelin and myelin-forming cells
  - distributed not only in oligodendrocytes and myelin but also in epithelial cells of the ependymal layer of the ventricle and choroid plexus
- Kir4.1 (Butt and Kalsi 2006; Olsen and Sontheimer 2008)
  - Kir establishes the high potassium (K+) selectivity of the glial cell membrane and strongly negative resting membrane potential (RMP)
  - specific expression of the Kir4.1 subtype, which is a major K+ conductance in glial cell membranes and has a key role in setting the glial RMP
- NG2 (Staugaitis and Trapp 2009; Trotter et al. 2010; Xu et al. 2011)
  - a novel distinct class of central nervous system (CNS) glial cells, characterized by the expression of the chondroitin sulfate proteoglycan NG2
  - is a type 1-transmembrane protein
  - express the NG2 chondroitin sulfate proteoglycan and platelet-derived growth factor receptor alpha
  - NG2 cells also called polydendrocytes
- Nkx2.2 (Briscoe et al. 1999; Fancy et al. 2004; Qi et al. 2001; Soula et al. 2001)
  - is a homeodomain-containing transcription factor

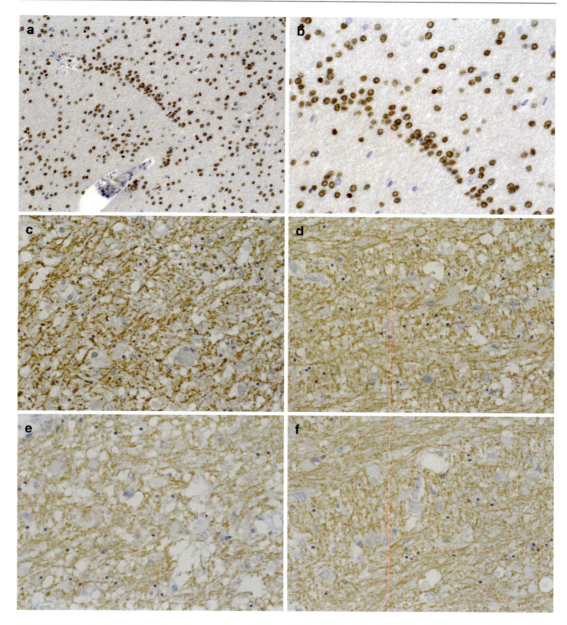

Fig. 3.20 Oligodendroglial markers: Immunohistochemical stain for Olig2 (**a**, **b**), Myelin-associated Glycoprotein (MAG) ©, Myelin Basic Protein (MBP) (**d**), Myelin Oligodendrocyte Glycoprotein (MOG) (**e**), proteolipid protein (PLP) (**f**)

- plays a critical role in neuroendocrine/glial differentiation
- NOGO-A (Grandpre and Strittmatter 2001; Huber and Schwab 2000; Schmandke et al. 2014)
  - integral membrane protein
  - localizes to CNS, but not peripheral nervous system, myelin
  - a potent inhibitor of axon elongation
  - stains oligodendrocyte cell bodies
- Proteolipid protein (PLP) (Campagnoni and Skoff 2001; Duncan 2005; Griffiths et al. 1998) (Fig. 3.20f)
  - major myelin protein of the CNS
  - PLP makes up to 50% of the CNS myelin proteins

- PLP is important for fusing the extracellular face of the myelin lamellae and for forming the intraperiod line
- Regulated intramembrane proteolysis (RIP) (Ebinu and Yankner 2002)
  - RIP processes SREBP-1, Notch-1, amyloid precursor protein (APP), and ErbB-4
- Tubulin polymerization promoting protein (TPPP/p25) (Kovacs et al. 2007; Preusser et al. 2007)
  - promotes tubulin polymerization
  - stains normal oligodendrocytes
- Transferrin
  - iron transport glycoprotein
  - in the oligodendrocyte cell body
- Myelin/oligodendrocyte-specific protein (MOSP) (Mu and Dyer 1994)
  - extracellular face of myelin
  - expressed exclusively by oligodendrocytes in the CNS
- Other proteins include
  - P2
  - OMgp (paranodal area)
  - Osp/claudin-11 (tight junctions of myelin sheaths)
  - Connexins (Cx32, Cx47)
  - Tetraspan

Myelin Markers (Bradl and Lassmann 2010)
- Myelin basic protein (MBP) (Fig. 3.20d)
  - MBP is a family of proteins with many isoforms
  - The main function of MBP is in the fusion of the cytoplasm interface of the myelin lamellae and the formation of the major dense line
- Myelin-associated glycoprotein (MAG) (Fig. 3.20c)
  - is a minor component of myelin but is the major glycoprotein
  - confined to the periaxonal cytoplasmic ridges of the myelin sheath in the CNS
  - plays a role in axon–myelin interactions
- Myelin oligodendrocyte glycoprotein (MOG) (Fig. 3.20e)
  - specific to oligodendrocytes
  - located on the cell surface and outermost lamellae of compacted myelin in the CNS
- 2′-3′-cyclic nucleotide 3′-phosphatase (CNP)
  - its function in myelin is unresolved
  - is specific to oligodendrocytes in the CNS and Schwann cells in the PNS
  - is localized to the cell body and processes
- MOBP
  - consists of several isoforms that are relatively abundant
  - located in the major dense line, where they play a similar role than MBP

Olig1, Olig2, Olig3 (Fig. 3.20a, b)
- encode basic helix-loop-helix (bHLH) transcription factors
- expressed in both the developing and mature vertebrate CNS
- critical functions during the formation of motor neurons and oligodendrocytes of the ventral neural tube
- unknown roles at later stages of development
- Olig expression continues to mark, and may regulate, the formation of oligodendroglia
- expression in human brain tumors and repair of demyelinating lesions (Ligon et al. 2006)
- Olig2 expression (Fig. 3.20a, b):
  - is restricted to glial tumors and non-tumoral oligodendrocytes
  - is higher in oligodendrogliomas as compared to astrocytomas and oligo-astrocytomas
  - is higher in grade III as compared to grade II tumors
  - Olig2 is absent or weakly expressed in glioblastoma (GBM)
  - strong expression was found in the oligodendroglial foci of GBM with oligodendroglial component (GBMO) (Mokhtari et al. 2005)

3.5.6 Microglial Markers

- Cr3/43 (HLA-DR II) (Graeber et al. 1994; Caffo et al. 2005) (Fig. 3.21a)
  - major histocompatibility complex Class II
  - Stains activated microglia

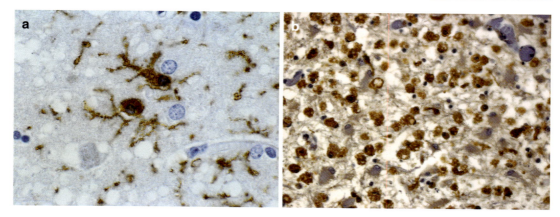

Fig. 3.21 Macrophage and microglia markers: macrophages are immunohistochemically stained for CD68 (**a**); microglia are immunohistochemically stained for HLA-DRII (Cr3/43) (**b**)

- CD68 (Fig. 3.21b)
  - Type I transmembrane glycoprotein
  - member of scavenger receptor family
  - stains macrophages, monocytes, mast cells
- Lectins
  - *Ricinus communis* agglutinin (RCA)
    - galactose-binding lectin
    - stains microglia
  - Ulex europeaus agglutinin I
    - specific lectin for alpha-linked fucose
    - stains microglia

3.5.7 Markers for Neurodegeneration

- Beta-amyloid (Kummer and Heneka 2014; Knowles et al. 2014; Hayden and Teplow 2013) (Fig. 3.22c)
  - Amyloid beta peptide is a 42-amino acid peptide.
  - It is processed from the precursor protein, amyloid beta precursor protein (APP).
  - Amyloid beta precursor protein is a transmembrane glycoprotein that spans the membrane once.
  - The gene for amyloid beta precursor protein is located on chromosome 21.
  - It is found as insoluble aggregates in senile plaques.
- Tau (Spillantini and Goedert 2013; Takashima 2013) (Fig. 3.22a)
  - microtubule-associated protein
  - sorted into neuronal axons
  - failed sorting mechanisms in Alzheimer disease with missorted tau into the somatodendritic compartment
- phosphorylated tau
  - hyperphosphorylated tau
- Tau 3 repeat (tau 3R)
  - 3R tandem repeat sequence of 31 amino acids defining one tau isoform
  - expression of the 3R isoform causes more profound axonal transport defects and locomotor impairments, culminating in a shorter life span than the 4R isoform (Di Giorgio et al. 2017).
- Tau 4 repeat
  - 4R tandem repeat sequence of 32 amino acids defining one tau isoform
  - the 4R isoform leads to greater neurodegeneration and impairments in learning and memory (Di Giorgio et al. 2017).
- Alpha-synuclein (Bates and Zheng 2014; Lamberts et al. 2014; Lee et al. 2014; Brown 2013; Al-Mansoori et al. 2013; George et al. 2013; Ozansoy and Basak 2013) (Fig. 3.22d)
  - involved in vesicular trafficking and release, related to its associations with the SNARE complex proteins
  - metal-binding protein
  - localizes to the nucleus and the presynaptic terminal
  - major component of protein inclusions Lewy bodies and Lewy neurites in Parkinson disease and Lewy body disease

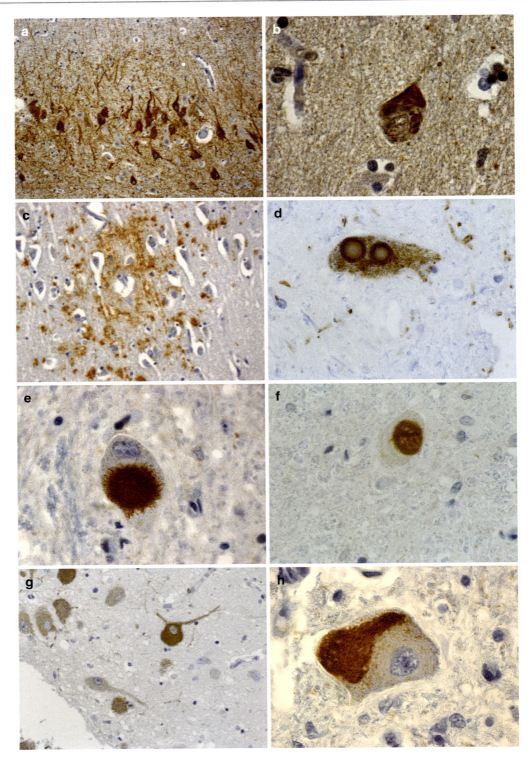

Fig. 3.22 Markers for neurodegenerative diseases: phosphorylated tau in Alzheimer disease (**a**), ubiquitin-positive neurofibrillary tangle in AD (**b**), beta-amyloid in Alzheimer disease (**c**), alpha-synuclein in Parkinson disease (**d**), FUS-positive inclusion in amyotrophic lateral sclerosis (ALS) (**e**)TDP-43-positive inclusion in amyotrophic lateral sclerosis (ALS) (**f**), p62-positive neuron in AD (**g**) and inclusion in ALS (**h**)

- TDP-43 (transactive response (TAR) DNA-binding protein of 43 kDa) (Baralle et al. 2013; Liu et al. 2013; Janssens and Van Broeckhoven 2013; Youmans and Wolozin 2012) (Fig. 3.22f)
  - is an hnRNP (heterogeneous nuclear ribonucleoprotein) protein
  - predominantly located in the nuclei
  - two RNA-recognition motifs (RRM) that allows it to bind to DNA and RNA
  - glycine-rich C-terminal domain in TDP-43, which allows it to bind to proteins
  - transcriptional regulation, mRNA processing, RNA splicing, and microRNA biogenesis
- FUS (Fused in Sarcoma) (Labbe et al. 2014; Orozco and Edbauer 2013; Dormann and Haass 2013; Lanson Jr and Pandey 2012) (Fig. 3.22e)
  - nuclear DNA/RNA-binding protein
  - regulates different steps of gene expression, including transcription, splicing, mRNA processing, and mRNA transport as well as microRNA biogenesis
- Ubiquitin (Atkin and Paulson 2014; Jansen et al. 2014) (Fig. 3.22b)
  - ubiquitin-proteasome system (UPS)
  - crucial for intracellular protein homeostasis and for degradation of aberrant and damaged proteins
- P62 (p62/SQSTM1/A170) (Geetha et al. 2012; Komatsu et al. 2012; Salminen et al. 2012) (Fig. 3.22g, h)
  - multifunctional protein
  - involved in the regulation of cellular signaling and protein trafficking
  - role in protein degradation and aggregation
  - is a stress-inducible intracellular protein

3.5.8 Tumor Markers

Tumor markers are used in neuropathology for the identification of the site of origin of brain metastases and to characterize other tumors affecting the nervous system and its coverings (Table 3.8) (Fig. 3.23a–h).

Table 3.8 Markers of differentiation in various tumors

Differentiation	Marker
Mesenchymal	- Vimentin
Epithelial	- Cytokeratins (CK) (Fig. 3.23b) - Epithelial membrane antigen (EMA) (Fig. 3.23a)
Smooth muscle	- Desmin - Muscle-specific actin - Smooth muscle actin - Calponin - H-caldesmon - Smooth muscle myosin heavy chain (MHC)
Skeletal muscle	- Desmin - Muscle-specific actin - Myogenin - MyoD
Myofibroblastic	- Actins (MSA, SMA) - Calponin
Myoepithelial	- Smooth muscle (SMA, calponin) - Neural (S100) - Glial (GFAP) - Epithelial (CK) - Basal/stem cell factor (p63) (Fig. 3.23h)
Endothelial	- CD34 - CD31 - Factor VIII - *Ulex europaeus* I - CD141 - Fli-1 - D2-40
Lipomatous	- S100
Melanocytic	- S100 - HMB45 (Fig. 3.23f) - Melan-A - MITF - Tyrosinase
Neuroendocrine	- Synaptophysin - Chromogranin A - Neuron-specific enolase - CD56 - CD57
Glial	- GFAP
Neuronal	- Neurofilament - NeuN - Synaptophysin - Chromogranin A
Nerve sheath	- S100
Serous acinar cells	- PAS - Trypsin - Chymotrypsin - Lipase

3.5 Immunohistochemistry

Table 3.8 (continued)

Differentiation	Marker
Hematopoietic	• CD45/LCA • CD3 (pan-T cell) • CD20 • CD79a • PAX5 (pan-Bcell) • CD138 (plasma cells)
Histiocytic	• CD68 • CD163 • HAM56 • MAC 387

Cytokeratins
- Intermediate filament proteins
- Present in epithelial cells
- Marker of epithelial differentiation
- Twenty distinct types of CKs
- Two categories of CKs based on 2D gel migration properties:
  - Basic (CK1–CK8)
  - Acidic (CK9–CK20)
- Each of the two categories (basic, acidic) contains two groups based on molecular weight:
  - Basic-high molecular weight (HMW): (CK1–CK6)
  - Basic-low molecular weight (LMW): (CK7, CK8)
  - Acidic-high molecular weight (HMW): (CK9–CK17)
  - Acidic-low molecular weight (LMW): (CK18–CK20)
- Distinction of CKs based on distribution:
  - HMW are squamous keratins (squamous epithelia and basal cells)
  - LMW are simple/non-squamous keratins (in the cytoplasm)
- Distribution patterns of CKs retained in carcinomas

Examples of often used CKs:

- AE1/AE3 (Fig. 3.23b)
  - Broad-spectrum CK
  - Reacts with HMW-CKs and LMW-CKs
  - Identifies virtually all types of epithelial neoplasms
- Cam5.2
  - LMW-CK cocktail
  - Reacts with all non-squamous epithelia
- CK5/6
  - HMW-CK cocktail
  - Reacts with squamous, urothelial, and few glandular epithelia
- CK7 and CK20
  - Distinctive patterns of expression in various organs
  - See Chap. 81
- Ber-EP4
  - Reacts with the majority of adenocarcinomas of various sites
- Epithelial membrane antigen (EMA)
  - Present in the majority of non-squamous carcinomas
  - Also present in non-epithelial tissues and neoplasms

3.5.9 Vascular Markers

- CD31
  - Identifies vascular endothelial adhesion molecule PECAM-1
  - Marker of endothelial cells but also of histiocytes and plasma cells
  - More sensitive and more specific
- CD34 (Fig. 3.24a, b)
  - Stains normal and neoplastic endothelial cells
  - Less sensitive and specific
- Factor VIII
  - Functional component of the antihemophiliac factor
- Collagen IV
  - Stains the basal membrane of vessels
- Ulex europaeus I
- CD141 (Thrombomodulin)
  - Endothelial cell-associated cofactor

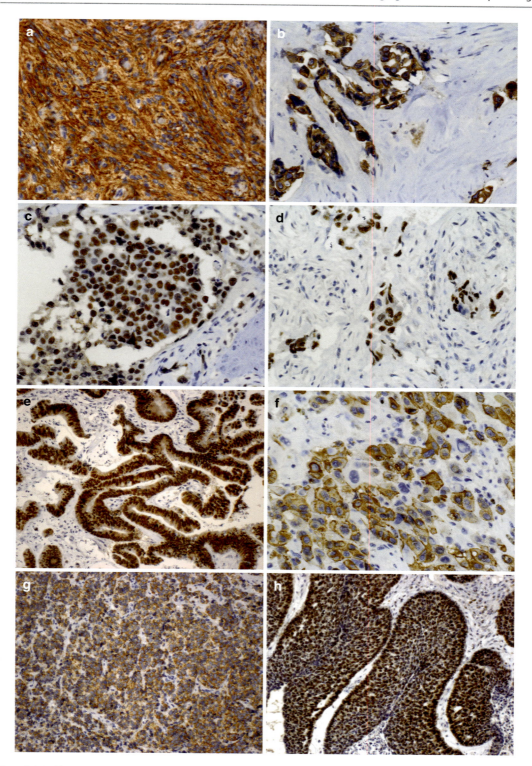

Fig. 3.23 Tumor markers: Immunohistochemical stains for epithelial membrane antigen (EMA) in meningioma (**a**), AE1/AE3 in a brain metastasis of a breast carcinoma (**b**), estrogen receptor in a metastasis of a breast carcinoma (**c**), thyroid transcription factor-1 (TTF1) in a metastasis of a lung carcinoma (**d**), CDX2 in a metastasis of colon carcinoma (**e**), HMB45 in a metastasis of melanoma (**f**), p504s in a metastasis of prostate carcinoma (**g**), and p63 in a metastasis of a squamous lung carcinoma (**h**)

3.5 Immunohistochemistry

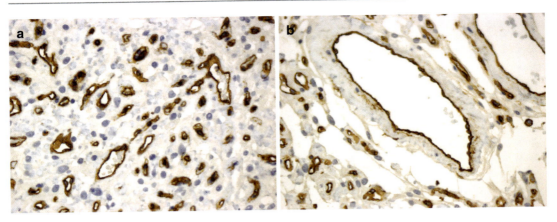

Fig. 3.24 Vascular marker: Immunostain of vessels stained for CD34 (**a**) and CD31 (**b**)

Table 3.9 Hematopoietic and lymphatic markers

Marker	Identification of
CD20	Mature B-lymphocyte (Fig. 3.25a)
CD79a	Mature B-lymphocyte, prolymphocyte, plasma cell
CD3	T-lymphocyte (Fig. 3.25b)
CD4	Helper T-lymphocyte
CD8	Cytotoxic T-lymphocyte
CD138	Plasma cell
CD5	Co-expressed in B-CLL/SLL
CD23	Co-expressed in B-CLL/SLL
Cyclin D1	Expressed in B-NHL, mantle cell lymphoma (Fig. 3.25c)
CD10	Co-expressed in follicular B-NHL
bcl6	Co-expressed in follicular B-NHL
Glycophorin A	Red blood cell and erythropoietic precursors
Myeloperoxidase	Neutrophils and granulopoietic precursors
CD61	Megakaryocyte
CD68	Histiocyte/macrophage
Fascin	Reed–Sternberg cells

- Located on cell membrane
- Expressed by endothelial cells
- Also expressed by mesothelial cells, epidermal keratinocytes
- Fli-1
  - Product of the *FLI*-gene, which is overexpressed in Ewing sarcoma/PNET
  - Endothelial cells
  - Marker for endothelial neoplasms
- D2-40 (Podoplanin)
  - transmembrane sialomucin-like glycoprotein
  - Lymphatic endothelial cells

3.5.10 Hematopoietic and Lymphatic Markers

Hematopoietic and lymphatic markers are used to identify among others lymphocytes, plasma cells in cases of encephalitis, vasculitis, lymphoma, or plasmacytoma (Table 3.9) (Fig. 3.25a–d).

3.5.11 Proliferation Markers in Tumors

- KI-67/MIB-1 (Fig. 3.26a, b)
  - Is a nuclear and nucleolar protein, which is tightly associated with somatic cell proliferation
  - Recognizes a core antigen present in proliferating cells and absent in quiescent cells
  - Ki-67 protein is present in every dividing cell (G1, S, G2/M phase) but is absent from the resting cells (G0 phase)
  - Identifies the proliferating fraction of cells
  - MIB-1 antibody recognizes the Ki-67 antigen in formalin-fixed and paraffin-embedded tissue sections
- Proliferating cell nuclear antigen (PCNA)
  - Is a cofactor of DNA polymerases that encircles DNA
  - Orchestrates several of these functions by recruiting crucial players to the replication fork

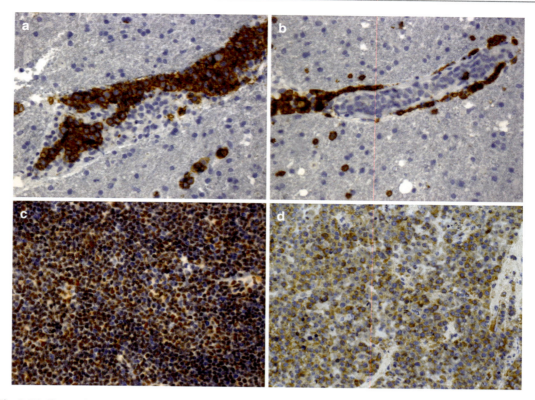

Fig. 3.25 Hematology markers: Immunohistochemical stains of B-lymphocytes (CD20) (**a**), T-lymphocytes (**b**), lymphoma cells (Cyclin D1) (**c**), and kappa chain in plasmacytoma (**d**)

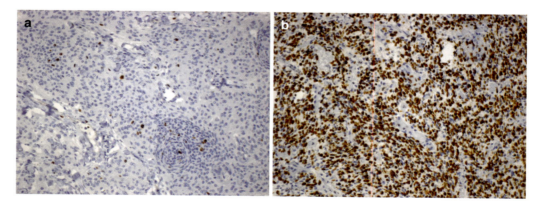

Fig. 3.26 Proliferation marker Ki-67 in brain tumors: low density in meningioma (WHO grade I) (**a**) and high density in glioblastoma (WHO grade IV) (**b**)

- Topoisomerase II α
  - Are ubiquitous enzymes that play essential roles in a number of fundamental DNA processes.
  - Its biological roles include the decatenation of newly replicated DNA and the relaxation of polymerase-driven supercoils.
  - Regulate DNA under- and overwinding, and resolve knots and tangles in the genetic material by passing an intact double helix through a transient double-stranded break that they generate in a separate segment of DNA.
  - Also implicated in gene expression.

3.5 Immunohistochemistry

- Minichromosome maintenance 2 (MCM2) protein
  - essential DNA replication factors crucial for initiating DNA synthesis once every cell cycle
  - regulates both the initiation and elongation phases of eukaryotic chromosome replication

3.5.12 Markers for Infectious Agents

- Prion
- Herpes simplex virus (HSV)
  - HSV1
  - HSV2
- Cytomegalovirus (CMV) (Fig. 3.27a)
- Epstein–Barr virus (EBV) (Fig. 3.27b)

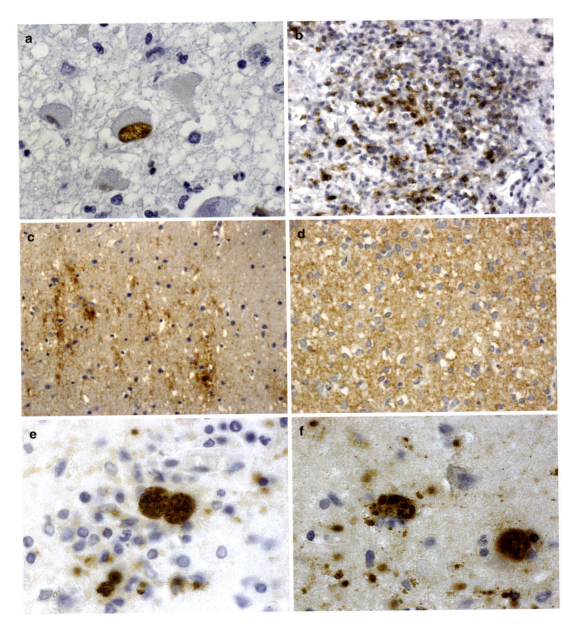

Fig. 3.27 Markers in infectious diseases: Immunohistochemical stains for cytomegalovirus (**a**), Epstein–Barr virus (**b**), prion protein (**c**, **d**), and toxoplasma gondii (**e**, **f**)

- Varicella-zoster virus (VZV)
- Human immunodeficiency virus (HIV)
  - p24
  - gp41
- Toxoplasma gondii (Fig. 3.27e, f)

3.5.13 Immunohistochemical Panels

The application of the following immunohistochemical panels proved to be useful in routine diagnostic neuropathology setting (Table 3.10).

3.6 Other Techniques

3.6.1 Electron Microscopy

In electron microscopy, electrons are used and either transmitted through or sweep over the surface of a specimen, allowing the distinction of:

- Transmission electron microscopy (Fig. 3.28a, b)
- Scanning electron microscopy

Magnification ranges between 1000 and 500,000.

3.6.2 Fluorescence Microscopy

In fluorescence microscopy (Fig. 3.29a–d)

- imaging is realized by exposing the tissue to short-wave ultraviolet light using a halogen or mercury lamp
- molecules absorb the energy and release it as visible light
- antibodies are labeled with a fluorescent dye (e.g., fluorescein isothiocyanate (FITC))
- distinguished are:
  - direct immunofluorescence
  - indirect immunofluorescence

3.6.3 Enzyme Histochemistry

Enzyme histochemistry is (Meier-Ruge and Bruder 2008) (Fig. 3.30a–f):

Table 3.10 Panel of markers used in the routine diagnostic setting

Panel	Antibodies used/required
Astroglial tumors	• IDH1 • GFAP • S100 • Olig2 • ATRX • p53
Oligodendroglial tumors	• IDH1 • GFAP • S100 • Olig2 • ATRX
Ependymal tumors	• GFAP • S100 • EMA (EMA dots)
Neuronal tumors	• Synaptophysin • NeuN • CD56
Embryonal tumors	• Synaptophysin • Class III ß-tubulin • Neurofilaments • S-100 • NSE • CD56 • Desmin • SMA • INI1 • EMA • Vimentin • GFAP • Keratins
Germ cell tumors	• PLAP • HCG • Alpha fetoprotein • C-kit (CD117)
Pituitary tumors	• ACTH • FSH • LH • TSH • P53 • Ki-67
Meningeal tumors	• EMA • S100
Metastatic carcinoma	• AE1/AE3 • CK7 • CK20 • TTF1 • CD45 • Melan-A
Epilepsy—hippocampal sclerosis	• NeuN • GFAP • HLA-DRII • CD34
Neurodegeneration	• ß-Amyloid • Tau • Phosphorylated tau • Tau 3R • Tau 4R • α-synuclein • TDP-43 • FUS • Ubiquitin • P62

3.6 Other Techniques

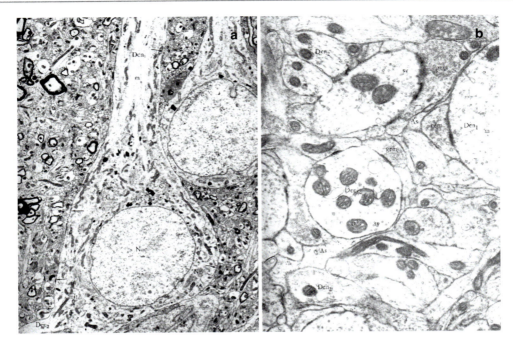

Fig. 3.28 Electron microscopy: neuron (**a**), and synaptic vesicles (**b**) (reproduced from Peters et al. (1991) with kind permission by Oxford Press)

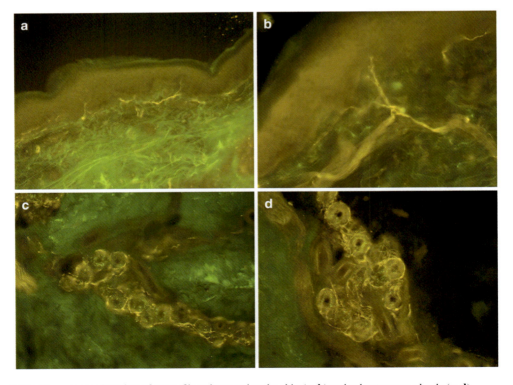

Fig. 3.29 Fluorescence imaging of nerve fibers innervating the skin (**a**, **b**) and subcutaneous glands (**c**, **d**)

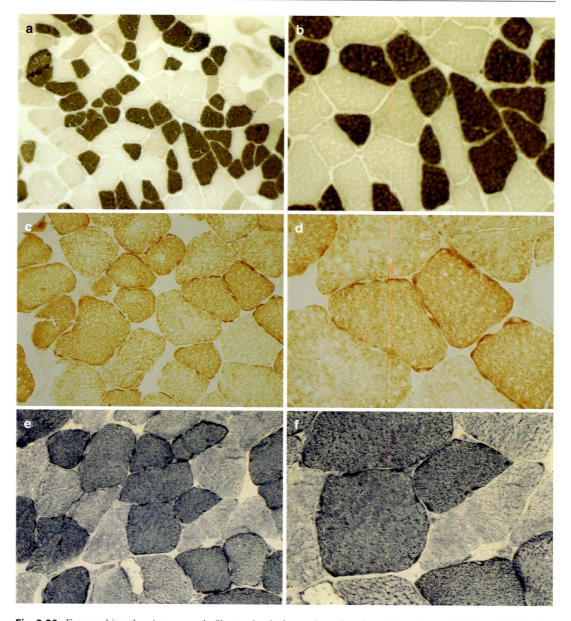

Fig. 3.30 Enzyme histochemistry: muscle fiber typing is done using adenosine triphosphatase (ATP) at pH 4.6 (**a**, **b**), cytochrome c oxidase (COX) (**c**, **d**), and nicotinamide adenine dinucleotide (NADH) (**e**, **f**)

- Based on metabolization of a substrate which is provided to a tissue enzyme in its orthotopic localization.
- A sensitive dynamic technique that mirrors even early metabolic imbalance of a pathologicaltissue lesion, combined with the advantage of histotopographic enzyme localization.
- Visualization is accomplished with an insoluble dye product.
- Serves as a link between biochemistry and morphology.
- Constitutes a valuable complement to conventional histology, immunohistochemistry, and molecular pathology for both diagnostic and experimental pathology.

- Applications:
  - Alkaline phosphatase represents tissue barrier functions in brain capillaries.
  - Decrease in enzyme histochemical alkaline phosphatase activity indicates serious functional impairment.
  - Enzyme histochemical increase in lysosomal acid phosphatase activity is an early marker of ischemic tissue lesions.
  - Acetylcholinesterase enzyme histochemistry has proven to be the gold standard for the diagnosis of Hirschsprung.

3.6.4 *In Situ* Hybridization (ISH)

In Situ Hybridization
- Is used to localize a specific DNA- or RNA sequence in a portion or section of tissue (in situ) within individual cells or on chromosomes.
- Uses a labeled complementary DNA strand ("DNA probe") or, now most commonly, a labeled complementary RNA strand ("riboprobe").
- Provides insights into
  - physiological processes
  - disease pathogenesis
  - understanding the organization, regulation, and function of genes
- Optimization for each tissue examined and for each probe used.
- The probe that is linked to either radio-, fluorescent-, or antigen-labeled molecules (e.g., digoxigenin) is localized and quantified in the tissue either by autoradiography, fluorescence microscopy, or immunohistochemistry, respectively.
- ISH can also use two or more probes, labeled with radioactivity or non-radioactive labels, to simultaneously detect two or more transcripts.

Major techniques in use include (Fig. 3.31a–d):

- *In situ* hybridization to mRNA with oligonucleotide and RNA probes.
- Whole mount *in situ* hybridization.
- Double detection of RNAs and RNA plus protein.
- Fluorescent in situ hybridization to detect chromosomal sequences, structure of chromosomes, and chromosomal integrity.
- RNA ISH (RNA *in situ* hybridization) is used to measure and localize RNAs (mRNAs, lncRNAs, and miRNAs) within tissue sections, cells, whole mounts, and circulating tumor cells (CTCs).
- Analysis with light and electron microscopes.

Basic steps for digoxigenin-labeled probes include:

- permeabilization of cells with proteinase K to open cell membranes (around 25 min, not needed for tissue sections or some early-stage embryos)
- binding of mRNAs to marked RNA probe (usually overnight)
- antibody-phosphatase binding to RNA probe (some hours)
- staining of antibody (e.g., with alkaline phosphatase)

In situ hybridization was invented by Joseph G. Gall

3.6.5 Molecular Biology

In the broadest sense of the word, molecular changes can also be visualized, i.e., imaged. *In situ* hybridization as described above is a classical molecular biology technique. Other techniques which provide images include:

- Western blot to visualize proteins (Fig. 3.32a–c)
- Northern blot to visualize RNA
- Southern blot to visualize DNA
- Imaging a mutation after sequencing (Fig. 3.32d)
- Imaging a deletion, duplication with Real Time-PCR
- Imaging single gene expression (Reverse Transcriptase-PCR)
- Imaging multiple gene expression (gene expression microarray)
- Imaging microRNA by array technology

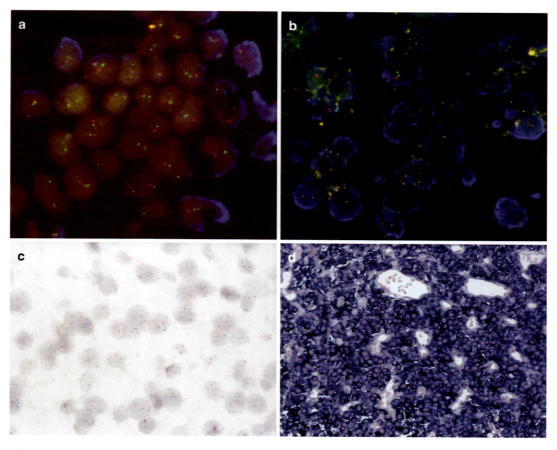

Fig. 3.31 *In situ* Hybridization: Fluorescence *in situ* hybridization (FISH) (**a**, **b**), chromogenic *in situ* hybridization (CISH) (**c**), and chromogenic in situ hybridization for lambda chain in plasmacytoma (**d**)

3.6.5.1 Blot Techniques

Basically, blotting techniques involve immobilization of proteins or nucleic acids on membrane sheets with high binding capacity, e.g., nitrocellulose or polyvinylidene difluoride (PVDF). The bound molecules are visualized by interaction with labeled binding partners (the "probes"), a process which is termed "staining." The following blotting techniques exist:

- Western blot to visualize proteins
- Northern blot to visualize RNA
- Southern blot to visualize DNA
- Dot blot

Western Blot

Proteins extracted from tissues or cells are separated according to molecular size by electrophoresis in an acrylamide gel. The proteins are then horizontally transferred from the gel onto a membrane, either electrophoretically or by diffusion, thus generating a 1:1 copy of the original gel. At this point, the protein bands on the membrane (generally termed "the blot") are still invisible. Imaging a molecule of interest is initiated by applying a specific, enzyme-linked antibody. In the subsequent enzymatic reaction, an insoluble visible product develops that precipitates at the position of the target protein on the blot.

Northern Blot

After electrophoresis in an agarose gel, cellular or tissue RNAs are transferred to a blotting membrane as described above. To detect specific RNA(s) on the blot, labeled DNA- or RNA probes are employed (e.g., cloned fragments or single-stranded oligonucleotides representing complementary sequences) that will hybridize to the

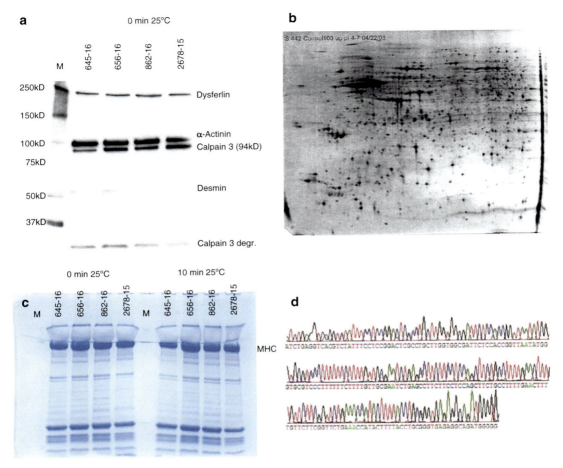

Fig. 3.32 Imaging in molecular biology: Western blot (**a**), 2D electrophoresis (**b**), Coomassie brilliant blue stain for proteins (**c**), and Sanger sequencing (**d**)

target RNA(s). Probes may be radioactively labeled or linked to fluorescent dyes to enable detection by autoradiography or on a fluorescence scanner.

Southern Blot
Southern blotting is principally performed as described above for Northern blots, except that RNA is replaced by DNA as the target to be analyzed. In the standard procedure, DNA restriction fragments are used for gel electrophoresis. Prior to blotting, an additional denaturing step is required to provide single-stranded DNA for hybridization with the specific probe(s).

Dot Blot
Dot blots provide a fast and simple alternative to Western-, Northern-, and Southern blotting and are mainly used to estimate relative concentrations of target molecules in protein-, DNA-, or RNA samples. Without preceding gel electrophoresis, samples are directly spotted onto the membrane as "dots." A molecule of interest bound in a dot area is detected by specific staining with labeled antibodies or probes. Assessment of the staining intensity allows a semi-quantification of the target molecule in the sample.

3.6.5.2 Molecular Imaging
- Imaging a mutation after sequencing
- Imaging a deletion, duplication with RT-PCR

The method relies on the PCR amplification of a region of interest from a DNA- or RNA template; in the latter case, a reverse transcription step is incorporated in the procedure to generate a single-stranded DNA copy for amplification (reverse transcription PCR [RT-PCR]). Detection/enhancement of the expected PCR product (amplicon) points to the presence/copy number gain of the target region. By contrast, absent amplicons are indicative of deletions.

3.6.5.3 Microarray Techniques

The basic principle of microarray technology is the simultaneous use of millions of individual oligonucleotides which—in combination—cover a representative portion of sequences from a given genome. The oligonucleotides are attached to the surface of a microchip in a defined grid pattern; thus, each spot on the grid corresponds to a specific sequence.

Investigating gene expression or chromosomal aberrations in a cell-/tissue sample requires extraction of cellular DNA or RNA from which fluorescence-labeled single-stranded fragments are generated. Hybridization of the labeled fragments to complementary sequences on the microarray produces a distinct image of the grid surface since only spots with bound fragments can be visualized by fluorescence. Dark spots indicate sequences that are absent in the analyzed sample.

Possible applications of microarray technology include:

- Imaging chromosomal gains/losses
- Imaging single gene expression
- Imaging multiple gene expression (gene expression microarray)
- Imaging microRNAs

Visualization of microarray images basically yields a confusing pattern of scattered fluorescence signals on a grid; elaborate software algorithms are needed to translate the raw data to reasonable genetic information.

3.6.6 Other Imaging Techniques

Other imaging techniques, developed during the last decades, include (Wouterlood 2012):

- Confocal laser scanning microscopy
- Multiphoton confocal fluorescence microscopy
- Nano resolution optical imaging
- Full-field optical coherence microscopy
- Atomic force microscopy (AFM)
- Cryo-electron tomography
- STED (stimulated emission depletion) microscopy
- CARS (coherent anti-Stokes Raman scattering) microscopy

Selected References

Alafuzoff I, Pikkarainen M, Parkkinen L (2015) Synucleinopathies. In: Kocvacs GG (ed) Neuropathology of neurodegenerative diseases. A practical guide. Cambridge University Press, Cambridge, pp 149–175

Al-Mansoori KM, Hasan MY, Al-Hayani A, El-Agnaf OM (2013) The role of alpha-synuclein in neurodegenerative diseases: from molecular pathways in disease to therapeutic approaches. Curr Alzheimer Res 10(6):559–568

Atkin G, Paulson H (2014) Ubiquitin pathways in neurodegenerative disease. Front Mol Neurosci 7:63. https://doi.org/10.3389/fnmol.2014.00063

Baralle M, Buratti E, Baralle FE (2013) The role of TDP-43 in the pathogenesis of ALS and FTLD. Biochem Soc Trans 41(6):1536–1540. https://doi.org/10.1042/bst20130186

Barinka F, Druga R (2010) Calretinin expression in the mammalian neocortex: a review. Physiol Res 59(5):665–677

Barnett P (2003) Somatostatin and somatostatin receptor physiology. Endocrine 20(3):255–264. https://doi.org/10.1385/endo:20:3:255

Bates CA, Zheng W (2014) Fluids Barriers CNS 11:17. https://doi.org/10.1186/2045-8118-11-17

Benarroch EE (2009) Neuropeptide Y: its multiple effects in the CNS and potential clinical significance. Neurology 72(11):1016–1020. https://doi.org/10.1212/01.wnl.0000345258.18071.54

Bradl M, Lassmann H (2010) Oligodendrocytes: biology and pathology. Acta Neuropathol 119(1):37–53. https://doi.org/10.1007/s00401-009-0601-5

Briscoe J, Sussel L, Serup P, Hartigan-O'Connor D, Jessell TM, Rubenstein JL, Ericson J (1999) Homeobox gene Nkx2.2 and specification of neuronal identity by graded Sonic hedgehog signalling. Nature 398(6728):622–627. https://doi.org/10.1038/19315

Brown DR (2013) alpha-Synuclein as a ferrireductase. Biochem Soc Trans 41(6):1513–1517. https://doi.org/10.1042/bst20130130

Selected References

Buffa R, Mare P, Salvadore M, Gini A (1990) Immunohistochemical detection of 28KDa calbindin in human tissues. Adv Exp Med Biol 269:205–210

Butt AM, Kalsi A (2006) Inwardly rectifying potassium channels (Kir) in central nervous system glia: a special role for Kir4.1 in glial functions. J Cell Mol Med 10(1):33–44

Caffo M, Caruso G, Germano A, Galatioto S, Meli F, Tomasello F (2005) CD68 and CR3/43 immunohistochemical expression in secretory meningiomas. Neurosurgery 57(3):551–557; discussion 551–7.

Cammer WB, Brion LP (2000) Carbonic anhydrase in the nervous system. EXS (90):475–489

Camp AJ, Wijesinghe R (2009) Calretinin: modulator of neuronal excitability. Int J Biochem Cell Biol 41(11):2118–2121. https://doi.org/10.1016/j.biocel.2009.05.007

Campagnoni AT, Skoff RP (2001) The pathobiology of myelin mutants reveal novel biological functions of the MBP and PLP genes. Brain Pathol (Zurich, Switzerland) 11(1):74–91

Cauli B, Zhou X, Tricoire L, Toussay X, Staiger JF (2014) Revisiting enigmatic cortical calretinin-expressing interneurons. Front Neuroanat 8:52. https://doi.org/10.3389/fnana.2014.00052

Clarke EJ, Allan V (2002) Intermediate filaments: vimentin moves in. Curr Biol 12(17):R596–R598

DeFelipe J (1997) Types of neurons, synaptic connections and chemical characteristics of cells immunoreactive for calbindin-D28K, parvalbumin and calretinin in the neocortex. J Chem Neuroanat 14(1):1–19

Dehmelt L, Halpain S (2005) The MAP2/Tau family of microtubule-associated proteins. Genome Biol 6(1):204. https://doi.org/10.1186/gb-2004-6-1-204

Di Giorgio ML, Esposito A, Maccallini P, Micheli E, Bavasso F, Gallotta I, Verni F, Feiguin F, Cacchione S, McCabe BD, Di Schiavi E, Raffa GD (2017) WDR79/TCAB1 plays a conserved role in the control of locomotion and ameliorates phenotypic defects in SMA models. Neurobiol Dis 105:42–50. https://doi.org/10.1016/j.nbd.2017.05.005

Donato R, Cannon BR, Sorci G, Riuzzi F, Hsu K, Weber DJ, Geczy CL (2013) Functions of S100 proteins. Curr Mol Med 13(1):24–57

Dormann D, Haass C (2013) Fused in sarcoma (FUS): an oncogene goes awry in neurodegeneration. Mol Cell Neurosci 56:475–486. https://doi.org/10.1016/j.mcn.2013.03.006

Duncan ID (2005) The PLP mutants from mouse to man. J Neurol Sci 228(2):204–205. https://doi.org/10.1016/j.jns.2004.10.011

Ebinu JO, Yankner BA (2002) A RIP tide in neuronal signal transduction. Neuron 34(4):499–502

Eng LF (1985) Glial fibrillary acidic protein (GFAP): the major protein of glial intermediate filaments in differentiated astrocytes. J Neuroimmunol 8(4–6):203–214

Eng LF, Ghirnikar RS (1994) GFAP and astrogliosis. Brain Pathol (Zurich, Switzerland) 4(3):229–237

Eng LF, Ghirnikar RS, Lee YL (2000) Glial fibrillary acidic protein: GFAP-thirty-one years (1969-2000). Neurochem Res 25(9–10):1439–1451

Epelbaum J, Dournaud P, Fodor M, Viollet C (1994) The neurobiology of somatostatin. Crit Rev Neurobiol 8(1–2):25–44

Evans RM (1998) Vimentin: the conundrum of the intermediate filament gene family. Bioessays 20(1):79–86. https://doi.org/10.1002/(sici)1521-1878(199801)20:1<79::aid-bies11>3.0.co;2-5

Fancy SP, Zhao C, Franklin RJ (2004) Increased expression of Nkx2.2 and Olig2 identifies reactive oligodendrocyte progenitor cells responding to demyelination in the adult CNS. Mol Cell Neurosci 27(3):247–254. https://doi.org/10.1016/j.mcn.2004.06.015

Fauser S, Haussler U, Donkels C, Huber S, Nakagawa J, Prinz M, Schulze-Bonhage A, Zentner J, Haas CA (2013) Disorganization of neocortical lamination in focal cortical dysplasia is brain-region dependent: evidence from layer-specific marker expression. Acta Neuropathol Commun 1(1):47. https://doi.org/10.1186/2051-5960-1-47

Friedrich P, Aszodi A (1991) MAP2: a sensitive cross-linker and adjustable spacer in dendritic architecture. FEBS Lett 295(1–3):5–9

Geetha T, Vishwaprakash N, Sycheva M, Babu JR (2012) Sequestosome 1/p62: across diseases. Biomarkers 17(2):99–103. https://doi.org/10.3109/1354750x.2011.653986

George S, Rey NL, Reichenbach N, Steiner JA, Brundin P (2013) alpha-Synuclein: the long distance runner. Brain Pathol (Zurich, Switzerland) 23(3):350–357. https://doi.org/10.1111/bpa.12046

Giacobini E (1987) Carbonic anhydrase: the first marker of glial development. Curr Top Dev Biol 21:207–215

Gottron F, Turetsky D, Choi D (1995) SMI-32 antibody against non-phosphorylated neurofilaments identifies a subpopulation of cultured cortical neurons hypersensitive to kainate toxicity. Neurosci Lett 194(1–2):1–4

Graeber MB, Bise K, Mehraein P (1994) CR3/43, a marker for activated human microglia: application to diagnostic neuropathology. Neuropathol Appl Neurobiol 20(4):406–408

Grandpre T, Strittmatter SM (2001) Nogo: a molecular determinant of axonal growth and regeneration. Neuroscientist 7(5):377–386

Griffiths I, Klugmann M, Anderson T, Thomson C, Vouyiouklis D, Nave KA (1998) Current concepts of PLP and its role in the nervous system. Microsc Res Tech 41(5):344–358. https://doi.org/10.1002/(sici)1097-0029(19980601)41:5<344::aid-jemt2>3.0.co;2-q

Hayden EY, Teplow DB (2013) Amyloid beta-protein oligomers and Alzheimer's disease. Alzheimers Res Ther 5(6):60. https://doi.org/10.1186/alzrt226

Heilig M, Widerlov E (1995) Neurobiology and clinical aspects of neuropeptide Y. Crit Rev Neurobiol 9(2–3):115–136

Heizmann CW (1999) Ca2+-binding S100 proteins in the central nervous system. Neurochem Res 24(9):1097–1100

Heizmann CW, Fritz G, Schafer BW (2002) S100 proteins: structure, functions and pathology. Front Biosci 7:d1356–d1368

Hendy GN, Bevan S, Mattei MG, Mouland AJ (1995) Chromogranin A. Clin Invest Med 18(1):47–65

Hof PR, Glezer II, Conde F, Flagg RA, Rubin MB, Nimchinsky EA, Vogt Weisenhorn DM (1999) Cellular distribution of the calcium-binding proteins parvalbumin, calbindin, and calretinin in the neocortex of mammals: phylogenetic and developmental patterns. J Chem Neuroanat 16(2):77–116

Hu H, Gan J, Jonas P (2014) Interneurons. Fast-spiking, parvalbumin(+) GABAergic interneurons: from cellular design to microcircuit function. Science (New York, NY) 345(6196):1255263. https://doi.org/10.1126/science.1255263

Huber AB, Schwab ME (2000) Nogo-A, a potent inhibitor of neurite outgrowth and regeneration. Biol Chem 381(5–6):407–419. https://doi.org/10.1515/bc.2000.053

Jackson P, Blythe D (2012) Immunohistochemical techniques. In: Suvarna KS, Layton C, Bancroft JD (eds) Bancroft's theory and practice of histological techniques, 7th edn. Churchill Livingstone, Edinburgh, pp 381–426

Jansen AH, Reits EA, Hol EM (2014) The ubiquitin proteasome system in glia and its role in neurodegenerative diseases. Front Mol Neurosci 7:73. https://doi.org/10.3389/fnmol.2014.00073

Janssens J, Van Broeckhoven C (2013) Pathological mechanisms underlying TDP-43 driven neurodegeneration in FTLD-ALS spectrum disorders. Hum Mol Genet 22(R1):R77–R87. https://doi.org/10.1093/hmg/ddt349

Jessen KR, Morgan L, Brammer M, Mirsky R (1985) Galactocerebroside is expressed by non-myelin-forming Schwann cells in situ. J Cell Biol 101(3):1135–1143

Johnstone M, Goold RG, Bei D, Fischer I, Gordon-Weeks PR (1997) Localisation of microtubule-associated protein 1B phosphorylation sites recognised by monoclonal antibody SMI-31. J Neurochem 69(4):1417–1424

Kawaguchi Y, Kondo S (2002) Parvalbumin, somatostatin and cholecystokinin as chemical markers for specific GABAergic interneuron types in the rat frontal cortex. J Neurocytol 31(3–5):277–287

Kligman D, Hilt DC (1988) The S100 protein family. Trends Biochem Sci 13(11):437–443. https://doi.org/10.1016/0968-0004(88)90218-6

Knowles TP, Vendruscolo M, Dobson CM (2014) The amyloid state and its association with protein misfolding diseases. Nat Rev Mol Cell Biol 15(6):384–396. https://doi.org/10.1038/nrm3810

Komatsu M, Kageyama S, Ichimura Y (2012) p62/SQSTM1/A170: physiology and pathology. Pharmacol Res 66(6):457–462. https://doi.org/10.1016/j.phrs.2012.07.004

Kovacs GG, Gelpi E, Lehotzky A, Hoftberger R, Erdei A, Budka H, Ovadi J (2007) The brain-specific protein TPPP/p25 in pathological protein deposits of neurodegenerative diseases. Acta Neuropathol 113(2):153–161. https://doi.org/10.1007/s00401-006-0167-4

Kummer MP, Heneka MT (2014) Truncated and modified amyloid-beta species. Alzheimers Res Ther 6(3):28. https://doi.org/10.1186/alzrt258

Labbe C, Rayaprolu S, Soto-Ortolaza A, Ogaki K, Uitti RJ, Wszolek ZK, Ross OA (2014) Investigating FUS variation in Parkinson's disease. Parkinsonism Relat Disord 20(Suppl 1):S147–S149. https://doi.org/10.1016/s1353-8020(13)70035-x

Lamberts JT, Hildebrandt EN, Brundin P (2015) Spreading of alpha-synuclein in the face of axonal transport deficits in Parkinson's disease: a speculative synthesis. Neurobiol Dis 77:276–283. https://doi.org/10.1016/j.nbd.2014.07.002

Lanson NA Jr, Pandey UB (2012) FUS-related proteinopathies: lessons from animal models. Brain Res 1462:44–60. https://doi.org/10.1016/j.brainres.2012.01.039

Lee HJ, Bae EJ, Lee SJ (2014) Extracellular alpha--synuclein-a novel and crucial factor in Lewy body diseases. Nat Rev Neurol 10(2):92–98. https://doi.org/10.1038/nrneurol.2013.275

Ligon KL, Fancy SP, Franklin RJ, Rowitch DH (2006) Olig gene function in CNS development and disease. Glia 54(1):1–10. https://doi.org/10.1002/glia.20273

Liu YC, Chiang PM, Tsai KJ (2013) Disease animal models of TDP-43 proteinopathy and their pre-clinical applications. Int J Mol Sci 14(10):20079–20111. https://doi.org/10.3390/ijms141020079

Lloyd RV (1987) Immunohistochemical localization of chromogranin in normal and neoplastic endocrine tissues. Pathol Annu 22(Pt 2):69–90

Loh YP, Cheng Y, Mahata SK, Corti A, Tota B (2012) Chromogranin A and derived peptides in health and disease. J Mol Neurosci 48(2):347–356. https://doi.org/10.1007/s12031-012-9728-2

Meier-Ruge WA, Bruder E (2008) Current concepts of enzyme histochemistry in modern pathology. Pathobiology 75(4):233–243. https://doi.org/10.1159/000132384

Middeldorp J, Hol EM (2011) GFAP in health and disease. Prog Neurobiol 93(3):421–443. https://doi.org/10.1016/j.pneurobio.2011.01.005

Minin AA, Moldaver MV (2008) Intermediate vimentin filaments and their role in intracellular organelle distribution. Biochemistry (Mosc) 73(13):1453–1466

Mokhtari K, Paris S, Aguirre-Cruz L, Privat N, Criniere E, Marie Y, Hauw JJ, Kujas M, Rowitch D, Hoang-Xuan K, Delattre JY, Sanson M (2005) Olig2 expression, GFAP, p53 and 1p loss analysis contribute to glioma subclassification. Neuropathol Appl Neurobiol 31(1):62–69. https://doi.org/10.1111/j.1365-2990.2004.00612.x

Morel A, Loup F, Magnin M, Jeanmonod D (2002) Neurochemical organization of the human basal ganglia: anatomofunctional territories defined by the distributions of calcium-binding proteins and SMI-32. J Comp Neurol 443(1):86–103

Morel L, Regan M, Higashimori H, Ng SK, Esau C, Vidensky S, Rothstein J, Yang Y (2013) Neuronal exosomal miRNA-dependent translational regulation of astroglial glutamate transporter GLT1. J Biol Chem 288(10):7105–7116. https://doi.org/10.1074/jbc.M112.410944

Mu QQ, Dyer C (1994) Developmental expression of MOSP in cultured oligodendrocytes. Neurochem Res 19(8):1033–1038

Mullen RJ, Buck CR, Smith AM (1992) NeuN, a neuronal specific nuclear protein in vertebrates. Development (Cambridge, England) 116(1):201–211

Nash DL, Bellolio MF, Stead LG (2008) S100 as a marker of acute brain ischemia: a systematic review. Neurocrit Care 8(2):301–307. https://doi.org/10.1007/s12028-007-9019-x

O'Connor DT, Mahata SK, Taupenot L, Mahata M, Livsey Taylor CV, Kailasam MT, Ziegler MG, Parmer RJ (2000) Chromogranin A in human disease. Adv Exp Med Biol 482:377–388. https://doi.org/10.1007/0-306-46837-9_31

Olsen ML, Sontheimer H (2008) Functional implications for Kir4.1 channels in glial biology: from K+ buffering to cell differentiation. J Neurochem 107(3):589–601. https://doi.org/10.1111/j.1471-4159.2008.05615.x

Orozco D, Edbauer D (2013) FUS-mediated alternative splicing in the nervous system: consequences for ALS and FTLD. J Mol Med (Berl) 91(12):1343–1354. https://doi.org/10.1007/s00109-013-1077-2

Ozansoy M, Basak AN (2013) The central theme of Parkinson's disease: alpha-synuclein. Mol Neurobiol 47(2):460–465. https://doi.org/10.1007/s12035-012-8369-3

Pekny M (2001) Astrocytic intermediate filaments: lessons from GFAP and vimentin knock-out mice. Prog Brain Res 132:23–30. https://doi.org/10.1016/s0079-6123(01)32062-9

Peters A, Palay SL, Webster HD (1991) The fine structure of the nervous system. Neurons and their supporting cells. Oxford University Press, New York

Preusser M, Lehotzky A, Budka H, Ovadi J, Kovacs GG (2007) TPPP/p25 in brain tumours: expression in non-neoplastic oligodendrocytes but not in oligodendroglioma cells. Acta Neuropathol 113(2):213–215. https://doi.org/10.1007/s00401-006-0173-6

Protas L, Qu J, Robinson RB (2003) Neuropeptide y: neurotransmitter or trophic factor in the heart? News Physiol Sci 18:181–185

Qi Y, Cai J, Wu Y, Wu R, Lee J, Fu H, Rao M, Sussel L, Rubenstein J, Qiu M (2001) Control of oligodendrocyte differentiation by the Nkx2.2 homeodomain transcription factor. Development (Cambridge, England) 128(14):2723–2733

Rauen T, Wiessner M (2000) Fine tuning of glutamate uptake and degradation in glial cells: common transcriptional regulation of GLAST1 and GS. Neurochem Int 37(2–3):179–189

Rhodes A (2012) Fixation of tissues. In: Suvarna KS, Layton C, Bancroft JD (eds) Bancroft's theory and practice of histological techniques, 7th edn. Churchill Livingstone, Edinburgh, pp 69–93

Rogers J, Khan M, Ellis J (1990) Calretinin and other CaBPs in the nervous system. Adv Exp Med Biol 269:195–203

Rostami A, Eccleston PA, Silberberg DH, Hirayama M, Lisak RP, Pleasure DE, Phillips SM (1984) Generation and biological properties of a monoclonal antibody to galactocerebroside. Brain Res 298(2):203–208

Salminen A, Kaarniranta K, Haapasalo A, Hiltunen M, Soininen H, Alafuzoff I (2012) Emerging role of p62/sequestosome-1 in the pathogenesis of Alzheimer's disease. Prog Neurobiol 96(1):87–95. https://doi.org/10.1016/j.pneurobio.2011.11.005

Sanchez C, Diaz-Nido J, Avila J (2000) Phosphorylation of microtubule-associated protein 2 (MAP2) and its relevance for the regulation of the neuronal cytoskeleton function. Prog Neurobiol 61(2):133–168

Schindler M, Humphrey PP, Emson PC (1996) Somatostatin receptors in the central nervous system. Prog Neurobiol 50(1):9–47

Schmandke A, Schmandke A, Schwab ME (2014) Nogo-A: multiple roles in CNS development, maintenance, and disease. Neuroscientist 20(4):372–386. https://doi.org/10.1177/1073858413516800

Schmidt H (2012) Three functional facets of calbindin D-28k. Front Mol Neurosci 5:25. https://doi.org/10.3389/fnmol.2012.00025

Schmitt A, Asan E, Puschel B, Jons T, Kugler P (1996) Expression of the glutamate transporter GLT1 in neural cells of the rat central nervous system: non-radioactive in situ hybridization and comparative immunocytochemistry. Neuroscience 71(4):989–1004

Schwaller B, Meyer M, Schiffmann S (2002) 'New' functions for 'old' proteins: the role of the calcium-binding proteins calbindin D-28k, calretinin and parvalbumin, in cerebellar physiology. Studies with knockout mice. Cerebellum (London, England) 1(4):241–258. https://doi.org/10.1080/147342202320883551

Shea TB, Beermann ML (1993) Evidence that the monoclonal antibodies SMI-31 and SMI-34 recognize different phosphorylation-dependent epitopes of the murine high molecular mass neurofilament subunit. J Neuroimmunol 44(1):117–121

Soula C, Danesin C, Kan P, Grob M, Poncet C, Cochard P (2001) Distinct sites of origin of oligodendrocytes and somatic motoneurons in the chick spinal cord: oligodendrocytes arise from Nkx2.2-expressing progenitors by a Shh-dependent mechanism. Development (Cambridge, England) 128(8):1369–1379

Spencer LT, Bancroft JD, Jones WG (2012) Tissue processing and microarray. In: Suvarna KS, Layton C, Bancroft JD (eds) Bancroft's theory and practice of histological techniques, 7th edn. Churchill Livingstone, Edinburgh, pp 105–123

Sperk G, Hamilton T, Colmers WF (2007) Neuropeptide Y in the dentate gyrus. Prog Brain Res 163:285–297. https://doi.org/10.1016/s0079-6123(07)63017-9

Spillantini MG, Goedert M (2013) Tau pathology and neurodegeneration. Lancet Neurol 12(6):609–622. https://doi.org/10.1016/s1474-4422(13)70090-5

Staugaitis SM, Trapp BD (2009) NG2-positive glia in the human central nervous system. Neuron Glia Biol 5(3–4):35–44. https://doi.org/10.1017/s1740925x09990342

Stoffel W, Korner R, Wachtmann D, Keller BU (2004) Functional analysis of glutamate transporters in excitatory synaptic transmission of GLAST1 and GLAST1/EAAC1 deficient mice. Brain Res Mol

Brain Res 128(2):170–181. https://doi.org/10.1016/j.molbrainres.2004.06.026

Takashima A (2013) Tauopathies and tau oligomers. J Alzheimers Dis 37(3):565–568. https://doi.org/10.3233/jad-130653

Tallent MK (2007) Somatostatin in the dentate gyrus. Prog Brain Res 163:265–284. https://doi.org/10.1016/s0079-6123(07)63016-7

Thiel G (1993) Synapsin I, synapsin II, and synaptophysin: marker proteins of synaptic vesicles. Brain Pathol (Zurich, Switzerland) 3(1):87–95

Trotter J, Karram K, Nishiyama A (2010) NG2 cells: properties, progeny and origin. Brain Res Rev 63(1–2):72–82. https://doi.org/10.1016/j.brainresrev.2009.12.006

Uchida T, Takahashi K, Yamaguchi H, Nagai Y (1981) Localization of galactocerebroside in oligodendrocytes, myelin sheath and choroid plexus. Jpn J Exp Med 51(1):29–35

Usman W, Asim A (2005) Histotechniques: laboratory techniques in histopathology: a handbook for medical technologists. LAP LAMPERT Academic Publishing

Voelker CC, Garin N, Taylor JS, Gahwiler BH, Hornung JP, Molnar Z (2004) Selective neurofilament (SMI-32, FNP-7 and N200) expression in subpopulations of layer V pyramidal neurons in vivo and in vitro. Cereb Cortex (New York, NY: 1991) 14(11):1276–1286. https://doi.org/10.1093/cercor/bhh089

Wiedenmann B (1991) Synaptophysin. A widespread constituent of small neuroendocrine vesicles and a new tool in tumor diagnosis. Acta Oncol (Stockholm, Sweden) 30(4):435–440

Willis M, Leitner I, Jellinger KA, Marksteiner J (2011) Chromogranin peptides in brain diseases. J Neural Transm 118(5):727–735. https://doi.org/10.1007/s00702-011-0648-z

Wouterlood FG (2012) Cellular imaging techniques for neuroscience and beyond. Elsevier, Amsterdam

Xu JP, Zhao J, Li S (2011) Roles of NG2 glial cells in diseases of the central nervous system. Neurosci Bull 27(6):413–421. https://doi.org/10.1007/s12264-011-1838-2

Yang Y, Gozen O, Watkins A, Lorenzini I, Lepore A, Gao Y, Vidensky S, Brennan J, Poulsen D, Won Park J, Li Jeon N, Robinson MB, Rothstein JD (2009) Presynaptic regulation of astroglial excitatory neurotransmitter transporter GLT1. Neuron 61(6):880–894. https://doi.org/10.1016/j.neuron.2009.02.010

Yang Y, Gozen O, Vidensky S, Robinson MB, Rothstein JD (2010) Epigenetic regulation of neuron-dependent induction of astroglial synaptic protein GLT1. Glia 58(3):277–286. https://doi.org/10.1002/glia.20922

Youmans KL, Wolozin B (2012) TDP-43: a new player on the AD field? Exp Neurol 237(1):90–95. https://doi.org/10.1016/j.expneurol.2012.05.018

Zimmer DB, Cornwall EH, Landar A, Song W (1995) The S100 protein family: history, function, and expression. Brain Res Bull 37(4):417–429

Part II
The Normal Human Brain

Subdivisions of the Nervous System

4.1 Central Nervous System (CNS) and Peripheral Nervous System (PNS)

From a topographical point of view, the human nervous system is subdivided into:

- the central nervous system (CNS)
- the peripheral nervous system (PNS)

However, there exists no functional partition between the CNS and the PNS. The PNS carries information from receptor organs of the periphery to the CNS. In the CNS, this information is processed, and responses are created which are carried back via the PNS to effector organs in the periphery.

The direction of information transduction to the CNS is called *afferent pathway*, and the opposite direction away from the CNS is called *efferent pathway* (Fig. 4.1).

4.1.1 Central Nervous System (CNS)

The central nervous system is composed of (Fig. 4.2):

- the brain
- the spinal cord

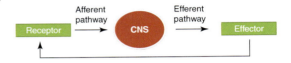

Fig. 4.1 Schematic illustration of the afferent and efferent pathways

All stimuli from the external environment, the periphery, and from the viscera are processed in the CNS. Adequate responses are produced and transmitted back to the periphery (Fig. 4.1). The incoming stimuli are processed at different levels in the CNS in the course of which the following reaction patterns are noted:

- *Level 1*: *Unconditioned reflex.* This reflex is inborn; a preformed reflex arc already exists.
- *Level 2*: *Conditioned reflex.* This reflex is formed after conditioning (classical Pavlovian conditioning).
- *Level 3*: *Instrumental reaction.* Problems are solved following the principle of "trial and error" (Skinner's operant conditioning).
- *Level 4*: *Cognitive processes.* They represent the highest level of neural information processing. After the stimuli are perceived, conscious reactions are created, e.g., the struggle of humans for life. In contrast to Level 2 and Level 3, a delay in time may exist between the stimulus and the generation of the reaction.

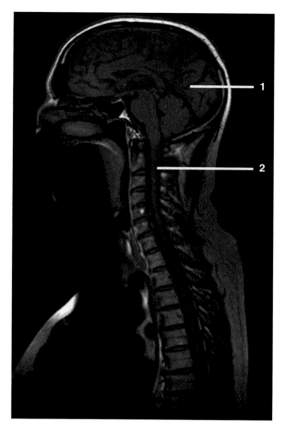

Fig. 4.2 Magnetic resonance image of the median-sagittal plane displaying the brain (1) and spinal cord (2)

4.1.2 Peripheral Nervous System (PNS)

The peripheral nervous system is composed of:

- 12 pairs of cranial nerves
- 31 pairs of spinal nerves

Information from peripheral receptors is conducted afferently through the cranial and spinal nerves to the CNS. The reaction of the CNS to the stimulus is conducted efferently via the PNS to the target organs of the periphery or the viscera. The following fiber types are found in the cranial and spinal nerves:

- *somatomotor*: nerve fibers abutting on striated muscles
- *somatosensory*: nerve fibers projecting from the skin or muscles (e.g., muscle spindle, tendon spindle) to the CNS
- *visceromotor*: nerve fibers abutting on smooth muscles of the viscera, blood vessels, and glands
- *viscerosensory*: nerve fibers projecting from the viscera to the CNS

4.2 Cerebrospinal and Autonomic Nervous System

Based on functional aspects, the nervous system can also be subdivided into:

- the cerebrospinal nervous system
- the autonomic nervous system

4.2.1 Cerebrospinal Nervous System

The cerebrospinal nervous system is under the control of the (conscious) will. It represents the level of cognitive processing of neural information (Level 4). Striated muscles are the only organ controlled by the cerebrospinal nervous system. In this way, the organism responds to its environment. The following types of nerve fibers are found:

- *afferent somatosensory nerve fibers* projecting from the skin and from the muscles of the trunk and limbs to the CNS
- *efferent somatomotor nerve fibers* supplying the muscles of the trunk and the limbs

4.2.2 Autonomic Nervous System

In contrast to the cerebrospinal nervous system, the autonomic nervous system cannot be controlled by the will. Nerve fibers of the autonomic nervous system innervate the smooth muscles of the intestines, as well as the vessels and the glands. The cardiac muscle is also innervated by the autonomic nervous system. The mechanisms of neural information processing occurring in the autonomic nervous system correspond to the previously described Levels 1, 2, and 3. Somatomotor, somatosensory, visceromotor, and viscerosensory fibers make up the autonomic nervous system.

4.3 Cortical Areas

The exact localization of specific functions to well-defined cortical regions in the human brain is quite challenging (see Chap. 14). When a lesion (e.g., hemorrhage, tumor, demyelination) is seen, one can only attempt to make a correlation between the morphological substrate and the functional deficits. This approach is quite limited since a lesion is never restricted to a specific functional area of the brain and a specific function is not restricted to a brain region.

Knowledge about functional relationships mostly stems from experimental animal studies and clinical studies. In experimental animal studies, neuronal activity may be registered electrophysiologically in specific brain regions. Electrical stimulation of brain regions is also possible. Furthermore, it is possible to produce a well-defined lesion and then observe the functional deficits.

In recent years, the application of fMRI and neuropsychology in humans led to an acquisition of knowledge about the topographical localization of specific functional systems (Chap. 14).

4.3.1 Somatotopic Organization

A brain region (cortical or subcortical) is somatotopically organized when different regions of the body are represented in different parts of this brain region. The best example is given by the motor cortex. The upper limb is represented at the superior margin, whereas the facial representation is located on the superolateral surface next to the lateral fissure. The picture of the "homunculus" (i.e. upside-down-man) is evoked to describe this somatotopic arrangement (Fig. 4.3a–c).

4.3.2 Primary Cortical Areas

Functional centers are localized in specific brain regions, i.e., the primary cortical areas. However, these centers do not operate independently from each other. The proper neuronal response is the result of the interplay of many primary and secondary centers which are closely interconnected with each other. Primary cortical areas are somatotopically organized. The primary motor cortex in the precentral gyrus is an example of a primary cortical area.

4.3.3 Secondary Cortical Areas

Secondary cortical regions are located in close proximity to primary cortical areas. In contrast, they are not somatotopically organized. In secondary cortical areas, mainly control and coordinative as well as associative functions are performed.

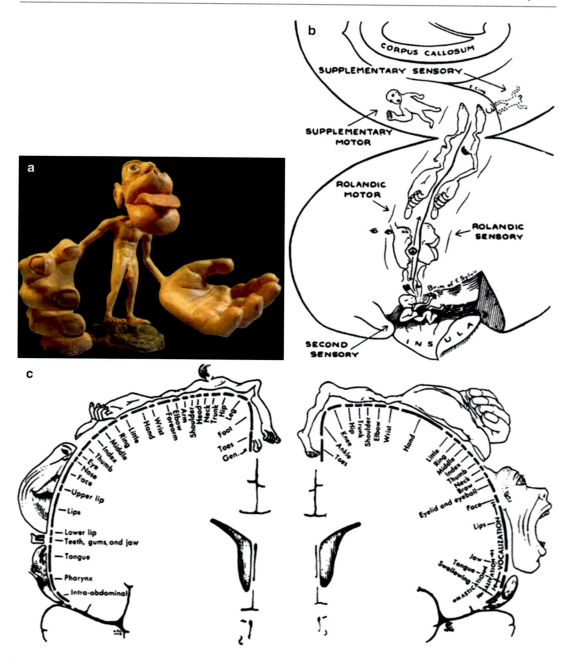

Fig. 4.3 "Homunculus" (i.e., upside-down-man) is evoked to describe the somatotopic arrangement of motor function (source: https://www.google.at/search?q=homunculus&source=lnms&tbm=isch&sa=X&ved=0ahUKEwjd98G08JDZAhUSnRQKHaByAW4Q_AUICigB&biw=1280&bih=878#imgrc=GX6J0Rx2oQcs3M:&spf=1517906005128) (**a**). The motor and sensory homunculus: the first map by Penfield and Rasmussen (1950) (Permission of Macmillan Publishing Company) (**b**). Multiple sets of homunculi (Penfield and Jasper 1954) (**c**)

4.4 Gray and White Matter

4.4.1 Gray Matter

The gray matter is composed of the perikarya of all neurons and their dendritic trees as well as of glial cells. Due to their staining properties, the constituents of the gray matter appear grayish-dark on sections, hence the name "gray matter" (Fig. 4.4).

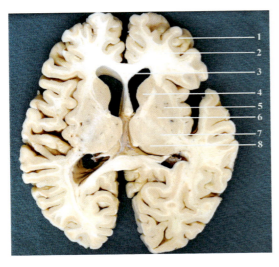

Fig. 4.4 Horizontal section of the brain showing (i) gray matter, i.e., cerebral cortex (1), (ii) white matter (2), (iii) nuclei, i.e., caudate nucleus (4), putamen (5), globus pallidus (6), and thalamus (8), and (iv) tracts, i.e., corpus callosum (3) and internal capsule with pyramidal tract (7)

4.4.2 White Matter

The white matter is composed of axons that arise from neurons located in the gray matter. Due to the staining properties of the myelin sheaths, this region stains light on sections, hence the name "white matter" (Fig. 4.4).

4.4.3 Nuclei and Ganglia

Groups of nerve cells form:

- nuclei in the CNS
  - for example, caudate nucleus (Fig. 4.5a–d)
- ganglia in the PNS
  - for example, spinal ganglia

4.4.4 Tracts

Nerve fibers (axons) connecting different brain regions with each other are referred to as tracts or fascicles (Fig. 4.6a–d).

4.4.5 Neuropil

All dendritic trees, axon terminals, and glial processes together form the neuropil.

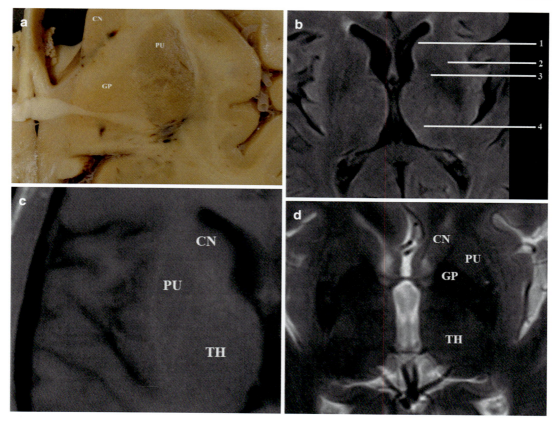

Fig. 4.5 Nuclei making up the basal ganglia, i.e., caudate nucleus (CN), globus pallidus (GP), and putamen (PU). Thalamus (TH). (1) CN, (2) PU, (3) GP, (4) TH. Autopsy brain (**a**), Flair (**b**), T1 (**c**), and T2 (**d**)

Selected References

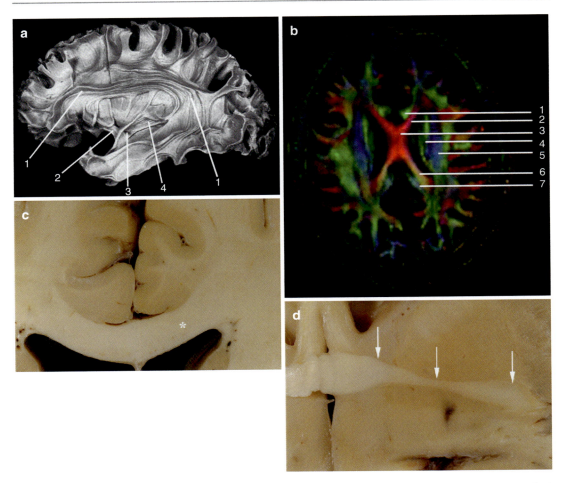

Fig. 4.6 Special tract preparation on an autopsy brain showing (1) superior longitudinal fascicle, (2) uncinate fascicle, (3) insular fascicle, (4) inferior occipito-frontal fascicle, and (5) superior longitudinal fascicle (preproduced from Ludwig and Klinger (1956) with permission by Karger Verlag) (**a**). Diffusion tensor imaging (DTI), horizontal plane with (1) caudate nucleus, (2) anterior limb of the internal capsule, (3) knee of the internal capsule, (4) globus pallidus, (5) putamen, (6) posterior limb of the internal capsule, (7) splenium of the corpus callosum) (**b**), corpus callosum (∗) (**c**), and anterior commissure → (**d**)

Selected References

Ludwig E, Klinger J (1956) Atlas Cerebri Humani. The inner structure of the brain. Little, Brown and Company, Karger Verlag, Boston, Toronto

Penfield W, Jasper H (1954) Epilepsy and the functional anatomy of the human brain. Churchill Livingstone, Edinburgh

Penfield W, Rasmussen T (1950) The cerebral cortex of man. Macmillan Publishing Company, New York

Gross Anatomy of the Nervous System

5.1 Subdivisions of the Central Nervous System

The human brain is subdivided along its rostrocaudal axis into the following parts (Fig. 5.1):

1. Prosencephalon
   - Telencephalon
   - Diencephalon
2. Mesencephalon
3. Rhombencephalon
   - Metencephalon
     – Pons
     – Cerebellum
   - Myelencephalon (medulla oblongata)

The term "*brain stem*" refers to the triad of mesencephalon, pons, and medulla oblongata. Although the cerebellum is part of the metencephalon, it does not belong to the brain stem. Several authors consider the diencephalon to be part of the brain stem. However, the diencephalon should be considered as a functional connection between the telencephalon and the brain stem.

5.2 Telencephalon

The telencephalon is composed of two cerebral *hemispheres* and of several nuclei contained within the hemispheres. These nuclei are termed the basal ganglia. The two cerebral hemispheres are partly separated by the *longitudinal fissure*. A dural duplication, the falx cerebri, enters the longitudinal fissure. In the depth of the longitudinal fissure, the cerebral hemispheres are connected by the corpus callosum. The occipital parts of the hemispheres are separated from the cerebellum by the transverse fissure. The tentorium cerebelli, another dural duplication, enters this fissure.

At each hemisphere, one can distinguish:

- a convex *superolateral surface*
- a *medial surface* running parallel to the longitudinal fissure
- an *inferior surface* which is divided into an orbital and a tentorial part

The following margins between the surfaces are defined for each hemisphere:

- *superior margin:* located between the superolateral and the medial surfaces
- *inferior margin:* located between the medial and the inferior surfaces
- *lateral margin:* located between the superolateral and the inferior surfaces

Three poles are distinguished:

- frontal pole
- occipital pole
- temporal pole

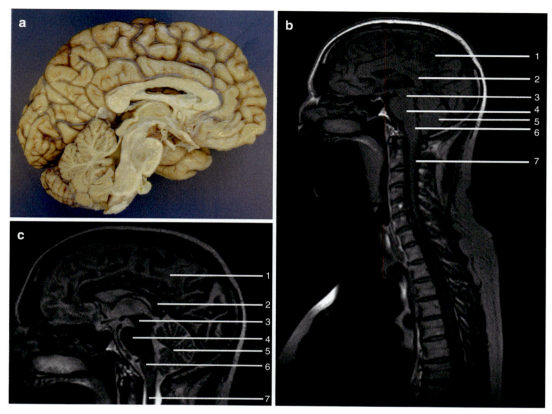

Fig. 5.1 Median-sagittal plane of the central nervous system. Autopsy specimen (**a**), MRI-T1 image showing the brain and spinal cord (**b**), MRI-T2 image showing the brain (**c**). (1) Telencephalon, (2) corpus callosum, (3) mesencephalon, (4) pons, (5) cerebellum, (6) medulla oblongata, (7) spinal cord

For further orientation, five lobes are defined (Fig. 5.2):

- frontal lobe
- parietal lobe
- occipital lobe
- temporal lobe
- insula

The insula lies as the fifth telencephalic lobe hidden beneath the frontal and temporal lobes in the depth of the lateral fissure (Fig. 5.2).

Three main sulci (fissures) serve as landmarks for the telencephalic lobes:

- The *lateral sulcus* traverses the superolateral surface horizontally and separates the frontal and parietal lobes from the temporal lobe (Fig. 5.3).
- The *central sulcus* originates from the superior margin and traverses the superolateral surface vertically towards the lateral sulcus without reaching it. Sometimes, the central sulcus sends a short ramification to the medial

5.2 Telencephalon

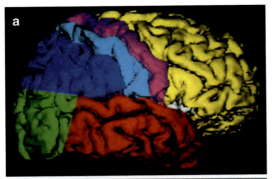

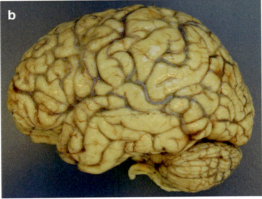

Fig. 5.2 View of the superolateral surface of the telencephalon (**a**, **b**). Frontal lobe (yellow), precentral gyrus (pink), postcentral gyrus (light blue), parietal lobe (dark blue), occipital lobe (green), temporal lobe (red), insula (white) (reproduced from Weis et al. (1992) with kind permission by Hogrefe Verlag)

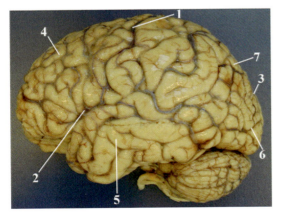

Fig. 5.3 The main sulci of the telencephalon. (1) Central sulcus, (2) lateral sulcus, (3) parieto-occipital sulcus, (4) frontal lobe, (5) temporal lobe, (6) occipital lobe, (7) parietal lobe

surface. The frontal lobe is separated from the parietal lobe by the central sulcus (Fig. 5.3).

- The *parieto-occipital sulcus* cuts the superior margin, sends a small ramification to the superolateral surface, and terminates at the medial surface. The parieto-occipital sulcus separates the parietal lobe from the occipital lobe (Fig. 5.3).

5.2.1 Superolateral Surface

5.2.1.1 Frontal Lobe

The frontal lobe is bounded on the superolateral surface as follows (Fig. 5.4):

- posteriorly by the central sulcus
- inferiorly by the lateral sulcus
- superiorly by the superior margin

The frontal lobe also extends to the medial surface (see also Sect. 5.2.2 and Fig. 5.9).

In the posterior part of the frontal lobe, the precentral gyrus runs parallel to the central sulcus (Fig. 5.4). The primary cortical motor area is located in this gyrus. Here, all information about locomotion is processed. This gyrus is somatotopically organized, i.e., all parts lying cranial in the body are represented in the inferior parts of the gyrus. The precentral gyrus is separated by the precentral sulcus from the other frontal gyri. Both precentral gyrus and sulcus show a more vertical topography as compared to the other gyri and sulci of the frontal lobe (Fig. 5.4).

The superolateral surface of the frontal lobe is organized as follows:

- The superior frontal gyrus runs horizontally and parallel to the superior margin.
- The superior frontal sulcus separates it from the middle frontal gyrus.
- The middle frontal gyrus runs horizontally and parallel to the superior frontal gyrus

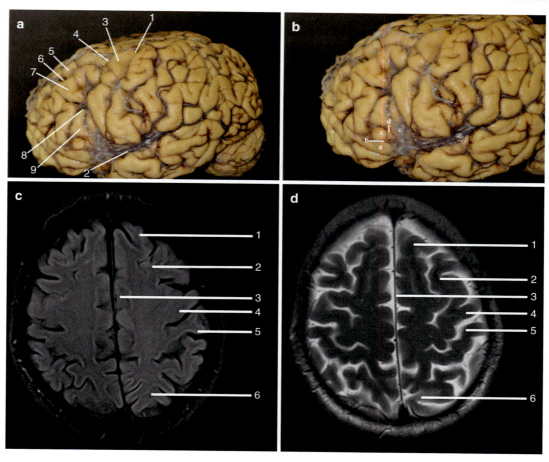

Fig. 5.4 Superolateral view of the frontal lobe. Autopsy brain (**a**, **b**): (1) Central sulcus, (2) lateral sulcus, (3) precentral gyrus, (4) precentral sulcus, (5) superior frontal gyrus, (6) superior frontal sulcus, (7) middle frontal gyrus, (8) inferior frontal sulcus, (9) inferior frontal gyrus with (a) pars orbitalis, (b) ramus anterior, (c) pars triangularis, and (d) ramus posterior, (e) pars opercularis. MRI Horizontal plane, Flair (**c**), T2 (**d**): (1) superior frontal gyrus, (2) middle frontal gyrus, (3) medial frontal gyrus, (4) precentral gyrus, (5) postcentral gyrus, (6) parietal lobe

- The inferior frontal sulcus extends between the middle frontal gyrus and the inferior frontal gyrus.
- The inferior frontal gyrus, being the largest of the three gyri, is subdivided into further parts.
  - An orbital part is separated from the triangular part by the anterior ramus, which is a ramification of the lateral sulcus.
  - The opercular part lies close to the ascending ramus.
  - The posterior ramus forms the occipital border of the posterior part. All these three rami are ramifications of the lateral sulcus (Fig. 5.4).

Notable functions:

- Motor control
- Expressive speech
- Personality
- Drive

The secondary cortical motor area for coordination of locomotion is located in the superior frontal gyrus, while that for the line of sight and head rotation is located in the middle frontal gyrus. Broca's speech area is localized mainly in the triangular part and partly in the opercular part of the inferior frontal gyrus. Lesions in this region

5.2 Telencephalon

lead to Broca's aphasia. This type of aphasia is characterized by decreased speech fluency with poor articulation as well as by phonetic paraphasias and agrammatism.

5.2.1.2 Parietal Lobe

The boundaries of the parietal lobe are the central sulcus anteriorly and, the superior margin superiorly (Fig. 5.5). The other boundaries (i.e., inferior and posterior) of the parietal lobe are not so distinct. Defining the inferior border is not possible since parts of the parietal lobe extend beyond the region of the lateral sulcus. The posterior border can only be described arbitrarily by drawing a line connecting the parieto-occipital sulcus with the preoccipital incisure. Parts of the parietal lobe also extend to the medial surface.

In the anterior part of the parietal lobe, the postcentral gyrus runs parallel to the central sulcus. This gyrus is separated by the postcentral sulcus from the other gyri of the parietal lobe (Fig. 5.5). The postcentral gyrus is recognized to be the primary somatosensory cortex. This gyrus is somatotopically organized. All pieces of information from superficial and deep receptors are processed in this brain region.

The superior parietal lobule runs parallel to the superior margin. It is separated by the intraparietal sulcus from the inferior parietal lobule. Two gyri of the inferior parietal lobule are distinguished as follows (Fig. 5.5):

- *Supramarginal gyrus* arches the lateral fissure.
- *Angular gyrus* lies close to the posterior end of the superior temporal gyrus.

Notable functions:

- sensory input and integration
- receptive speech

In the superior and inferior parietal lobules, neuronal information concerned with the understanding and interpretation of sensory signals is processed. Thus, in both lobules secondary cortical regions concerned with the processing of superficial and deep sensations as well as orientation are localized. In the supramarginal and angular gyri, the secondary centers of the optic speech region as well as the centers for writing and reading are localized.

5.2.1.3 Occipital Lobe

The boundaries of the occipital lobe are indistinct (Fig. 5.6). The occipital lobe extends posteriorly from the parieto-occipital sulcus, which forms its anterior border. The border with the temporal lobe is not distinct. The superior border is formed by the superior margin and the inferior border is formed by the inferior margin. Several irregularly

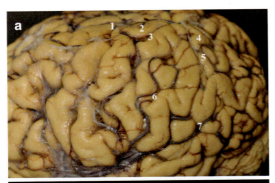
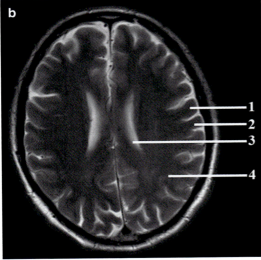

Fig. 5.5 Superolateral view of the parietal lobe. Autopsy brain (**a**): (1) Central sulcus, (2) postcentral gyrus, (3) postcentral sulcus, (4) superior parietal lobule, (5) inferior parietal lobule, (6) supramarginal gyrus, (7) angular gyrus. MRI horizontal plane T2 (**b**): (1) precentral gyrus, (2) postcentral gyrus, (3) lateral ventricular system, (4) parietal lobe

The primary visual center is located in the posterior aspects of the occipital lobe, and abuts on the calcarine fissure of the medial surface.

5.2.1.4 Temporal Lobe

The upper boundary of the temporal lobe is formed by the lateral sulcus, whereas the lower boundary is formed by the inferior margin (Fig. 5.7). The temporal lobe extends along the inferior margin towards the preoccipital incisure. The anterior boundary is formed by the temporal pole, while the boundary with the occipital lobe is indistinct.

The superior temporal gyrus runs parallel to the lateral sulcus. It is separated by the superior temporal sulcus from the middle temporal gyrus. The border between the middle temporal gyrus and the inferior temporal gyrus is formed by the inferior temporal sulcus (Fig. 5.7).

Notable functions:

- auditory input
- memory integration

Deep in the lateral sulcus and superior to the superior temporal gyrus, several gyri run transversely. These transverse gyri are separated by a transverse sulcus. In these transverse gyri, the primary auditory center is located.

In the superior temporal gyrus, the secondary auditory center is located, in which acoustic memory is processed. In the posterior part of this gyrus, the Wernicke speech center is located. A lesion in the latter region leads to Wernicke's aphasia, which is characterized by phonetic and/or semantic paraphasias, neologisms, disturbed speech understanding, and restricted communicative abilities.

5.2.1.5 Insula

Within the depth of the lateral sulcus lies a hidden cortical area, the insula (Fig. 5.8). The temporal, parietal, and frontal opercula have to be removed in order to visualize the insula. At its surface, several short and long gyri are seen. The insula is bordered by the circular insular fissure. However, the anterior part is open towards the medial aspect through the limen insulae.

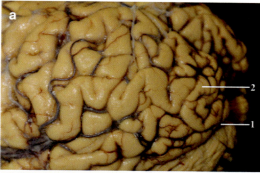
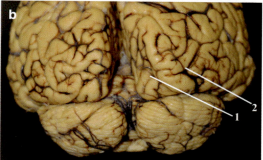
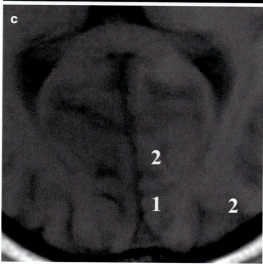

Fig. 5.6 Superolateral view of the occipital lobe. Autopsy brain (**a**, **b**). (1) Calcarine sulcus, (2) occipital gyri. MRI horizontal plane T1 (**c**)

shaped occipital gyri are distinguished. The transverse occipital sulcus, which is a continuation of the intraparietal sulcus, separates the occipital gyri, thus forming an upper and a lower part.

Notable function:

- visual input and processing

5.2 Telencephalon

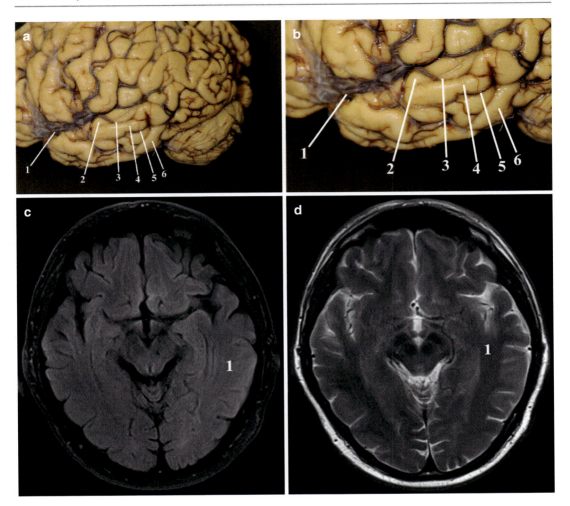

Fig. 5.7 Superolateral view of the temporal lobe. Autopsy brain (**a, b**). (1) Lateral sulcus, (2) superior temporal gyrus, (3) superior temporal sulcus, (4) middle temporal gyrus, (5) inferior temporal sulcus, (6) inferior temporal gyrus. MRI horizontal plane, Flair (**c**), T2 (**d**). (1) temporal lobe

5.2.2 Medial Surface

The cortical regions constituting the medial surface are arranged in such a way that they form a two-storied structure (Fig. 5.9).

In the "upper floor," the medial frontal gyrus extends from the frontal pole posteriorly. It ends at the point where the precentral sulcus reaches the medial surface. The region extending between the precentral and the postcentral sulci is termed paracentral lobule. The region between the postcentral sulcus and the parieto-occipital sulcus is the precuneus. Posterior to the precuneus, the cuneus extends between the parieto-occipital sulcus and the calcarine fissure. At the medial surface, the calcarine fissure forms the boundary between the occipital and the parietal lobes (Fig. 5.9).

The "lower floor" is separated from the "upper floor" by the cingulate sulcus. The cingulate sulcus joins posteriorly with the marginal sulcus. This lower floor is made up of the cingulate gyrus. The anterior part of the cingulate gyrus is termed paraterminal lobe; its posterior part is narrow and is called isthmus of the cingulate gyrus. The sulcus corporis callosi separates the cingulate gyrus from the corpus callosum. Along its anterior-posterior axis, different parts

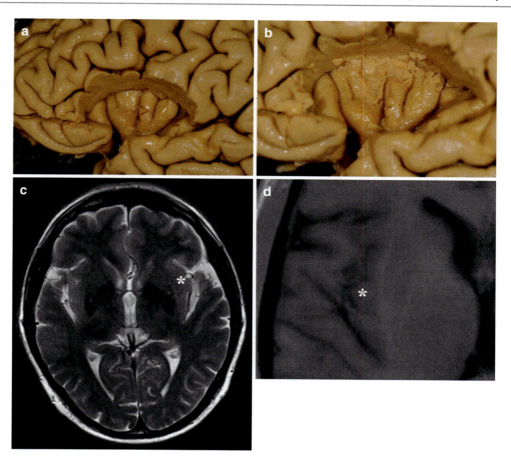

Fig. 5.8 Insula (**a**, **b**) is seen after removal of the opercular part of the inferior frontal gyrus. MRI horizontal plane T2 (**c**), T1 (**d**): the insula (∗) is covered by parts of the frontal and temporal lobes (**c**, **d**)

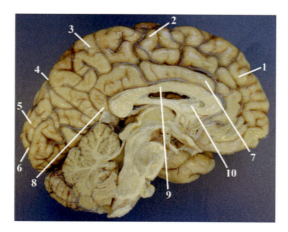

Fig. 5.9 View of the medial surface. Autopsy specimen. (1) Medial frontal gyrus, (2) paracentral lobule, (3) precuneus, (4) parieto-occipital sulcus, (5) cuneus, (6) calcarine fissure, (7) cingulate gyrus, (8) paraterminal lobe, (9) isthmus of cingulate gyrus, (10) corpus callosum, (11) septum pellucidum

of the corpus callosum are distinguished: (a) rostrum, (b) knee, (c) trunk, and (d) splenium. The superior surface of the corpus callosum is entirely covered by the indusium griseum, on which the medial longitudinal stria and the two lateral longitudinal striae can be seen. The septum pellucidum is attached to the inferior surface of the corpus callosum. The former forms the medial wall of the lateral ventricle (Fig. 5.10).

5.2.3 Inferior Surface

The inferior surface of the telencephalon rests on the anterior and middle cranial fossae as well as on the cerebellar tentorium. An orbital and a tentorial part are discerned (Fig. 5.11). The orbital part is mainly formed by the frontal lobe and lies within the anterior cranial fossa.

5.3 Limbic System

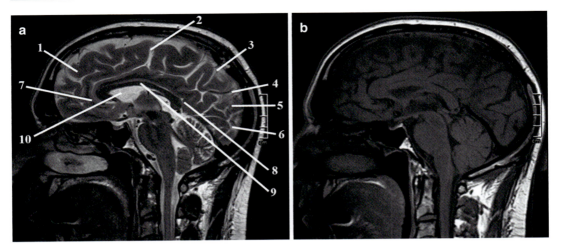

Fig. 5.10 View of the medial surface. MRI-T2 (**a**), MRI-T1 (**b**). (1) Medial frontal gyrus, (2) paracentral lobule, (3) precuneus, (4) parieto-occipital sulcus, (5) cuneus, (6) calcarine fissure, (7) cingulate gyrus, (8) isthmus of cingulate gyrus, (9) corpus callosum, (10) septum pellucidum

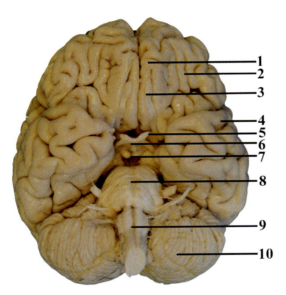

Fig. 5.11 View of the inferior surface. (1) Straight gyrus, (2) fronto-orbital gyri, (3) olfactory nerve, (4) temporal pole, (5) optic nerve, (6) pituitary stalk, (7) mammillary bodies, (8) pons, (9) medulla oblongata, (10) cerebellum

The following structures are seen in the orbital part. First, the straight gyrus runs parallel to the median-sagittal axis. The olfactory sulcus is located at its lateral border. Along this sulcus the olfactory tract, which is part of the olfactory nerve (first cranial nerve), runs. In the anterior part of the sulcus lies the olfactory bulb. Several irregularly shaped gyri, the orbital gyri, constitute the remaining part of the inferior surface of the frontal lobe (orbital part). These are separated from each other by orbital sulci (Fig. 5.11).

The inferior surface of the temporal lobe rests on the middle cranial fossa. Towards the midline, the lateral occipito-temporal gyrus, the occipito-temporal sulcus, the medial occipito-temporal gyrus, the collateral sulcus, and the parahippocampal gyrus are seen. Because of its hooked shape, the anterior part of the parahippocampal gyrus is called uncus. Occipitally, the parahippocampal gyrus blends with the lingual gyrus. The lingual gyrus is separated from the occipital lobe by the calcarine fissure. The posterior and inferior parts of the cerebral hemispheres rest on the cerebellar tentorium and represent the tentorial part of the inferior telencephalic surface.

5.3 Limbic System

Under the term "limbic system" or "limbic gyrus" various phylogenetically old regions of the medial surface, which also share the same functions, are grouped together.

The limbic system is composed of the:

- Cingulate gyrus
- Parahippocampal gyrus
- Dentate gyrus
- Amygdala
- Hypothalamus
- Epithalamus
- Subthalamus

The limbic system plays a major role in maintaining homeostasis by activating visceral effector mechanisms, by modulating the secretion of hypophyseal hormones, and by regulating sexual and reproductive behavior.

5.4 Hippocampal Formation

The hippocampal formation consists of the following structures:

- Dentate gyrus
- Hippocampus (proper)
- Subiculum
- Presubiculum
- Parasubiculum
- Entorhinal cortex

The hippocampus lies buried deep in the temporal lobe, protruding as a bulb-like structure into the temporal horn of the lateral ventricle (Fig. 5.12a–s). Based on its development, it is a curved cortical structure that is rolled into (inner rotation) the depths of the temporal lobe. It forms an arc whose anterior part is enlarged and whose posterior part narrows like a comma. It is bordered anteriorly by the amygdala; its posterior end is located near the splenium corporis callosi. Inferiorly, it constitutes the floor of the inferior horn of the lateral ventricle.

Hippocampal anatomy is complex. Roughly, the hippocampus can be subdivided into:

- Hippocampal head (anterior segment)
  - Transversally oriented and dilated
  - Shows elevations: the digitationes hippocampi
  - Extraventricular or uncal part
- Hippocampal body (middle segment)
  - Oriented sagittally
  - Extraventricular or superficial part
- Hippocampal tail (posterior segment)
  - Transversally oriented
  - Posteriorly narrowing and disappearing beneath the splenium corporis callosi

An intraventricular as well as an extraventricular part of each hippocampal part is distinguished.

The parahippocampal gyrus is divided into the following two segments:

- The *subiculum:* The narrow posterior segment and its flat superior surface. It is separated from the hippocampus by the hippocampal sulcus.
- The *piriform lobe:* The more voluminous anterior segment consisting of the *uncus* and the *entorhinal area*.

The *uncus* rests on the parahippocampal gyrus itself from which it is separated by the uncal sulcus. The posterior part of the uncus which belongs to the hippocampus; the anterior part displays two protrusions: the *semilunar gyrus* and the *ambient gyrus*, which are separated by the *semianular sulcus*, both covering a deep nucleus, the amygdala.

The *entorhinal area* is the lower part of the piriform lobe extending to the posterior segment of the parahippocampal gyrus.

The *indusium griseum* covers as a neuronal lamina the corpus callosum up to its splenium.

The *subiculum* is a strip of cortical tissue situated between the hippocampus and the entorhinal cortex in the parahippocampal gyrus.

5.4 Hippocampal Formation

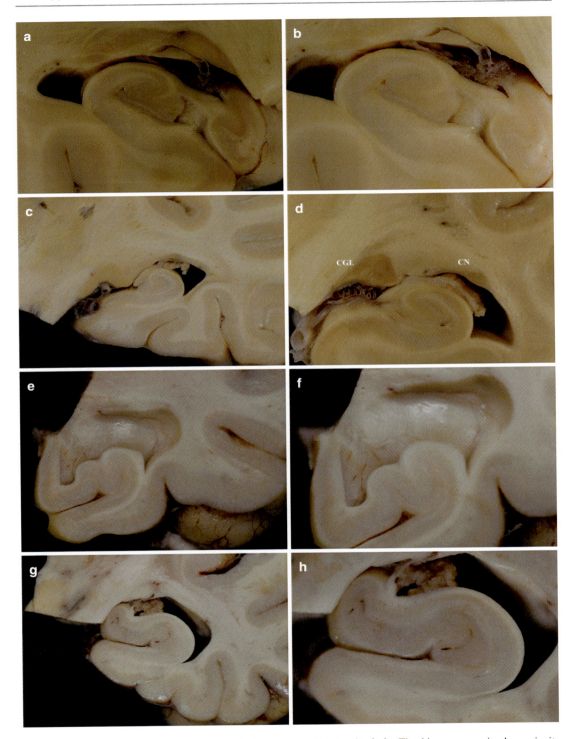

Fig. 5.12 Hippocampus. Typical structure of the hippocampus as cut at a level along its anterior-posterior axis (**a–d**), as cut at anterior levels along its anterior-posterior axis (**e–h**), as cut at a posterior level along its anterior-posterior axis (**i**, **j**). The hippocampus is shown in its anterior-posterior length (**k–m**). MRI frontal plane T2 (**n–p**), sagittal plane T2 (**q–s**)

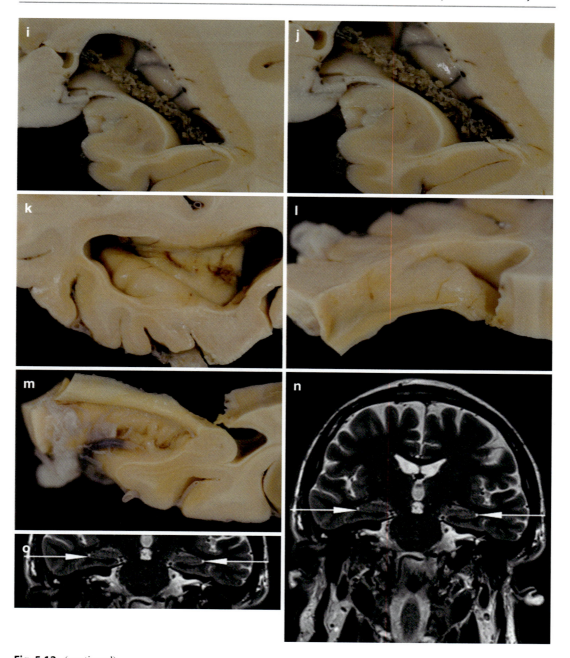

Fig. 5.12 (continued)

5.4 Hippocampal Formation

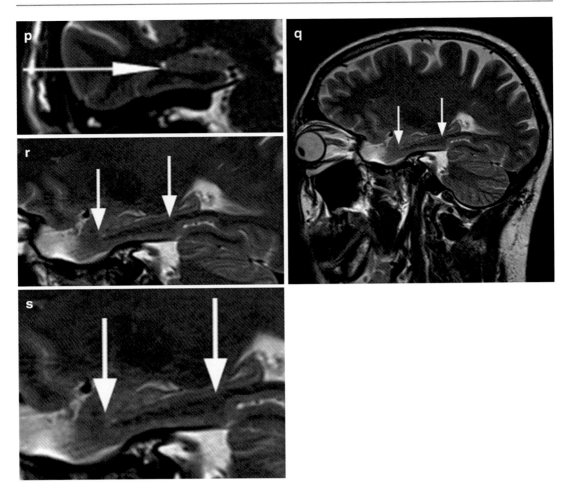

Fig. 5.12 (continued)

5.5 Amygdala

The amygdala is located in the anterior dorsomedial region of the temporal lobe below the uncus gyri parahippocampalis and in front of the inferior horn of the lateral ventricle. It is part of the rhinencephalon (Fig. 5.13).

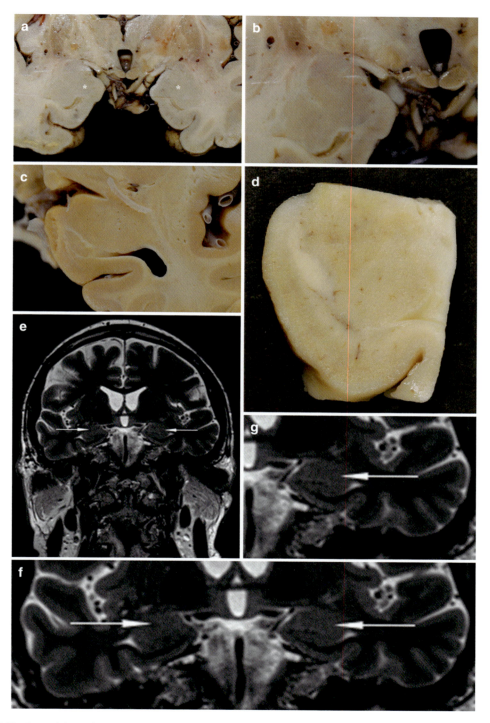

Fig. 5.13 Amygdala (**a–d**) as seen on frontal sections. MRI frontal plane T2 (**e–g**)

5.6 Basal Ganglia

Several distinct nuclear masses of the telencephalon are termed basal ganglia (Figs. 5.14, 5.15, and 5.16). These nuclear masses include the following:

- Caudate nucleus
- Putamen
- Globus pallidus

The term "corpus striatum" refers collectively to the caudate nucleus, putamen, and globus pallidus, whereas the term "lentiform nucleus" refers to both putamen and globus pallidus.

In order to maintain clarity the designations "corpus striatum" and "lentiform nucleus" should be avoided. The basal ganglia represent individual entities which are connected with each other in a very complicated way.

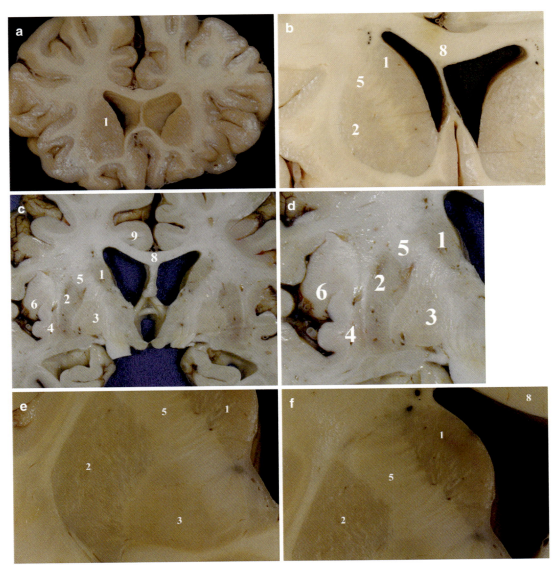

Fig. 5.14 Basal ganglia seen on frontal brain slices along the anterior-posterior length (**a–j**). (1) caudate nucleus, (2) putamen, (3) globus pallidus, (4) claustrum, (5) internal capsule, (6) insula, (7) thalamus, (8) corpus callosum, (9) cingulate gyrus

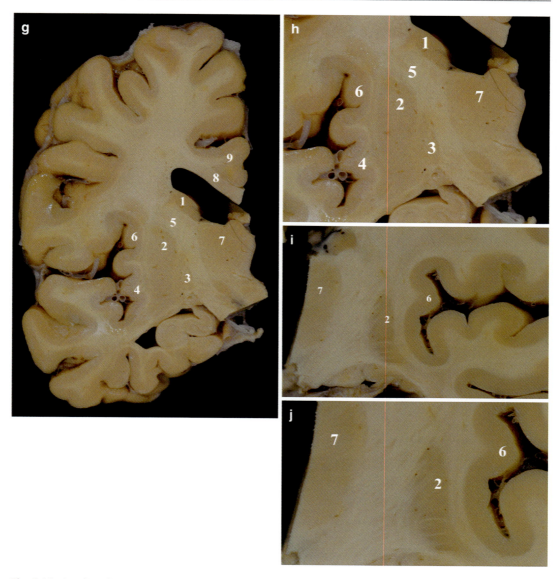

Fig. 5.14 (continued)

The function of the basal ganglia is complex and many aspects are not yet clearly understood. They are concerned with initiation and coordination of motor activities.

5.6.1 Caudate Nucleus

The caudate nucleus consists of three parts:

- The *head of the caudate nucleus* (caput nuclei caudati) is the anterior part and forms the lateral border of the anterior horn of the lateral ventricle.
- The *body of the caudate nucleus* (corpus nuclei caudati) is the continuation of the head. This part forms the lateral border of the lateral ventricles. The body of the caudate nucleus lies close to the thalamus dorsolaterally.
- The *tail of the caudate nucleus* (cauda nuclei caudati) lines the curvature of the inferior horn of the lateral ventricle and forms its roof in the temporal lobe. The tail of the caudate nucleus ends at the amygdala.

5.6 Basal Ganglia

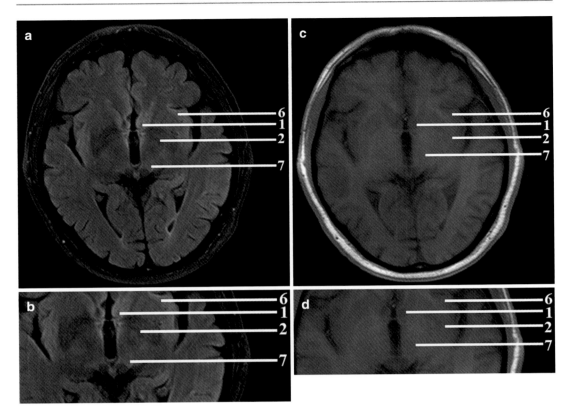

Fig. 5.15 Basal ganglia seen on MRI horizontal brain slices, Flair (**a**, **b**), T1 (**c**, **d**). (1) caudate nucleus, (2) putamen, (3) globus pallidus, (4) claustrum, (5) internal capsule, (6) insula, (7) thalamus

5.6.2 Globus Pallidus

The globus pallidus appears pale on sections. It constitutes the medial part of the lentiform nucleus.

The globus pallidus is composed of two parts:

- The pars interna.
- The pars externa.
- These parts are separated by the lamina medullaris medialis.

5.6.3 Putamen

The putamen is the largest and most lateral part of the lentiform nucleus. It is separated from the globus pallidus by the lamina medullaris lateralis.

The putamen and the caudate nucleus are interconnected by bundles of white matter. The area of white matter between the globus pallidus and putamen on the one hand and the caudate nucleus on the other hand is called the internal capsule. Laterally, the putamen is separated by the external capsule from the claustrum. The claustrum is an accumulation of gray matter and is separated from the insula by the extreme capsule.

5.6.4 Nucleus Accumbens

- It is situated between the caudate and putamen.
- It is divided into two structures:
  - the nucleus accumbens core
  - the nucleus accumbens shell

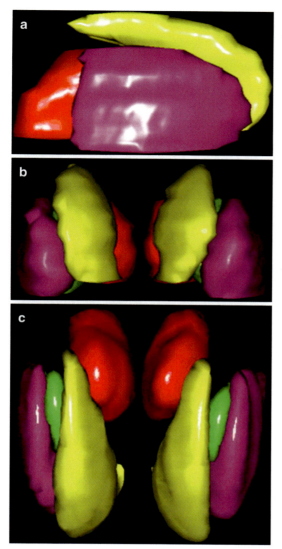

Fig. 5.16 Basal ganglia and thalamus as seen on 3D reconstruction (method: triangulation). Caudate nucleus (yellow), putamen (pink), globus pallidus (green), thalamus (red). Lateral view (right hemisphere) (**a**), anterior view (**b**), top view (**c**) (reproduced from Weis et al. (1992) with kind permission by Hogrefe Verlag)

5.7 White Matter

Due to its oval form on horizontal sections of the brain, the white matter of the telencephalon is called centrum semiovale (Fig. 5.17). By blunt dissection, different fiber systems of the white matter

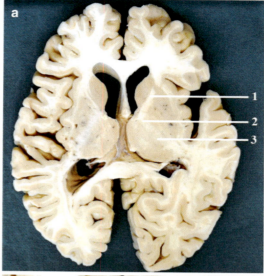

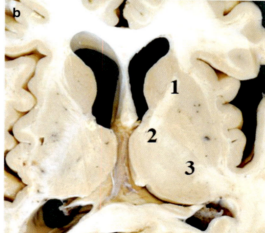

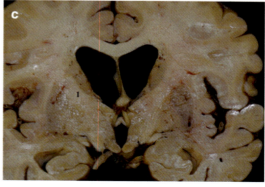

Fig. 5.17 Internal capsule seen on a horizontal section (**a**, **b**) and frontal section (**c**). Anterior limb (1), knee (2), posterior limb (3)

5.7 White Matter

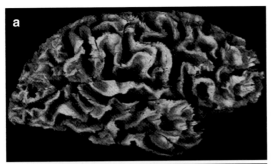
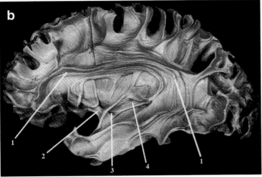

Fig. 5.18 Association fibers as seen on the superolateral face (**a**, **b**) after removal of the cerebral cortex (**a**) and after blunt dissection of white matter (**b**). (1) superior longitudinal fascicle, (2) uncinate fascicle, (3) insular fascicle, (4) inferior occipito-frontal fascicle, and (5) superior longitudinal fascicle (reproduced with kind permission from Ludwig and Klinger (1956))

become apparent (Fig. 5.18a, b). The fiber systems of the white matter are distinguished as follows:

- Projection fibers
- Association fibers
- Commissural fibers

5.7.1 Projection Fibers

Projection fibers conduct impulses from the cortex to centers located deep in the brain and vice versa. Projection fibers that project fan-like from inferior centers to the cortex are called corona radiata. At the rostral end of the brain stem, these fibers lie close together and form the internal capsule. The fibers which form the anterior limb of the internal capsule project horizontally, vertically, and laterally to the frontal lobe. Those fibers forming the posterior limb terminate in the parietal lobe. The fibers which project most posteriorly to the calcarine sulcus are called optic radiation.

The thalamocortical fascicle is the fiber system that contains all fibers connecting the thalamus with nearly all cortical areas. Other fiber systems connecting cortical regions with deeply located brain centers are the corticothalamic, corticopontine, corticobulbar, and corticospinal fascicles.

5.7.1.1 Internal Capsule

The area between the caudate nucleus and both the putamen and globus pallidus is called internal capsule (Fig. 5.17). The internal capsule contains all fiber systems that project from the cerebral cortex to deep brain centers as well as fibers that connect these deep brain centers with the cerebral cortex.

The internal capsule is made up of five parts which are best seen on horizontal sections (Fig. 5.17):

- The *anterior limb* of the internal capsule lies between the head of the caudate nucleus and both the putamen and globus pallidus.
- The *knee* of the internal capsule lies between the anterior and the posterior limb.
- The *posterior limb* of the internal capsule lies between the thalamus and both the putamen and globus pallidus.
- The *sublentiform part* of the internal capsule lies below the putamen and the globus pallidus.
- The *retrolentiform part* of the internal capsule lies behind the putamen and the globus pallidus.

5.7.2 Association Fibers

Association fibers connect cortical gyri within the same hemisphere. Short and long association fiber tracts are distinguished:

- Short association fibers connect adjacent gyri, but may sometimes skip one gyrus.
- Long association fibers connect distant gyri within the same hemisphere.

The following fascicles have been described (Fig. 5.18a, b):

- The *uncinate fascicle* is composed of fibers connecting the limen insulae with orbital gyri of the frontal lobe, as well as fibers which connect the middle and inferior frontal gyri with the anterior parts of the temporal lobe.
- The *arcuate fascicle* contains fibers that connect the middle and superior frontal gyri with the temporal lobe. Connection between Broca's expressive and Wernicke's receptive language areas.
- The *superior longitudinal fascicle* is composed of fibers that connect regions of the parietal lobe with regions of the occipital lobe.
- The *inferior longitudinal fascicle* contains fiber tracts that run from the occipital lobe to the temporal lobe.
- The *cingulum* is composed of fibers that are located in the cingulate gyrus. These fibers connect regions of the frontal lobe with the parahippocampal gyrus.

The external and extreme capsules also contain association fibers.

5.7.3 Commissural Fibers

Commissural fibers connect cortical regions of one hemisphere with the corresponding regions of the contralateral hemisphere as homotopic fibers, and non-corresponding regions of the contralateral hemisphere as heterotopic fibers.

5.7.3.1 Corpus Callosum

The corpus callosum is the largest commissural fiber system of the human brain (Fig. 5.19). Four

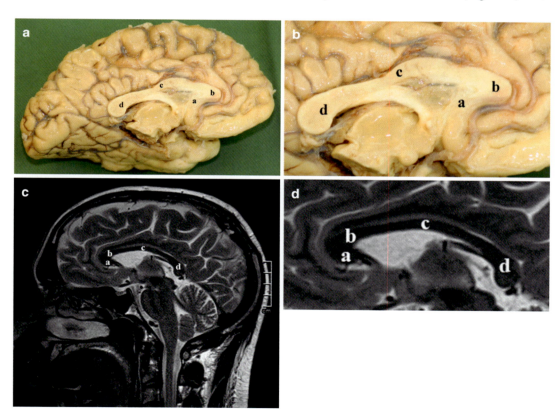

Fig. 5.19 The corpus callosum displayed on a median-sagittal plane (autopsy specimen, **a**, **b**) and MRI T2 (**c**, **d**). Rostrum (a), genu (b), trunk (c), splenium (d). Corpus callosum as seen on frontal slices (**e–l**) with genu corporis callosi (**e**, **f**), trunk (**g**, **h**), posterior parts of the trunk with underlying fornix (**i**, **j**), and splenium corporis callosi (**k**, **l**) with pineal gland

5.7 White Matter

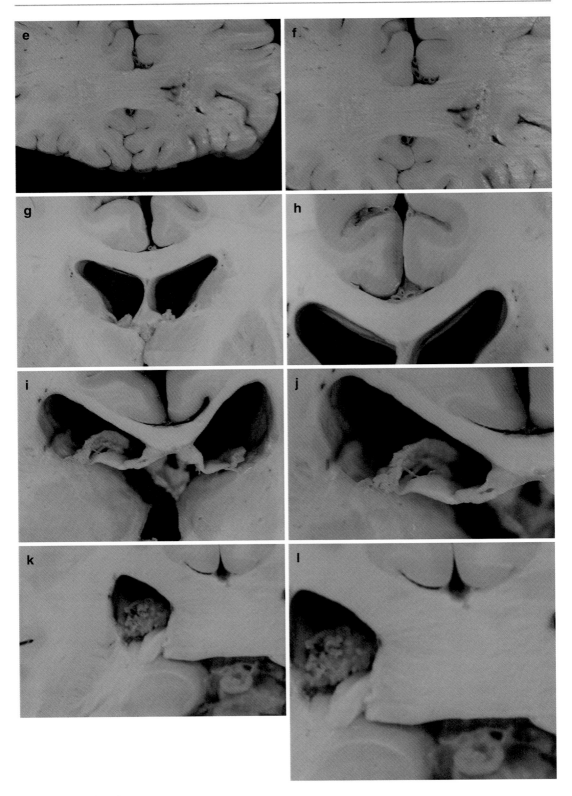

Fig. 5.19 (continued)

parts of the corpus callosum are distinguished from rostral towards the caudal end:

- Rostrum
- Genu
- Truncus
- Splenium

There exists no distinct boundary between these different parts. Callosal fibers also radiate fan-like to the telencephalon, called the radiatio corporis callosi.

The connections between the different cortical regions by callosal fibers are described as follows:

- *Rostrum:* Contains fibers from regions of the orbital surface of the frontal lobe and from deep layers of the extreme capsule.
- *Genu* (knee): Fibers from other regions of the frontal lobe cross through the knee.
- *Truncus* (trunk): The fibers connect the middle frontal gyrus, opercular part of the inferior frontal gyrus, inferior parietal lobule, superior and inferior temporal gyri, insula, cingulate gyrus, precentral gyrus, paracentral lobule, and precuneus.
- *Splenium:* Fibers from the occipital lobe, precuneus, and cuneus cross here and run to the contralateral hemisphere.

Fibers which cross through the splenium and run occipitally to separate the posterior horn of the lateral ventricle from the optic radiation are called tapetum. On horizontal sections, the fibers that connect both frontal lobes and both occipital lobes are called anterior forceps and posterior forceps, respectively.

It is covered on each side of the midline by two small white fascicules, the medial and lateral longitudinal striae.

5.7.3.2 Anterior Commissure

The anterior commissure contains 2–3 million fibers that interconnect regions of the frontal lobes and mainly the medial and inferior temporal gyri with the corresponding regions of the contralateral hemisphere (Fig. 5.20). Connections between the anterior olfactory nucleus to its contralateral olfactory bulb cross through the anterior commissure.

5.7.3.3 Ansa Lenticularis

The ansa lenticularis is a fiber pathway connecting the internal segment of the globus pallidus to the ventral lateral thalamic nuclei. It is involved in motor function.

5.8 Diencephalon

5.8.1 Thalamus

The thalamus is the largest part of the diencephalon (Figs. 5.21a–j and 5.22a–f). The thalamus extends from the lateral border of the third ventricle medially to the internal capsule. Ventrally, the thalamus is separated by the hypothalamic sulcus from the hypothalamus. The thalamus extends rostrally to the interventricular foramen, and posteriorly to the posterior commissure. The posterior part of the thalamus is broadened, and is called pulvinar. Sometimes, the right and the left thalami are connected by the interthalamic adhesion.

The medial geniculate body is located below and lateral to the pulvinar. It is connected by the brachium colliculi inferioris with the inferior colliculus and contains fibers of the auditory tract. Close and lateral to the medial geniculate body lies the lateral geniculate body. This is connected by the brachium colliculi superioris with the superior colliculus and contains fibers of the optic tract. The inferior and superior colliculi are part of the mesencephalon. The stratum zonale is a thin layer of fibers covering the thalamus. Another layer of fibers found close to the caudate nucleus is called lamina affixa. This is part of the floor of the lateral ventricle. The stria terminalis and the terminal vein are located where the thalamus and

5.8 Diencephalon

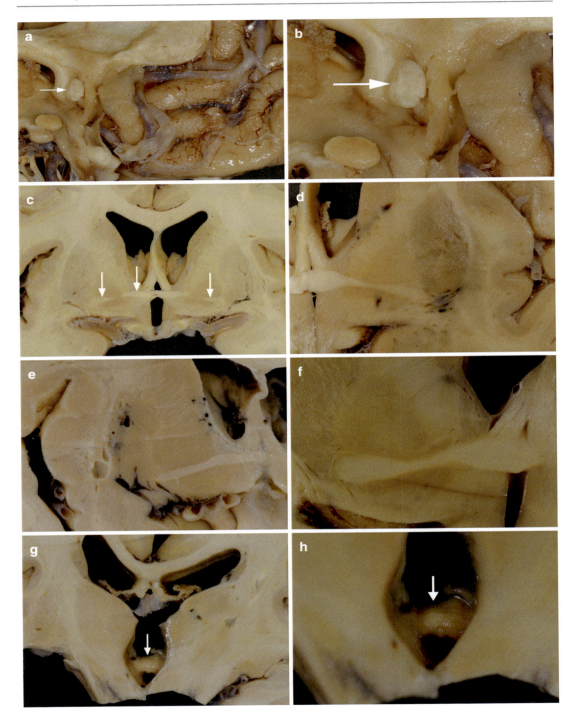

Fig. 5.20 The anterior commissure shown on a median-sagittal plane (→) (**a**, **b**), on frontal sections through the brain at the level of basal ganglia (**c–f**) and in the third ventricle at the level of the thalamus (**g**, **h**)

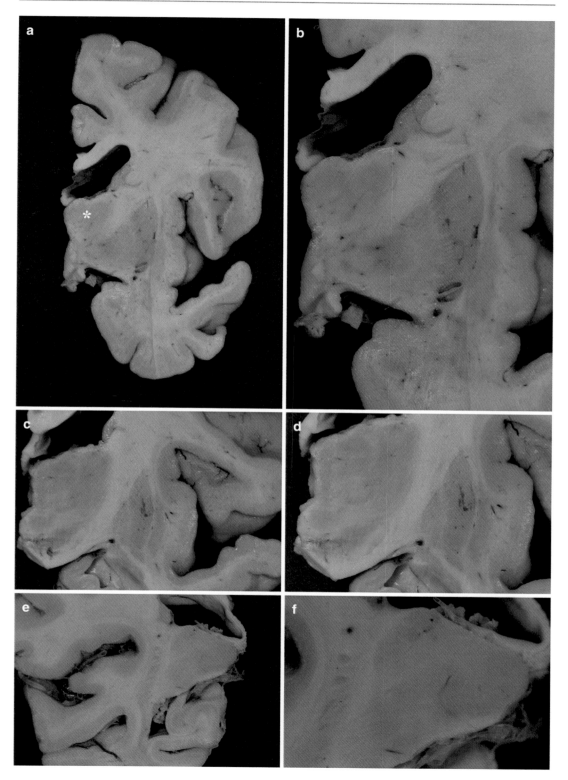

Fig. 5.21 Thalamus (∗) seen on frontal sections (**a–h**) and displayed on a median-sagittal plane (**i, j**) with the fornix running above it

5.8 Diencephalon

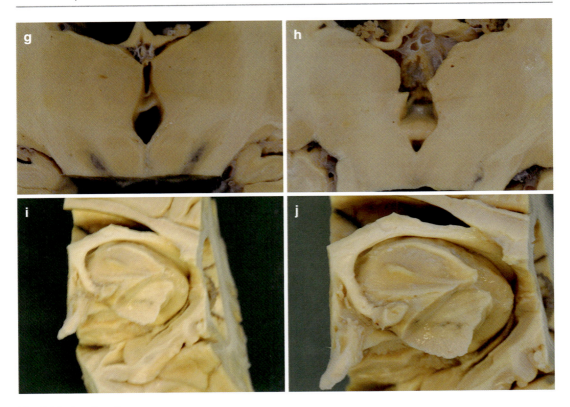

Fig. 5.21 (continued)

caudate nucleus lie next to each other. The stria medullaris is located dorsomedially.

Important functions of the organism are regulated by and coordinated in the thalamus. It is a relay station for afferent nerve fibers. The information carried by these fibers is filtered and processed in the thalamus and, subsequently, conducted to the cerebral cortex. Thus, the electrical activity of the cortex is regulated. Furthermore, the thalamus contains relay stations for nerve fibers from the basal ganglia and the cerebellum. It also fulfills some integrative functions of the motor system.

5.8.2 Hypothalamus

The hypothalamus lies beneath the thalamus and is separated from the latter by the hypothalamic sulcus. The hypothalamus forms part of the inferior and lateral walls of the third ventricle. The following structures are seen at its basal surface:

- Optic chiasm
- Infundibulum
- Tuber cinereum
- Mammillary bodies

The hypothalamus regulates functions of metabolism, body temperature, sleep, and emotional behavior.

5.8.2.1 Optic Chiasm

The optic chiasm represents that part of the optic tract where both optic nerves exchange fibers. In the optic chiasm, nasal fibers cross to the contralateral side, whereas temporal fibers project uncrossed to the ipsilateral side (Fig. 5.23a, b).

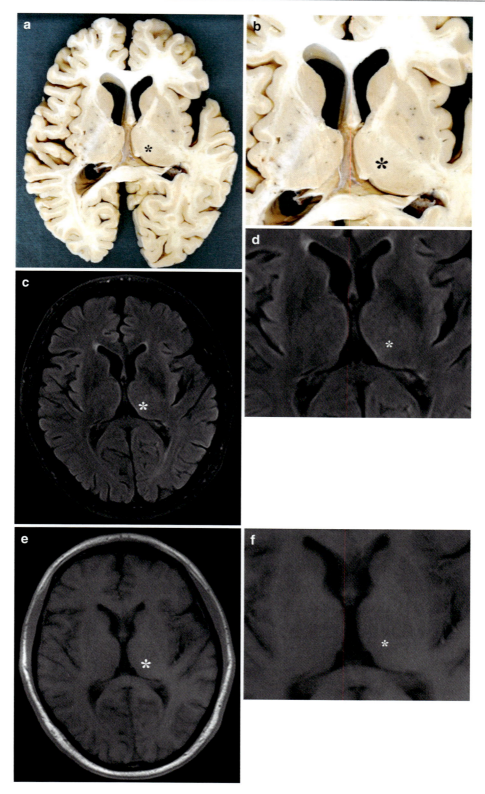

Fig. 5.22 Thalamus (∗) seen on a horizontal section (**a**, **b**). (1) Thalamus, (2) parietal lobe, (3) temporal lobe. MRI horizontal plane, Flair (**c**, **d**), T1 (**e**, **f**)

5.8 Diencephalon

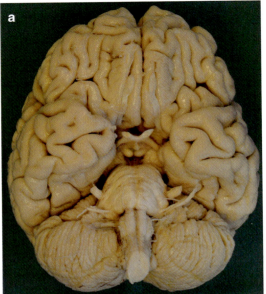

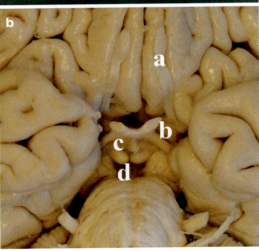

Fig. 5.23 View of the basal aspect of the brain (**a**, **b**) displaying the optic chiasm (a), infundibulum (b), the tuber cinereum (c), and the mammillary bodies (d)

5.8.2.2 Infundibulum
The infundibulum is the funnel-shaped connection between the hypothalamus and the hypophysis.

5.8.2.3 Tuber Cinereum
The tuber cinereum is composed of masses of gray matter which are located dorsal to the infundibulum.

5.8.2.4 Mammillary Bodies
The mammillary bodies are paired elevations at the floor of the diencephalon. They are connected with the thalamus, mesencephalon, and hippocampus (Fig. 5.23a, b).

5.8.2.5 Anterior Perforated Substance
The anterior perforated substance is a region near the optic chiasm where branches of the anterior cerebral artery perforate into the brain to supply the basal ganglia and internal capsule.

5.8.2.6 Olfactory Tubercle
The olfactory tubercle is a collection of neurons located in the anterior aspects of the anterior perforated substance.

5.8.3 Subthalamus

The subthalamus lies inferior to the thalamus, lateral to the hypothalamus, and medial to the internal capsule. The subthalamus is composed of various nuclear masses and contains several important fiber tracts.

5.8.4 Epithalamus

The epithalamus lies dorsally and is composed of:

- Taenia thalami
- Stria medullaris
- Habenula
- Pineal gland

5.8.4.1 Taenia Thalami
The taenia thalami is the tear-off area of the tela choroidea at the superior border of the third ventricle.

5.8.4.2 Stria Medullaris
The stria medullaris lies at the medial surface of the thalamus beneath the taenia thalami. The stria medullaris contains fiber tracts of the limbic system and of the fornix.

5.8.4.3 Habenula
The habenula is the dorsal continuation of the stria medullaris.

5.8.4.4 Pineal Gland

The pineal gland as part of the epithalamus lies between the laterally positioned thalamic bodies behind the habenular commissure in the quadrigeminal cistern near to the quadrigeminal plate and behind the third ventricle (Fig. 5.24a, b). The pineal gland is composed of a stroma rich in vessels and nerve cells, in which the pinealocytes are embedded. Pinealocytes produce the hormones serotonin and melatonin. The pineal gland regulates the diurnal-nocturnal biorhythm by endogenous secretion of its products.

5.9 Mesencephalon

The mesencephalon forms the rostral part of the brain stem (Figs. 5.25 and 5.26). On its posterior surface, the superior colliculus and the inferior colliculus are seen. The superior and inferior colliculi are collectively termed quadrigeminal bodies (lamina quadrigemina or tectum mesencephali). The superior colliculus is an important relay station for the visual pathway, whereas the inferior colliculus is a nuclear mass where fiber tract of the auditory pathway are switched. Large fiber tracts, the cerebral peduncles, are seen on the lateral surface of the mesencephalon. The cerebral peduncles contain projection fibers that connect regions of the telencephalon with deeply located centers. The following fiber tracts compose the cerebral peduncles: fibrae pontinae, fibrae corticonucleares, tractus corticospinalis, fibrae parietotemporopontinae. The region that is located between the crura cerebri and below the mammillary bodies is the fossa interpeduncularis. On horizontal sections, the tegmentum is recognized to be that part of the mesencephalon that lies anterior to the cerebral aqueduct, which in turn is surrounded by a gray mass: the substantia centralis grisea.

The tegmentum and the crura cerebri are separated by a pigmented nuclear mass, the substantia nigra. In the tegmentum medial to the substantia nigra lies the oval nucleus ruber, which is also a pigmented mass displaying on fresh sections a red color owing to its rich blood supply. The substantia nigra and the nucleus ruber are both important relay stations for the locomotor system.

5.10 Pons

The pons is continuous with the mesencephalon (Figs. 5.27 and 5.28). The anterior view of the pons displays a slightly corrugated surface showing no major details. In the midline, a small

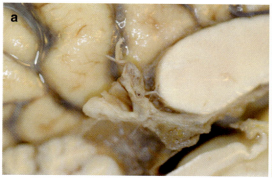 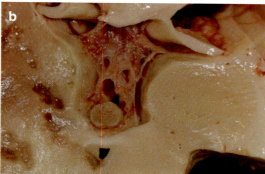

Fig. 5.24 Pineal gland seen on a median-sagittal plane (**a**) and frontal slice (**b**)

5.10 Pons

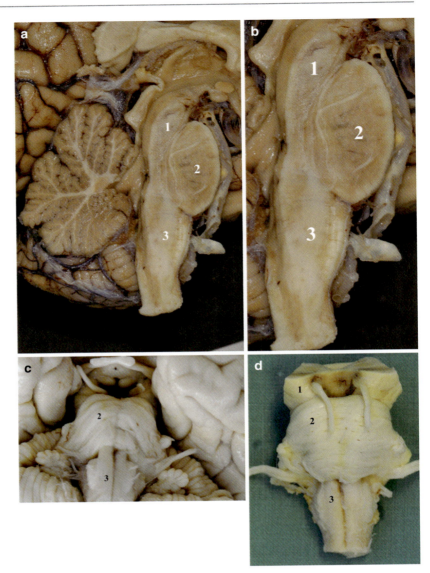

Fig. 5.25 Median-sagittal (**a**, **b**) and anterior (**c**, **d**) view of the brain stem. (1) mesencephalon, (2) pons, (3) medulla oblongata

impression, the basilar fissure, is sometimes seen, which harbors the basilar artery.

After removing the cerebellum from the brain stem, the rhomboid fossa is seen. This is divided into two symmetrical parts by the median fissure. The fossa is further divided into an upper and a lower part by the transversely running striae medullares. The surface of the rhomboid fossa appears bumpy due to the nuclear masses lying underneath. Lateral to the median fissure, the medial eminence protrudes in the upper part of the rhomboid fossa; this

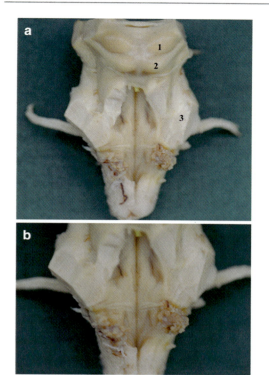

Fig. 5.26 Posterior view of the brain stem. (1) Superior colliculus, (2) inferior colliculus, (3) cerebellar peduncle

elongated bulging structure is laterally bounded by the sulcus limitans. Below the medial eminence the facial colliculus is found. It is formed by the knee of the facial nerve and the abducens nucleus. The facial colliculus abut upon the striae medullares.

Below the striae medullares, from the midline lateralwards, the trigonum of the hypoglossal nerve, the trigonum of the vagal nerve, and the vestibular area are seen. The lateral recess ends through the lateral aperture into the outer cerebrospinal fluid spaces.

The area postrema is located at the inferolateral border of the rhomboid fossa. The former is a small triangular field composed of highly vascularized tissue containing many glial cells. In this region, there is no blood–brain barrier.

Many fiber tracts as well as nuclear masses (nuclei pontes) are found in the pons. These fiber tracts connect different areas of the telencephalon with the cerebellum, the spinal cord, and the motor cranial nerves. The nuclei pontes represent the relay station of these fiber tracts.

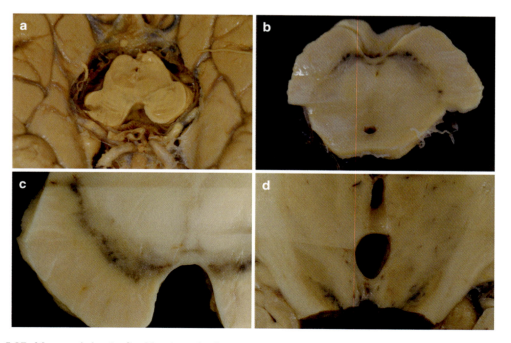

Fig. 5.27 Mesencephalon (**a**–**d**) with substantia nigra seen on a horizontal section (**b**, **c**) and on a frontal section (**d**). MRI horizontal plane, Flair (**e**, **f**), T1 (**g**, **h**)

5.10 Pons

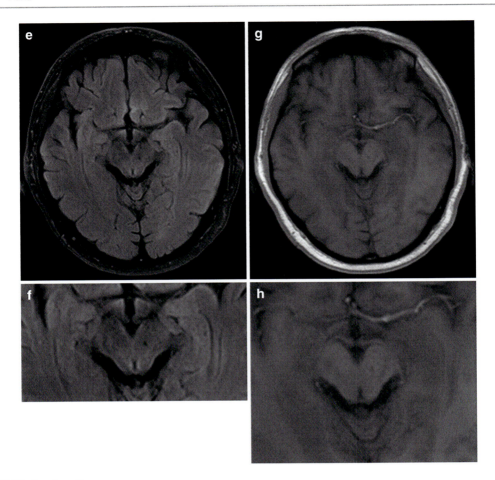

Fig. 5.27 (continued)

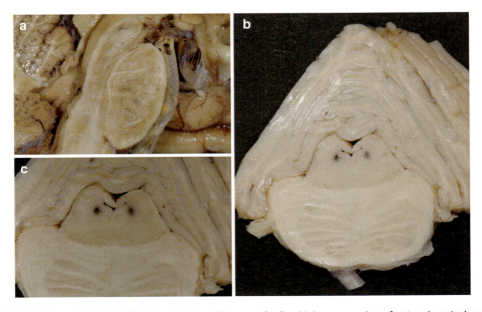

Fig. 5.28 Median-sagittal (**a**) and horizontal view of the pons (**b–d**) with locus coeruleus (**b, c**) and vertical and horizontal fiber tracts and nuclei (**d**). MRI horizontal plane, Flair (**e, f**), T1 (**g**)

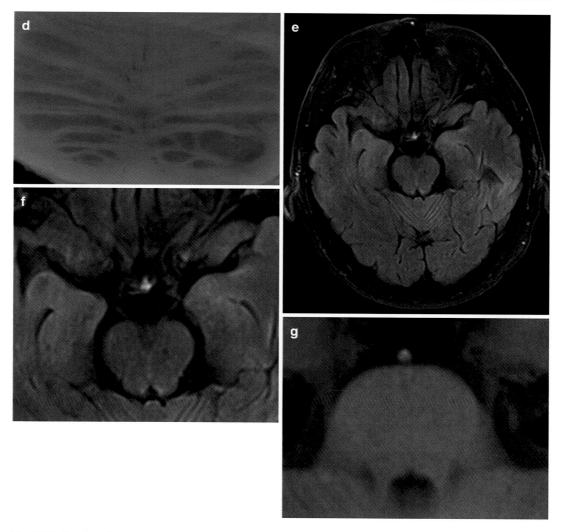

Fig. 5.28 (continued)

5.11 Medulla Oblongata

The medulla oblongata is the lowest part of the brain stem (Figs. 5.29 and 5.30). There is no strict boundary between the medulla oblongata and the spinal cord. However, for practical purposes, this border is drawn at the foramen magnum and at the decussatio pyramidum. The anterior view displays the medulla oblongata to be divided by the anterior median fissure into symmetrical halves. Lateral to this fissure is located the pyramid. The pyramid contains fibers of the pyramidal tract, which connect the precentral gyrus with the spinal cord and are concerned with motion. Several millimeters below the pyramid, the decussatio pyramidum is seen, where 90% of the fibers of the pyramidal tract cross the midline to the contralateral side. The pyramid is laterally separated by the ventrolateral sulcus from the olive, which contains the olivary nucleus. The lateral border of the olive is formed by the retroolivary sulcus. Caudal to the pyramid and the olive, the anterior external arcuate fibers run transversely.

The posterior view of the medulla oblongata displays the posterior median fissure, which

5.11 Medulla Oblongata

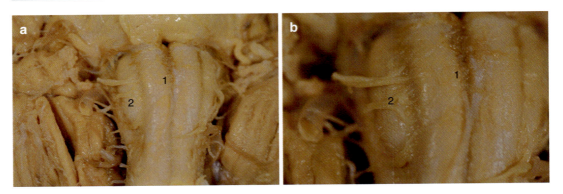

Fig. 5.29 Anterior view of the medulla oblongata with (1) pyramis and (2) inferior olivary nucleus (**a**, **b**)

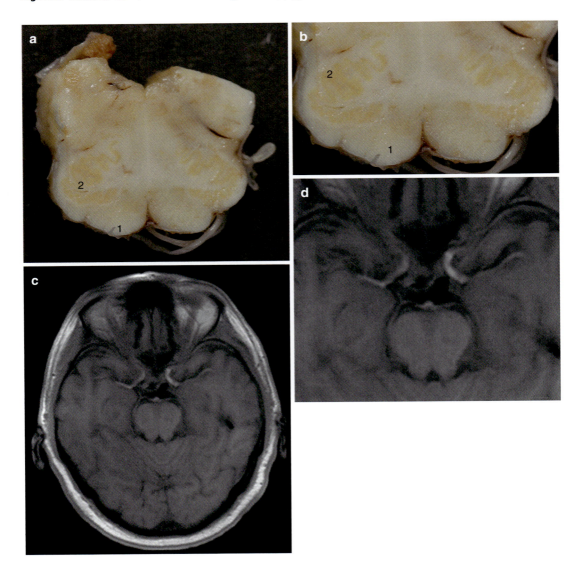

Fig. 5.30 Cross-sectional view of the medulla oblongata with (1) pyramis and (2) inferior olivary nucleus (**a**, **b**). MRI horizontal plane T1 (**c**, **d**)

divides the medulla into symmetrical halves. Lateral to the posterior median fissure is located the gracile fascicle which ends in the gracile tubercle. Beneath the bulge of the gracile tubercle is located the gracile nucleus. Lateral to the gracile fascicle lies the cuneate fascicle, which ends cranially in the cuneate tubercle. The bulge of the cuneate tubercle contains the cuneate nucleus. Both tubercles contain nuclear masses where sensory fibers of the spinal cord synapse.

The medulla oblongata contains the nuclei of the VIIIth, IXth, Xth, XIth, and XIIth cranial nerves. The XIIth cranial nerve leaves the medulla at the level of the ventrolateral sulcus, whereas the VIIIth, IXth, Xth, and XIth cranial nerves leave at the level of the retroolivary sulcus.

5.12 Cerebellum

The cerebellum is located in the posterior cranial fossa posterior to the pons and medulla oblongata (Figs. 5.31 and 5.32). The cerebellum is composed of two cerebellar hemispheres which are connected by an unpaired structure, the vermis. Many sulci and small gyri, called cerebellar foliae, are seen at its surface. A few deep fissures subdivide the cerebellar surface into lobes and lobules.

At the cerebellar surface, a cranial surface lying adjacent to the tentorium cerebelli and a caudal surface lying at the floor of the posterior cranial fossa are discerned. At the cranial surface, the fissura prima and the superior posterior fissure are seen. The fissura prima borders the anterior lobe. The posterior quadrangular lobule extends between the fissura prima and the superior anterior fissure. The superior semilunar lobule is adjacent to the superior posterior fissure. This lobule is separated by the horizontal fissure from the inferior semilunar lobule. Caudally, the gracile lobule, lobulus biventer, the tonsil, and the flocculus are seen. Distinct fissures separating these lobuli are regularly present but difficult to discern.

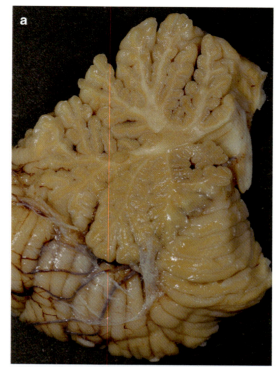

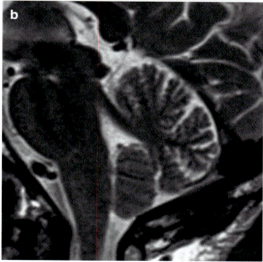

Fig. 5.31 Cerebellum-Vermis. Median-sagittal view (**a**, **b**). MRI median-sagittal plane T2 (**b**)

In summary, the cerebellum is composed of two lobes, i.e., the anterior and posterior lobes (Fig. 5.32a, b). The anterior lobe is separated by the fissura prima from the posterior lobe.

5.13 Spinal Cord

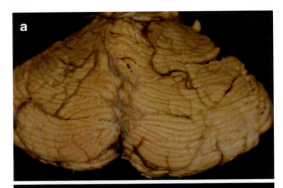

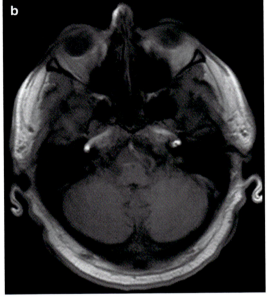

Fig. 5.32 View of the surface of the cerebellum

The anterior lobe is formed by the ala lobuli centralis and the lobulus quadrangularis anterior. The posterior lobe is formed by the lobulus quadrangularis posterior, lobulus semilunaris superior, lobulus semilunaris inferior, lobulus gracilis, lobulus biventer, the cerebellar tonsil, and the flocculus.

After cutting the cerebral hemispheres at the level of the vermis, the picture of the "arbor vitae" is displayed at the median-sagittal plane (Fig. 5.33). The following parts of the vermis are distinguished caudalwards:

- Lingula
- Lobulus centralis
- Culmen
- Declive
- Folium
- Tuber
- Pyramis
- Uvula
- Nodulus

The correspondence of various parts of the vermis to the cerebellar lobules is given in Table 5.1.

Within the cerebellar hemispheres four nuclear masses are noted (Fig. 5.34a, b):

- Dentate nucleus
- Emboliform nucleus
- Globose nucleus
- Fastigial nucleus

The cerebellum is connected by the superior, middle, and inferior cerebellar peduncles with the brain stem.

The cerebellum is functionally concerned with the coordination of locomotion, the control of muscle tone, and the regulation of equilibrium.

5.13 Spinal Cord

The spinal cord is a long cylindrical structure lying within the vertebral canal that extends from the medulla oblongata to the level of the first and second lumbar vertebrae. On average, the spinal cord is 45 cm long and has a diameter of 6–12 mm (Fig. 5.35).

The caudal end of the spinal cord is called conus medullaris (Fig. 5.35). From the conus medullaris the filum terminal arises. The latter is a filamentous thread of non-neural tissue extending from the conus medullaris and anchoring the spinal cord and the dural sac to the base of the vertebral canal.

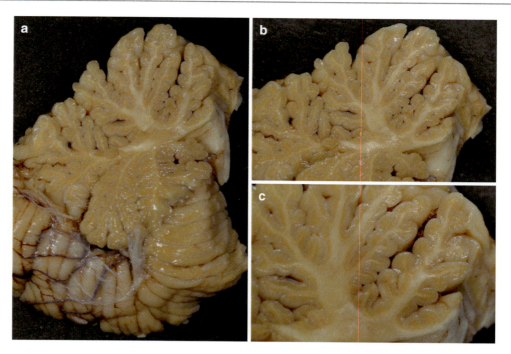

Fig. 5.33 View of the cerebellar vermis (a–c)

Table 5.1 The various parts of the vermis correspond to the various lobules of the cerebellar hemispheres

Cerebellar hemisphere	Vermis
Ala lobuli centralis	Lobulus centralis
Lobulus quadrangularis anterior	Culmen
Lobulus quadrangularis posterior	Declive
Lobulus semilunaris superior	Folium
Lobulus semilunaris inferior	Tuber
Lobulus gracilis	Tuber
Lobulus biventer	Pyramis
Tonsilla cerebelli	Uvula
Flocculus	Nodulus

The following enlargements are noted along the spinal cord:

- cervical enlargement at the level of C4-Th1
- lumbosacral enlargement at the level of L1-S2

On the surface of the spinal cord, the following fissures are noted:

- ventromedian fissure at the anterior surface
- ventrolateral sulcus
- dorsolateral sulcus
- dorso-median sulcus at the posterior surface

At the level of the upper cervical and mid-thoracic spinal cord, a dorsal-intermediate sulcus might be noted at the posterior surface.

Thirty-one pairs of spinal nerves are connected to the spinal cord. Dorsal roots as part of the spinal nerve contain sensory nerve fibers from the neuronal perikarya located in the dorsal root ganglia into the spinal cord. Motor nerve fibers from neurons located in the ventral portion of the spinal cord leave via the ventral roots (composition of peripheral nerve, see chapter) (Fig. 5.36).

5.14 Pituitary Gland

Synonym used: hypophysis.

The pituitary gland is a bean-shaped organ located in the sella turcica of the sphenoid bone (Fig. 5.37). It weighs approximately 0.6 g. The size of the pituitary gland is given as follows: 13 mm in its transverse axis, 9 mm in its anterior-posterior axis, and 6 mm in its vertical axis. The size of the gland is larger in pregnant and postpartum females.

5.14 Pituitary Gland

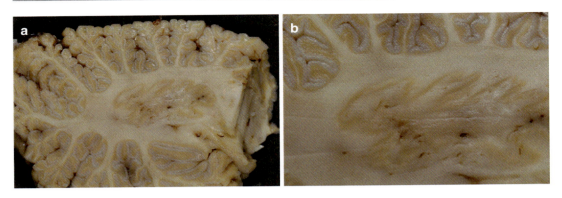

Fig. 5.34 Cerebellar dentate nucleus (**a**, **b**)

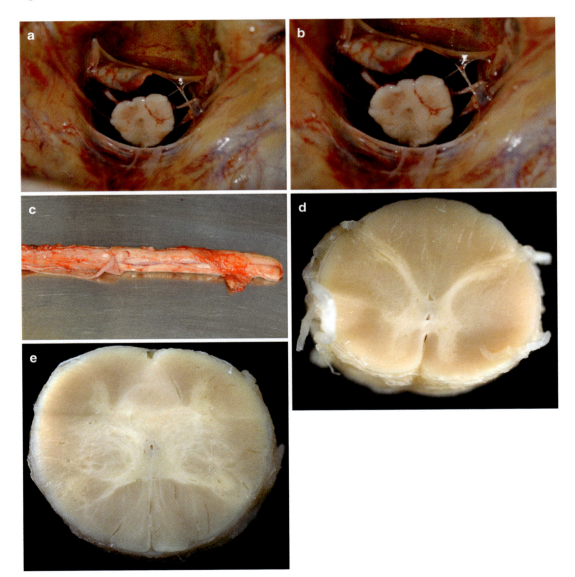

Fig. 5.35 Spinal cord (**a–e**) within the spinal canal (**a**, **b**), after removal (**c**), horizontal sections through the fixed spinal cord (**d**, **e**)

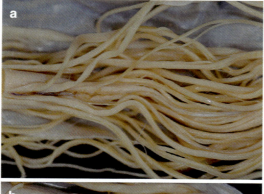

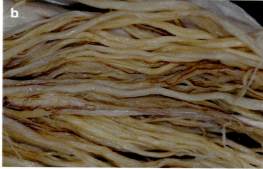

Fig. 5.36 Conus medullaris, cauda equina, and filum terminale (**a**, **b**)

Two parts can be distinguished:

- Adenohypophysis (red-brown epithelial gland)
  - Anterior lobe of the pituitary
- Neurohypophysis (firm gray neural structure)

The diaphragma sellae, a reflection of the dura mater, constitutes the roof the sella turcica. The hypophyseal stalk passes through the opening of the diaphragm and connects the pituitary with the hypothalamus.

5.15 3D Reconstructions of the Brain and Cutplanes

The 3D reconstructions and cutplanes shown in Figs. 5.38, 5.39, 5.40, and 5.41 were rendered by R. Thaler and E. Wenger within the frame work of the published book of Weis et al. (1992) but never published in this form. They serve to test the acquired knowledge about the topographical arrangements of the various brain structures.

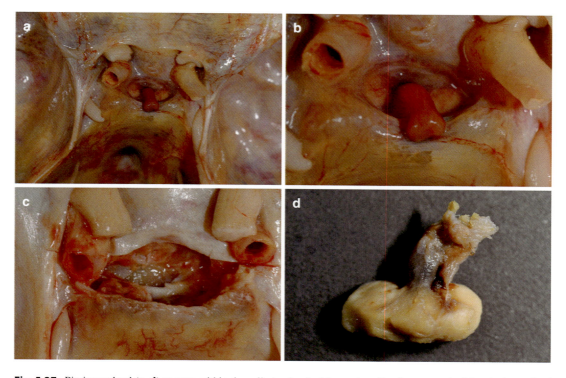

Fig. 5.37 Pituitary gland (**a–d**) as seen within the sella turcica (**a**, **b**), empty sella after removal of the pituitary gland (**c**), removed pituitary gland with stalk (**d**)

5.15 3D Reconstructions of the Brain and Cutplanes

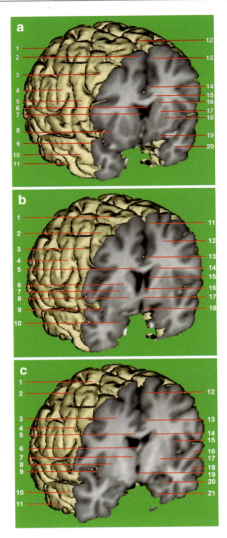
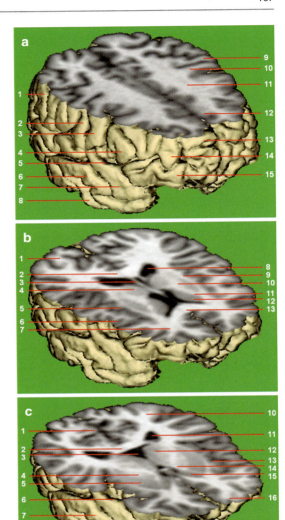

Fig. 5.38 Frontal cutplanes (**a**): (1) parietal lobe, (2) superior frontal gyrus, (3) middle frontal gyrus, (4) postcentral gyrus, (5) precentral gyrus, (6) septum pellucidum, (7) lateral ventricle, (8) insula, (9) superior temporal gyrus, (10) middle temporal gyrus, (11) inferior temporal gyrus, (12) longitudinal fissure, (13) medial frontal gyrus, (14) cingulate gyrus, (15) corpus callosum, (16) caudate nucleus, (17) internal capsule, (18) putamen, (19) orbital frontal gyri, (20) temporal white matter. (**b**): (1) superior frontal gyrus, (2) middle frontal gyrus, (3) precentral gyrus, (4) postcentral gyrus, (5) corpus callosum, (6) internal capsule, (7) putamen, (8) globus pallidus, (9) insula, (10) amygdala, (11) medial frontal gyrus, (12) centrum semiovale, (13) cingulate gyrus, (14) caudate nucleus, (15) lateral ventricle, (16) septum pellucidum, (17) anterior commissure, (18) optic chiasm. (**c**): (1) precentral gyrus, (2) postcentral gyrus, (3) centrum semiovale, (4) central sulcus, (5) corpus callosum, (6) fornix, (7) thalamus, (8) putamen, (9) lateral sulcus, (10) middle temporal gyrus, (11) inferior temporal gyrus, (12) medial frontal gyrus, (13) cingulate gyrus, (14) caudate nucleus, (15) insula, (16) superior temporal gyrus, (17) globus pallidus, (18) middle temporal gyrus, (19) third ventricle, (20) hippocampus, (21) parahippocampal gyrus

Fig. 5.39 Horizontal cutplanes. (**a**): (1) parietal lobe, (2) postcentral gyrus, (3) precentral gyrus, (4) inferior frontal gyrus, (5) lateral sulcus, (6) middle temporal gyrus, (7) superior frontal gyrus, (8) inferior temporal gyrus, (9) postcentral gyrus, (10) precentral gyrus, (11) centrum semiovale, (12) medial frontal gyrus, (13) superior frontal gyrus, (14) middle frontal gyrus, (15) inferior frontal gyrus. (**b**): (1) occipital lobe, (2) corpus callosum, splenium, (3) septum pellucidum, (4) thalamus, (5) insula, (6) inferior frontal gyrus, (7) frontal white matter, (8) lateral ventricle, posterior horn, (9) external capsule, (10) globus pallidus, (11) internal capsule, (12) caudate nucleus, (13) corpus callosum, knee. (**c**): (1) calcarine cortex, (2) corpus callosum, splenium, (3) third ventricle, (4) globus pallidus, (5) putamen, (6) lateral sulcus, (7) middle temporal gyrus, (8) superior temporal gyrus, (9) inferior temporal gyrus, (10) occipital white matter, (11) lateral ventricle, posterior horn, (12) thalamus, (13) insula, (14) internal capsule, (15) caudate nucleus, (16) frontal lobe

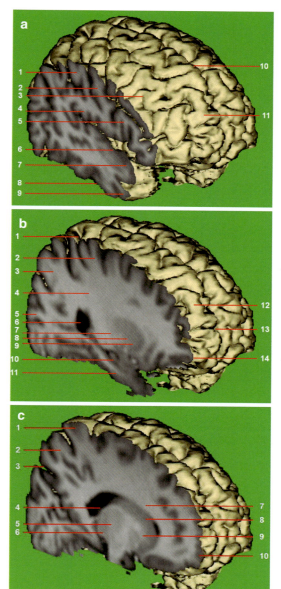

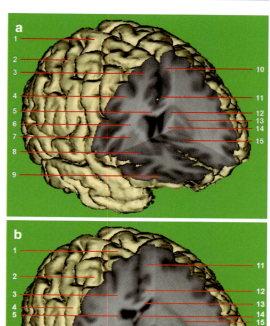

Fig. 5.40 Sagittal cutplanes. (**a**): (1) postcentral gyrus, (2) precentral gyrus, (3) middle frontal gyrus, (4) insula, (5) inferior frontal gyrus, (6) lateral sulcus, (7) superior temporal gyrus, (8) inferior temporal gyrus, (9) middle temporal gyrus, (10) longitudinal cerebral fissure, (11) superior frontal gyrus. (**b**): (1) central sulcus, (2) precentral gyrus, (3) parietal lobe, (4) centrum semiovale, (5) occipital lobe, (6) lateral ventricle, (7) thalamus, (8) globus pallidus, (9) putamen, (10) hippocampus, (11) parahippocampal gyrus, (12) superior frontal gyrus, (13) longitudinal cerebral fissure, (14) middle frontal gyrus. (**c**): (1) postcentral gyrus, (2) parietal lobe, (3) parieto-occipital sulcus, (4) lateral ventricle, (5) thalamus, (6) quadrigeminal bodies, (7) corpus callosum, (8) caudate nucleus, (9) putamen, (10) superior frontal gyrus

Fig. 5.41 Combined cutplanes. (**a**): (1) precentral gyrus, (2) postcentral gyrus, (3) superior frontal gyrus, (4) middle frontal gyrus, (5) corpus callosum, (6) centrum semiovale, (7) putamen, (8) putamen, (9) orbital frontal gyri, (10) medial frontal gyrus, (11) cingulate gyrus, (12) caudate nucleus, (13) caudate nucleus, (14) internal capsule, (15) caudate nucleus. (**b**): (1) superior frontal gyrus, (2) precentral gyrus, (3) centrum semiovale, (4) postcentral gyrus, (5) caudate nucleus, (6) thalamus, (7) internal capsule, (8) globus pallidus, (9) insula, (10) frontal orbital gyri, (11) medial frontal gyrus, (12) cingulate gyrus, (13) corpus callosum, (14) septum pellucidum, (15) caudate nucleus, (16) caudate nucleus

Selected References

Ludwig E, Klinger J (1956) Atlas Cerebri Humani. The inner structure of the brain. Little, Brown and Company, Karger Verlag, Boston, Toronto

Weis S, Thaller R, Villringer A, Wenger E (1992) Das Gehirn des Menschen. Morphologie, Kernspintomographie und 3D-Computerrekonstruktion. Hogrefe Verlag für Psychologie, Göttingen, Torornto, Zürich

Ventricular System: Cerebrospinal Fluid (CSF)—Barriers

6.1 Introduction

The ventricles are filled by a colorless, watery liquid called cerebrospinal fluid (CSF). CSF buffers the brain from mechanical injury by reducing its effective weight from 1400 g to less than 50 g.

6.2 Ventricular System

The ventricular system is composed of hollow cavities which are located in the telencephalon, diencephalon, and mesencephalon and extend via the pons to the medulla oblongata (Figs. 6.1 and 6.2). Four communicating compartments of the ventricles and their connections are distinguished:

- Lateral ventricles (ventricle 1 and 2)
- Third ventricle
- Fourth ventricle
- Interventricular foramen (connecting the lateral and the third ventricles)
- Cerebral aqueduct (connecting the third and the fourth ventricles)
- Central canal (an extension of the ventricular system into the medulla oblongata and spinal cord)

6.2.1 Lateral Ventricles

The lateral ventricles are located in the telencephalon (Figs. 6.3 and 6.4). The following parts of the lateral ventricles and their corresponding locations are noted:

- Anterior horn in the frontal lobe
- Posterior horn in the occipital lobe
- Central part (the communicating part between the anterior and posterior horns)
- Inferior horn in the temporal lobe

The boundaries of the lateral ventricles are made up of the following structures:

- *Anterior horn*:
  - superiorly, anteriorly, and inferiorly by the corpus callosum
  - laterally by the head of the caudate nucleus
  - medially by the thin septum pellucidum
- *Posterior horn*:
  - medially by the splenium of the corpus callosum
  - laterally by calcar avis and optic radiation
- *Central part*:
  - superiorly by the trunk of the corpus callosum
  - inferiorly and medially by the thalamus

Fig. 6.1 Drawing of the brain displaying the ventricular system (lateral ventricles) in a horizontal plane (**a**) and in a posterior-lateral plane (**b**) (reproduced from Heimer (1983) with kind permission by Springer Nature)

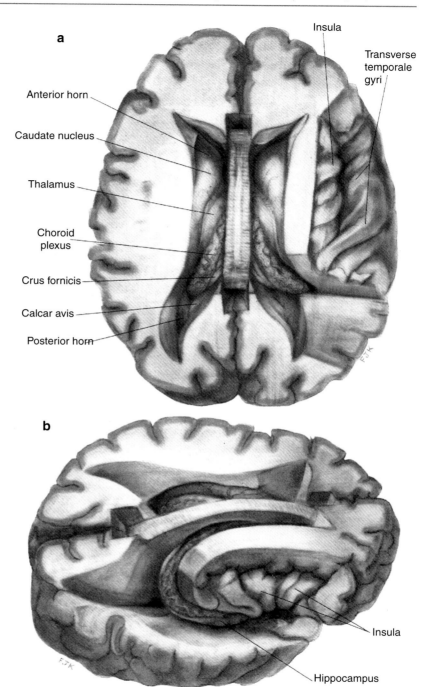

6.2 Ventricular System

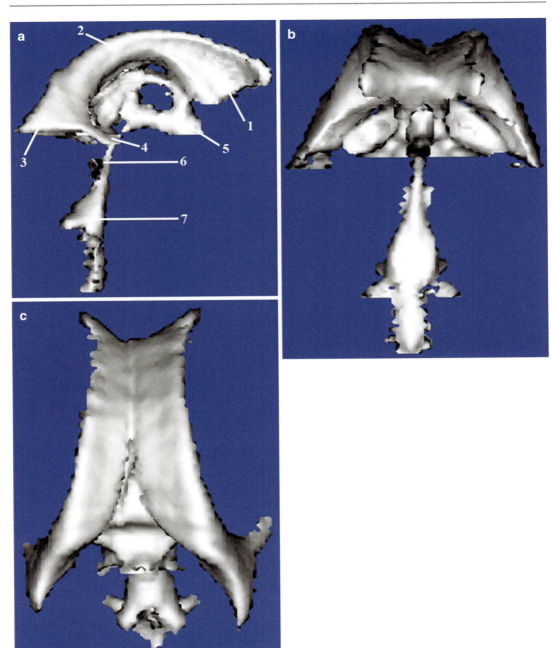

Fig. 6.2 3D reconstruction of the ventricular system: lateral view (**a**), anterior view (**b**), view from above (**c**). (1) anterior horn of the lateral ventricle, (2) central part of the lateral ventricle, (3) posterior horn of the lateral ventricle, (4) inferior horn of the lateral ventricle, (5) Location of the interthalamic adhesion, (5) third ventricle (6) cerebral aqueduct, (7) fourth ventricle (reproduced from Weis et al. (1992) with kind permission by Hogrefe Verlag)

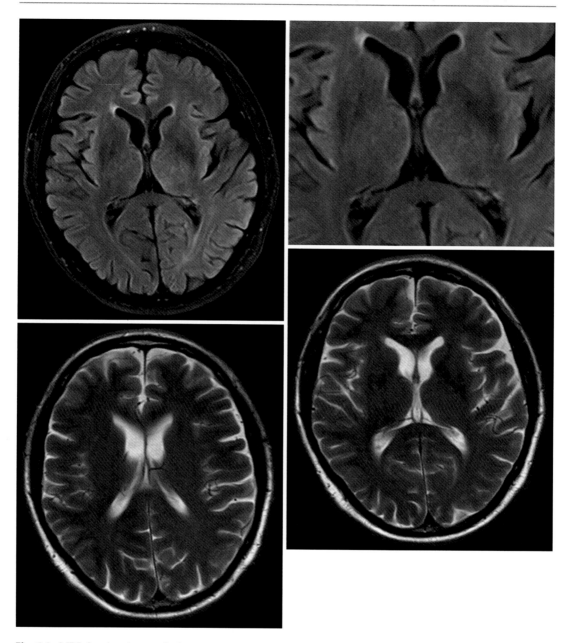

Fig. 6.3 MRI showing the ventricular system

6.2 Ventricular System

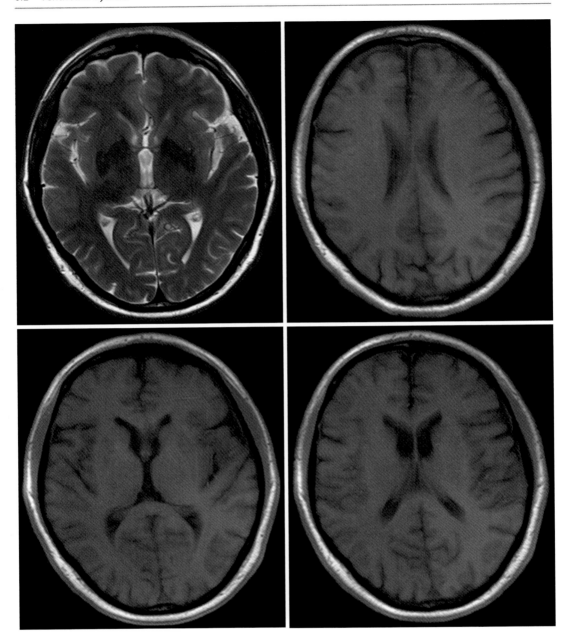

Fig. 6.3 (continued)

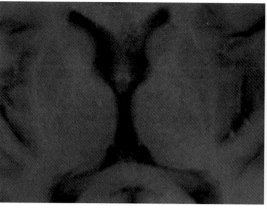
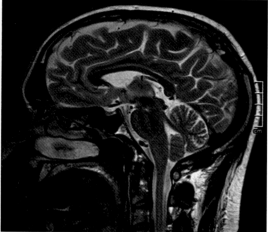

Fig. 6.3 (continued)

- *Inferior horn*:
  - inferiorly by the hippocampus
  - superiorly by the cauda of the caudate nucleus
  - laterally by the optic radiation
  - medially by the choroid plexus

6.2.2 Third Ventricle

The lateral ventricles drain via the interventricular foramen below the septum pellucidum into the unpaired third ventricle. The latter is located at the level of the diencephalon and is bounded by thalami as well as by the hypothalamus. The third ventricle communicates via the cerebral aqueduct with the fourth ventricle. The cerebral aqueduct is located in the posterior part of the mesencephalon.

6.2.3 Fourth Ventricle

The fourth ventricle is located at the level of the rhomboid fossa. Its anterior border is formed by the structure underlying the rhomboid fossa. The roof of the fourth ventricle is formed by the superior medullary velum which extends between both superior cerebellar peduncles. Its connection with the lamina quadrigemina is called frenulum veli medullare. The inferior medullary velum connects the flocculus with the cerebellar nodule. A communication between the fourth ventricle and the external cerebrospinal fluid spaces is formed by the two lateral apertures and the medial aperture. The medial aperture is located at the level of the obex which forms the inferior medial border of the rhomboid fossa.

6.3 Cerebrospinal Fluid (CSF)

All ventricles contain the cerebrospinal fluid (CSF) which is produced by the choroid plexuses found in the lateral and the fourth ventricles. The cerebrospinal fluid fulfills a nutritive and protective function of the brain. Approximately 140 mL of CSF are contained within the ventricular system and the subarachnoidal spaces. In humans, the turnover in the production of CSF is approximately 700 mL per day. As compared to serum, CSF is composed mainly of water and contains higher levels of sodium chloride but lower levels of proteins, glucose, and potassium.

Most of the CSF is passively absorbed by the arachnoidal villi and drained into the venous

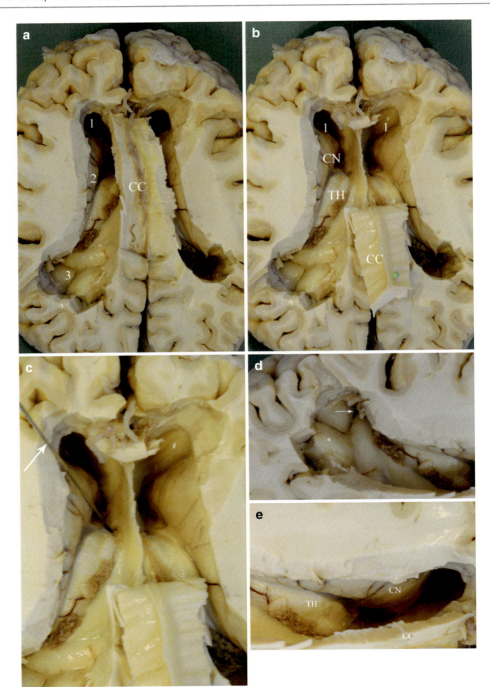

Fig. 6.4 Gross-anatomical preparation of the ventricular system. After removal of a slab of brain tissue at the lower level of the interhemispheric fissure, the lateral ventricle with its anterior horn (1), central part (2), and posterior horn (3) becomes apparent (**a**). Corpus callosum (CC) is seen in (**a**). After partial removal of the anterior parts of the corpus callosum (CC), the anterior horns (1) are seen (**b**) the head of the caudate nucleus (CN) and the thalamus (TH) are seen. Enlarged view of (**b**) in (**c**). The probe (→) is placed in the interventricular foramen. View of the posterior horn (∗) and route to the inferior horn (→) (**d**). View into the central part displaying the corpus callosum (CC), caudate nucleus (CN), and the thalamus (TH) (**e**). View of the third ventricle on a median-sagittal section (1) thalamus, (2) interthalamic adhesion, (3) commissural anterior, (4) optic chiasm, interventricular foramen (→) (**f**). Fourth ventricle with parts of the cerebellum and pons. Cerebral aqueduct (→) (**g**)

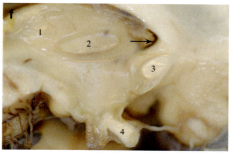
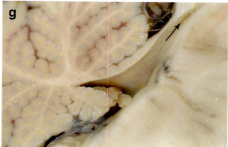

Fig. 6.4 (continued)

system. An overproduction of CSF or an obstruction of the draining routes lead to an intraventricular accumulation of CSF which can be associated with the clinical signs and symptoms of hydrocephalus.

6.4 Choroid Plexus

The choroid plexus is the production site for the cerebrospinal fluid (Fig. 6.5).

It is found in the following locations:

- body and inferior horns of the lateral ventricle
- interventricular foramen of Monro
- roof of the third ventricle
- roof and lateral recesses of the fourth ventricle

It is absent in the following locations:

- anterior and posterior horns of the lateral ventricles
- aqueduct

6.5 Barriers

The brain is protected from the surrounding structures by barriers. The exchange of chemical substances between the arterial blood, the CSF, and the brain is regulated by the barrier system. Thus, a stabilization of the physical and chemical milieu of the CNS is achieved and the normal functioning of the neurons is granted.

The following barriers may be distinguished:

- blood–brain barrier BBB
- brain–liquor barrier BLB
- blood–liquor barrier

6.5.1 The Blood–Brain Barrier (BBB)

The blood–brain barrier is composed of the endothelial cells of the capillaries, the basal lamina, and the astrocytic foot processes and separates the blood plasma from the intercellular spaces of the CNS. Only several substances can cross the BBB through a special filtration system. This is of great importance for applied pharmacology since drugs have to be developed which are small enough to cross the BBB but still develop therapeutic effects.

6.5.2 The Brain–Liquor Barrier (BLB)

The brain–liquor barrier is formed by the ependymal layer of the ventricular system and the adjacent glial elements. Chemical substances are filtrated on their route from the cerebrospinal fluid to the interstitial fluid of the CNS.

6.5.3 The Blood–Liquor Barrier

The epithelium of the choroid plexus and the pia mater constitute the blood–liquor barrier. The differences in the concentration of the cerebrospinal fluid and the blood plasma are indicative of an intact blood–liquor barrier. The

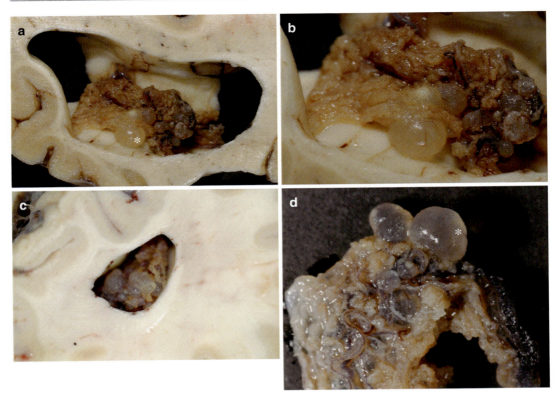

Fig. 6.5 Choroid plexus located in the lateral ventricle. The choroid plexus is well seen in a widened central part of the lateral ventricle. The choroid plexus displays focally a cystic lesion (∗) (**a, b**). Choroid plexus with two cysts in the posterior horn of the lateral ventricle (**c**). Two well-discernible choroid plexus cysts (the cysts have no space-occupying character) (**d**)

transport of substances at the blood–liquor barrier is unidirectional, i.e., into the ventricular system and into the subarachnoidal cisterns. In cases of meningitis, the blood–liquor barrier is disturbed.

Selected References

Benarroch EE (2016) Choroid plexus—CSF system: recent developments and clinical correlations. Neurology 86(3):286–296. https://doi.org/10.1212/wnl.0000000000002298

Heimer L (1983) The human brain and spinal cord: functional neuroanatomy and dissection guide. Springer, Berlin, Heidelberg

Kaur C, Rathnasamy G, Ling EA (2016) The choroid plexus in healthy and diseased brain. J Neuropathol Exp Neurol 75(3):198–213. https://doi.org/10.1093/jnen/nlv030

Lehtinen MK, Bjornsson CS, Dymecki SM, Gilbertson RJ, Holtzman DM, Monuki ES (2013) The choroid plexus and cerebrospinal fluid: emerging roles in development, disease, and therapy. J Neurosci 33(45):17553–17559. https://doi.org/10.1523/jneurosci.3258-13.2013

Lun MP, Monuki ES, Lehtinen MK (2015) Development and functions of the choroid plexus-cerebrospinal fluid system. Nat Rev Neurosci 16(8):445–457. https://doi.org/10.1038/nrn3921

Marques F, Sousa JC, Brito MA, Pahnke J, Santos C, Correia-Neves M, Palha JA (2017) The choroid plexus in health and in disease: dialogues into and out of the brain. Neurobiol Dis 107:32–40. https://doi.org/10.1016/j.nbd.2016.08.011

McLone DG (2004) The anatomy of the ventricular system. Neurosurg Clin N Am 15(1):33–38. https://doi.org/10.1016/s1042-3680(03)00073-1

Mortazavi MM, Adeeb N, Griessenauer CJ, Sheikh H, Shahidi S, Tubbs RI, Tubbs RS (2014a) The ventricular system of the brain: a comprehensive review of its history, anatomy, histology, embryology, and surgical considerations. Childs Nerv Syst 30(1):19–35. https://doi.org/10.1007/s00381-013-2321-3

Mortazavi MM, Griessenauer CJ, Adeeb N, Deep A, Bavarsad Shahripour R, Loukas M, Tubbs RI, Tubbs RS (2014b) The choroid plexus: a comprehensive review of its history, anatomy, function, histology, embryology, and surgical considerations. Childs Nerv Syst 30(2):205–214. https://doi.org/10.1007/s00381-013-2326-y

Spector R, Keep RF, Robert Snodgrass S, Smith QR, Johanson CE (2015) A balanced view of choroid plexus structure and function: focus on adult humans. Exp Neurol 267:78–86. https://doi.org/10.1016/j.expneurol.2015.02.032

Stratchko L, Filatova I, Agarwal A, Kanekar S (2016) The ventricular system of the brain: anatomy and normal variations. Semin Ultrasound CT MR 37(2):72–83. https://doi.org/10.1053/j.sult.2016.01.004

Weis S, Thaller R, Villringer A, Wenger E (1992) Das Gehirn des Menschen. Morphologie, Kernspintomographie und 3D-Computerrekonstruktion. Hogrefe, Göttingen

Wolburg H, Paulus W (2010) Choroid plexus: biology and pathology. Acta Neuropathol 119(1):75–88. https://doi.org/10.1007/s00401-009-0627-8

Meninges

7.1 Introduction

The meninges cover the brain and spinal cord and, thus, provide protection and support for these fragile structures.

The following meninges are characterized:

- *Dura mater*, a connective tissue membrane
- *Arachnoidea*, a thin layer of reticular fibers
- *Pia mater*, a thin translucent membrane

The pia mater and the arachnoidea are also called the leptomeninges while the synonym used for the dura mater is the pachymeninx.

The following table gives a schematic representation of the topographical arrangement of the meninges and the spaces located between them.

Bone	Pachymeninx	Epidural space	
↓		Dura mater	Outer surface next to bone
		Subdural space	
	Leptomeninges	Arachnoidea	
		Subarachnoidal space	
Brain		Pia mater	Inner surface next to brain
		Subpial space	

7.2 Dura Mater

The dura mater is composed of the following two layers:

- an outer periosteal layer, i.e., stratum periostale
- an inner meningeal layer, i.e., stratum meningeale

The periostal layer contains blood vessels and nerves. Both layers can separate at certain places to form venous sinuses, i.e., the dural sinus (see Chap. 9 on venous drainage of the nervous system).

The meningeal layer gives rise to the following septae which subdivide the cranial cavity into the various compartments:

- The *cerebral falx* extends in the sagittal direction from the crista galli to the internal occipital protuberans (Figs. 7.1 and 7.2). The cerebral falx extends between both hemispheres and reaches the corpus callosum.
- The *cerebellar tentorium* rises from the petrosal part of the temporal bone and merges into the cerebellar falx (Fig. 7.1). It covers the posterior cranial fossa. The cerebellar tentorium separates the telencephalon from the cerebellum.
- The *cerebellar falx* separates the cerebellar hemispheres.
- The *sellar diaphragm* covers the hypophyseal fossa and is pierced by the infundibulum of the pituitary gland.

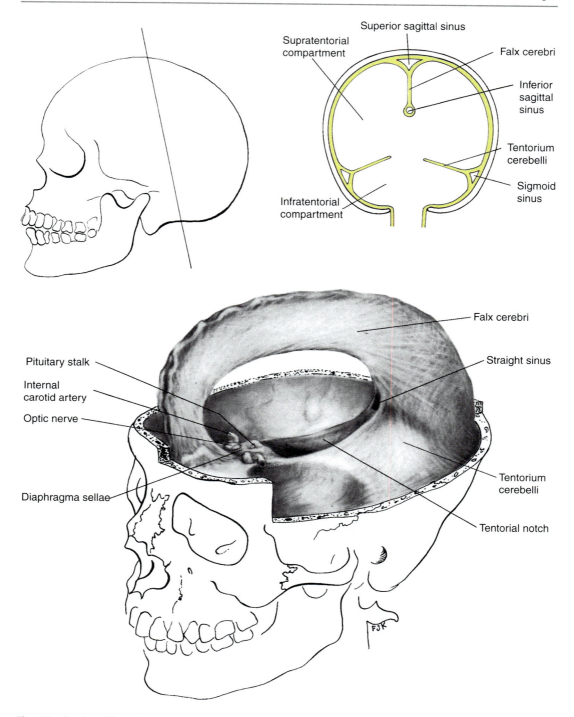

Fig. 7.1 Cerebral falx and cerebellar tentorium (reproduced from Heimer (1983) with kind permission by Springer Nature)

7.2 Dura Mater

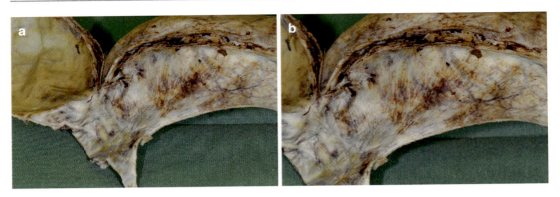

Fig. 7.2 Falx cerebri (**a, b**)

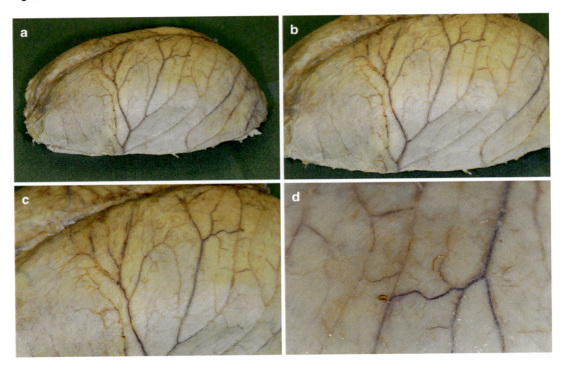

Fig. 7.3 Dura mater (**a, b**) and meningeal arteries in the dura (**c, d**)

The dura mater receives blood supply from the following vessels (Fig. 7.3a–d):

- the medial meningeal artery originating from the maxillary artery
- the anterior meningeal branches originating from the ophthalmic artery
- the posterior meningeal branches originating from the occipital artery and the vertebral artery

The innervation of the dura mater is realized by the trigeminal nerve (N. V), the vagal nerve (N. X), and by cervical spinal nerves.

The meningeal layer of the encephalic dura mater is continuous with the spinal dura mater, whereas the periostal layer of the cranial dura becomes the periost of the vertebral canal between the periost and the dura mater there is a space containing a venous plexus and which is called the epidural space. The spinal dura mater extends as a closed tube from the foramen magnum till the second sacral vertebra. It narrows at its caudal end to form a thin, fibrous structure, the coccygeal ligament, covering the filum terminale of the spinal cord.

7.3 Dural Sinuses

The veins drain the blood through the following sinuses into the extracranial venous system (Fig. 7.4a, b):

- Postero-superior group
  - Superior sagittal sinus
  - Inferior sagittal sinus
  - Straight sinus

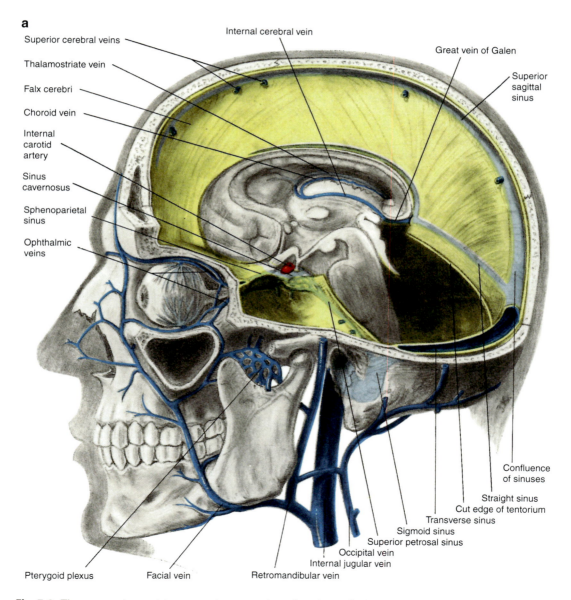

Fig. 7.4 The venous sinuses (**a**), venous sinuses on the base of the skull cavity (**b**) (reproduced from Heimer (1983) with kind permission by Springer Nature). Superior sagittal sinus seen from above (**c**, **d**), cut up as seen from above (**e**, **f**), cut up as seen from the midline (**g**), seen as a lumen on a horizontal cut (**h**)

7.3 Dural Sinuses

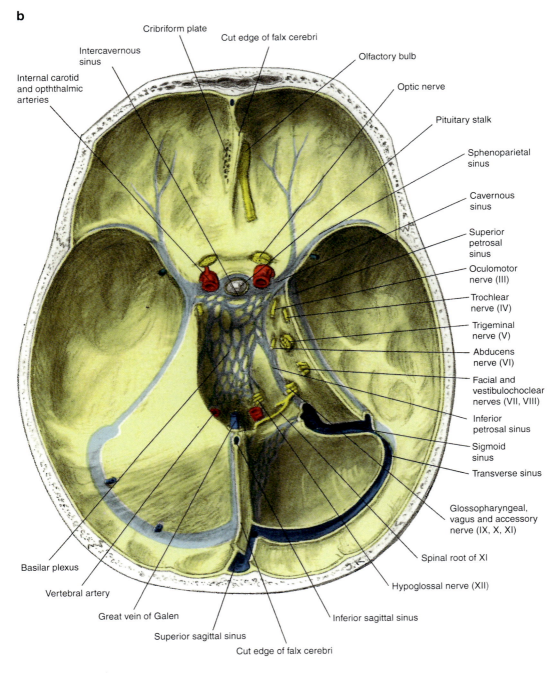

Fig. 7.4 (continued)

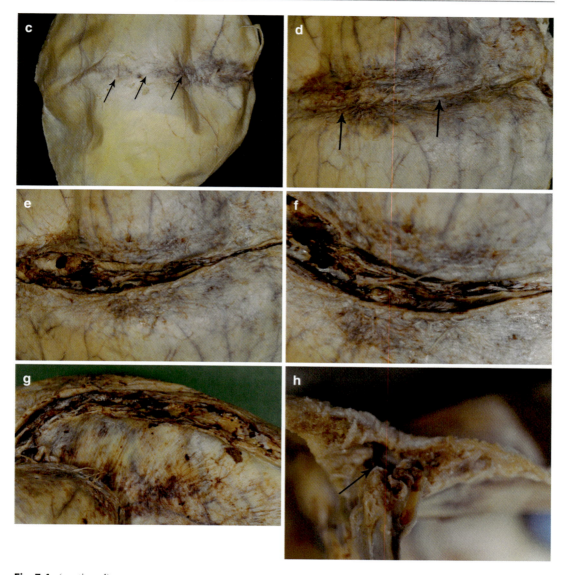

Fig. 7.4 (continued)

- Transverse sinus
- Occipital sinus
- Sigmoid sinus
- Antero-inferior venous sinuses
  - Cavernous sinus
  - Sphenoparietal sinus
  - Superior and inferior petrosal sinuses
- Postero-superior group
  - Superior sagittal sinus (Fig. 7.4c–h)
    - Runs along the superior margin of the falx cerebri
    - Receives from the superior cerebral veins
    - Empties into the confluence of the sinuses
  - Inferior sagittal sinus
    - Runs along the inferior margin of the falx cerebri
    - Merges with the vein of Galen
    - Continues as the straight sinus
  - Straight sinus
    - Extends from the falx cerebri to the tentorium cerebelli
    - Empties into the confluence of the sinuses

7.3 Dural Sinuses

- Occipital sinus
  - Lies within the falx cerebelli
  - Drains into the confluence of the sinuses
- Transverse sinus (Fig. 7.5a, b)
  - Receives venous blood from the confluence of the sinuses
  - Pass laterally and anteriorly along the tentorium cerebelli in the occipital bone
  - Runs inferiorly and medially of the petrous part of the temporal bone to form the sigmoid sinus
- Sigmoid sinus
  - Drains into the internal jugular vein in the jugular foramen
- Antero-inferior venous sinuses
  - Cavernous sinus
    - Middle cranial fossa
    - Lateral surface of the body of the sphenoid bone
    - Drains the inferior and superficial middle cerebral veins, ophthalmic vein
    - Empties into the superior and inferior petrosal sinuses
  - Intercavernous sinus
    - Communication between both cavernous sinuses
  - Sphenoparietal sinus
    - Lesser wing of the sphenoid bone
    - Empties into the cavernous sinus
  - Superior and inferior petrosal sinuses
    - On the superior and inferior borders of the petrous portion of the temporal bone
    - Drain the cavernous sinus
    - Superior petrosal sinus empties into the transverse and sigmoid sinuses
    - Inferior petrosal sinus empties into the internal jugular vein

There exists a strong trabecular network between the falx cerebri and the superior sagittal sinus (Fig. 7.6a, b). The veins draining into the superior sagittal sinus are shown in Fig. 7.7a, b.

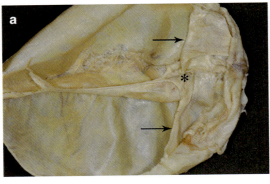
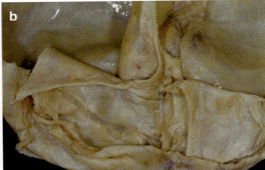

Fig. 7.5 Transverse sinuses (→) and confluens sinuum (∗) as seen from below (**a**, **b**)

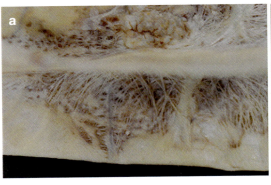
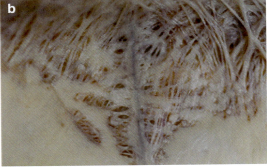

Fig. 7.6 Trabecular network for the fixation of the falx (**a**, **b**)

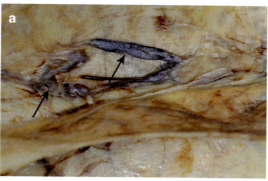 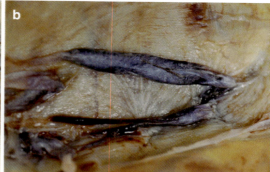

Fig. 7.7 Drainage of veins into the superior sagittal sinus (**a, b**)

7.4 Arachnoidea

The arachnoidea is not vascularized and arches the various sulci (Fig. 7.8a, b). Between the arachnoidea and the pia mater a space spreads and contains cerebrospinal fluid: the subarachnoidal space. The extension of the subarachnoidal space is variable depending on the topography. Thus at the surface of the cerebral hemispheres it is narrow, whereas it is wide at the basal aspect of the brain. Here, it forms several subarachnoidal cisterns.

Subarachnoidal cisterns are areas where the subarachnoidal space is widened forming the following cavities (Fig. 7.9):

- The *cerebellomedullary cistern* extends between the cerebellum and the medulla oblongata. The cerebrospinal fluid of the fourth ventricle drains through the median aperture and both lateral apertures into this cistern.
- The *chiasmatic cistern* is located around the optic chiasm.
- The *interpeduncular cistern* extends between the cerebral peduncles and contains the oculomotor nerve (N. III).
- The *pontine cistern* is located at the level of the pons.
- The *ambiens cistern* surrounds the mesencephalon except its occipital part and contains the great vein, the posterior cerebral artery, and the superior cerebral artery.
- The *cistern of the lateral fossa* arches the lateral sulcus.
- The *lumbal cistern* extends from the medullary conus (at the lower border of the first lumbal vertebra) till the second sacral vertebra and contains the terminal filum as well as the cauda equina.

7.5 Pia Mater

The pia mater is composed of the following two layers:

- inner, membranous layer, or the pia mater intima
- superficial epipial layer

The pia mater intima follows exactly the curvature of the brain. It is not vascularized and, thus, takes its nutrients from the cerebrospinal fluid. It accompanies the vessels which penetrate the CNS.

The epipial layer contains vessels. The epipial layer also forms the denticulate ligaments which connect the spinal cord with the dura mater. These ligaments are triangular; the basis of the triangle is fixed to the pia mater and the tip anchors at the arachnoid and the dura mater. In contrast, the pia mater intima rests upon the spinal cord.

7.5 Pia Mater

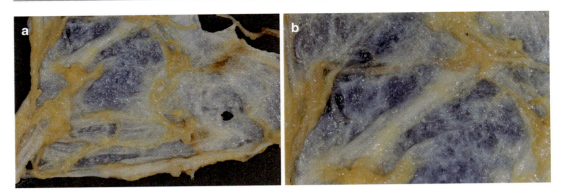

Fig. 7.8 Arachnoidea (**a**, **b**)

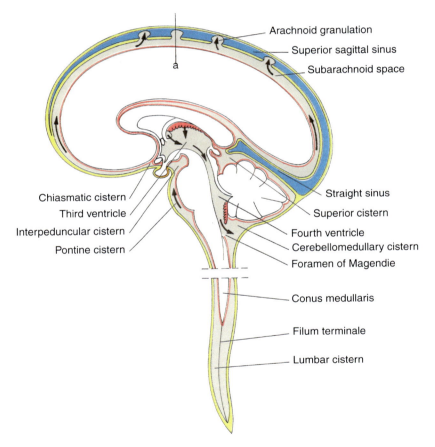

Fig. 7.9 Arachnoidal cisterns (reproduced from Heimer (1983) with kind permission by Springer Nature)

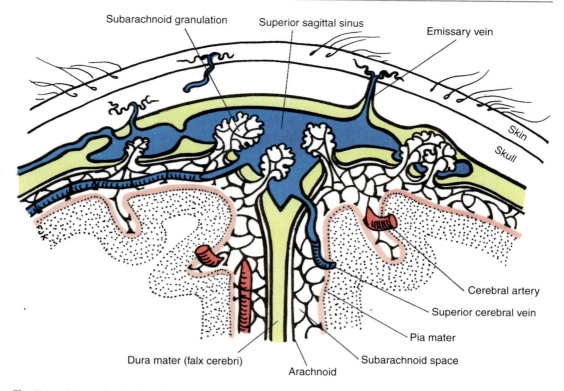

Fig. 7.10 Schematic drawing of the meningeal spaces (reproduced from Heimer (1983) with kind permission by Springer Nature)

7.6 The Meningeal Spaces

The following meningeal spaces can be defined:

- Epidural space
  - Space between bone and dura mater
- Subdural space
  - Space between dura mater and arachnoidea
- Subarachnoidal space
  - Space between arachnoidea and pia mater
- Subpial space
  - Space between pia mater and brain surface

Accumulation of blood with clinical relevance is encountered in the meningeal spaces as follows (Fig. 7.10):

- Epidural space
  - Epidural hematoma due to rupture of meningeal artery
- Subdural space
  - Subdural hemorrhage (SDH) due to trauma
- Subarachnoidal space
  - Subarachnoidal bleeding (SAB) due to rupture of aneurysms

7.7 Arachnoidal Granulations

Extensions of the pia-arachnoidea piercing the meningeal layer of the dura mater are termed arachnoidal granulations (Fig. 7.11a, b). These granulations are composed of numerous arachnoidal villi. The arachnoidal villi and the granulations are the place where the cerebrospinal fluid drains from the subarachnoidal space into the venous system. This is executed along a gradient of pressure. Furthermore, the granulations react to changes of the pressure by changes of their permeability.

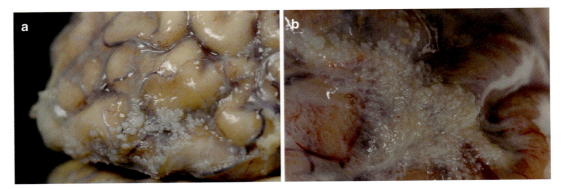

Fig. 7.11 Arachnoidal granulations in an autopsy brain (**a**, **b**)

Selected References

Balak N (2014) The Sylvian fissure, cistern and arachnoid membrane. Br J Neurosurg 28(1):98–106. https://doi.org/10.3109/02688697.2013.815324

Greenberg RW, Lane EL, Cinnamon J, Farmer P, Hyman RA (1994) The cranial meninges: anatomic considerations. Semin Ultrasound CT MR 15(6):454–465

Heimer L (1983) The human brain and spinal cord: functional neuroanatomy and dissection guide. Springer, Berlin, Heidelberg

Lu J (2015) Arachnoid membrane: the first and probably the last piece of the roadmap. Surg Radiol Anat 37(2):127–138. https://doi.org/10.1007/s00276-014-1361-z

Maurizi CP (2010) Arachnoid granules: Dandy was Dandy, Cushing and Weed were not. Med Hypotheses 75(2):238–240. https://doi.org/10.1016/j.mehy.2010.02.030

McKinnon SG (1998) Anatomy of the cerebral veins, dural sinuses, sella, meninges, and CSF spaces. Neuroimaging Clin N Am 8(1):101–117

Meltzer CC, Fukui MB, Kanal E, Smirniotopoulos JG (1996) MR imaging of the meninges. Part I. Normal anatomic features and nonneoplastic disease. Radiology 201(2):297–308. https://doi.org/10.1148/radiology.201.2.8888215

Patel N, Kirmi O (2009) Anatomy and imaging of the normal meninges. Semin Ultrasound CT MR 30(6):559–564

Tubbs RS, Hansasuta A, Stetler W, Kelly DR, Blevins D, Humphrey R, Chua GD, Shoja MM, Loukas M, Oakes WJ (2007) Human spinal arachnoid villi revisited: immunohistological study and review of the literature. J Neurosurg Spine 7(3):328–331. https://doi.org/10.3171/spi-07/09/328

Weller RO (2005) Microscopic morphology and histology of the human meninges. Morphologie 89(284):22–34

Weller RO, Sharp MM, Christodoulides M, Carare RO, Mollgard K (2018) The meninges as barriers and facilitators for the movement of fluid, cells and pathogens related to the rodent and human CNS. Acta Neuropathol 135(3):363–385. https://doi.org/10.1007/s00401-018-1809-z

Arterial Supply of the Brain

8.1 Introduction

Although the weight of the brain (1250–1350 g) amounts for approximately 2% of the body weight (80–120 kg), the brain receives 15% of the cardiac output and accounts for 20% of total resting oxygen, and 25–35% of glucose utilization.

The arterial supply of the brain is provided by the following two systems (Fig. 8.1a, b):

- Carotid system (anterior circulation)
- Vertebro-basilar system (posterior circulation)

Both systems form a complex anastomoses, i.e., circulus arteriosus, circle of Willis.

8.2 Carotid System

The carotid artery possesses the following major portions:

- Common carotid artery
- External carotid artery
- Internal carotid artery

In the following, the major arterial branches are given in a schematic way, illustrated by classical angiograms (Figs. 8.1, 8.2, 8.3, 8.4, 8.5, and 8.6) as well as images of vessels of autopsy brains (Fig. 8.7a–r). The regions that they supply are given in Table 8.1.

- Common carotid artery
  - Bifurcates at the level of the thyroid cartilage
- External carotid artery
  - Superior thyroid artery
  - Lingual artery
  - Facial artery
  - Maxillary artery
    - Middle meningeal artery
  - Superficial temporal artery
  - Ascending pharyngeal artery
  - Occipital artery
  - Posterior auricular artery
  - Terminates as two branches:
    - Maxillary artery
    - Superficial temporal artery
- Internal carotid artery (ICA) (Figs. 8.2a–f and 8.3a–f)
  - C1: Cervical segment (extracranial portion)
    - none
  - C2: Petrous segment (lies within the carotid canal)
    - Artery of the pterygoid canal (vidian artery)
    Caroticotympanic artery
  - C3: Lacerum segment (from the petrous apex to the cavernous sinus)
    none
  - C4: Cavernous segment
    - Meningohypophyseal trunk
      - Tentorial basal branch
      - Tentorial marginal branch

© Springer-Verlag GmbH Austria, part of Springer Nature 2019
S. Weis et al., *Imaging Brain Diseases*, https://doi.org/10.1007/978-3-7091-1544-2_8

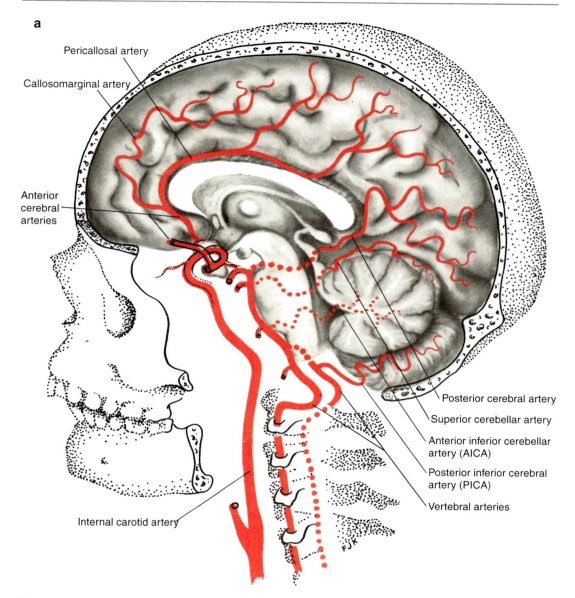

Fig. 8.1 Survey of the arterial supply of the brain (with kind permission from Heimer (1983)) (**a**). Orthogonal frontal (**a**) and sagittal (**b**) projections of the main cranial arteries (carotid and vertebro-basilar systems). Note trifurcation of the MCA (**b**) (with kind permission from ten Donkelaar (2011)). *Abbreviations: ACA* anterior cerebral artery, *acalc* calcarine artery, *acmg* callosomarginal artery, *aocl*, *aocm* lateral and medial occipital arteries, *apc* pericallosal artery, *ap-o* parieto-occipital artery, *AICA* anterior inferior cerebellar artery, *BA* basilar artery, *C1–C4* cervical, petrous, cavernous, and cerebral parts of internal carotid artery, *MCA* middle cerebral artery, *mma* middle meningeal artery, *PCA* posterior cerebral artery, *pcma* posterior communicating artery, *PICA* posterior inferior cerebellar artery, *SCA* superior cerebellar artery, *VA* vertebral artery; in (**a**) *1–3* refer to the trifurcation of the MCA; in (**b**) *1–6* are branches of the ACA: *1* orbitofrontal artery; *2* frontopolar artery; *3–5* anterior, middle, and posterior frontal arteries; *6* paracentral artery

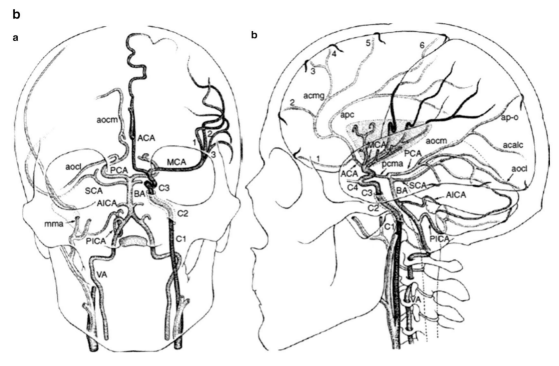

Fig. 8.1 (continued)

- Meningeal branch—helps supply blood to the meninges of the anterior cranial fossa
- Clivus branches—tiny branches that supply the clivus
- Inferior hypophyseal artery
  - Capsular branches
  - Infero-lateral trunk
    - Branches to trigeminal ganglion— provide blood to trigeminal ganglion
    - *Artery of the foramen rotundum*
    - Branches to nerves
- C5: Clinoid segment (intradural)
  - Posterior communicating artery
- C6: Ophthalmic segment (subarachnoid space)
  - Ophthalmic artery
  - Superior hypophyseal artery
- C7: Communicating (terminal) segment
  - Posterior communicating artery
  - Anterior choroidal artery
  - Anterior cerebral artery (a terminal branch)
  - Middle cerebral artery (a terminal branch)
- Bifurcation of ICA (Carotid T) into ACA and MCA
  - Anterior choroidal artery
- Anterior cerebral artery (ACA)
  - A1 segment (horizontal segment, precommunicating segment)
    - Medial lenticulostriate arteries
    - Recurrent artery of Heubner (medial striate artery)
  - A2 segment (vertical segment, postcommunicating segment)
    - Frontopolar artery
  - A3 segment (callosal segment)
  - Anterior communicating artery
- Middle cerebral artery (MCA)
  - M1 segment (sphenoidal/horizontal segment)
    - Thalamostriate arteries
    - Lateral lenticulostriate arteries
    - Anterior temporal artery

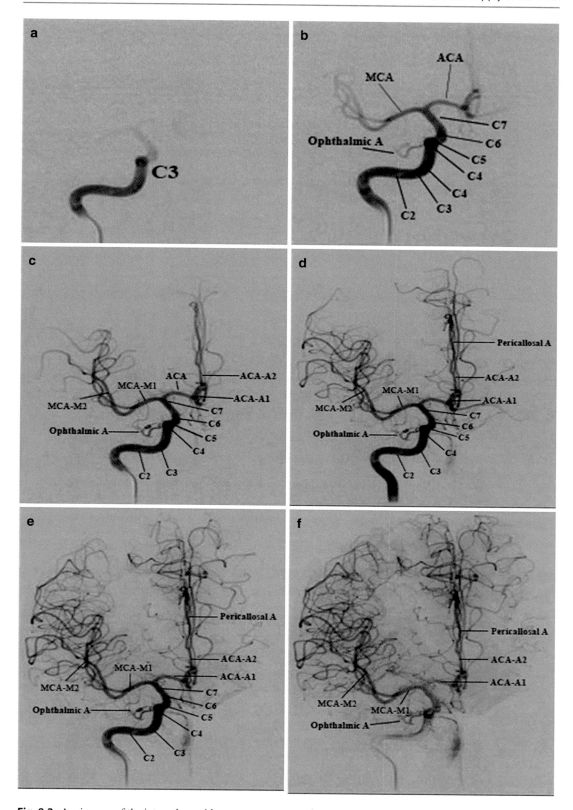

Fig. 8.2 Angiogram of the internal carotid artery system—anterior-posterior view (a–f)

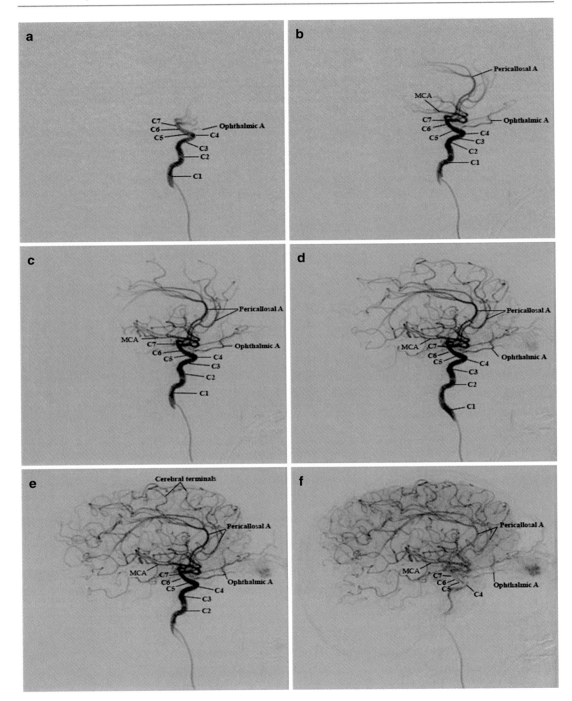

Fig. 8.3 Angiogram of the internal carotid artery system—lateral-posterior view (**a–f**)

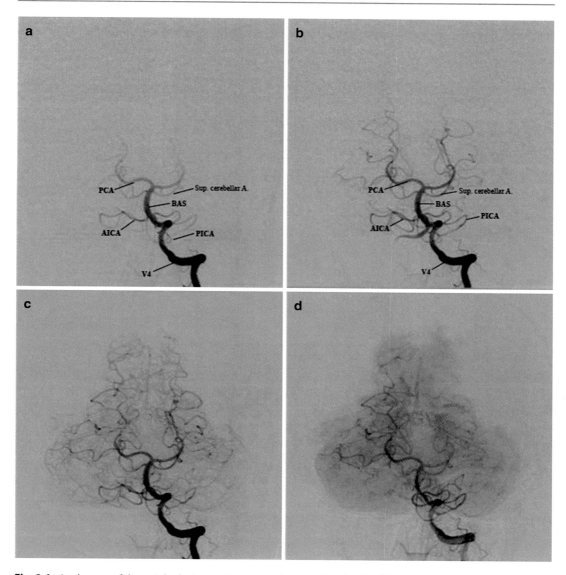

Fig. 8.4 Angiogram of the vertebral artery system—anterior-posterior view (a–d)

- M2 segment (insular segment)
    - Insular arteries
- M3 segment (opercular segment)
    - Insular arteries
    - Frontobasal arteries
    - Temporal arteries
- M4 segment (terminal segment)
    - Arteries of the precentral and triangular sulci
    - Anterior and posterior parietal arteries
    - Arteries of the central and postcentral sulci

8.2 Carotid System

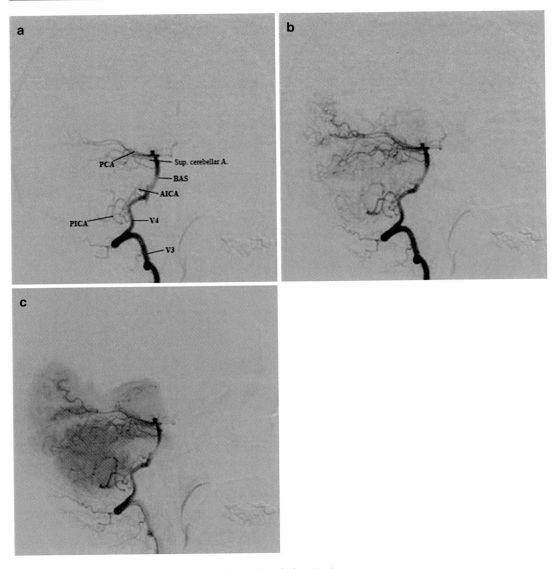

Fig. 8.5 Angiogram of the vertebral artery system—lateral view (**a–c**)

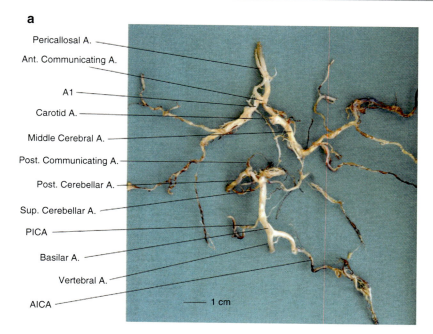

Fig. 8.6 MRI angiogram. *M1* sphenoidal/horizontal segment (M1), *M2* insular segment (M2), *M3* opercular segment (M3), *M4* terminal segment (M4) of the middle cerebral artery, *ACA* anterior cerebral artery, *A1* horizontal segment, precommunicating segment (A1), *A2* vertical segment, postcommunicating segment (A2) of the anterior cerebral artery (ACA), *P1* precommunicating segment (P1), *P2* ambient segment (P2) of the posterior cerebral artery (PCA), *SCA* superior cerebellar artery, *AICA* anterior inferior cerebellar artery, *PICA* posterior inferior cerebellar artery, *C1* cervical segment (C1), *C2* petrous segment (C2), *C3* lacerum segment (C3), *C4* cavernous segment (C4), *C5* clinoid segment (C5), *C6* ophthalmic segment (C6), *C7* communicating (terminal) segment (C7) of the internal carotid artery, *V4* segment 4 of the vertebral artery

8.3 Vertebro-Basilar System

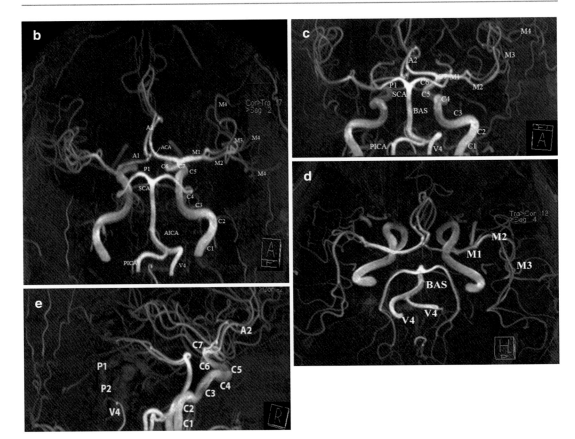

Fig. 8.6 (continued)

8.3 Vertebro-Basilar System

The vertebro-basilar system consists of:

- Vertebral artery, extracranial portion
- Vertebral artery, intracranial portion
- Basilar artery

In the following, the major arterial branches are given in a schematic way, illustrated by classical angiograms (Figs. 8.4a–d and 8.5a–c). The regions that they supply are given in Table 8.1.

- Vertebral artery, extracranial portion
  - V0 point of exit from subclavian artery
  - V1 extraosseous prevertebral segment (from V0 to foramen of the transverse process of C6)
    - segmental branches
  - V2 foraminal transversarial segment (through the foraminae transversaria C6 to C2)
    - Branches to cervical nerves
    - Branches to vertebrae and intervertebral joints
    - Branches to neck muscle
    - Branches to spinal cord
    - Anterior meningeal artery
  - V3 extraspinal segment (Atlas C1 loop)
    - posterior meningeal artery
- Vertebral artery, intracranial segment
  - V4 intradural segment
    - anterior spinal arteries
    - posterior spinal arteries
    - medullary perforating branches
  - Posterior inferior cerebellar artery (PICA)
    - Forms with the contralateral vertebral artery the basilar artery

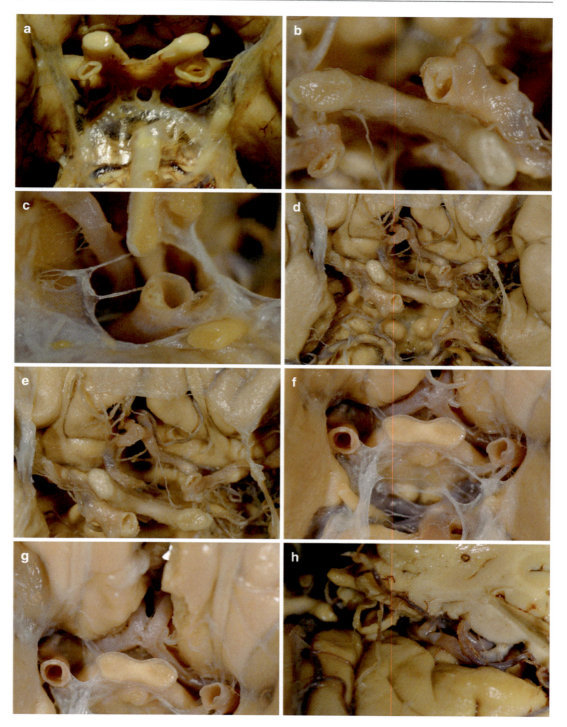

Fig. 8.7 Arteries of the brain, autopsy specimen. Carotid artery (**a–c**) with optic chiasm, anterior cerebral artery (**d, e**), anterior communicating artery (**f, g**), middle cerebral artery (**h, i**), insular artery (**j**), pericallosal artery (**k**), posterior communicating artery, basilar artery (**l–n**), basilar artery (**o, p**), posterior inferior cerebellar artery (PICA) (**q**), vertebral arteries (**r**)

8.3 Vertebro-Basilar System

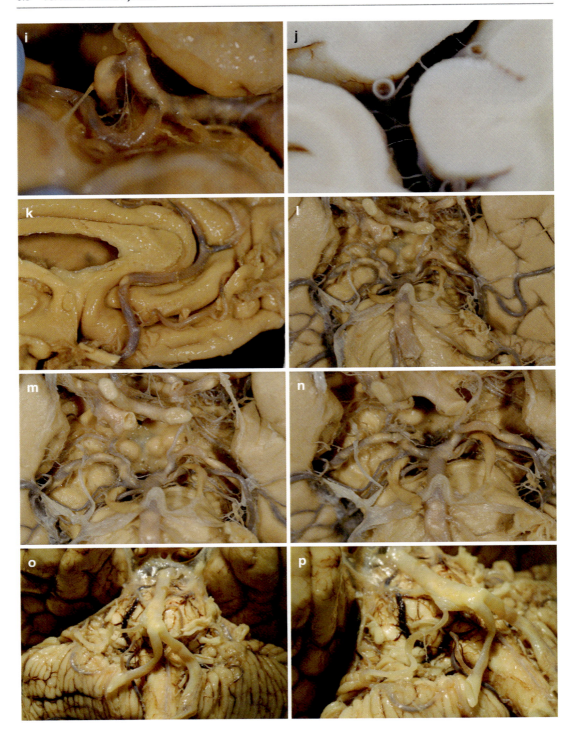

Fig. 8.7 (continued)

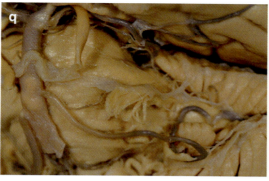
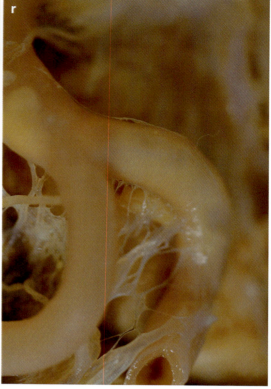

Fig. 8.7 (continued)

- Basilar artery
  - Anterior inferior cerebellar artery (AICA)
    - Labyrinthine artery
  - Basilar perforating arteries
  - Superior cerebellar artery (SCA) bifurcates to form the
- Posterior cerebral arteries (PCA)
  - P1 precommunicating segment
    - Posterior thalamoperforating arteries
  - P2 ambient segment
    - anterior and posterior temporal arteries
    - thalamogeniculate arteries
    - peduncular perforating arteries
    - medial posterior choroidal artery
    - lateral-posterior coroidal artery
  - P3 quadrigeminal
  - P4 calcarine segment
    - parieto-occipital artery
    - calcarine artery
    - posterior splenial arteries
    - lateral occipital artery

8.4 Clinical Vascular Syndromes

The clinical vascular syndromes resulting from lack of blood supply in the various territories (Fig. 8.8a–c) are briefly described and listed in Table 8.2.

8.4.1 Anterior Cerebral Artery Syndrome

Strokes that occur in a part of the artery prior to the anterior communicating usually do not produce many symptoms because of collateral circulation. If a blockage occurs in the A2 segment or later, the following signs and symptoms may be noted.

Table 8.1 The vascular territories supplied by the arteries are given as follows

Artery	Territory
External carotid artery (ECA)	
ECA-Superior thyroid artery	• Thyroid
ECA-Lingual artery	• Upper portion of the mucosa and the inner laryngeal muscles • Gland • Muscles • Gingiva
ECA-Facial artery	• Lower lip • Upper lip • Palatine tonsil • Posterior part of tongue • Ala of the nose • Nasal septum
ECA-Maxillary artery	• Deep structures of the face
ECA-Middle meningeal artery	• Dura mater • Bone
ECA-Superficial temporal artery	• Parotid gland • Auricle • Forehead region of the scalp • Temporal region of the scalp
ECA-Ascending pharyngeal artery	• Wall of the pharynx • Auditory tube • Palatine tonsil
ECA-Occipital artery	• Mastoid • Auricle • Sternocleidomastoid muscle • Scalp overlying the occiput
ECA-Posterior auricular artery	• Muscles attached to mastoid process • Muscles attached to styloid process
Internal carotid artery (ICA)	
ICA-C1 Cervical segment C1 (extracranial portion)	
ICA-C2 Petrous segment	• Middle ear
ICA-C3 Lacerum segment	
ICA-C4 Cavernous segment	• Pituitary gland • Tentorium • Clival dura
ICA-C5 Clinoid segment	

Table 8.1 (continued)

ICA-C6 Ophthalmic segment	• Retina • Optic nerve • Anterior pituitary lobe • Infundibular stalk • Optic chiasm
ICA-C7 Communicating (terminal) segment	
Anterior choroidal artery (AChA)	• Globus pallidus (internal) • Internal capsule (posterior limb) • Head of caudate nucleus • Optic radiation • Medial temporal lobe • Choroid plexus
Anterior cerebral artery (ACA)	• Anterior medial frontal lobe • Superior medial frontal lobe • Parietal lobe • Paramedian hemisphere • Rostral corpus callosum • Internal capsule (anterior limb) • Putamen (rostral) • Caudate nucleus
ACA-A1-Basal perforating arteries	• Medial basal ganglia
ACA-A1-Heubner artery	• Inferomedial basal ganglia • Anterior limb of the internal capsule
ACA-A2	• Inferomedial aspect of the frontal lobe
ACA-A3 (callosal segment)	• Corpus callosum
Anterior communicating artery	• Connects the two anterior cerebral arteries
Middle cerebral artery (MCA)	
Middle cerebral artery (MCA)	• Frontal lobe • Parietal lobe • Superior temporal lobe
M1-Thalamostriate arteries	• Thalamus • Putamen • Globus pallidus (external) • Caudate nucleus • Internal capsule (posterior limb)

(continued)

Table 8.1 (continued)

Artery	Territory
M1-Lenticulostriate arteries	• Putamen • Globus pallidus (external) • Caudate nucleus • Internal capsule (posterior limb) • Corona radiata • Cortical and subcortical frontoparietal hemisphere • Lateral temporal lobe
M2-Insular arteries	• Lateral frontal hemispheres • Corona radiata
M3-Insular arteries	• Insular cortex • Extreme capsule • Claustrum • External capsule • Putamen • Amygdala
M3-Frontobasal arteries	• Frontal lobe, lateral side • Orbital gyri • Inferior frontal gyrus
M3-Temporal arteries	• Temporal lobe • Transverse gyri • Wernicke region
M4-Arteries of the precentral and triangular sulci	• Precentral gyrus • Frontal lobe
M4-Anterior and posterior parietal arteries	• Posterior gyrus • Anterior parts of the parietal lobe • Posterior parts of the parietal lobe
M4-Arteries of the central and postcentral sulci	• Postcentral suclus • Parietal lobe
Vertebral artery, extracranial portion (VA-EP)	
VA-EP-V0 point of exit from subclavian artery	
VA-EP-V1 prevertebral segment	• Cervical muscles • Lower cervical spinal cord
VA-EP-V2 transversarial segment	• Branches to cervical nerves • Branches to vertebrae and intervertebral joints • Branches to neck muscle • Branches to spinal cord
VA-EP-V2—V3 segment (Atlas C1 loop)	• Meninges

Table 8.1 (continued)

Artery	Territory
VA-IP-V4 segment	• Medulla oblongata • Choroid plexus • Cerebellar tonsils • Inferior cerebellum
VA-Posterior inferior cerebellar artery (PICA)	• Lateral medulla (spinothalamic tract, descending sympathetic tract) • Inferior/posterior aspects of cerebellum • Inferior vermis • Inferior cerebellar peduncle
Basilar artery (BA)	
BA-Anterior inferior cerebellar artery (AICA)	• Lateral pontine tegmentum • Rostral medulla • Anterior/inferior aspects of cerebellum • Middle cerebral peduncle • Cochlea • Vestibule • Paramedian pons
BA-Labyrinthine artery	• Internal ear
BA-Superior cerebellar artery (SCA)	• Upper pontine tegmentum • Part of midbrain • Upper surface of cerebellar hemispheres • Upper portion of vermis • Cerebellar nuclei (dentate) • Choroid plexus
Posterior cerebral artery (PCA)	
PCA-Pars circularis-precommunicating—P1	• Mammillary bodies • Thalamus • Lateral wall of third ventricle • Posterior part of the internal capsule
PCA-Pars circularis-ambient—P2 t	• Posterior thalamus • Tectal plate • Pineal body • Medial geniculate body
PCA-Pars circularis-quadrigeminal—P3 Lateral occipital artery	• Basilar surface of the posterior occipital lobe • Posterior temporal lobe
PCA-Pars terminalis-calcarine—P4 Medial occipital artery	• Medial surface of the posterior occipital lobe • Splenium corporis callosum • Cuneus • Precuneus • Occipital pole

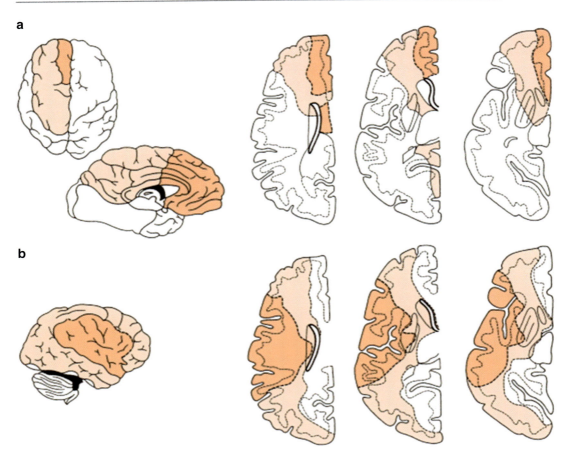

Fig. 8.8 Vascular territories of the main cerebral arteries and variations in the vascularization of the cerebral cortex (**a–c**) (with kind permission from ten Donkelaar (2011)). Minimal and maximal areas of vascularization are shown in *red* and *light red*, respectively, for (**a**) the anterior cerebral artery, (**b**) the middle cerebral artery and (**c**) the posterior cerebral artery on dorsal, medial, and lateral surfaces of the cerebrum and in three horizontal sections. Two adjacent horizontal sections of the cerebrum with the vascular territories of the main cerebral arteries (**d**). The vascular territories are indicated as follows: *light red* for the ACA, *light gray* for the MCA, and *red* for the PCA. Central structures are supplied by perforating branches of the ACA (*medium red*) and the MCA (*gray*), the anterior choroidal artery (*dotted area*), perforating branches of the posterior communicating artery (*a*), posterior choroidal arteries (*d*) and the anterior communicating artery (*f*). The *arrows* indicate the variability of the vascular territories of the ACA, MCA, and PCA. *Abbreviations*: *ac* anterior commissure, *Acc* nucleus accumbens, *AM* amygdala, *aos* anterior occipital sulcus, *APS* anterior perforated substance, *cals* calcarine sulcus, *cp* cerebral peduncle, *crc* crus cerebri, *cs* colliculus superior, *FMG* frontomarginal gyrus, *fx* fornix, *GR* gyrus rectus, *H* hippocampus, *lgb* lateral geniculate body, *LOG* lateral orbital gyrus, *ls* lateral sulcus, *mgb* medial geniculate body, *MOG* medial orbital gyrus, *O2* middle occipital gyrus, *O5* lingual gyrus, *O6* cuneus, *POG* posterior orbital gyrus, *T2*, *T3* middle and inferior temporal gyri, *T5* parahippocampal gyrus

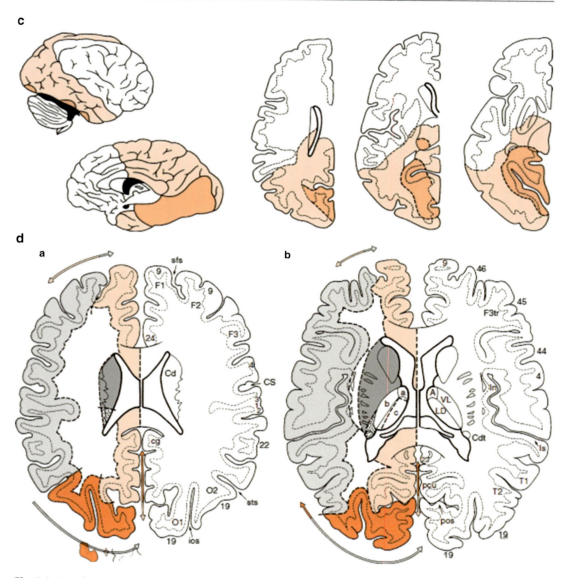

Fig. 8.8 (continued)

8.4 Clinical Vascular Syndromes

Table 8.2 Clinical syndromes resulting from pathology of the respective artery and involved structures

Territory	Artery	Clinical syndrome
Carotid	Ophthalmic	• Monocular blindness • Altitudinal field defect
	Anterior choroidal	• Contralateral hemiparesis • Hemisensory loss • Homonymous hemianopia with sparing of horizontal segment
	Anterior cerebral	• Contralateral foot and leg weakness • Hemiparesis • Abulia • Incontinence • Grasp reflexes • Mutism • Left hand apraxia • Transcortical motor aphasia • Frontal release signs • Urinary incontinence
	Middle cerebral	• Contralateral central facial weakness • Hemiparesis • Global aphasia
	Medial lenticulostriate	• Contralateral pure motor hemiparesis
	Lateral lenticulostriate	• Contralateral hemiparesis • Dysphasia • Visual-spatial-perceptual dysfunction • Contralateral hemisensory/motor syndrome (face/arm/leg) • Global aphasia with dominant hemisphere involvement • Visuospatial neglect (nondominant hemisphere) • Contralateral gaze paresis • Contralateral homonymous hemianopia
Vertebral	Posterior inferior cerebellar	• Ipsilateral Horner syndrome • Ipsilateral facial sensory loss • Vertigo • Nystagmus • Ataxia • Dysphagia • Dysarthria • Gaze paresis • Pain/temperature deficits face (ipsilateral), trunk/extremities (contralateral)
Basilar	Anterior inferior cerebellar	• Ipsilateral Horner syndrome • Ipsilateral facial sensory loss • Ipsilateral nuclear facial and abducens palsy • Vertigo • Vomiting • Nystagmus • Ipsilateral facial anesthesia • Weakness • Ipsilateral deafness • Contralateral decrease in temperature/pain sensation in limbs • Ipsilateral ataxia
	Paramedian and circumferential basilar penetrators	• Lacunar syndromes
	Superior cerebellar artery	• Ipsilateral Horner syndrome • Ipsilateral limb ataxia • Vertigo • Nystagmus • Contralateral IVth nerve palsy • Ipsilateral tremor/dyskinesia • Contralateral decreased sensation to pain/temperature in the trunk

Table 8.2 (continued)

Territory	Artery	Clinical syndrome
Posterior	Posterior cerebellar	• Contralateral homonymous hemianopia with macular sparing (if purely cortical) • If bilateral: Balint syndrome or cortical blindness with or without denial of blindness (Anton syndrome) • Dysnomic aphasia with alexia without agraphia (dominant hemisphere) • Memory disturbance • Color dysnomia • Agitated delirium • Hemisensory deficits with thalamic stroke

- Paralysis or weakness of the foot and leg on the opposite side, due to involvement of leg part of the motor cortex
- Cortical sensory loss in the opposite foot and leg
- Gait apraxia (impairment of gait and stance)
- Abulia, akinetic mutism, slowness, and lack of spontaneity
- Urinary incontinence which usually occurs with bilateral damage in the acute phase
- Frontal cortical release reflexes: Contralateral grasp reflex, sucking reflex, paratonic rig

8.4.2 Middle Cerebral Artery Syndrome

1. Paralysis (-plegia) or weakness (-paresis) of the contralateral face and arm (faciobrachial).
2. Sensory loss of the contralateral face and arm.
3. Damage to the dominant hemisphere (usually the left hemisphere) results in aphasia, i.e., Broca's or Wernicke's.
4. Damage to the nondominant hemisphere (usually the right hemisphere) results in contralateral neglect syndrome.
5. Large MCA infarcts often have déviation conjuguée, a gaze preference towards the side of the lesion, especially during the acute period. Contralateral homonymous hemianopsia is often present.

MCA occlusion site and resulting aphasia

- Global—trunk of MCA
- Broca—anterior branch of MCA
- Wernicke—posterior branch of MCA

8.4.3 AICA Syndrome (Lateral Pontine Syndrome)

Occlusion of AICA is considered rare, but generally results in

- Sudden onset of vertigo and vomiting
- Nystagmus
- Dysarthria
- Falling to the side of the lesion (due to damage to vestibular nuclei)
- Variety of ipsilateral features including
  - Hemiataxia
  - Loss of all modalities of sensation of the face (due to damage to the principal sensory trigeminal nucleus)
  - Facial paralysis (due to damage to the facial nucleus)
  - Hearing loss and tinnitus (due to damage to the cochlear nuclei)
- Loss of pain and temperature sensation from the contralateral limbs and trunk
- DD lateral medullary syndrome
  - "crossed" neurological signs
  - does not usually cause cochlear symptoms, severe facial palsy, or multimodal facial sensory loss

8.4.4 Posterior Inferior Cerebellar Artery Syndrome (PICA Syndrome)

- Known as *lateral medullary syndrome*, or *Wallenberg syndrome*.

- Severe occlusion of this or vertebral arteries could lead to Horner syndrome as well.

8.4.5 Posterior Cerebral Artery Syndrome

- Stroke
  - Contralateral loss of pain and temperature sensations
  - Visual field defects (contralateral hemianopia with macular sparing)
  - Prosopagnosia with bilateral obstruction of the lingual and fusiform gyri
  - Superior Alternating Syndrome (Weber's syndrome)
  - Ipsilateral deficits of oculomotor nerve
  - Contralateral deficits of facial nerve (only lower face, upper face receives bilateral input), vagus nerve, and hypoglossal nerve
  - Horner syndrome
- Peripheral territory (Cortical branches)
  - Homonymous hemianopia (often upper quadrantic): Calcarine cortex or optic radiation nearby.
  - Bilateral homonymous hemianopia, cortical blindness, awareness, or denial of blindness; tactile naming, achromatopsia (color blindness), failure to see to-and-fro movements, inability to perceive objects not centrally located, apraxia of ocular movements, inability to count or enumerate objects, tendency to run into things that the patient sees and tries to avoid: Bilateral occipital lobe with possibly the parietal lobe involved.
  - Verbal dyslexia without agraphia, color anomia: Dominant calcarine lesion and posterior part of corpus callosum.
  - Memory defect: Hippocampal lesion bilaterally or on the dominant side only.
  - Topographic disorientation and prosopagnosia: Usually with lesions of non-dominant, calcarine, and lingual gyrus.
  - Simultanagnosia, hemivisual neglect: Dominant visual cortex, contralateral hemisphere.
  - Unformed visual hallucinations, peduncular hallucinosis, metamorphopsia, teleopsia, illusory visual spread, palinopsia, distortion of outlines, central photophobia: Calcarine cortex.
  - Complex hallucinations: Usually non-dominant hemisphere.
- Central territory (Ganglionic branches)
  - Thalamic syndrome: sensory loss (all modalities), spontaneous pain and dysesthesias, choreoathetosis, intention tremor, spasms of hand, mild hemiparesis, contralateral hemianethesia: Posteroventral nucleus of thalamus; involvement of the adjacent subthalamus body or its afferent tracts.
  - Thalamoperforate syndrome: Crossed cerebellar ataxia with ipsilateral third nerve palsy (Claude's syndrome): Dentatothalamic tract and issuing third nerve.
  - Weber's syndrome: Third nerve palsy and contralateral hemiplegia: Third nerve and cerebral peduncle.
  - Contralateral hemiplegia: Cerebral peduncle.
  - Paralysis or paresis of vertical eye movement, skew deviation, sluggish pupillary responses to light, slight miosis and ptosis (retraction nystagmus and "tucking" of the eyelids may be associated): Supranuclear fibers to third nerve, interstitial nucleus of Cajal, nucleus of Darkschewitsch, and posterior commissure.
  - Contralateral rhythmic, ataxic action tremor; rhythmic postural or "holding" tremor (rubral tremor): Dentatothalamic tract.

Selected References

Heimer L (1983) The human brain and spinal cord: functional neuroanatomy and dissection guide. Springer, Berlin, Heidelberg

Krayenbühl H, Yaşargil MG, Huber P, Bosse G (1982) Cerebral angiography. Thieme, London

Moore KL, Dalley AR (1999) Clinically oriented anatomy, 4th edn. Lippincott Williams & Wilkins, Philadelphia

Osborn AG, Jacobs JM (1999) Diagnostic cerebral angiography. Lippincott Williams & Wilkins, Philadelphia

ten Donkelaar HJ (2011) Clinical neuroanatomy. Brain circuitry and its disorders. Springer, Berlin, Heidelberg

Venous Drainage of the Brain

9.1 Introduction

The venous drainage of the brain is schematically illustrated in Figs. 9.1 and 9.6a–c.

9.2 Venous System

The cortical veins:

- Lie superficially.
- Are adherent to the deep surface of the arachnoid mater so that they keep the sulci open.
- Drain to the nearest dural venous sinus.
- The cerebral venous system does not even remotely follow the cerebral arterial system.

Cerebral veins have

- Thin walls with no muscular tissue.
- Possess no valves.
- Emerge from the brain.
- Pierce the meninges.
- Lie in the subarachnoid space.
- Coursing over the surface of the brain.
- Aggregating into larger channels until they pierce the arachnoid mater and the meningeal layer of the dura mater.
- Drain into the dural venous sinuses.
- Superficial cortical veins drain the outer 1–2 cm from the brain surface to the dural sinuses.
- Deep cerebral veins drain blood from the hemispheric white matter, basal ganglia, corpus callosum, choroid plexus, and cortical areas.
- Anastomoses between superficial and deep veins exist.

The cerebral venous system can be divided into (Table 9.1):

- Superficial (cortical) cerebral veins
  - The superficial venous system is comprised of the sagittal sinuses and cortical veins.
  - The cortical veins course along the cortical sulci, drain the cortex and some of the adjacent white matter.
  - There are numerous cortical veins, and most of them are unnamed; however, the large cortical veins can be identified according to their locations, the cortical venous system can be subdivided into superior, middle, and inferior groups.
  - Important veins of the superficial cerebral venous system are:
    o Superficial middle cerebral vein
    o Superior anastomotic vein of Trolard
    o Vein of Labbé

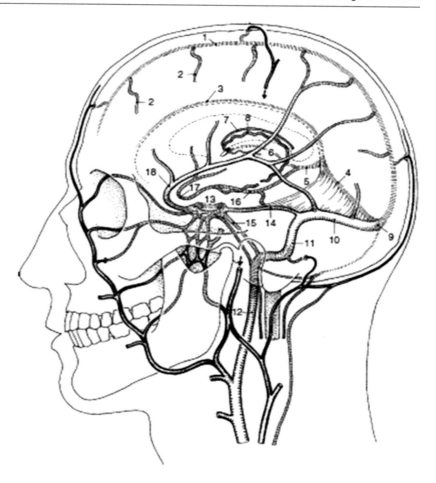

Fig. 9.1 Venous system and sinuses (with kind permission form ten Donkelaar (2011)). *1* superior sagittal sinus; *2* superior cerebral veins; *3* inferior sagittal sinus; *4* straight sinus; *5* great cerebral vein; *6* internal cerebral vein; *7* superior thalamostriate vein; *8* superior choroid vein; *9* confluens sinuum; *10* transverse sinus; *11* sigmoid sinus; *12* internal jugular vein; *13* cavernous sinus; *14* superior petrous sinus; *15* inferior petrous sinus; *16* basal vein; *17* deep middle cerebral vein; *18* superficial middle cerebral vein

- Deep (subependymal) cerebral veins
  - The deep venous system consists of the lateral sinuses, sigmoid sinuses, straight sinus, and draining deep cerebral veins (subependymal and medullary veins).
    - *Medullary veins*: They are numerous and originate 1–2 cm below cortical gray matter and pass through deep medullary white matter and drain into subependymal veins. The medullary veins are arranged in a wedge-shaped manner and distributed at a right angle to subependymal veins.
    - *Subependymal veins*: They receive medullary veins and aggregate into greater tributaries, mainly into septal veins, thalamostriate veins, internal cerebral veins, basal vein of Rosenthal and vein of Galen.

The venous blood is collected by the veins, drained into the dural sinuses, and emptied into the jugular vein in the following way:

- Emissary veins
- Cerebral veins
- Dural sinuses
- Internal jugular vein
- Brachicephalic vein
- Superior vena cava
- Right cardiac atrium

The venous system consists of (Table 9.1):

- Emissary veins (connections between a venous sinus, diploic veins, and superficial cranial veins)
  - Parietal emissary veins
  - Mastoid emissary veins
  - Condylar emissary veins
  - Occipital emissary veins

9.2 Venous System

Table 9.1 List of veins with their anatomical specifics, the drained territory, and their draining

Vein	Specifics	Drained territory	Drains into
Cerebral veins—Cortical supratentorial veins			
Superficial cortical veins	• Travel over the surface of the brain	• Frontal • Temporal • Parietal	• Superior sagittal sinus
Bridging veins	• Pierce the arachnoid membrane • Bridge subdural space	• Underlying neural tissue	• Sinus
Superficial middle cerebral vein	• Follows the posterior part of the fissure lateralis (Sylvian)	• Temporopolar region	• Cavernous sinus • Transverse sinus
Cerebral veins—Central supratentorial veins			
Central supratentorial veins		• Cerebrum	• Great cerebral vein of Galen
Internal cerebral vein	• Interventricular foramen	• Deep parts of the hemisphere	• Basal vein
Venous angle	• Junction of the internal jugular and subclavian veins		
Great cerebral vein of Galen	• Formed by the two internal cerebral veins • Under splenium corporis callosi	• Cerebrum	• Straight sinus
Basal vein of Rosenthal	• Paired Paramedian vein	• Perforated substance • Optic tract • Brain stem	• Great cerebral vein
Cerebral veins—Infratentorial veins			
Cerebellar veins	• Superior cerebellar veins • Inferior cerebellar veins	• Cerebellum	• Straight sinus • Transverse sinus • Superior petrosal sinus • Great cerebral veins • Internal cerebral veins
Extracerebral veins			
Diploic veins		• Diploë between the inner and outer layers of the cortical bone in the skull	• Extracranial veins of the scalp • Intracranial veins • Dural venous sinuses
Emissary veins	• Connect the sinuses, diploic veins, and superficial veins of the skull	• Veins outside of the cranium	• Venous sinuses
Cranial veins			
Facial vein		• Face • Anterior portion of the scalp	• Internal jugular vein
Retromandibular vein		• Temporal region • External ear	• Facial veins • Internal jugular vein
Pterygoid vein		• Deep portions of the face • External ear	• Internal jugular vein
Cervical veins			
Deep cervical veins		• Occipital vein • Suboccipital plexus	• Brachiocephalic vein
Vertebral veins		• Occipital vein • Suboccipital plexus	• Brachiocephalic vein

- Venous plexus of hypophyseal canal
- Venous plexus of formane ovale
- Internal carotid venous plexus
- Portal veins of pituitary gland
• Cerebral veins (located in the subarachnoid space, have no valves, empty into dural venous sinuses)
  - Superficial cortical veins (Cortical supratentorial veins)
    o Superior cortical veins
      • Superior anastomotic vein of Trolard
        - connects the superior sagittal sinus and the superficial middle cerebral vein (of Sylvius)

- Middle cortical veins
  - Superficial middle cerebral vein
    - Passes along the Sylvian fissure postero-anteriorly.
    - Collects numerous small tributaries which drain the opercular areas around the lateral sulcus.
    - Curves anteriorly around the tip of the temporal lobe and drains into the sphenoparietal sinus or cavernous sinus.
    - It may have connections to other dural venous sinuses by anastomotic veins:
      - to the superior sagittal sinus by the great anastomotic vein of Trolard
      - to the transverse sinus by the posterior anastomotic vein of Labbé
  - Inferior cortical veins
  - Deep middle cerebral vein
  - Basal vein of Rosenthal
  - Inferior anastomotic vein of Labbé
    - The largest vein crossing the temporal lobe between the Sylvian fissure and the transverse sinus.
    - Connects the superficial middle cerebral vein and the transverse sinus.
    - Highly variable location:
      - mid-temporal region: 60%
      - posterior temporal: 30%
      - anterior temporal: 10%
    - Gathers draining tributaries from the medial, antero-inferior, and postero-inferior temporal lobe.
    - There is a relationship between the size of the terminal superficial middle cerebral vein, the anastomotic vein of Trolard and the vein of Labbé, as all three share a similar drainage territory.
- Suzuki classification of the superficial Sylvian venous drainage pathways:
  - Sphenoparietal type: (54%)
    - drains into the sphenoparietal sinus
  - Emissary type: (12%)
    - courses along the lesser wing of sphenoid
    - turns inferiorly to reach the floor of the middle cranial fossa
    - joins the sphenoidal emissary veins
    - passes through the floor to reach the pterygoid plexus
  - Cavernous type: (7%)
    - directly drains into the anterior end of the cavernous sinus
  - Superior petrosal type: (54%)
    - runs along the lesser wing and just before reaching the cavernous sinus
    - turns downward along the anterior inner wall of the middle cranial fossa
    - runs along its floor medially to the foramen ovale to join the superior petrosal sinus
  - Basal type: (2%)
    - runs along the lesser wing
    - turns downward along the anterior wall of the middle cranial fossa
    - runs along its floor laterally to the foramen ovale over the petrous pyramid, presumably to join the transverse sinus through the lateral tentorial sinus or superior petrosal sinus
  - Squamosal type: (2%)
    - turns directly backward along the inner aspect of the temporal squama
    - runs posteriorly to join the transverse sinus or lateral tentorial sinus
  - Undeveloped type: (9%)
    - absent
    - superficial Sylvian drainage is through a large channel that extends forward, upward, upward and backward, or downward and backward into the superior sagittal sinus or transverse sinus
  - Deep cerebral veins (Central supratentorial veins)
    - Medullary veins
    - Subependymal veins
      - septal veins
      - thalamostriate veins
    - Deep paramedian veins
      - internal cerebral veins
      - great cerebral vein of Galen
  - Brain stem/Posterior Fossa Veins (Infratentorial veins)

9.2 Venous System

- Superior (Galenic) group
  - precentral cerebellar vein
  - superior vermian veins
  - anterior pontomesencephalic veins
- Anterior (petrosal) group
  - petrosal vein
- posterior (tentorial) group
  - inferior vermian veins
- Dural sinuses
  - Superior sagittal sinus
  - Inferior sagittal sinus
  - Straight sinus
  - Transverse sinus
  - Occipital sinus
  - Sigmoid sinus
- Extracerebral veins
  - Diploic veins
  - Emissary veins
- Cranial veins
  - Facial vein
  - Retromandibular vein
  - Pterygoid vein
- Cervical veins
  - Deep cervical veins
  - Vertebral veins

The venous drainage of the territories supplied by the carotid system are shown in Figs. 9.2a–d and 9.3a–d, while the venous drainage of the territories supplied by the vertebro-basilar system are shown in Figs. 9.4a–c and 9.5a–c.

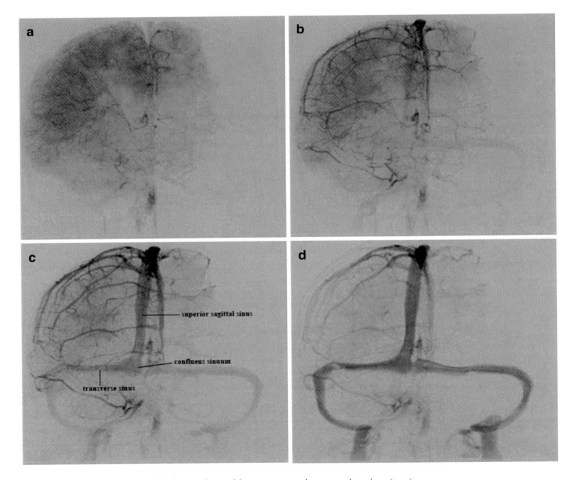

Fig. 9.2 Venous drainage of the internal carotid artery—anterior-posterior view (a–c)

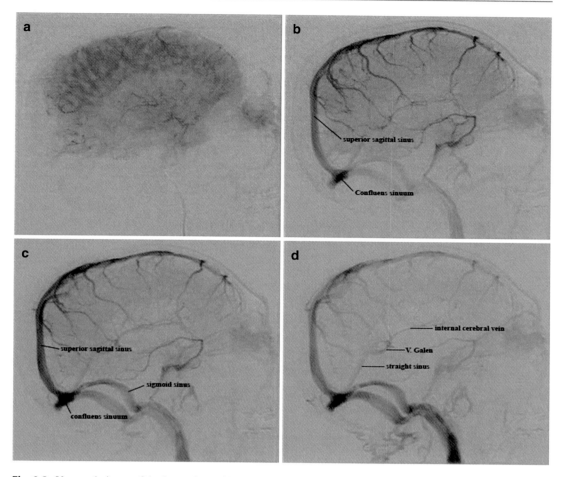

Fig. 9.3 Venous drainage of the internal carotid artery—lateral view (**a–d**)

9.2 Venous System

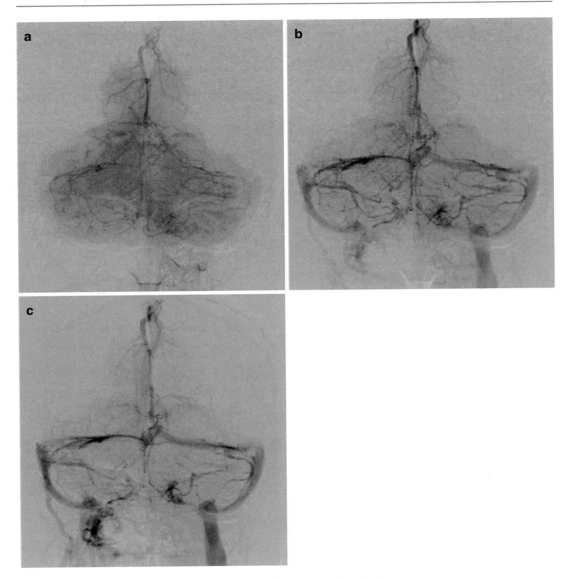

Fig. 9.4 Venous drainage of the vertebral artery—anterior-posterior view (**a–c**)

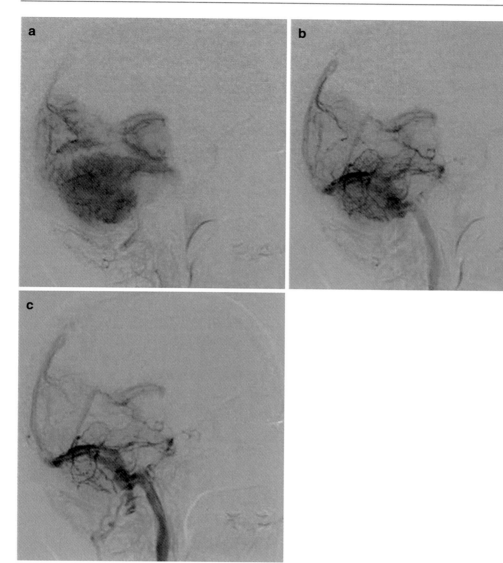

Fig. 9.5 Venous drainage of the vertebral artery—lateral view (**a–c**)

9.3 Dural Venous Sinuses

The system of dural venous sinuses is illustrated in Fig. 9.6a–c and pictured in Figs. 9.7, 9.8, and 9.9.

Dural venous sinuses are:

- venous channels
- located intracranially
- between the two layers of dura mater (endosteal layer and meningeal layer)
- "trapped epidural veins"
- run alone, not parallel to arteries
- valveless → bidirectional blood flow in intracranial veins
- the draining territories of intracranial veins are different from those of major cerebral arteries
- form the major drainage pathways from the brain, predominantly to the internal jugular veins

The venous sinuses are (Table 9.2):

9.3 Dural Venous Sinuses

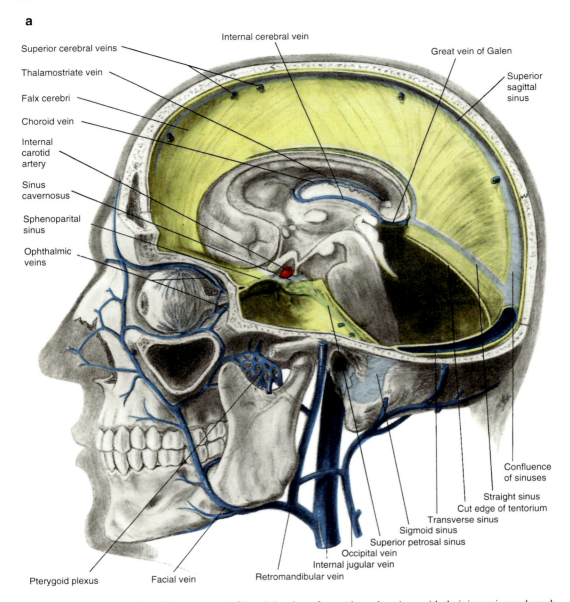

Fig. 9.6 Schematic drawing of the sinuses (**a**, **b**) and drawing of a cut through a sinus with draining veins and arachnoidal granulations (**c**) (reproduced from Heimer (1983) with kind permission by Springer Nature)

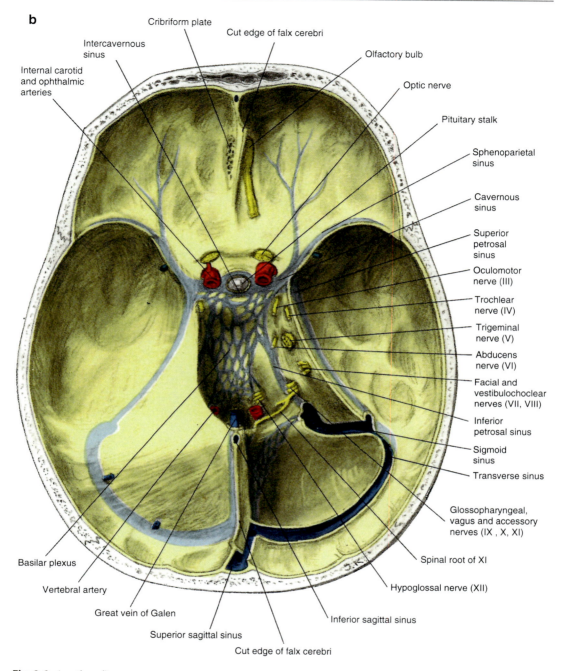

Fig. 9.6 (continued)

9.3 Dural Venous Sinuses

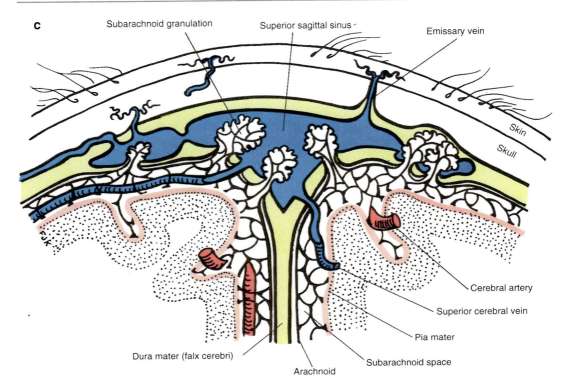

Fig. 9.6 (continued)

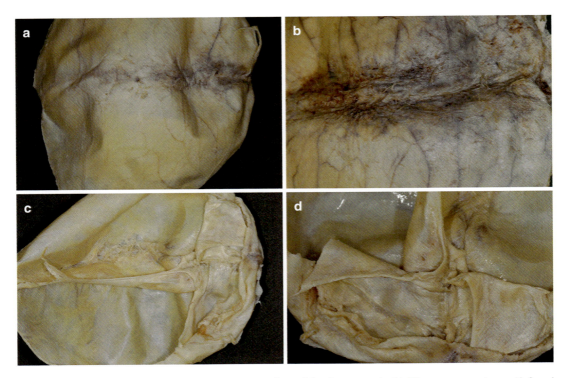

Fig. 9.7 Superior sagittal sinus as seen on the outer surface of the dura mater (**a**, **b**). The transverse sinuses (left and right) as seen on the inner surface of the dura mater (**c**, **d**)

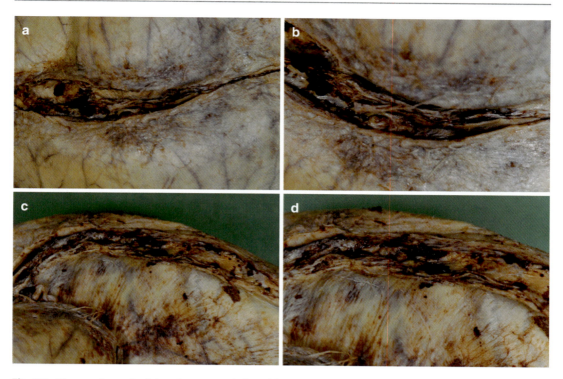

Fig. 9.8 The superior sagittal sinus is cut up and viewed from above (**a, b**) and from the side (**c, d**)

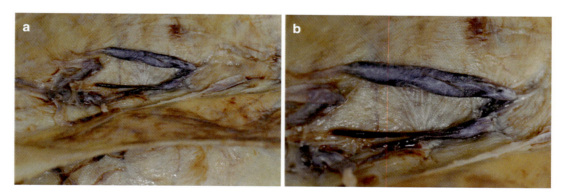

Fig. 9.9 Veins draining into the superior sagittal sinus (**a, b**)

Table 9.2 List of unpaired and paired venous sinuses

Unpaired	• Superior sagittal sinus
	• Inferior sagittal sinus
	• Straight sinus
	• Occipital sinus
	• Intercavernous sinus
Paired	• Transverse sinus
	• Sigmoid sinus
	• Inferior petrosal sinus
	• Superior petrosal sinus
	• Cavernous sinus
	• Sphenoparietal sinus
	• Basilar venous plexus

- unpaired
- paired

The veins drain the blood through the following sinuses into the extracranial venous system:

- Postero-superior group
  - Superior sagittal sinus (Figs. 9.7a–d and 9.8a–d)
    ○ Is the largest dural venous sinus
    ○ Runs in a sagittal plane along the superior margin of the falx cerebri

9.3 Dural Venous Sinuses

- Terminates at the confluence of sinuses at the occipital protuberance
- Receives from the superior cerebral veins
- Empties into the confluence of the sinuses at the occipital protuberance
- Inferior sagittal sinus
  - Runs along the inferior margin of the falx cerebri
  - Merges with the vein of Galen
  - Continues as the straight sinus
  - Receives tributaries from the falx itself as well as some small veins from the medial surface of the cerebral hemispheres
- Straight sinus
  - Extends from the falx cerebri to the tentorium cerebelli.
  - Is triangular in cross-section.
  - It receives the inferior sagittal sinus, the vein of Galen at its anterior end and some superior cerebellar veins along its course.
  - Empties into the confluence of the sinuses.
  - Exact drainage is variable:
    - confluence of sinuses (56%)
    - left transverse sinus (21%)
    - right transverse sinus (13%)
- Occipital sinus
  - Smallest of the dural venous sinuses
  - Lies within the falx cerebelli on the inner surface of the occipital bone
  - Tributaries from the margins of the foramen magnum, some of which connect with the sigmoid sinus and internal vertebral plexus, coalesce to pass in the attached margin of the falx cerebelli to drain postero-superiorly at the confluence of the sinuses
  - Drains into the confluence of the sinuses
- Transverse sinus
  - Receives venous blood from the confluence of the sinuses
  - Drains the superior sagittal sinus, the occipital sinus, and the straight sinus
  - Passes laterally and anteriorly along the tentorium cerebelli in the occipital bone
  - Runs inferiorly and medially of the petrous part of the temporal bone to form the sigmoid sinus
  - Empties into the sigmoid sinus which in turn reaches the jugular bulb
- Sigmoid sinus
  - Is a paired structure
  - Is the continuation of the transverse sinus
  - Becomes the sigmoid sinus as the tentorium ends
  - Receives the superior petrosal sinus.
  - Passes inferiorly in an S shaped groove posteromedial to the mastoid air-cells to the jugular foramen, where it ends in the jugular bulb, in the posterior half of the foramen (pars vascularis)
  - Drains into the internal jugular vein in the jugular foramen
- Antero-inferior venous sinuses
  - Cavernous sinus
    - Is a paired structure
    - Lies in the middle cranial fossa
    - Is located
      - On either side of the pituitary fossa and body of the sphenoid bone.
      - Between the endosteal and meningeal layers of the dura.
      - Anteriorly it is bounded by the superior orbital fissure and posteriorly by the petrous apex and Meckel's cave.
      - Superior relations include the middle cerebral artery and the optic chiasm.
      - Inferiorly it is bound by the sphenoid sinus.
      - The pituitary gland is medial to the cavernous sinus and the temporal lobes sit laterally.
    - Drains the inferior and superficial middle cerebral veins, ophthalmic vein.
    - It receives venous blood from:
      - inferior and superior ophthalmic veins
      - intercavernous sinus
      - sphenoparietal sinus
      - superficial middle cerebral vein
      - occasionally
        - central retinal vein

- a frontal tributary of the middle meningeal vein
  o Drainage of the cavernous sinus is via:
    - superior petrosal sinus to the transverse sinus
    - inferior petrosal sinus directly to the jugular bulb
    - venous plexus on the internal carotid artery (ICA) to the clival (basilar) venous plexuses
    - emissary veins passing through the sphenoidal foramen
      - foramen ovale: communicates between the CS and pterygoid plexuses
      - foramen lacerum
  o Empties into the superior and inferior petrosal sinuses
- Intercavernous sinus (anterior and posterior)
  o Are the communication between both cavernous sinuses
  o Lie in the anterior and posterior borders of the diaphragma sellae
  o Drain into the intercavernous sinuses
  o Are a cause of bleeding during transphenoidal hypophysectomy
- Sphenoparietal sinus
  o located along the postero-inferior ridge of the lesser wing of the sphenoid bone
  o receives tributaries from:
    - superficial middle cerebral vein
    - middle meningeal vein (frontal ramus)
    - anterior temporal diploic vein
  o empties into the cavernous sinus
- Superior petrovsal sinuses
  o It runs along superior aspect of the petrous temporal bone
  o It receives:
    - cerebellar veins
    - inferior cerebral veins
    - labyrinthine vein: draining the inner ear structures
  o Drains the cavernous sinus, posterolaterally to the transverse sinus
- Inferior petrosal sinus
  o Is often a venous channels rather than a true sinus.
  o Runs in a shallow groove between the petrous temporal bone and basilar occipital bone (on either side of the clivus). It is connected across the midline by the basilar plexus.
  o Receives tributaries from the medulla oblongata, pons, and inferior surface of the cerebellum as well as labyrinthine veins (via the cochlear canaliculus and the vestibular aqueduct).
  o Drains blood from the cavernous sinus to the jugular foramen (pars nervosa) or sometimes via a vein which passes through the hypoglossal canal to the suboccipital venous plexus.
  o Empties into the internal jugular vein.
- Basilar venous plexus
  o Lies between the endosteal and visceral layers of the dura on the inner surface of the clivus
  o It connects the:
    - inferior petrosal sinuses
    - cavernous sinuses
    - intercavernous sinuses
    - superior petrosal sinuses
    - internal vertebral venous plexus
    - marginal sinus (around the margins of foramen magnum)

Selected References

Arslan OE (2015) Neuroanatomical basis of clinical neurology, 2nd edn. CRC Press, Boca Raton

Heimer L (1983) The human brain and spinal cord: functional neuroanatomy and dissection guide. Springer, Berlin, Heidelberg

ten Donkelaar HJ (2011) Clinical neuroanatomy. Brain circuitry and its disorders. Springer, New York

Histological Constituents of the Nervous System

10.1 Neuron

The *neuron (nerve cell)* is the basic morphological, functional, and trophic unit of the nervous system (Fig. 10.1). There exist at least 100 billion of neurons in the human brain. Although the size, shape, and form of neurons are highly variable (Fig. 10.2a, b), a general description of the constituents of the nerve cell can be given.

The neuronal *cell membrane* corresponds in its structural composition to the well-known unit membrane. This membrane is 7–9 nm thick and is composed of three layers, i.e., two dark lines separated by a lucent central zone. The neuronal membrane is one of those sites at which the electric processes for the information transfer take place.

The *cell body (perikaryon or soma)* is embedded in the cytoplasm and contains the nucleus and several organelles including mitochondria, Golgi apparatus, lysosomes, as well as endoplasmic reticulum and free ribosomes (Fig. 10.3). The free ribosomes are the morphologic substrate of the Nissl substance which is seen at the light-microscopic level.

Many *processes* originate from the cell body: the dendrites and the axon.

- The *dendrites* originate in a variable number. The dendrites are highly ramified forming the so-called dendritic tree. At the site of the dendrites, the neuron receives the information from other neurons. The dendrites form the receptor zone (input zone) of the neuron. Along the dendrites, small knop-like extensions of the cytoplasm are seen: the dendritic spines. Both, the ramifications and the dendritic spines serve to augment the surface area of the dendrites and, thus, the receptor zone for input of neuronal information is tremendously increased.

- One *axon* usually originates from the cell body. The site of origin of the axon on the soma is called axon hillock. The axon hillock is characterized by the lack of Nissl substance. The length of the axon is highly variable and may amount between several μm up to 1.5 m. Small processes, the axonal collaterals, originate from the axon and abut on other neurons. The axon ramifies at its distal part in axonal terminals. The roundly thickened ends of the axonal terminals are called boutons terminaux. They participate in the formation of synapses. At these sites, the neuronal information is transmitted either to other neurons or to effector organs (i.e., glands, muscle). The axon forms the through-put zone of the neuron while the axonal collaterals and the axonal terminals constitute the output zone.

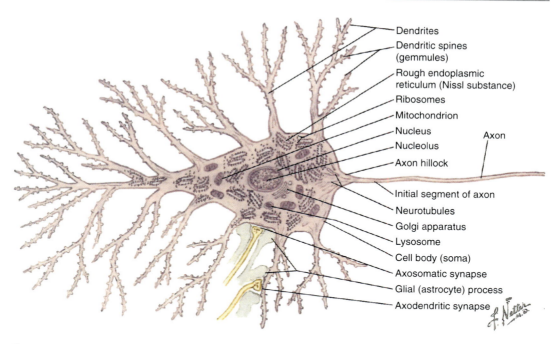

Fig. 10.1 Neuron with dendrites, perikaryon, nucleus, axon, myelin sheath, and axon (reproduced with kind permission from Felten and Shetty (2010))

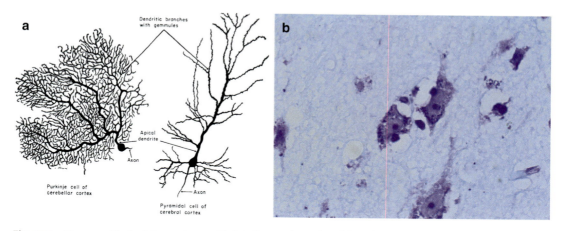

Fig. 10.2 Neuron with dendrites and axon (Golgi silver impregnation) (**a**) (left side: Purkinje cell of the cerebellum, right side: pyramidal cell of the cerebral cortex) (reproduced from Parent (1996) with kind permission by). Nerve cells with nucleus and nucleolus (Nissl stain) (**b**)

The axon is encased by a lipoprotein-containing substance, the ***myelin sheath***.

The *nucleus* is centrally located in the soma and is poor in chromatin. The nuclear membrane contains nuclear pores and is made up of two unit membranes. The latter are thought to be part of the endoplasmic reticulum (ER).

The *nucleolus* shows a compact shape and relatively large size. It contains high amounts of RNA. Although no mitotic figures are encoun-

10.1 Neuron

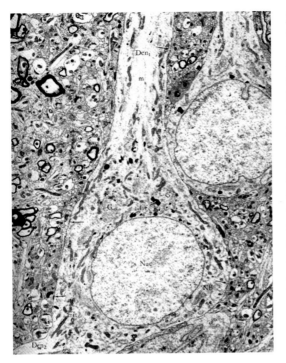

Fig. 10.3 Electron micrograph of a neuronal soma (reproduced from Peters et al. (1991) with kind permission by Oxford University Press)

tered in histological preparations, centrosomes can be seen the function of which are not yet clarified.

The *neuroplasm* is the structureless cytoplasm of neurons. It contains high concentrations of K^+-ions as well as other substances which participate in the information processing and the metabolism of the nerve cell.

The *mitochondria* are present in high amounts and can be even found in the finest cell processes. They function as "power supply" of the cell by being the sites of oxidative phosphorylation and providing the energy in the form of adenosine triphosphatase.

The *Golgi apparatus* is located next to the nucleus. Here, transmitter substances and peptide hormones are packaged as granula, which are then transported along the axon into the synaptic boutons. The Golgi apparatus also serves in the production of lysosomes and in the synthesis of cell membranes.

The *endoplasmic reticulum* is present in the cell in the form of smooth endoplasmic reticulum and rough endoplasmic reticulum. In the soma, both forms of endoplasmic reticulum are found whereas only smooth endoplasmic reticulum is present in the axon.

The *Nissl substance* is found in each cell body as well as in the dendrites. However, the axon hillock and the axon are devoid of it. The Nissl substance is composed of ribosomes as well as densely packed endoplasmic reticulum. They are responsible for the protein synthesis. In case of cell damage, a special reaction can be observed: chromatolysis. The Nissl substance is dissolved in such a way that the ribonucleoproteins can be used for the increased protein synthesis.

Lysosomes contain enzymes with hydrolytic activity. They are released in case of cell death and lead to autolysis. They are also called "suicide-bags." Lysosomes originate from the Golgi apparatus.

In the cytoplasm, various *pigments* may be present. They are believed to be side-products of the cellular metabolism. Of importance are lipofuscin, melanin, and iron.

- Lipofuscin is found in the cytoplasm closely apposed to the nucleus as well as at the axon hillock. The amount of lipofuscin deposits is proportionally increased with age. Melanin is localized in the substantia nigra and the locus coeruleus.
- Melanin deposits are already found in the developing brain. They are increased in adulthood and remain unchanged during life. There is no relationship to aging processes.
- Small amounts of iron deposits are found in various brain regions. It is believed that iron plays a certain role in the catalysis of the respiratory chain in the cell.

The cytoskeleton is made up of a highly interconnected network of filaments (Fig. 10.4):

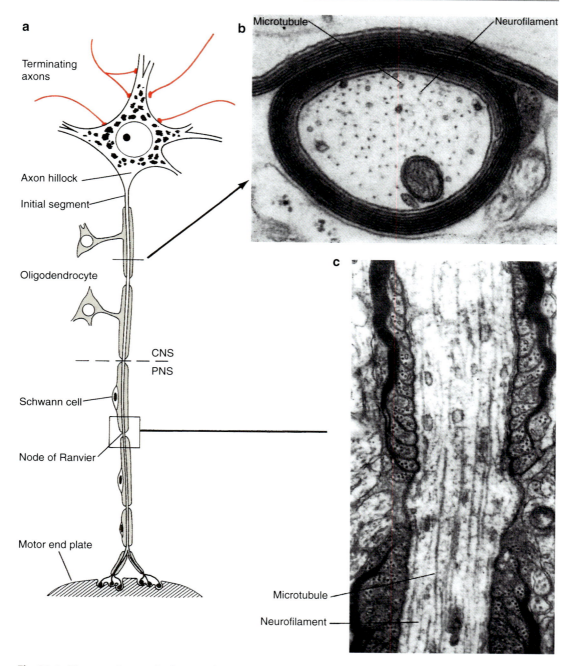

Fig. 10.4 Electron micrograph of neuronal processes. Nerve fiber of the CNS with axon (**a**, **b**) and myelin sheath and node of Ranvier (**c**) (reproduced from Heimer (1983) with kind permission by Springer Nature)

- Microtubules
  - Are made up of polymers of tubulin
  - Tubulin: globular protein forming a heterodimer between α and ß tubulin
  - Microtubule-associated proteins (MAPs): play roles in the assembly of microtubules, in cross-linking them to other filaments and in transport function
    - MAP 2 in dendrites
    - Tau in axons
- Intermediate filaments
  - Three polypeptide subunits: low weight, middle weight, high weight
- Actin filaments
  - Actin: globular protein that self-assembles into a linear polymer
  - Concentrated in dendritic spines and growth cones

Neurofibrils are seen at the light-microscopic level and are composed of neurofilaments and neurotubules.

- Neurotubules: are only identified at the electron microscopic level. They are made up of fine threads with a specific orientation in space. They are found in axons and in dendrites. Neurotubules have a diameter of 20–30 nm
- Neurofilaments: The diameter of neurofilaments is 6–10 nm

Neurofilaments play an eminent role in the transport of substances within the cell and the cell processes:

- The cellulifugal transport is directed from the soma to the axon and operates at a various speed:
  - slow axoplasmic flow at a rate of some 0.1–3.0 mm per day
  - fast axoplasmic flow at some 100–400 mm per day
- The cellulipetal transport or retrograde transport operates in the opposite direction.

The fast axonal transport is derived from the following force-generating proteins:

- Kinesin
  - Moves proteins towards the plus end of microtubules
  - Is the motor for fast anterograde transport

- Dynein
  - Moves proteins towards the minus end of microtubules
  - Is the motor for fast retrograde transport

Neurosecretory products are granular substances with a diameter of 100–700 µm. Examples are oxytocin and vasopressin.

10.1.1 Classification of Neurons

10.1.1.1 Classification of Neurons Based on Cell Processes

Based on the number of cell processes, the following subdivision of neurons is possible (Fig. 10.5):

- unipolar neuron
- bipolar neuron
- pseudounipolar neuron
- multipolar neuron

Unipolar Neuron

A unipolar neuron possesses a long axon. The information is mainly received at the surface of the perikaryon and transported along the axon. Unipolar neurons are found in the olfactory mucosa.

Bipolar Neuron

The bipolar neuron possesses two processes whereby one serves as the receptor (dendrite) and the other as the medium for information transport (axon). Bipolar nerve cells are found in the retina or in the ganglion of the eighth cranial nerve, i.e., vestibular ganglion and spiral ganglion.

Pseudounipolar Neuron

The pseudounipolar neuron possesses like the bipolar neuron two processes. However, the axon and the dendrite are lined against each other along a certain distance before reaching the

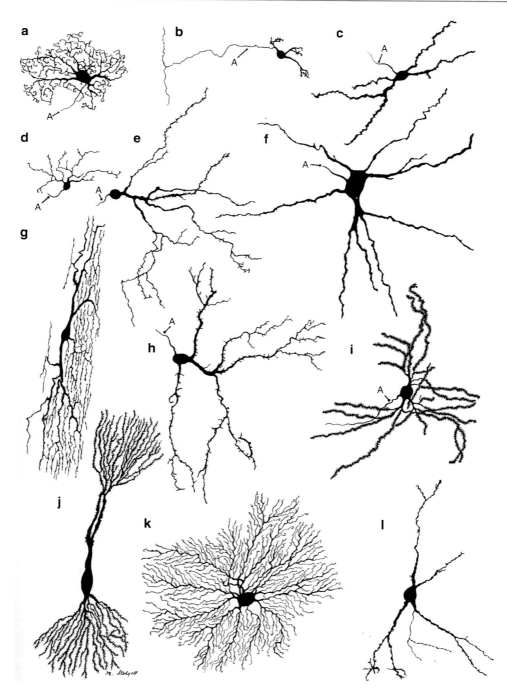

Fig. 10.5 The various types of neurons (reproduced from Parent (1996) with kind permission), neuron of the inferior olivary nucleus (**a**), granule cell of the cerebellum (**b**), small cell of reticular formation (**c**), small gelatinosa cell of spinal cord (**d**), ovoid cell of nucleus tractus solitaries (**e**), large cell of reticular formation (**f**), spindle-shaped cell of substantia gelatinosa of spinal cord (**g**), large cell of spinal trigeminal nucleus (**h**), neuron of putamen (**i**), double pyramidal cell in Ammon's horn of hippocampal formation (**j**), cell from thalamic nucleus (**k**), cell from globus pallidus (**l**)

perikaryon. Pseudounipolar neurons are found in, e.g., the spinal ganglion.

It has to be mentioned that in English-speaking countries a distinction between bipolar neurons and pseudounipolar neurons is not made.

Multipolar Neuron

The multipolar neuron possesses a multitude of processes serving as receptor organ (dendritic tree) and one structure for information conduction, i.e., the axon. The description of a neuron as given previously (Sect. 10.1) is that of a multipolar neuron. Multipolar neurons can be found throughout the nervous system, e.g., motor neurons in the anterior horn of the spinal cord.

10.1.1.2 Classification of Neurons Based on Axonal Length

Based on the length of the axon, the following subdivision of neurons is possible (Fig. 10.6a, b):

- Type I neuron
- Type II neuron

Type I Neuron

Type I neurons or Golgi I neurons have a long axon. The cells are identified as pyramidal cells in the cerebral cortex or as the Purkinje cells of the cerebellar cortex (Fig. 10.6a).

Type II Neuron

Type II neurons or Golgi II neurons have a small axon. They are identified as interneurons of the gray matter of the spinal cord or as granular cells in the granular layer of the cerebellar cortex (Fig. 10.6b).

10.1.2 Size of Neurons

The size neurons vary from region to region (Fig. 10.7a, b). There exist no relationship between the size and the functional determination of the nerve cell. The granular cells of the cerebellar cortex display the smallest diameter amounting 4 m. The largest diameters of 130 μm were measured on neurons of the primary motor area of the cerebral cortex, i.e., Betz cells.

10.1.3 Types of Neuronal Connection

- Projection neurons
  - Send axons to other regions of the CNS
  - Axon can reach a length of 1 m
  - Axon is myelinated
- Interneurons
  - Axons remain within the CNS region
  - Axon length less than 1 mm
  - Axon is not myelinated

Based on embryonic origin the following interneurons are distinguished (Table 10.1): (Wamsley and Fishell 2017):

- Medial ganglionic eminence (MGE)
  - Parvalbumin (PV)
  - Somatostatin (SST)
- Caudal ganglionic eminence (CGE)
  - Vasoactive intestinal peptide (VIP)
  - Reelin (RELN)

A selection of genes associated with neurons is given in Table 10.2.

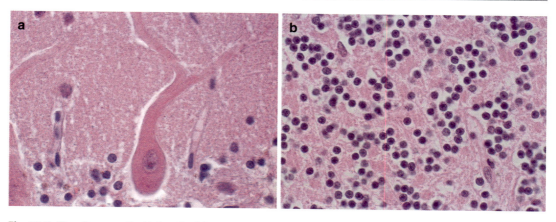

Fig. 10.6 Type I neuron: Purkinje cell of the cerebellum (**a**), Type II neuron: granular cells in layer 3 of the cerebellar cortex (**b**)

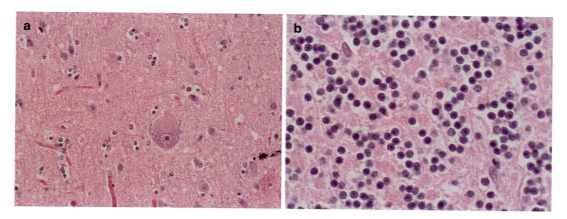

Fig. 10.7 Neurons of various sizes: Betz cell in the precentral gyrus (**a**), granular cell of the cerebellar layer 3 (**b**)

10.2 Synapse

The synapse is the zone of contact between two neurons or between the neuron and the effector cell. At the site of the synapse, the information is transduced. Certain cells like Purkinje cells of the cerebellum might form more than 100,000 synapses. There might be more than 100 trillion of synapses in the human brain.

The synapse is composed of (Fig. 10.8):

- presynaptic membrane
- synaptic cleft
- postsynaptic membrane

10.2.1 The Presynaptic Membrane

The presynaptic membrane is part of the bouton terminal of the distal axonal ramifications.

Table 10.1 Characteristics of various interneurons

Cell type	Layers	Markers	Characteristics
Parvalbumin (PV)			
Basket	• Present in L2–6 • Highest density in L4 and L5	• Tachykinin 1 (TAC) • Cholecystokinin (CCK)	• Multipolar dendrites • Soma and proximal dendrites • Mainly target cortical pyramidal neurons and PV+ cortical interneurons • Intra- and interlaminar arbors • Intra- and intercolumnar arbors • Low input resistance • High firing frequency • Fast, strong, and depressing excitatory inputs and inhibitory output
Chandelier	• Mainly in L2–6	• Tachykinin 1 (TAC) • Cholecystokinin (CCK)	• Multipolar dendrites • Axonal initial segment • Mainly target cortical pyramidal neurons • Axonal arbor mainly local • Fast spiking pattern but slower than basket cells • Potentially depolarizing
Somatostatin (SST)			
Martinotti	• Present in L2–6 • Highest density in L5	• Calretinin (CR) • Neuronal nitric oxide synthase (nNOS) • Reelin (RELN) • Neuropeptide Y (NPY)	• Multipolar and bitufted dendrites • L1 axonal arbor plexus • Local axonal arbors • Translaminar and columnar axon • High input resistance • LTS adapting or burst firing
Non-Martinotti	• Present in L2–6 • Highest density in L5	• Calretinin (CR) • Neuronal nitric oxide synthase (nNOS) • Reelin (RELN) • Neuropeptide Y (NPY)	• Multipolar and bitufted dendrites • Local axonal arbors • L4 cells: PV+ cortical interneurons targeting preference • L5 cells: axon plexus in both L4 and L5 • Low input resistance • Potentially fast spiking
Vasoactive intestinal peptide (VIP)			

Bipolar	• Present in L2–3 and L5–6
	• Highest density in L2 and L3
		• Calretinin (CR)
		• ChAT
		• Cholecystokinin (CCK)
			• Vertical intralaminar dendrites
			• Soma and dendrite targeting
			• Intralaminar and columnar axon arbor
			• Cortical interneurons targeting (i.e., SST+ c cortical interneurons)
			• High input resistance
			• Many firing patterns:
			  – irregular
			  – bursting
			  – adapting

Multipolar	• Present in L2–3 and L5–6 • Highest density in L2 and L3	• Calretinin (CR) • ChAT • Cholecystokinin (CCK)	• Vertical intralaminar dendrites
Reelin (RELN) (non-SST)			
Small basket cells (SBC)	• L1	• Neuronal nitric oxide synthase (nNOS) • Neuron-derived neurotrophic factor (NDNF) • Cholecystokinin (CCK)	• Multipolar dendrites • Narrow translaminar axon arbor • Cortical interneurons targeting

(continued)

Table 10.1 (continued)

Cell type	Layers	Markers	Characteristics
Neurogliaform cell (NGFC)	• Present in L1–6	• Neuronal nitric oxide synthase (nNOS) • Neuron-derived neurotrophic factor (NDNF) • Cholecystokinin (CCK)	• Multipolar dendrites • Dense axon arbor plexus • Synaptic and volume transmission • High input resistance • Commonly LS firing • Electronically coupled to other cortical interneurons

Table 10.2 Selection of genes associated with neurons

Cell type	Gene
Neuron	• DLX1—distal-less homeobox 1 • DLX2—distal-less homeobox 2 • GRM2—glutamate metabotropic receptor 2 • ISLR2—immunoglobulin superfamily-containing leucine-rich repeat 2 • SLC17A6—solute carrier family 17 member 6 • TBR1—T-box, brain 1

10.2.2 The Postsynaptic Membrane

The postsynaptic membrane is part of the dendritic tree or part of the perikaryon of the second neuron to which the information is conducted. This membrane can also be part of the effector organ, i.e., muscle cell or glandular cells.

10.2.3 The Synaptic Cleft

The synaptic cleft is located between the presynaptic and the postsynaptic membrane. Neurotransmitter substances are released in the synaptic cleft. The width of the synaptic cleft varies between 10 and 40 nm.

10.2.4 Types of synapses

Two types of synapses may be distinguished:

- the electrical synapse
- the chemical synapse

10.2.4.1 The Electrical Synapse

The electrical synapse is seldom found in the mammalian brain. The synaptic cleft of an electric synapse is 2 nm wide. The presynaptic and postsynaptic membranes lie closely together and form a gap junction. The impulse jumps from one cell to the other, whereby the impulse conduction can be executed in both directions, i.e., forwards and backwards. In contrast to the chemical synapse, neurotransmitters do not

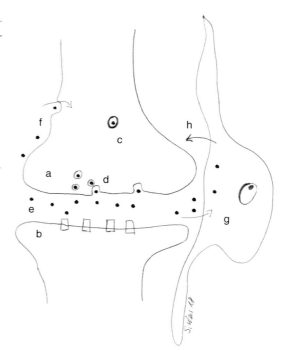

Fig. 10.8 Schematic drawing of the components of a synapse. Presynaptic bouton (**a**) with neurotransmitter in microvesicles (**b**), release of the neurotransmitter into the synaptic cleft (**c**), postsynaptic bouton with receptors and/or channels for neurotransmitter uptake (**d**), uptake of neurotransmitter from the synaptic cleft into glial cells (**e**) or into neurons (**f**). Neurotransmitter is also released from glial cells into neurons (**g**)

play a role in the transmission of neuronal information.

10.2.4.2 The Chemical Synapse

The impulse conduction in a chemical synapse can only be effected in one direction: unidirectional conduction. After the impulse reaches the synapse via the axon, neurotransmitters are released into the synaptic cleft. The transmitter substances are stored in small vesicles before they are released into the cleft. Depending on the nature of the transmitter, the information may be transmitted to the other cell or the transmission may be inhibited:

- At *excitatory synapses*, the transmitter produces at the level of the membrane of the second neuron an excitatory postsynaptic potential (EPSP).
- At *inhibitory synapses*, the transmitter produces at the level of the membrane of the second neuron an inhibitory postsynaptic potential (IPSP).

10.2.5 Classification of synapses

Based on the thickness of the postsynaptic density, the following synapses might be distinguished:

- asymmetric synapse, Gray type I
  - prominent postsynaptic density
- symmetric synapse, Gray type II
  - thin, less prominent postsynaptic density

The synapses may be classified as follows:

- *Interneuronal synapse*: A synapse between two neurons.
- *Myoneuronal synapse*: A synapse between a neuron and a muscle cell.
- *Neuroglandular synapse*: A synapse between a neuron and a gland.
- *Synapse á distance*: A synapse composed of a free ending presynaptic bouton terminal and a very wide synaptic cleft. The transmitter is released into the intercellular space. An example of a synapse á distance is the postganglionic axon of the sympathetic nervous system.

Based on their zones of contact, the synapses can be subdivided into the following types:

- *Axo-dendritic synapse*: The synapse contacts a dendrite of the second neuron.
- *Axo-somatic synapse*: The synapse contacts the perikaryon of the second neuron or the perikaryon of the same neuron.
- *Axo-axonal synapse*: The synapse contacts the axon of the second neuron or the axon of the same neuron.

The correlation between the type of synapse and its function is given as follows:

- Axo-dendritic synapses—excitatory
- Axo-somatic synapses—inhibitory
- Axo-axonal synapses—inhibitory

Recently, the synapse is not seen as being only the connection between two neurons, but includes other cellular and tissue elements as follows:

- *Tripartite synapse* composed of:
  - presynaptic element
  - postsynaptic element
  - endfeet of glial cells
- *Tetrapartite synapse* or "synaptic quadriga" composed of:
  - presynaptic element
  - postsynaptic element
  - endfeet of glial cells
  - extracellular matrix (ECM) structures
    ○ ECM structures are produced by both astrocytes and neurons and contribute to the functional synaptic complex.

The synaptic vesicles are also called synaptosomes. They can be marked immunohistochemically with the anti-synaptophysin antibody.

Based on their ultrastructural features, various types of synaptic vesicles may be distinguished:

- Round, pale vesicles with a diameter of 40–60 nm. They often contain the transmitter acetylcholine.
- Ellipsoid vesicles.
- Small dense core vesicles with a diameter of 50 nm. They often contain the transmitters, noradrenalin, and dopamine.

Synaptic proteins can be grouped as follows:

- small synaptic vesicle proteins
  - include among others syntaxin, synaptobrevin, synaptophysin, synaptoporin, synaptogamin, synapsins, SV-2, Rab 3, amphiphysin
- large dense core vesicles
  - comprise chromogranin A and secretogranin II
- synaptic plasma membrane proteins
  - include GAP-43 and PKC
- synaptic mitochondria membrane proteins
  - include SNAP 25
- synaptic skeletal proteins
  - include brain spectrin, actin, and actin-binding proteins

Genes involved in the regulation of synaptic proteins include:
- Presynaptic neurotransmitter release
  - SV2A (synaptic vesicle glycoprotein 2A), SYNs (synapsin), STX1B (syntaxin 1B), SNP25 (synaptosomal-associated protein 25kDa), STXBP1 (syntaxin-binding protein 1), CACNA1A (calcium voltage-gated channel subunit alpha 1A), DNM-1KCNA1 (dynamin 1), KCNA2 (potassium voltage-gated channel subfamily A member 2), CHRNA4 (cholinergic receptor nicotinic alpha 4 subunit)
- Postsynaptic proteins
  - GRIN2A (glutamate ionotropic receptor NMDA type subunit 2A), GRIN2B (glutamate ionotropic receptor NMDA type subunit 2B), CACNG2 (calcium channel, voltage-dependent, gamma subunit 2), SYNGAP1 (synaptic Ras GTPase-activating protein 1), PLPPR4 (phospholipid phosphatase related 4), SLC12A5 (solute carrier family 12, member 5), GABRA1 (gamma-aminobutyric acid (GABA) A receptor, subunit alpha 1), GABRB3 (gamma-aminobutyric acid type A receptor beta 3 subunit), GABRG2 (gamma-aminobutyric acid type A receptor gamma 2 subunit), IQSEC2 (IQ motif and Sec7 domain 2)
- Trans-synaptic communication
  - NRXN1 (neurexin 1), DAG1 (dystroglycan 1), CNTNAP2 (contactin-associated protein like 2), SRPX (sushi repeat-containing protein, X-linked), ADAM22-ADAM23 (ADAM metallopeptidase domain 22 - ADAM metallopeptidase domain 23), C1Q (complement C1q A chain), endocannabinoid (2-AG)

10.3 Nerve Fibers and Peripheral Nerve

10.3.1 Morphological Features of Nerve Fibers

An axon with its myelin sheath is called nerve fiber. Schwann cells ensheath the axons of the peripheral nervous system, while oligodendrocytes produce the myelin sheath of axons in the central nervous system.

Axons are ensheathed in different ways which allows to distinguish (Figs. 10.9 and 10.10):

- non-myelinated nerve fibers
- myelinated nerve fibers

10.3.1.1 Non-myelinated Nerve Fibers

The name is not exact since there is a very thin sheath; however, the name is commonly used (Fig. 10.9a, b). Non-myelinated nerve fibers constitute cables of axons which are ensheathed by one single Schwann cell. The mesaxon is that part where the plasmalemma of the Schwann cells is in contact with each other. Since one Schwann cells is too small to ensheath an axon along its whole distance, many Schwann cells are lined up to fulfill this task.

10.3 Nerve Fibers and Peripheral Nerve

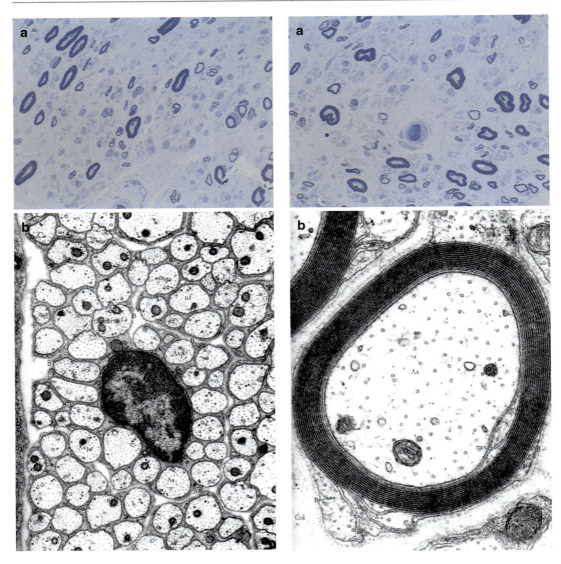

Fig. 10.9 Non-myelinated nerve fibers. Semithin section (**a**), electron microscopy (**b**) (**b** reproduced from Peters et al. (1991) with kind permission by Oxford University Press)

Fig. 10.10 Myelinated nerve fibers. Semithin section (**a**), electron microscopy (**b**) (**b** reproduced from Peters et al. (1991) with kind permission by Oxford University Press)

Non-myelinated fibers display diameters of about 1–2 μm.

10.3.1.2 Myelinated Nerve Fibers

Myelinated nerve fibers are wrapped by a big myelin sheath (Fig. 10.10a, b). The Schwann cells are arranged in such a way that they form at a distance of 1 mm incisures, the node of Ranvier. That part of the axon extending between two nodes of Ranvier is called internodium. This part is not covered by Schwann cells and, thereby, forms a region devoid of electrical isolation. Thus, it is the place at which the electrical phenomena of impulse conduction can take place. The impulse jumps from one internodium to the other: the saltatory impulse conduction. In this way, the neuronal information can be transmitted at a high speed.

The myelin sheath is biochemically composed of lipids and proteins. Ultrastructurally, a lamellar organization into dark and bright lines is noted corresponding to the alternating assembly of lipids and proteins. The impulse conduction velocity is proportionally correlated with the myelin sheath thickness. The thicker the myelin sheath the higher is the speed of impulse conduction. At the light-microscopic examination of longitudinal sections, incisures into the myelin sheath are described, the Schmidt-Lanterman incisures. They are interpreted to be structural figure of plasma movements.

Myelinated display diameters of about 20 mm.

10.3.2 Classification of Nerve Fibers

The classification of nerve fibers is done following the degree of myelin formation and results grossly into three groups:

- Group A
- Group B
- Group C

10.3.2.1 Group A Nerve Fibers
Characteristics of group A nerve fibers are given in Tables 10.3 and 10.4.

Table 10.3 Group A fibers are characterized by the following features

Myelination	Strong
Diameter	3–20 µm
Conduction velocity	15–120 m/s
Localization	Motor fibers

10.3.2.2 Group B Nerve Fibers
Characteristics of group B nerve fibers are given in Table 10.5.

10.3.2.3 Group C Nerve Fibers
Characteristics of group A nerve fibers are given in Table 10.6.

10.3.3 Structure of Peripheral Nerves

A peripheral nerve is composed of many bundles of non-myelinated and myelinated nerve fibers. An exchange of nerve fibers between bundles is possible. Efferent and afferent nerve fibers are contained with nerves.

The following three layers of connective tissue give support to the nerve (Fig. 10.11a–d):

- Endoneurium
- Perineurium
- Epineurium

10.3.3.1 The Endoneurium
The endoneurium is a layer of connective tissue holding together many nerve fibers forming a single bundle. The endoneurium contains capillaries and lymphatics.

10.3.3.2 The Perineurium
The perineurium is made up of connective tissue and fills the space between several fiber bundles.

Table 10.4 Subdivision of nerve fibers of group A based on their diameter, conduction velocity, and specific functions

Aα	10–20 µm	60–120 m/s	• Motoric fibers for skeletal muscles	• Proprioception • Stretch • Primary muscle spindle afferents • Motor efferents to muscles
Aβ	7–10 µm	40–60 m/s	• Sensory fibers originating in the skin (receptors for touch)	• Mechanoreception • Discriminative touch • Pressure • Joint rotation • Secondary muscle spindle afferents
Aγ	4–7 µm	30–40 m/s	• Motor fibers for muscle spindles	• Muscle spindle (intrafusal) efferents
Aδ	3–4 µm	15–30 m/s	• Sensory fibers originating in the skin (receptors for heat, cold, and pain)	• Mechanoreception: touch • Nociception: discriminative pain

10.4 Glial Cells

Table 10.5 Group B fibers are characterized by the following features

Myelination	Mild
Diameter	3 μm
Conduction velocity	Approximately 15 m/s
Localization	Visceral afferents of the vegetative system
Function	Sympathetic preganglionic axons

Table 10.6 Group C fibers are characterized by the following features

Myelination	None
Diameter	Less than 1 ìm
Conduction velocity	Approximately 0.5–2 m/s
Localization	Postganglionic fibers of the vegetative system
Function	Nociception: inflammatory or visceral pain, thermal sense

10.3.3.3 The Epineurium

The epineurium is composed of loose connective tissue and surrounds the fiber bundles and perineurium.

10.4 Glial Cells

The glial cells are the non-neural elements of the nervous system. Since they form the interstitial tissue of the nervous system and were thought to hold together the nervous tissue, they were called glia, i.e., glue by Rudolf Virchow.

Among the glial cells, the following types are identified:

- Astrocytes
- Oligodendrocytes
- Microglia

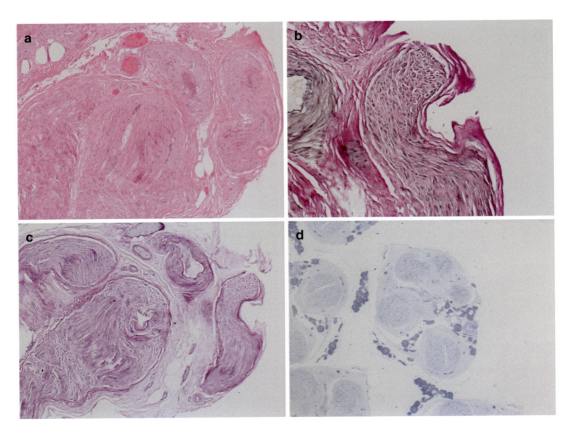

Fig. 10.11 Connective tissue of a peripheral nerve. Fascicles are discernible (**a**, stain: H&E, **b**, stain: EvG, **c**, stain: PAS, **d**, semithin section, stain: toluidine blue)

- Ependymal cells
- Tanycytes
- Choroid epithelium

In former times, people liked to group together astrocytes and oligodendrocytes into macroglia and compared this group to microglia. These classifications should not anymore be considered. Each type of glial cell has its own identity and fulfills specific functions in the cellular interplay of the nervous system.

10.5 Astroglia (Astrocytes)

Astrocytes fulfill trophic, plasticity, and reparatory functions. Through their processes, they bridge the gap between neurons and capillaries, thus allowing the diffusion of various nutritive substances from the blood stream to the nerve cells. Damaged neuronal tissue is replaced by a scar which is mainly formed by astrocytic processes containing glial fibrillary acidic protein (GFAP).

Two major types of astrocytes are distinguished (Fig. 10.12a–d):

- protoplasmic astrocytes, which are mainly found in the gray matter
- fibrillary astrocytes, which are most numerous in the white matter

Protoplasmic astrocytes
- have irregular and profusely branching processes

Fibrous/fibrillary astrocytes
- Have long processes (up to 300 μm).
- However, they are less elaborate than protoplasmatic astrocytes.

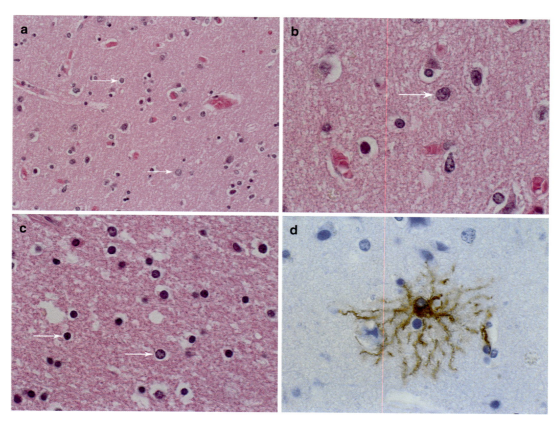

Fig. 10.12 Astrocytes. Astrocytes in the cerebral cortex (**a**, **b**), and white matter (**c**) immunohistochemistry for GFAP of a fibrillary astrocyte (**d**) (astrocytes are marked →)

10.5 Astroglia (Astrocytes)

- They establish several perivascular or subpial endfeet.
- Fibrous astrocytes possess numerous extensions (perinodal processes) that contact axons at the nodes of Ranvier.
- The numerical density of fibrous astrocytes in the white matter is approximately 200,000/mm^3.

Radial glia
- Elongated fibers span the width of the cerebral wall during development.
- Direct neuroblasts from the germinal matrix to the cerebral cortex.

Stains for astrocytes
- Older stains:
  - Holzer
  - Phosphotungstic acid hematoxylin (PTAH)
- Immunohistochemical
  - GFAP (not all astrocytes are stained) (Fig. 10.12d)
  - S100ß
  - Vimentin (not very specific)
  - Expression of growth factors
    - Epidermal growth factor
    - Basic fibroblast growth factor

Electron microscopy
- Abundant intermediate filaments
- Cytoplasmic dense bodies
- Gap junctions
- Multiple cellular processes

The functions of astrocytes are manifold and include:
- Development
  - regulation of neuro- and gliogenesis
  - neural path finding
  - regulation of synaptogenesis
- Structural
  - scaffold of the nervous system
  - continuous syncytium
- Vascular
  - glial-vascular interface
  - regulation of cerebral microcirculation
  - formation of the blood–brain barrier
- Metabolic
  - providing energy substrates for neurons
  - collecting neuronal waste
- Maintenance of the extracellular milieu and control of CNS environment
  - regulation of extracellular ion concentrations
  - regulation of extracellular pH
  - removal of transmitters
  - brain water homeostasis
- Signaling
  - modulation of synaptic transmission
  - release of neurotransmitter
  - long-range signaling within glial syncytium
  - integration of neuronal-glial network
- Response to injury

Astrogliosis is:
- Isomorphic
  - Astrocytes arrange themselves along anatomical structures.
- Anisomorphic
  - Astrocytes arranged haphazardly at the edges of infarcts.
- Associated with proliferation of Rosenthal fibers.
  - Protein aggregates in astrocytic processes.
    - Contain ubiquitin, αß-crystallin, heat shock protein HSP27.

A selection of genes associated with astrocytes is given in Table 10.7.

A summary of astroglial functions is given in Table 10.8 while its involvement in disease states is shown in Table 10.9.

Table 10.7 A selection of genes associated with astrocytes

Gene
• ALDH1L1—aldehyde dehydrogenase 1 family member L1
• EGFR—epidermal growth factor receptor
• ENTPD2—ectonucleoside triphosphate diphosphohydrolase 2
• GDPD2—glycerophosphodiester phosphodiesterase domain-containing 2
• ITGA7—integrin subunit alpha 7
• KIAA1161—KIAA1161 ortholog
• NWD1—NACHT and WD repeat domain-containing 1
• SOX9—SRY-box 9

Table 10.8 Physiological functions of astrocytes (Verkhratsky et al. 2017) reproduced with kind permission from Wiley-Blackwell

Functional group	Function	Molecular pathways
Ion homeostasis	K$^+$ buffering and homeostasis	• Na$^+$-K$^+$ pump, NKA • Na$^+$-K$^+$-Cl$^-$ co-transporter 1 NKCC1/SLC12A2 (operational at high Kl loads) • Inward rectifier K$^+$ channels Kir4.1 • Connexins Cx43, Cx30
	Cl$^-$ homeostasis	• GABAA receptors • Anion channels, ClC-2, • Volume-regulated anion channels VRAC/SWELL1 • Best1 Cl$^-$ channels • Na$^+$-K$^+$-Cl$^-$ co-transporter 1 NKCC1/SLC12A2
	H$^+$ homoeostasis and control of extracellular pH	• Na$^+$-H$^+$ exchanger NHE1/SLC9A1 • Na1-HCO– • 3 transporter NBCe1/SLC4A4 • Plasmalemmal V-type H1 pump
	Na$^+$, Ca2$^+$ homoeostasis	• Plasmalemmal Ca^{2+} pump PMCA • Na$^+$-Ca2$^+$ exchanger NCX1/SLC8A1, NCX2/SLC8A2, and NCX3/SLC8A3
Neurotransmitter homoeostasis	Glutamate	• Na$^+$-dependent glutamate transporters EAAT1/ • SLC1A6 and EAAT2/SLC1A2 • Cystine/glutamate antiporter Sxc– composed of • xCT/SCL7A11 and 4F2hc/SLC3A2 proteins
	GABA	• Na$^+$-dependent GABA transporter GAT3/SLC6A11 (148, 223) shuttle
	Glutamate/GABA-glutamine	• Glutamine synthetase GS • Na$^+$-dependent glutamine transporters
	Glycine	• Na$^+$-dependent glycine transporters GlyT1/SLC6A9
	Monoamines	• Norepinephrine transporter NET/SLC6A2 (which transports both noradrenaline and dopamine) • Monoamine oxidase B MAO-B
	Adenosine	• Na$^+$-dependent concentrative nucleoside transporters • CNT2/SLC28A2 and CNT3/SLC28A3 • Adenosine kinase ADK
Metabolic support	Uptake of glucose, synthesis of glycogen	• Glucose transporter
	Aerobic glycolysis, shuttling of lactate to neurones	• Monocarboxylate transporters 1 and 4 (MCT1/ SLC16A1, MCT4/SLC16A3)
Network homeostasis and synaptic transmission	Synaptogenesis	• Cholesterol, thrombospondins, hevin, secreted protein acidic and rich in cysteine SPARC
	Synaptic maturation	• Activity-dependent neurotrophic factor, tumor necrosis factor-a (TNFa), cholesterol, astroglia-derived glypicans 4 and 6
	Synaptic extinction	• Complement factor C1q

10.5 Astroglia (Astrocytes)

Table 10.8 (continued)

Functional group	Function	Molecular pathways
Organ homeostasis	Regulation of the formation and permeability of blood–brain and CSF–brain barriers	
	Formation of glial-vascular interface and regulation of microcirculation	• Epoxyeicosatrienoic acids EETs, 20-hydroxyeicosatetraenoic acid 20-HETE, prostaglandin E2 PGE2 • Ca21-dependent K channels KCa3.1
	Functional operation of the glymphatic system	• Water channel aquaporin-4 AQP4
	Gliocrine system, astrocytes act as secretory cells of the brain	• Neurotransmitters • Neuromodulators • Neurohormones • Cytokines • Neurotrophic factors
Systemic homeostasis	Central chemoreception of plasma Na^+ concentration	• Na^+-activated Nax channels
	Central chemoreception of oxygen, pH, and CO_2	• Oxygen sensor associated with mitochondria in cortical astrocytes pH sensor in brain stem astrocytes • Na1-Ca21 exchanger. Kir4.1 K^+ channels
	Regulation of sleep	• Astrocytes are linked to the sleep homeostat through an elevation of brain adenosine content in the wake state. Astrocytes may also regulate sleep through dynamic control over ion composition of the interstitium

Table 10.9 Astrocytopathology modified after Verkhratsky et al. (2017) reproduced with kind permission from Wiley-Blackwell

Nosological forms	Astrocytopathy
Leukodystrophies	
Alexander disease	• Sporadic mutations of glial fibrillary acidic protein (GFAP) with pathological remodeling of astrocytes and severe white matter lesions • Decrease in astroglial glutamate uptake
Megalencephalic leukoencephalopathy with subcortical cysts (MLC)	• Mutations in the MLC1 gene • Often in combination with mutations in the hepatic and glial cell adhesion molecule gene (Hepacam/Glialcam) • The MLC1 protein is predominantly expressed in astrocytic endfeet • MLC1 is a part of membrane signaling complex which includes Na1-K1- pump, inward rectifier Kir4.1 channels, aquaporin4 (AQP4), caveolin-1, and TRPV4 channels • Involves a loss of astroglial control over fluid homoeostasis and cell volume
Vanishing white matter syndrome (VWM) or childhood ataxia with central nervous system hypomyelination (CACH)	• Mutations in the eukaryotic translation initiation factor 2 (EIF-2B) gene • The disease is associated with atrophic (dysmorphic) astrocytes • Altered GFAP filaments • Deficient astroglial reactivity • Impaired astrocytic differentiation • Pathologically remodeled astrocytes secret factors inhibiting oligodendroglial maturation

(continued)

Table 10.9 (continued)

Nosological forms	Astrocytopathy
Demyelinating diseases	
Neuromyelitis optica (NMO)	• Autoantibodies-induced loss of AQP4 and GFAP • Astroglial atrophy and demise
Balós disease	• Downregulation of expression of Cx43 and AQP4 • Mislocalization of MLC1 • Astroglial hypertrophy • Loss of astroglial function is considered to be a primary cause for oligodendroglial lesions and demyelination
Neurotoxic encephalopathies	
Hepatic encephalopathy	• Pathological remodeling of astrocytes; failure of K1 and glutamate homeostasis with ensuing excitotoxicity • Pathological Ca21 signaling • Aberrant glutamate release • Deficient operation of glutamate-glutamine shuttle because of excessive ammonium obliterating the GS pathway
Heavy metal (lead, manganese mercury, aluminum)-induced encephalopathies	• Astroglial loss-of-function: accumulation of heavy metal into astrocytes instigated significant downregulation of plasmalemmal glutamate transporters with ensuing excitotoxicity
Wilson disease	• Pathological remodeling of astrocytes • Failure of astroglial regulation of copper homoeostasis
Psychiatric diseases	
Wernicke–Korsakoff encephalopathy	• Loss of astroglial function: substantial (up to 80%) downregulation of astroglial plasmalemmal glutamate transporters with ensuing glutamate excitotoxicity
Major depressive disorder	• Reduction in astroglial densities in cortex and amygdala • Reduced expression of GFAP • Decrease in expression of plasmalemmal glutamate transporters, connexins Cx43 and Cx30, glutamine synthetase, and AQP4 • Impaired astroglial homeostatic capabilities may underlie aberrant neurotransmission responsible for depressive symptoms
Schizophrenia	• Astrodegeneration and astroglial atrophy • Downregulation of homeostatic molecular pathways, including plasmalemmal glutamate transporters, AQP4, GS, thrombospondins • Upregulation of plasmalemmal cystine/glutamate exchanger • Increased production of kynurenic acid
Addictive disorders	• Combination of astrodegeneration and astroglial reactivity • Impaired astroglial glutamate homoeostasis • Ablation of astrocytes from the prelimbic area of the prefrontal cortex, as well as inhibition of astroglial gap junctions increased alcohol seeking behavior • Atrophic astrocytes (nucleus accumbens)
Neurodegenerative diseases	
Alzheimer disease	• Astroglial atrophy at the early stages • Reactive remodeling of senile plaque-associated astrocytes • Reduced astrogliosis at the terminal stages • Decreased astroglial synaptic coverage • Loss of astroglial homeostatic support • Impairment of water transport, glutamate uptake, and glutamate-glutamine shuttle • Astrocytes associated with senile plaques display Ca21 hyperexcitability and generate abnormal propagating intercellular Ca21 waves
Aging-related tau astrogliopathy	• Exclusive expression of pathological tau in astrocytes

Table 10.9 (continued)

Nosological forms	Astrocytopathy
Amyotrophic lateral sclerosis (ALS)	• Early astrodegeneration • Astroglial death (through apoptosis) • Loss glutamate clearance function • Subsequent excitotoxicity and neuronal demise • Selective silencing of human SOD1-mutated gene in astrocytes delays ALS progression • Neuronal death, occurring at later stages of ALS triggers astrogliotic response
Parkinson disease	• Astrocytes provide protection of dopaminergic neurones • Astrocytes may accumulate α-synuclein • Evidence for suppressed astroglial reactivity, which may indicate decrease in neuroprotection
Huntington disease (HD)	• Progressive astroglial reactivity • No signs of astrogliosis • In HD mouse model • Decrease in glutamate uptake • Deficient K1 buffering • Pathologically increased release of glutamate
Other diseases	
Glioblastoma	• Cancer developed from astrocytes or their precursors
Traumatic brain injury	• Reactive astrogliosis prevails with a gradient of phenotypes from the lesion to the healthy tissue • Astrocytes move towards the lesion site (anisomorphic astrogliosis) • Form the scar • Reactive astrocytes control post-lesion regeneration
Ischemia and stroke	• Reactive astrocytes surround the area of the infarction core and define survival or demise of neurons in the penumbra • Astrocytes may also convey death signals
Epilepsy	• Reactive astrogliosis • Pathological remodeling of astroglia • Downregulation of expression of Kir4.1 channels • Changes in astroglial morphology • Disappearance of gap junction coupling (in mesial temporal lobe epilepsy)
Migraine	• Loss-of-function mutation of astroglia-specific a2 subunit of Na1-K1 pump • Decrease of expression of astroglial plasmalemmal glutamate transporters
Autistic spectrum disorders (ASD)	• Pathological remodeling of astrocytes

10.6 Oligodendroglia (Oligodendrocytes)

Oligodendrocytes which are found closely apposed to neuronal perikarya in the gray matter are known as the perineuronal satellite cells, while the interfascicular oligodendrocytes are those seen in the white matter (Fig. 10.13a–d). Oligodendrocytes form the myelin sheath of axons in the central nervous system. In the peripheral nervous system, the cells fulfilling the same function are called Schwann cells.

Oligodendrocytes show on H&E-stained sections a round, dark nucleus without prominent cytoplasm small processes. The available immunohistochemical markers are problematic in such a way that they do not allow a reliable and reproducible demonstration of this cell type.

Oligodendrocytes were first described in 1928 by Del Rio-Hortega who classified them into four types:

- *Type I oligodendrocytes* have small round cell bodies and produce four to six primary processes which branch and myelinate 10–30

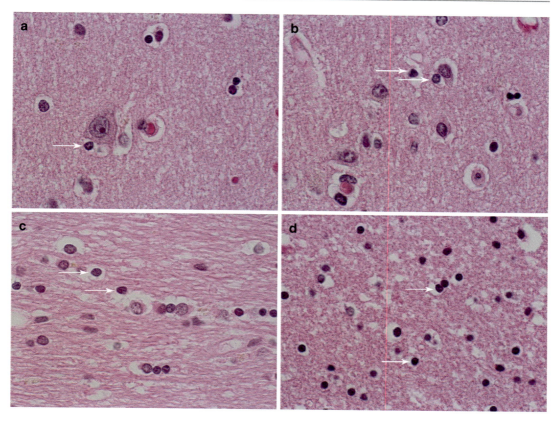

Fig. 10.13 Oligodendrocytes. Perineuronal satellite cell (**a**), oligodendrocyte in the cerebral cortex (**b**), oligodendrocytes in the white matter (**c**, **d**) (oligodendrocytes are marked →)

axons with a diameter of <2 μm. They form a single internodal myelin segment of approximately 100–200 μm length. They are found in the forebrain, cerebellum, and spinal cord.
- *Type II oligodendrocytes* are similar to type I; they have small round cell bodies and produce four to six primary processes which branch and myelinate 10–30 axons with a diameter of <2 μm. They form a single internodal myelin segment of approximately 100–200 μm length. They are found only in the white matter (e.g., corpus callosum, optic nerve, cerebellar white matter).
- *Type III oligodendrocytes* have larger cell bodies and several thick primary processes which myelinate up to five thick axons (4–15 μm in diameter). They produce myelin sheaths with approximately 200–500 μm internodal length. They are found in the cerebral and cerebellar peduncles, the medulla oblongata, and spinal cord.
- *Type IV oligodendrocytes* don't have processes. They form a single long myelin sheath up to 1000 μm internodal length on the largest diameter axons. They are found around the entrances of the nerve roots into the CNS.

A cautionary approach in the analysis of oligodendrocytes is advised. A clear-cut distinction of oligodendrocytes and their product, myelin, has to be drawn between gray and white matter. Moreover, the myelin sheath in the white matter is much thicker than that found in the gray matter. Also, the volume density of myelin differs from layer to layer, being highest in layers IV–VI and scant in layers I–III. Although reliable data on the number/numerical density of oligodendrocytes in specific layers do not exist, one might assume that

10.7 Microglia

an equal or varying number of oligodendrocytes have to produce varying amounts of myelin.

A selection of genes associated with oligodendrocytes is given in Table 10.10.

10.7 Microglia

Microglia function as defense cells of the nervous system secluded behind the blood–brain barrier. Microglia are highly specialized tissue macrophages of the brain (Fig. 10.14a, b).

Table 10.10 Selection of genes associated with oligodendrocytes

Cell type	Gene
Oligodendrocytes	• BCAS1—breast carcinoma amplified sequence 1 • ERBB3—erb-b2 receptor tyrosine kinase 3 • FA2H—fatty acid 2-hydroxylase • GAL3ST1—galactose-3-O-sulfotransferase 1 • GJB1—gap junction protein beta 1 • GSN—gelsolin • MYRF—myelin regulatory factor • NINJ2—ninjurin 2 • PLLP—plasmolipin • PLXNB3—plexin B3 • PRKCQ—protein kinase C theta • SOX10—SRY-box 10 • UGT8—UDP glycosyltransferase 8

Resting microglia are scattered throughout the CNS and form networks of immunoeffector cells that are activated by different stimuli (nerve injury, infection, mechanical brain trauma). Activated microglia are proliferating and immunophenotypically changed cells that have not yet undergone transformation into macrophages. Confirmed as a distinctive cell type by Rio-Hortega and Penfield (1927) and Gill and Binder (2007). Microglia make up 15% of cells in certain parts of the CNS.

The following types of microglia based on different functional states are distinguished:
- Ramified microglia
  - Highly branched processes
  - Exploring surrounding microenvironment
- Activated microglia (Fig. 10.14a, b)
  - Retracted processes
  - Enlarged cytoplasm due to organelle buildup
  - Rod shape
  - Increased metabolic activity
- Phagocytic microglia
  - Rounded brain macrophages

The activation pathways of microglia are (Franco and Fernandez-Suarez 2015)**:**
- M1 classical pathway
  - Mediators of pro-inflammatory responses
    - Cytokines (IL-1ß, IL-2, IL-6, IL12, IFNγ, TNFα)
    - Chemokines (CCL5, CCL8, CCL11, CCL15, CXCL1)

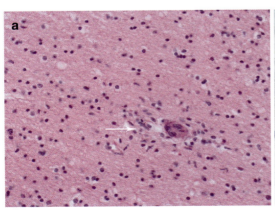
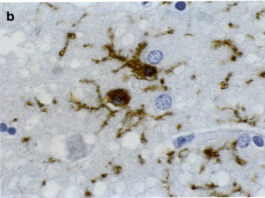

Fig. 10.14 Microglia. Elongated cells with scant cytoplasm (→) (**a**; stain: H&E), immunostained for HLA-DRII (**b**)

- Surface receptors (CD16, CD32, CD36, CD68, MHC-II)
- M2 alternative pathway
  - For resolution and cleanup
    ○ Cytokines (IL-4Rα, IL-10, IL1-RA, TGFß, CD301, etc.)
    ○ Chemokines (CCL17, CCL18, CCL22, CCL26, CXCL13)
    ○ Surface receptors (CD206, CD163, etc.)
    ○ Sensory proteins, growth factors, transcription factor

Pathologic changes of microglia are designated as dystrophic microglia with breaded, twisted, or fragmented processes.

Dual functions:
- "Housekeeping" maintaining tissue homeostasis under non-inflammatory conditions
  - Neuronal development
  - Maintenance irregardless of immune challenge
  - Immune surveillance
- Inflammatory and pathological setting
- Immunological sensors within the CNS
- Antigen-presenting cells
- Produce cytokines and chemokines
  - Cytokines:
    ○ low molecular weight proteins
    ○ modulate inflammatory and immune responses
    ○ interleukins, tumor necrosis factors, interferons, transforming growth factors, colony-stimulating factors
  - Chemokines:
    ○ Small (8–10 kDa) inducible, secreted pro-inflammatory molecules
    ○ Activate leukocytes
    ○ Act as chemoattractant
- Express transcripts for
  - Cytokine receptors
  - Ciliary neurotrophic factor
  - Chemokine receptor CXCR4
- Synthesis of
  - Neurotrophins
  - Nerve growth factor
  - Brain-derived neurotrophic factor
  - Hepatocyte growth factor
  - Basic fibroblast growth factor

- Phagocytose and secrete soluble factors in a regulated manner with minimum inflammatory changes.
- Unique transcriptome among other macrophages.
- Microglia require a characteristic gene expression.
- Modify their structure and repertoire of expressed cell surface antigens in response to their ambient microenvironment.
- Progression of lesions in primarily non-inflammatory diseases (Alzheimer disease).
- Harbor for the HIV-1 virus, productively infected by it.

Development
- Interaction with neurons.
- Phagocytosis of
  - Apoptotic neurons
  - Synaptic material
  - Cellular debris
- Induction of phagocytosis.
- Secretion of soluble factors.
- Ontogenetically and functionally related to their peripheral counterparts of the mononuclear phagocytic system.
- Develop early during embryogenesis from immature yolk sac progenitors.
- Microglia are established before the formation of the blood–brain barrier.
- After birth, microglia remain independent from input from bone marrow-derived monocytes and hematopoiesis.
- Maintain themselves by longevity and limited self-renewal.

Immunohistochemical markers:
- CD45 (nonspecific)
- CD68
- HAM-56 (human alveolar macrophage 56)
- CD11b (Mac1)
- CD11c (LeuM5)
- CD64 (immunoglobulin receptor)
- MHC Class I antigen
- MHC Class II antigen (HLA-DR-II, clone Cr3/43) (Fig. 10.14b)
- Ricinus communis agglutinin I lectin (RCA)
- Iba1

Ultrastructural features include:
- Sparse microtubules and intermediate filaments
- Numerous cytoplasmic dense bodies
- Cell surface with pseudopodia and filopodia

A selection of genes associated with microglia is given in Table 10.11 while Table 10.12 depicts microglial genes activated in disease pathways.

Table 10.11 Selection of genes associated with microglia

Cell type	Gene
Microglia	• GPR84—G-protein-coupled receptor 84 • IRF8—interferon regulatory factor 8 • LRRC25—leucine-rich repeat-containing 25 • NCF1—neutrophil cytosolic factor 1 • TLR2—toll-like receptor 2 • TNF—tumor necrosis factor • AIF1—allograft inflammatory factor 1 • TMEM119—transmembrane protein 119 • ITGAM—integrin subunit alpha M • CX3CR1—C-X3-C motif chemokine receptor 1 • P2RY12—purinergic receptor P2Y12 • SPI1—Spi-1 proto-oncogene

Table 10.12 Microglial genes and pathways implicated in health and disease (Salter and Stevens 2017) reproduced with kind permission from Springer Nature

Health and disease	Genes and/or pathways of interest
Synaptic pruning	C3R, C1A, CR3, and CX3CR1
Neuronal programmed cell death	CR3, TAM-receptor kinases (AXL, Mer), DAP12, NGF, and TNF
Synaptic plasticity	Tlr4, TGF-b, CX3CR1, BDNF, and TNF
Nasu–Hakola disease	TREM2
Rett syndrome	MECP2
Alzheimer disease	TREM2, DAP12, APOE, APOJ, CD33, CR1, C1q, C3, and classical-complement cascade
Frontal temporal dementia	Progranulin and C1qA
Neuropathic pain	P2RX4, P2RX7, P2RY12, BDNF, DAP12, IRF5, and IRF8

10.8 Ependymal Cells

Ependymal cells are (Fig. 10.15a, b):
- Line the ventricular system
- Cuboidal or columnar epithelium
- No well-defined basal lamina
- Prominent apical cilia beating in a coordinated fashion
- Connected to each other by gap junctions with presence of connexins (Cx26, Cx30, Cx43, Cx45)
- Immunopositive for GFAP
- Play a role in fluid homeostasis between brain parenchyma and CSF
- Are rich in membrane water channel protein aquaporin-4
- Have electrophysiological properties

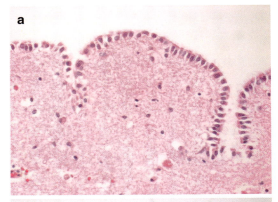

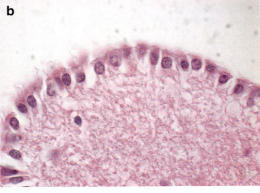

Fig. 10.15 Ependyma. Cuboidal ependymal lines the ventricular wall (**a**; **b**: stain: H&E)

10.9 Tanycytes

Tanycytes:
- Are a special form of ependymal cells.
- Are found in
  - the third ventricle
- Are found in floor of the fourth ventricle.
- Circumventricular organs share morphological features with radial glia and astrocytes.
- Are genealogical descendants of radial glia that do not develop into astrocytes.
- Are radially directed basal processes extending into the periventricular neuropil.
- Enwrap blood vessels.
- Terminate on neurons, glia, external glia limitans.
- Bridge via cerebrospinal fluid the gap between the central nervous system and the hypophyseal portal blood.
- Participate in the release of gonadotropin-releasing hormone.

10.10 Molecular Composition of White Matter Myelin

Myelin is mainly made of lipids (70% of its dry weight) and of proteins (30% of its dry weight). Lipids provide myelin with its insulating properties, while proteins serve to fuse and stabilize myelin lamellae and to mediate membrane–membrane interactions between myelin lamellae, and between the axon and myelin sheath.

10.10.1 Lipids

- The major component of myelin is cholesterol followed by phospholipids and glycolipids.
- Myelin lipids are rich in glycosphingolipids, particularly in galactocerebrosides (GalC) and their sulfated derivatives, sulfatides.
- Other galactolipids include fatty esters of cerebroside and a number of gangliosides.
- Galactolipids play an essential role in axon–glial interactions.
- Animals lacking GalC display abnormalities of internodal myelin spacing and complete absence of transverse bands at the paranodal axo-glial junction.

10.10.2 Myelin Basic Protein (MBP)
(Fig. 10.16a, b)

- MBP is a family of proteins with many isoforms.
- The main function of MBP is in the fusion of the cytoplasm interface of the myelin lamellae and the formation of the major dense line.
- Multiple isoforms of MBP are differentially expressed in oligodendrocytes somata and myelin, indicating that they have multiple functions.
- The shiverer mutant mouse, resulting from a large deletion of the MBP, shows loss of the major dense line.

10.10.3 Proteolipid Protein (PLP)

- PLP makes up to 50% of the CNS myelin proteins two isoforms PLP and DM20.
- PLP is important for fusing the extracellular face of the myelin lamellae and for forming the intraperiod line.
- Absence of PLP/DM20 results in axonal degeneration.
- Animals with spontaneous mutations include the jimpy mouse, myelin deficient rat, and the shaking pup.

10.10.4 Myelin-Associated Glycoprotein (MAG)

- MAG is a minor component of myelin but is the major glycoprotein.
- MAG is confined to the periaxonal cytoplasmic ridges of the myelin sheath in the CNS.
- Two isoforms are known:
  - L(large)-MAG is expressed during early myelination and declines during development.
  - S(small)-MAG is the predominant form in the adult.
- MAG plays a role in axon–myelin interactions.
- Its absence is associated with abnormal formation of the paranodal loops and periaxonal cytoplasmic ridge.

10.10.5 Myelin Oligodendrocyte Glycoprotein (MOG)
(Fig. 10.16c, d)

- MOG is specific to oligodendrocytes.
- It is located on the cell surface and outermost lamellae of compacted myelin in the CNS.
- The function of MOG is not clearly resolved.
  - It might have similar adhesive and intracellular functions as MAG and P0.

10.10.6 2′,3′-Cyclic Nucleotide 3′-Phosphodiesterase (CNP)

- Two isoforms of CNP exists, i.e., CNP1 and CNP2.
- CNP is specific to oligodendrocytes in the CNS and Schwann cells in the PNS.
- CNP is localized to the cell body and processes.
- CNP function in myelin is unresolved.
  - CNP might interact with the actin cytoskeleton and microtubule to regulate the outgrowth of processes.

10.10.7 Myelin Oligodendrocyte Basic Protein (MOBP)

- MOBP consists of several isoforms that are relatively abundant.
- They are located in the major dense line.
- They play a similar role then MBP.
- MBP isoforms are differentially expressed within oligodendrocyte somata and myelin.

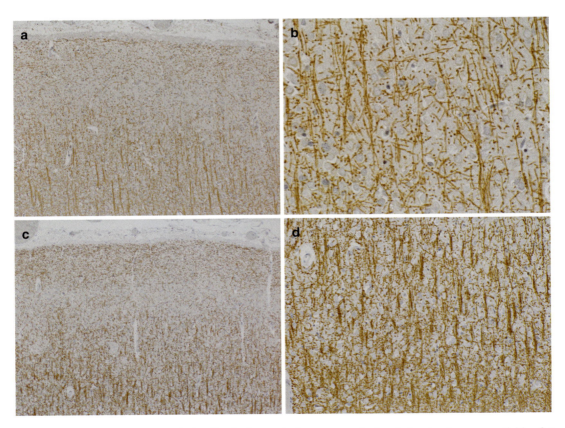

Fig. 10.16 Myelin proteins: Myelin bundles in the cerebral cortex are displayed showing immunoreactivities for myelin basic protein (MBP) (**a**, **b**), and myelin oligodendrocyte glycoprotein (MOG) (**c**, **d**)

10.10.8 Other CNS Myelin Proteins

Other proteins include
- P2
- OMgp (paranodal area)
- Nogo-A (oligodendrocyte cell bodies)
- MOSP (extracellular face of myelin)
- Transferrin (iron transport glycoprotein in the oligodendrocyte cell body)
- Carbonic anhydrase
- OSp/claudin-11 (tight junctions of myelin sheaths)
- Connexins (Cx32, Cx47)
- Tetraspan

10.11 Meninges

10.11.1 Dura mater

- Consists of two tightly annealed fibrous connective tissue (Fig. 10.17a, b).
  - outer layer: periosteum of the cranium
  - inner layer:
    - joins the arachnoid membrane by weak intercellular junctions
    - forms the dural duplications (i.e., falx cerebri, falx cerebelli, tentorium cerebelli, diaphragma sellae)
- Most of the fibers are collagen fibers.
- The collagen fibers run in the direction of lines of tension in the dural folds and form interlacing bundles.
- Elastic fibers are scant.
- Subdural surface lined by elongated flattened mesothelial cells.

10.11.2 Arachnoidea

The arachnoidea (Fig. 10.18a–d):
- Is composed of several layers of flattened, polygonal cells (fibroblasts) with
  - several long and delicate processes
  - linked by tight junctions
- Sends inward projections ("spider's web"): the arachnoid trabeculae.
- The cells are called arachnoidal or meningothelial or mesothelial.

10.11.3 Pia Mater

The pia mater (Fig. 10.19a, b):
- Cells of the pia resemble those of arachnoidea.
- Irregularly oval with long delicate processes.
- Share basal lamina with subpial glial cells.

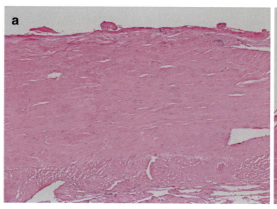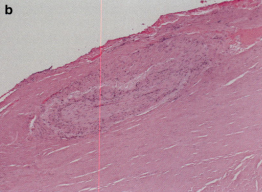

Fig. 10.17 Dura mater: The dura mater is made up of connective tissue (**a**) and might contain the branch of a supplying nerve (**b**)

10.11 Meninges

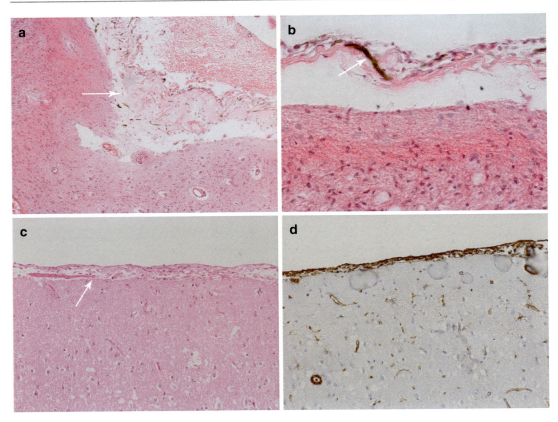

Fig. 10.18 Arachnoidea: The arachnoidea can be widened and fibrosed (→) (**a**), contains melanocytes (→) (**b**) and lines the cortical surface (→) (**c**) immunophenotype: positive for vimentin (**d**)

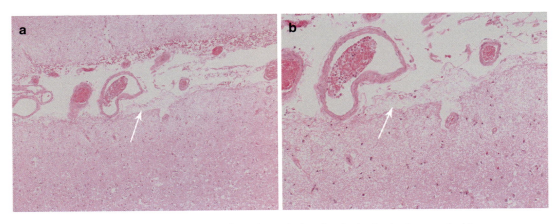

Fig. 10.19 Pia mater. The thin membrane (→) lines the cortical surface in the depth of a gyrus (**a, b**)

10.11.4 Sinuses

Sinuses are (Fig. 10.20a, b):
- Formed by the separation of the two dural layers to accommodate the dural venous sinuses.
- Inner layer is pierced by draining veins and arachnoid villi.

10.12 Choroid Plexus

The choroid plexus consists of (Fig. 10.21a–d):
- Invaginated fronds of vascular leptomeninges.
- Covered by a highly secretory epithelium (modified ependyma).
- Made up of large cobblestoned cells.
- Epithelial cells rest on a basal lamina adjacent to fenestrated blood vessels.
- Tight junctions between choroid plexus epithelial cells.
  - contain occludin, claudin-3, claudin-5, endothelial selective adhesion molecule (ESAM)
- Presence of small nests of meningothelial cells.

10.13 Vessels

The following types of vessels are distinguished:
- artery
  - elastic artery (conducting artery) (i.e., common carotid artery)
  - muscular arteries (distributing arteries)
  - arteriole
- capillary
- vein
  - venule
  - muscular (medium-sized) vein
  - large veins

Arteries are efferent vessels that function in a high-pressure system, while veins are afferent vessels that function under normal pressure.

- Large elastic arteries are conducting vessels.
- Medium-sized muscular arteries are distributing vessels.
- Arterioles are resistance vessels.
- Capillaries are exchange vessels.
- Veins are capacitance, or reservoir, vessels.

In general, with the exception of capillaries, the wall of vessels is made from the lumen towards the outer surface of:

- Intima (Tunica intima)
  - Endothelial layer
  - Subendothelial layer
- Media (Tunica media)
- Adventitia

The cellular components of the vessel wall comprise:
- Endothelium

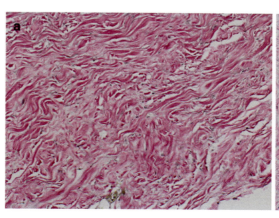
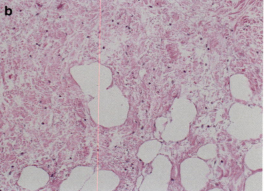

Fig. 10.20 Sinus: The wall of the superior sagittal sinus is made up of connective tissue (**a**, stain: EvG) which contains thin-walled cavities (**b**)

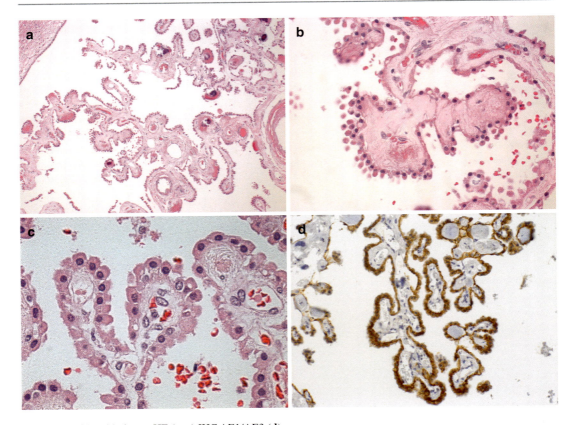

Fig. 10.21 Choroid plexus. HE (**a–c**) IHC AE1/AE3 (**d**)

- Barrier between intravascular and extravascular space
- Smooth muscle cells
  - Responsible for the resistance
  - Produce extracellular matrix
- Extracellular matrix composed of:
  - Collagen fibers
  - Elastic fibers
  - Proteoglycans

Determine the mechanic properties of vessel wall

10.13.1 Artery

The wall of an *elastic artery* is composed of the following layers from the lumen towards the outer surface of the vessel (Fig. 10.22a–f):

- Endothelial cells
- Basal lamina
- Subendothelial layer of connective tissue consisting of:
  - Collagen fibers, elastic fibers, and fibroblasts
- Internal elastic lamina
- Tunica media composed of:
  - Elastic fibers
  - Smooth muscle fibers
- Tunica adventitia
  - Longitudinally oriented collagen fibers
  - Scattered fibroblasts
  - Vasa vasorum (small nutritive blood vessels)

10.13.2 Arteriole

The arteriole has (Fig. 10.23a, b):
- Outer diameter <100 μm
- Inner diameter ~ 30 μm
- Thick relative to the lumen
- Intima

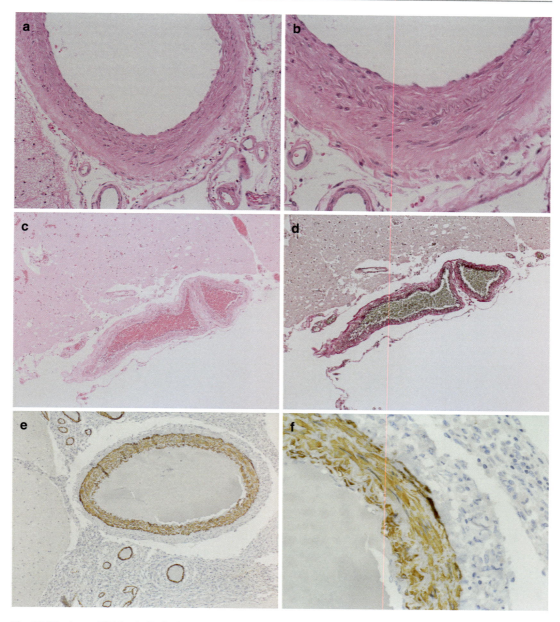

Fig. 10.22 Artery HE (**a**–**c**), EvG (**d**). The vessel wall stains for actin (**e**, **f**)

- Endothelial cells resting on
- Basal lamina
- Internal elastic lamina
- Media with one or two layers of closely packed, helically arranged smooth muscle cells
- Adventitia
    - Loosely arranged collagen and elastic fibers

10.13.3 Capillary

The capillaries of the nervous system have the same structure as those found elsewhere in the body. A capillary is a vessel with a diameter varying between 5 and 12 μm and is composed of the following elements (Fig. 10.24):

10.13 Vessels

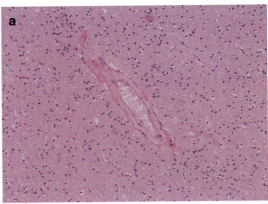
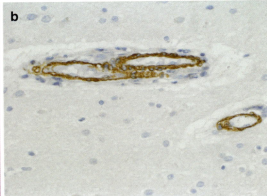

Fig. 10.23 Arterioles in the white matter (**a**). The vessel wall stains for actin (**b**)

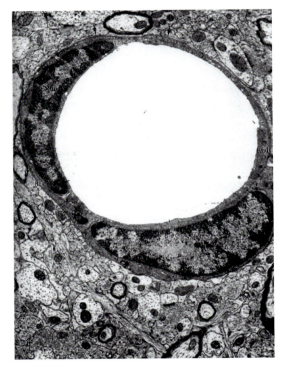

Fig. 10.24 Electron micrograph of a capillary (reproduced from Peters et al. (1991) with kind permission by Oxford University Press)

- endothelial cell
  - is a flattened cell with an oval nucleus
  - uninterrupted endothelium
- basal lamina
  - is 20–50 nm thick
  - surrounds pericytes

Classification of capillaries into:
- Continuous capillary
- Fenestrated capillary
- Discontinuous capillary

Pericytes
- mesenchymally derived pluripotent stem cells
- can give rise to endothelial cells, fibroblasts, or smooth muscle cells

Functions of pericytes (Sweeney et al. 2016)
- Under physiological conditions:
  - BBB integrity, i.e., tight or adherens junctions and transcytosis across the BBB
  - angiogenesis, i.e., microvascular remodeling, stability, and architecture
  - phagocytosis, i.e., clearance of toxic metabolites from the CNS
  - CBF and capillary diameter
  - neuroinflammation, i.e., leukocyte trafficking into the brain
  - multipotent stem cell activity
- Pericyte dysfunction
  - BBB breakdown causing leakage of neurotoxic blood-derived molecules into the brain (e.g., fibrinogen, thrombin, plasminogen, erythrocyte-derived free iron, and anti-brain antibodies)
  - aberrant angiogenesis
  - impaired phagocytosis causing CNS accumulation of neurotoxins
  - CBF dysfunction and ischemic capillary obstruction

- increased leukocyte trafficking promoting neuroinflammation

impaired stem cell-like ability to differentiate into neuronal and hematopoietic cellsAstrocytes send their process which reach the abluminal part of the basal lamina and participate thus in the formation of the blood–brain barrier.

10.13.4 Venule and Vein

Venules are postcapillary small veins (Fig. 10.25a, b). Diameter 10-50 µm

Veins are composed of:
- Endothelium
  - 0.2–0.4 µm wide
  - Intercellular junctions
- Media
  - One or two layers of smooth muscle cells
- Adventitia
  - Thickest layer
  - Consists of longitudinally oriented collagen fibers

10.13.5 Endothelium

- Endothelium forms the inner cellular lining of blood vessels.
- Maintains a selectively permeable, antithrombotic barrier.
- semipermeable barrier between blood plasma and interstitial tissue fluid
- Secretes paracrine factors for vessel dilatation, constriction, and growth of adjacent cells.
- Determines when and where white blood cells leave the circulation for the interstitial space of tissues.
- Plays roles in inflammation and local immune responses.
- Cells are simple squamous, polygonal, and elongated epithelial cells with long axis in the direction of blood flow.
- Cells are linked by intercellular junctions (selective permeability barrier).
- Rests on basal lamina.
- Cytoplasm contains small Golgi complex, scattered free ribosomes, a few mitochondria, and sparse rough endoplasmic reticulum.
- Membrane-bound vesicles or caveolae, 70–90 nm diameter.
- Unique Weibel–Palade bodies, 3 µm in diameter, contain tubular arrays and store von Willebrand protein.
- Luminal surface coated by negatively charged glycocalyx rich in proteoglycans and glycoproteins.

Junctional complexes between endothelial cells are:
- tight
  - barrier function created by claudin family molecules

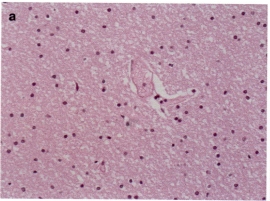 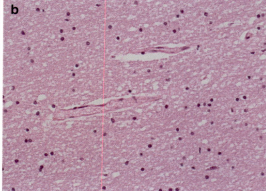

Fig. 10.25 Venules in the white matter (**a, b**)

Table 10.13 Selection of genes associated with endothelial cells

Cell type	Gene
Endothelial cells	• CLDN5—claudin 5 • EMCN—endomucin • ESAM—endothelial cell adhesion molecule • FLT1—fms-related tyrosine kinase 1 • ICAM2—intercellular adhesion molecule 2 • LSR—lipolysis-stimulated lipoprotein receptor • MYCT1—MYC target 1 • NOSTRIN—nitric oxide synthase trafficking • TIE1—tyrosine kinase with immunoglobulin-like and EGF-like domains 1

- adherens
  - regulate permeability to white cells and soluble molecules
- gap junctions
  - form channels between adjacent cells
  are assembled from connexinsA selection of genes associated with endothelial cells is given in Table 10.13.

10.13.6 Glymphatic System

The glia-lymph or "glymphatic" system is responsible for waste clearance from the brain (Fig. 10.26) (Abbott et al. 2018).

The glymphatic system
- links a bulk (convective) flow of CSF into the brain
  - along the outside of penetrating arteries
  - glia-mediated convective transport of fluid and solutes through the brain extracellular space (ECS) involving the aquaporin-4 (AQP4) water channel
- final delivery of fluid to venules for clearance along perivenous spaces

New concept of a perivascular fluid system, whereby
- CSF enters the brain via
  - perivascular space (PVS) convective flow or
  - dispersion along larger caliber arteries/arterioles
- diffusion predominantly regulates CSF/ISF exchange at the level of the neurovascular unit associated with CNS microvessels, and, finally
- a mixture of CSF/ISF/waste products is normally cleared
  - along the PVS of venules/veins as well as
  - other pathways
  - such a system may or may not constitute a true "circulation"

10.14 Neurovascular Unit

The neurovascular unit is composed of (McConnell et al. 2017):
- neurons
- glia
- endothelial cells
- vascular smooth muscle
- immune cells

The neurovascular unit:
- reflects the communication between components of the blood–brain barrier and cells in the brain parenchyma
- triggers the hemodynamic responses of neuronal activity
- regulates nutrient influx to support neuronal metabolism
- modulates neuronal modeling

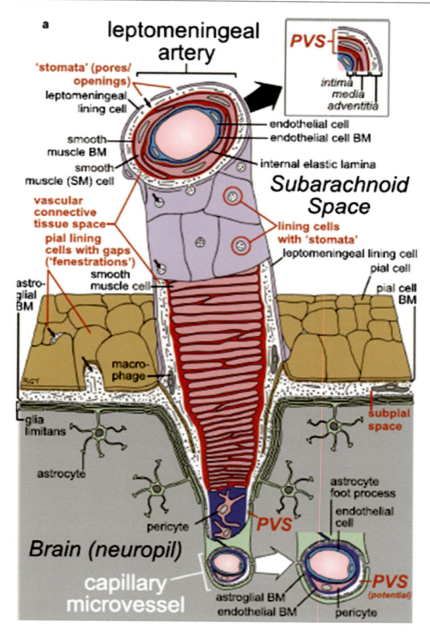

Fig. 10.26 Gliolymphatic system (reproduced from Abbott et al. (2018) with kind permission by Springer Nature). Perivascular space (PVS). A leptomeningeal artery in the subarachnoid space penetrates into the brain parenchyma (neuropil), with a gradually thinning smooth muscle cell layer (tunica media) and narrowing lumen diameter. Key locations of potential CSF and ISF exchange are labeled with red text: (1) stomata/pores present on the CSF-facing leptomeningeal lining cells that have been identified on the outer surfaces of arteries in the subarachnoid space; (2) fenestrations/gaps/clefts on the CSF-facing pial lining cells of the brain surface; and (3) the PVS, a fluid compartment within the outer walls of blood vessels that includes the vascular connective tissue space of the arterial/arteriolar adventitia, the basement membrane (BM) surrounding smooth muscle cells in the tunica media, and potentially extends all the way down to a pericapillary fluid space between astroglial and endothelial BM of microvessels

Selected References

Abbott NJ, Pizzo ME, Preston JE, Janigro D, Thorne RG (2018) The role of brain barriers in fluid movement in the CNS: is there a 'glymphatic' system? Acta Neuropathol 135(3):387–407. https://doi.org/10.1007/s00401-018-1812-4

Aird WC (2012) Endothelial cell heterogeneity. Cold Spring Harb Perspect Med 2(1):a006429. https://doi.org/10.1101/cshperspect.a006429

Allen NJ (2014) Astrocyte regulation of synaptic behavior. Annu Rev Cell Dev Biol 30:439–463. https://doi.org/10.1146/annurev-cellbio-100913-013053

Azpurua J, Eaton BA (2015) Neuronal epigenetics and the aging synapse. Front Cell Neurosci 9:208. https://doi.org/10.3389/fncel.2015.00208

Azzarelli R, Guillemot F, Pacary E (2015) Function and regulation of Rnd proteins in cortical projection neuron migration. Front Neurosci 9:19. https://doi.org/10.3389/fnins.2015.00019

Baldwin KT, Eroglu C (2017) Molecular mechanisms of astrocyte-induced synaptogenesis. Curr Opin Neurobiol 45:113–120. https://doi.org/10.1016/j.conb.2017.05.006

Bankston AN, Mandler MD, Feng Y (2013) Oligodendroglia and neurotrophic factors in neurodegeneration. Neurosci Bull 29(2):216–228. https://doi.org/10.1007/s12264-013-1321-3

Bayraktar OA, Fuentealba LC, Alvarez-Buylla A, Rowitch DH (2014) Astrocyte development and heterogeneity. Cold Spring Harb Perspect Biol 7(1):a020362. https://doi.org/10.1101/cshperspect.a020362

Bazargani N, Attwell D (2016) Astrocyte calcium signaling: the third wave. Nat Neurosci 19(2):182–189. https://doi.org/10.1038/nn.4201

Bernardinelli Y, Muller D, Nikonenko I (2014) Astrocyte-synapse structural plasticity. Neural Plast 2014:232105. https://doi.org/10.1155/2014/232105

Birey F, Kokkosis AG, Aguirre A (2017) Oligodendroglia-lineage cells in brain plasticity, homeostasis and psychiatric disorders. Curr Opin Neurobiol 47:93–103. https://doi.org/10.1016/j.conb.2017.09.016

Blanco-Suarez E, Caldwell AL, Allen NJ (2017) Role of astrocyte-synapse interactions in CNS disorders. J Physiol 595(6):1903–1916. https://doi.org/10.1113/jp270988

Brown GC, Vilalta A (2015) How microglia kill neurons. Brain Res 1628(Pt B):288–297. https://doi.org/10.1016/j.brainres.2015.08.031

Cardenas A, Kong M, Alvarez A, Maldonado H, Leyton L (2014) Signaling pathways involved in neuron-astrocyte adhesion and migration. Curr Mol Med 14(2):275–290

Carmen J, Magnus T, Cassiani-Ingoni R, Sherman L, Rao MS, Mattson MP (2007) Revisiting the astrocyte-oligodendrocyte relationship in the adult CNS. Prog Neurobiol 82(3):151–162. https://doi.org/10.1016/j.pneurobio.2007.03.001

Cerutti C, Ridley AJ (2017) Endothelial cell-cell adhesion and signaling. EMBO J 358(1):31–38. https://doi.org/10.1016/j.yexcr.2017.06.003

Chatton JY, Magistretti PJ, Barros LF (2016) Sodium signaling and astrocyte energy metabolism. Glia 64(10):1667–1676. https://doi.org/10.1002/glia.22971

Ch'ng TH, Martin KC (2011) Synapse-to-nucleus signaling. Curr Opin Neurobiol 21(2):345–352. https://doi.org/10.1016/j.conb.2011.01.011

Choquet D, Triller A (2013) The dynamic synapse. Neuron 80(3):691–703. https://doi.org/10.1016/j.neuron.2013.10.013

Chung WS, Barres BA (2012) The role of glial cells in synapse elimination. Curr Opin Neurobiol 22(3):438–445. https://doi.org/10.1016/j.conb.2011.10.003

Chvatal A, Anderova M, Neprasova H, Prajerova I, Benesova J, Butenko O, Verkhratsky A (2008) Pathological potential of astroglia. Physiol Res 57(Suppl 3):S101–S110

Corty MM, Freeman MR (2013) Cell biology in neuroscience: architects in neural circuit design: glia control neuron numbers and connectivity. J Cell Biol 203(3):395–405. https://doi.org/10.1083/jcb.201306099

Davila D, Thibault K, Fiacco TA, Agulhon C (2013) Recent molecular approaches to understanding astrocyte function in vivo. Front Cell Neurosci 7:272. https://doi.org/10.3389/fncel.2013.00272

De Bock K, Georgiadou M, Carmeliet P (2013) Role of endothelial cell metabolism in vessel sprouting. Cell Metab 18(5):634–647. https://doi.org/10.1016/j.cmet.2013.08.001

De Vos KJ, Hafezparast M (2017) Neurobiology of axonal transport defects in motor neuron diseases: opportunities for translational research? Neurobiol Dis 105:283–299. https://doi.org/10.1016/j.nbd.2017.02.004

Dejana E, Hirschi KK (2017) The molecular basis of endothelial cell plasticity. Nat Commun 8:14361. https://doi.org/10.1038/ncomms14361

del Zoppo GJ (2012) Aging and the neurovascular unit. Ann N Y Acad Sci 1268:127–133. https://doi.org/10.1111/j.1749-6632.2012.06686.x

Dickerson K, Gerhardstein P, Moser A (2017) The role of the human mirror neuron system in supporting communication in a digital world. Front Psychol 8:698. https://doi.org/10.3389/fpsyg.2017.00698

Dickins EM, Salinas PC (2013) Wnts in action: from synapse formation to synaptic maintenance. Front Cell Neurosci 7:162. https://doi.org/10.3389/fncel.2013.00162

Dieterich DC, Kreutz MR (2016) Proteomics of the synapse—a quantitative approach to neuronal plasticity. Mol Cell Proteomics 15(2):368–381. https://doi.org/10.1074/mcp.R115.051482

Dityatev A, Rusakov DA (2011) Molecular signals of plasticity at the tetrapartite synapse. Curr Opin

Neurobiol 21(2):353–359. https://doi.org/10.1016/j.conb.2010.12.006

Domingues HS, Portugal CC, Socodato R, Relvas JB (2016a) Oligodendrocyte, astrocyte, and microglia crosstalk in myelin development, damage, and repair. Front Cell Dev Biol 4:71. https://doi.org/10.3389/fcell.2016.00071

Domingues HS, Portugal CC, Socodato R, Relvas JB (2016b) Oligodendrocyte, astrocyte, and microglia crosstalk in myelin development, damage, and repair. Glia 4:71. https://doi.org/10.3389/fcell.2016.00071

Domingues HS, Cruz A, Chan JR, Relvas JB, Rubinstein B, Pinto IM (2017) Mechanical plasticity during oligodendrocyte differentiation and myelination. Glia 66(1):5–14. https://doi.org/10.1002/glia.23206

Dugas JC, Notterpek L (2011) MicroRNAs in oligodendrocyte and Schwann cell differentiation. Dev Neurosci 33(1):14–20. https://doi.org/10.1159/000323919

Dzyubenko E, Gottschling C, Faissner A (2016) Neuron-glia interactions in neural plasticity: contributions of neural extracellular matrix and perineuronal nets. Neural Plast 2016:5214961. https://doi.org/10.1155/2016/5214961

Eelen G, de Zeeuw P, Simons M, Carmeliet P (2015) Endothelial cell metabolism in normal and diseased vasculature. Nat Commun 116(7):1231–1244. https://doi.org/10.1161/circresaha.116.302855

Eelen G, de Zeeuw P, Treps L, Harjes U, Wong BW, Carmeliet P (2018) Endothelial cell metabolism. Physiol Rev 98(1):3–58. https://doi.org/10.1152/physrev.00001.2017

ElAli A, Theriault P, Rivest S (2014) The role of pericytes in neurovascular unit remodeling in brain disorders. Int J Mol Sci 15(4):6453–6474. https://doi.org/10.3390/ijms15046453

Emery B (2010) Regulation of oligodendrocyte differentiation and myelination. Science 330(6005):779–782. https://doi.org/10.1126/science.1190927

Ettle B, Schlachetzki JCM, Winkler J (2016) Oligodendroglia and myelin in neurodegenerative diseases: more than just bystanders? Mol Neurobiol 53(5):3046–3062. https://doi.org/10.1007/s12035-015-9205-3

Fan Y, Xie L, Chung CY (2017) Signaling pathways controlling microglia chemotaxis. Mol Cells 40(3):163–168. https://doi.org/10.14348/molcells.2017.0011

Farmer WT, Murai K (2017) Resolving astrocyte heterogeneity in the CNS. Front Cell Neurosci 11:300. https://doi.org/10.3389/fncel.2017.00300

Felten DL, Shetty AN (2010) Netter's atlas of neuroscience. Elsevier, Amsterdam

Ferrari PF, Gerbella M, Coude G, Rozzi S (2017) Two different mirror neuron networks: the sensorimotor (hand) and limbic (face) pathways. Nat Neurosci 358:300–315. https://doi.org/10.1016/j.neuroscience.2017.06.052

Fitzpatrick JM, Anderson RC, McDermott KW (2015) MicroRNA: key regulators of oligodendrocyte development and pathobiology. Int J Biochem Cell Biol 65:134–138. https://doi.org/10.1016/j.biocel.2015.05.021

Frade JM, Ovejero-Benito MC (2015) Neuronal cell cycle: the neuron itself and its circumstances. Cell Cycle 14(5):712–720. https://doi.org/10.1080/15384101.2015.1004937

Franco R, Fernandez-Suarez D (2015) Alternatively activated microglia and macrophages in the central nervous system. Prog Neurobiol 131:65–86. https://doi.org/10.1016/j.pneurobio.2015.05.003

Gill AS, Binder DK (2007) Wilder Penfield, Pio del Rio-Hortega, and the discovery of oligodendroglia. Neurosurgery 60(5):940–948.; discussion 940-948. https://doi.org/10.1227/01.neu.0000255448.97730.34

Hakim NH, Majlis BY, Suzuki H, Tsukahara T (2017) Neuron-specific splicing. Biosci Trends 11(1):16–22. https://doi.org/10.5582/bst.2016.01169

Han KA, Jeon S, Um JW, Ko J (2016) Emergent synapse organizers: LAR-RPTPs and their companions. Int Rev Cell Mol Biol 324:39–65. https://doi.org/10.1016/bs.ircmb.2016.01.002

Hattori R, Kuchibhotla KV, Froemke RC (2017) Functions and dysfunctions of neocortical inhibitory neuron subtypes. Nat Neurosci 20(9):1199–1208. https://doi.org/10.1038/nn.4619

Heimer L (1983) The human brain and spinal cord: functional neuroanatomy and dissection guide. Springer, Berlin

Heller JP, Rusakov DA (2015) Morphological plasticity of astroglia: understanding synaptic microenvironment. J Neurosci Res 63(12):2133–2151. https://doi.org/10.1002/glia.22821

Herculano-Houzel S (2014) The glia/neuron ratio: how it varies uniformly across brain structures and species and what that means for brain physiology and evolution. Glia 62(9):1377–1391. https://doi.org/10.1002/glia.22683

Holtman IR, Skola D, Glass CK (2017) Transcriptional control of microglia phenotypes in health and disease. J Clin Invest 127(9):3220–3229. https://doi.org/10.1172/jci90604

Hu Z, Li Z (2017) miRNAs in synapse development and synaptic plasticity. Glia 45:24–31. https://doi.org/10.1016/j.conb.2017.02.014

Iacoangeli A, Tiedge H (2013) Translational control at the synapse: role of RNA regulators. Trends Biochem Sci 38(1):47–55. https://doi.org/10.1016/j.tibs.2012.11.001

Iadecola C (2017) The neurovascular unit coming of age: a journey through neurovascular coupling in health and disease. Neuron 96(1):17–42. https://doi.org/10.1016/j.neuron.2017.07.030

Johnson MB, Walsh CA (2017) Cerebral cortical neuron diversity and development at single-cell resolution. Curr Opin Neurobiol 42:9–16. https://doi.org/10.1016/j.conb.2016.11.001

Kabba JA, Xu Y, Christian H, Ruan W, Chenai K, Xiang Y, Zhang L, Saavedra JM, Pang T (2018) Microglia: housekeeper of the central nervous system. Cell Mol Neurobiol 38(1):53–71. https://doi.org/10.1007/s10571-017-0504-2

Khakh BS, Sofroniew MV (2015) Diversity of astrocyte functions and phenotypes in neural circuits. Nat

Neurosci 18(7):942–952. https://doi.org/10.1038/nn.4043

Kierdorf K, Prinz M (2017) Microglia in steady state. J Clin Invest 127(9):3201–3209. https://doi.org/10.1172/jci90602

Kim SK, Nabekura J, Koizumi S (2017) Astrocyte-mediated synapse remodeling in the pathological brain. Glia 65(11):1719–1727. https://doi.org/10.1002/glia.23169

Komiyama T, Lecrux C, Hamel E (2011) The neurovascular unit in brain function and disease. Acta Physiol 203(1):47–59. https://doi.org/10.1111/j.1748-1716.2011.02256.x

Li D, Agulhon C, Schmidt E, Oheim M, Ropert N (2013) New tools for investigating astrocyte-to-neuron communication. Front Cell Neurosci 7:193. https://doi.org/10.3389/fncel.2013.00193

Liu J, Moyon S, Hernandez M, Casaccia P (2016) Epigenetic control of oligodendrocyte development: adding new players to old keepers. Curr Opin Neurobiol 39:133–138. https://doi.org/10.1016/j.conb.2016.06.002

Liu B, Teschemacher AG, Kasparov S (2017) Neuroprotective potential of astroglia. J Neurosci Res 95(11):2126–2139. https://doi.org/10.1002/jnr.24140

Lloyd AF, Davies CL, Miron VE (2017) Microglia: origins, homeostasis, and roles in myelin repair. Curr Opin Neurobiol 47:113–120. https://doi.org/10.1016/j.conb.2017.10.001

Lodato S, Shetty AS, Arlotta P (2015) Cerebral cortex assembly: generating and reprogramming projection neuron diversity. Trends Neurosci 38(2):117–125. https://doi.org/10.1016/j.tins.2014.11.003

MacVicar BA, Newman EA (2015) Astrocyte regulation of blood flow in the brain. Cold Spring Harb Perspect Biol 7(5):a020388. https://doi.org/10.1101/cshperspect.a020388

Maki T, Hayakawa K, Pham LD, Xing C, Lo EH, Arai K (2013) Biphasic mechanisms of neurovascular unit injury and protection in CNS diseases. CNS Neurol Disord Drug Targets 12(3):302–315

Marcelo KL, Goldie LC, Hirschi KK (2013) Regulation of endothelial cell differentiation and specification. Circ Res 112(9):1272–1287. https://doi.org/10.1161/circresaha.113.300506

Marin-Padilla M (2015) Human cerebral cortex Cajal-Retzius neuron: development, structure and function. A Golgi study. Front Neuroanat 9:21. https://doi.org/10.3389/fnana.2015.00021

McCarthy MM (2017) Location, location, location: microglia are where they live. Neuron 95(2):233–235. https://doi.org/10.1016/j.neuron.2017.07.005

McConnell HL, Kersch CN, Woltjer RL, Neuwelt EA (2017) The translational significance of the neurovascular unit. J Biol Chem 292(3):762–770. https://doi.org/10.1074/jbc.R116.760215

Mena MA, de Bernardo S, Casarejos MJ, Canals S, Rodriguez-Martin E (2002) The role of astroglia on the survival of dopamine neurons. Mol Neurobiol 25(3):245–263. https://doi.org/10.1385/mn:25:3:245

Meyer K, Kaspar BK (2017) Glia-neuron interactions in neurological diseases: testing non-cell autonomy in a dish. Brain Res 1656:27–39. https://doi.org/10.1016/j.brainres.2015.12.051

Miron VE (2017) Microglia-driven regulation of oligodendrocyte lineage cells, myelination, and remyelination. J Leukoc Biol 101(5):1103–1108. https://doi.org/10.1189/jlb.3RI1116-494R

Morrison BM, Lee Y, Rothstein JD (2013) Oligodendroglia: metabolic supporters of axons. Trends Cell Biol 23(12):644–651. https://doi.org/10.1016/j.tcb.2013.07.007

Mosser CA, Baptista S, Arnoux I, Audinat E (2017) Microglia in CNS development: shaping the brain for the future. Prog Neurobiol 149-150:1–20. https://doi.org/10.1016/j.pneurobio.2017.01.002

Muoio V, Persson PB, Sendeski MM (2014) The neurovascular unit—concept review. Acta Physiol 210(4):790–798. https://doi.org/10.1111/apha.12250

Okabe S (2012) Molecular dynamics of the excitatory synapse. Adv Exp Med Biol 970:131–152. https://doi.org/10.1007/978-3-7091-0932-8_6

Olsen ML, Khakh BS, Skatchkov SN (2015) New insights on astrocyte ion channels: critical for homeostasis and neuron-glia signaling. Nat Neurosci 35(41):13827–13835. https://doi.org/10.1523/jneurosci.2603-15.2015

Ornelas IM, McLane LE, Saliu A, Evangelou AV, Khandker L, Wood TL (2016) Heterogeneity in oligodendroglia: Is it relevant to mouse models and human disease? J Neurosci Res 94(12):1421–1433. https://doi.org/10.1002/jnr.23900

Ovsepian SV (2017) The birth of the synapse. Brain Struct Funct 222(8):3369–3374. https://doi.org/10.1007/s00429-017-1459-2

Papa S, Caron I, Rossi F, Veglianese P (2016) Modulators of microglia: a patent review. Expert Opin Ther Pat 26(4):427–437. https://doi.org/10.1517/13543776.2016.1135901

Parent A (1996) Carpenter's human neuroanatomy, 9th edn. Williams & Wilkins, Baltimore

Park YK, Goda Y (2016) Integrins in synapse regulation. Nat Rev Neurosci 17(12):745–756. https://doi.org/10.1038/nrn.2016.138

Park C, Kim TM, Malik AB (2013) Transcriptional regulation of endothelial cell and vascular development. Circ Res 112(10):1380–1400. https://doi.org/10.1161/circresaha.113.301078

Patani R (2016) Generating diverse spinal motor neuron subtypes from human pluripotent stem cells. Neural Plast 2016:1036974. https://doi.org/10.1155/2016/1036974

Peferoen L, Kipp M, van der Valk P, van Noort JM, Amor S (2014) Oligodendrocyte-microglia cross-talk in the central nervous system. Immunology 141(3):302–313. https://doi.org/10.1111/imm.12163

Pekny M, Pekna M (2014) Astrocyte reactivity and reactive astrogliosis: costs and benefits. Physiol Rev 94(4):1077–1098. https://doi.org/10.1152/physrev.00041.2013

Perea G, Sur M, Araque A (2014) Neuron-glia networks: integral gear of brain function. Front Cell Neurosci 8:378. https://doi.org/10.3389/fncel.2014.00378

Perez-Alvarez A, Araque A (2013) Astrocyte-neuron interaction at tripartite synapses. Curr Drug Targets 14(11):1220–1224

Peters A, Palay SL, Webster HD (1991) The fine structure of the nervous system. Neurons and their supporting cells. Oxford University Press, Oxford

Pfisterer U, Khodosevich K (2017) Neuronal survival in the brain: neuron type-specific mechanisms. Cell Death Dis 8(3):e2643. https://doi.org/10.1038/cddis.2017.64

Philips T, Rothstein JD (2017) Oligodendroglia: metabolic supporters of neurons. J Clin Invest 127(9):3271–3280. https://doi.org/10.1172/jci90610

Pirttimaki TM, Parri HR (2013) Astrocyte plasticity: implications for synaptic and neuronal activity. Neuroscientist 19(6):604–615. https://doi.org/10.1177/1073858413504999

Ramaswamy S, Markram H (2015) Anatomy and physiology of the thick-tufted layer 5 pyramidal neuron. Front Cell Neurosci 9:233. https://doi.org/10.3389/fncel.2015.00233

Rio-Hortega PD, Penfield W (1927) Cerebral cicatrix: the reaction of neuroglia and microglia to brain wounds. Bull Johns Hopkins Hosp 41:278–303

Rohlenova K, Veys K, Miranda-Santos I, De Bock K, Carmeliet P (2018) Endothelial cell metabolism in health and disease. Trends Cell Biol 28(3):224–236. https://doi.org/10.1016/j.tcb.2017.10.010

Rose CR, Chatton JY (2016) Astrocyte sodium signaling and neuro-metabolic coupling in the brain. Neuroscience 323:121–134. https://doi.org/10.1016/j.neuroscience.2015.03.002

Rusakov DA (2015) Disentangling calcium-driven astrocyte physiology. Nat Rev Neurosci 16(4):226–233. https://doi.org/10.1038/nrn3878

Salter MW, Stevens B (2017) Microglia emerge as central players in brain disease. Nat Med 23(9):1018–1027. https://doi.org/10.1038/nm.4397

Santello M, Cali C, Bezzi P (2012) Gliotransmission and the tripartite synapse. Adv Exp Med Biol 970:307–331. https://doi.org/10.1007/978-3-7091-0932-8_14

Sa-Pereira I, Brites D, Brito MA (2012) Neurovascular unit: a focus on pericytes. Mol Neurobiol 45(2):327–347. https://doi.org/10.1007/s12035-012-8244-2

Schreiner D, Savas JN, Herzog E, Brose N, de Wit J (2017) Synapse biology in the 'circuit-age'-paths toward molecular connectomics. Curr Opin Neurobiol 42:102–110. https://doi.org/10.1016/j.conb.2016.12.004

Seong E, Yuan L, Arikkath J (2015) Cadherins and catenins in dendrite and synapse morphogenesis. Cell Adh Migr 9(3):202–213. https://doi.org/10.4161/19336918.2014.994919

Shemer A, Erny D, Jung S, Prinz M (2015) Microglia plasticity during health and disease: an immunological perspective. Trends Immunol 36(10):614–624. https://doi.org/10.1016/j.it.2015.08.003

Simons M, Siskova Z, Tremblay ME (2013) Microglia and synapse: interactions in health and neurodegeneration. Neural Plast 2013:425845. https://doi.org/10.1155/2013/425845

Sousa C, Biber K, Michelucci A (2017) Cellular and molecular characterization of microglia: a unique immune cell population. Biomed Res Int 8:198. https://doi.org/10.3389/fimmu.2017.00198.eCollection.2017

Stanimirovic DB, Friedman A (2012) Pathophysiology of the neurovascular unit: disease cause or consequence? J Cereb Blood Flow Metab 32(7):1207–1221. https://doi.org/10.1038/jcbfm.2012.25

Staszel T, Zapala B, Polus A, Sadakierska-Chudy A, Kiec-Wilk B, Stepien E, Wybranska I, Chojnacka M, Dembinska-Kiec A (2011) Role of microRNAs in endothelial cell pathophysiology. Pol Arch Med Wewn 121(10):361–366

Sweeney MD, Ayyadurai S, Zlokovic BV (2016) Pericytes of the neurovascular unit: key functions and signaling pathways. Nat Neurosci 19(6):771–783. https://doi.org/10.1038/nn.4288

Taber KH, Hurley RA (2008) Astroglia: not just glue. J Neuropsychiatry Clin Neurosci 20(2):iv-129. https://doi.org/10.1176/appi.neuropsych.20.2.iv

Tai Y, Jia Y (2017) TRPC channels and neuron development, plasticity, and activities. Adv Exp Med Biol 976:95–110. https://doi.org/10.1007/978-94-024-1088-4_9

Tang BL (2016) Rab, Arf, and Arl-regulated membrane traffic in cortical neuron migration. J Cell Physiol 231(7):1417–1423. https://doi.org/10.1002/jcp.25261

Tauheed AM, Ayo JO, Kawu MU (2016) Regulation of oligodendrocyte differentiation: Insights and approaches for the management of neurodegenerative disease. Pathophysiology 23(3):203–210. https://doi.org/10.1016/j.pathophys.2016.05.007

Terni B, Lopez-Murcia FJ, Llobet A (2017) Role of neuron-glia interactions in developmental synapse elimination. Brain Res Bull 129:74–81. https://doi.org/10.1016/j.brainresbull.2016.08.017

Thompson KK, Tsirka SE (2017) The diverse roles of microglia in the neurodegenerative aspects of central nervous system (CNS) autoimmunity. Int J Mol Sci 18(3):E504. https://doi.org/10.3390/ijms18030504

Treps L, Tse KH, Herrup K (2017) DNA damage in the oligodendrocyte lineage and its role in brain aging. Mech Ageing Dev 161(Pt A):37–50. https://doi.org/10.1016/j.mad.2016.05.006

Verkhratsky A, Parpura V (2010) Recent advances in (patho)physiology of astroglia. Acta Pharmacol Sin 31(9):1044–1054. https://doi.org/10.1038/aps.2010.108

Verkhratsky A, Rodriguez JJ, Parpura V (2012) Calcium signalling in astroglia. Mol Cell Endocrinol 353(1-2):45–56. https://doi.org/10.1016/j.mce.2011.08.039

Verkhratsky A, Zorec R, Parpura V (2017) Stratification of astrocytes in healthy and diseased brain. Brain Pathol 27(5):629–644. https://doi.org/10.1111/bpa.12537

von Bernhardi R, Heredia F, Salgado N, Munoz P (2016) Microglia function in the normal brain. Adv

Exp Med Biol 949:67–92. https://doi.org/10.1146/annurev-physiol-022516-034406

Wamsley B, Fishell G (2017) Genetic and activity-dependent mechanisms underlying interneuron diversity. Nat Rev Neurosci. https://doi.org/10.1038/nrn.2017.30

Weber B, Barros LF (2015) The astrocyte: powerhouse and recycling center. Cold Spring Harb Perspect Biol 7(12). https://doi.org/10.1101/cshperspect.a020396

Wolf SA, Boddeke HW, Kettenmann H (2017) Microglia in physiology and disease. Annu Rev Physiol 79:619–643. https://doi.org/10.1146/annurev-physiol-022516-034406

Wong BW, Marsch E (2017) Endothelial cell metabolism in health and disease: impact of hypoxia. EMBO J 36(15):2187–2203. https://doi.org/10.15252/embj.201696150

Wu Y, Dissing-Olesen L, MacVicar BA, Stevens B (2015) Microglia: dynamic mediators of synapse development and plasticity. Trends Immunol 36(10):605–613. https://doi.org/10.1016/j.it.2015.08.008

Wu F, Liu L, Zhou H (2017) Endothelial cell activation in central nervous system inflammation. J Leukoc Biol 101(5):1119–1132. https://doi.org/10.1189/jlb.3RU0816-352RR

Xiao Q, Hu X, Wei Z, Tam KY (2016) Cytoskeleton molecular motors: structures and their functions in neuron. Int J Biol Sci 12(9):1083–1092. https://doi.org/10.7150/ijbs.15633

Xie J, Wang H, Lin T (2017) Microglia-synapse pathways: promising therapeutic strategy for Alzheimer's disease. Cell Mol Neurobiol 2017:2986460. https://doi.org/10.1155/2017/2986460

Xing C, Hayakawa K, Lok J, Arai K, Lo EH (2012) Injury and repair in the neurovascular unit. Neurol Res 34(4):325–330. https://doi.org/10.1179/1743132812y.0000000019

Yuste R (2015) From the neuron doctrine to neural networks. Nat Rev Neurosci 16(8):487–497. https://doi.org/10.1038/nrn3962

Zhou M, Lee CJ, Rouach N, Jahn HM, Scheller A, Kirchhoff F (2015) Genetic control of astrocyte function in neural circuits. J Neurosci 9:310. https://doi.org/10.3389/fncel.2015.00310.eCollection.2015

Zuchero JB, Barres BA (2013) Intrinsic and extrinsic control of oligodendrocyte development. Curr Opin Neurobiol 23(6):914–920. https://doi.org/10.1016/j.conb.2013.06.005

Microscopical Buildup of the Nervous System

11

In the following chapter, the light-microscopic features of the constituents of the nervous system are described. The description proceeds in the following way: (1) cerebral cortex, (2) white matter, (3) basal ganglia, (4) cerebellum, (5) diencephalon, (6) mesencephalon, (7) medulla oblongata, (8) spinal cord, and (9) ventricular system.

11.1 Cerebral Cortex

The neurons of the cerebral cortex are grouped into (Fig. 11.1):
- Pyramidal cells
- Spiny non-pyramidal cells
- Aspiny non-pyramidal cells

Another classification distinguishes between:
- Pyramidal cells
- Stellate or granule cells
- Fusiform cells
- Horizontal cells of Cajal
- Cells of Martinotti

Pyramidal cells
- In all layers except layer I
- 10–70 μm in diameter
- Synapses:
  - 200 on cell body from other neurons
  - 40,000 on axon and dendrites
- Many intracortical collaterals
- Glutaminergic neurons
- Source of excitatory synapses
- Communicate with other neurons as:
  - Projection neurons
  - Association neurons
  - Commissural neurons

Spiny non-pyramidal neurons
- Short axon cells
- Located in the middle layers of the cortex
- Glutaminergic neurons

Aspiny non-pyramidal neurons (smooth interneurons)
- Short axon cells
- Few or no dendritic spines
- In all layers
- 15–30% of all cortical neurons
- GABA-ergic
- Main source of inhibitory synapses
- Expression of
  - cotransmitters
  - neuroactive peptides
  - calcium-binding proteins
- Classification into:
  - Axo-dendritic
  - Axo-somatodendritic
  - Axo-axonic or chandelier cells

Stellate cells
- Interneurons
- Present in the cerebral cortex

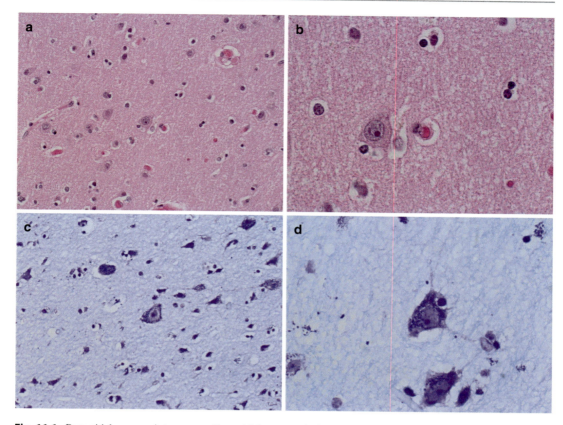

Fig. 11.1 Pyramidal neuron, interneuron: Pyramidal neurons (→) and interneurons (∗) in the cerebral cortex (**a**, **b**; stain: H&E; **c**, **d**; stain: cresyl violet)

- Similar in size
- Polygonal shape
- Possess many dendrites
- Short axon
- Excitatory interneurons using glutamate

Fusiform cells
- Interneurons
- Concentrated in the deepest layers of the cortex
- Send dendrites towards the surface of the cortex
- Influence neurons in the superficial cortical layers

Horizontal cells (of Cajal)
- Confined to the most superficial layer of the cortex (layer I)
- Are small fusiform cells
- Are horizontally oriented
- Axons run parallel to the cortical surface
- Contact with ascending dendrites of pyramidal neurons

Cells of Martinotti
- Present throughout the cerebral cortex
- Send axons to the most superficial layers of the cortex

Subdivision of the cortex into:
- Neocortex (=isocortex)
- Allocortex (Hippocampal formation and olfactory system)
- Transition zone (mesocortex)

The neocortex (neopallium or isocortex), which forms 90% of the hemispheric surface, has six fundamental layers. Some of these layers are divided into sublayers.

11.1.1 Architectonics

The cerebral cortex is a highly organized structure. Based on the observation that the telencephalic cortex is not a uniformly built structure, attempts were undertaken to describe a number of distinct cortical areas (parcellation, architectonics) which differed due to:

- Arrangement of cells
- Packing density
- Size and shape of various components
- Types of neurons
- Arrangements of neurons

A long-standing and fundamental hypothesis in neuroscience states:

- Differences in the microarchitecture of cell bodies across cortical layers (referred to as cytoarchitecture) also contribute to the cortical location and functionality of brain regions (Brodmann 1909; Amunts and Zilles 2015; Zilles and Amunts 2010; Van Essen et al. 1992; Hubel and Wiesel 1977; von Economo and Koskinas 1925).

Thus, based on the cell structure examined the following approaches are distinguished:

- Cytoarchitectonics
- Myeloarchitectonics
- Pigmentarchitectonics
- Angioarchitectonics
- Chemoarchitectonics
- Dendrite architectonics
- Glia architectonics
- Receptor architectonics

Using these different approaches, cortical maps were drawn by the following people:

- Cytoarchitectonics (Fig. 11.2a–f)
  - Campbell Alfred: 16 cortical areas (Campbell 1905)
  - Smith Grafton Elliot:, 50 subdivisions (Smith 1907)
  - Brodmann Korbinian: 52 cortical areas, BA Brodmann areas (Brodmann 1909)
  - Von Economo Constantin and Koskinas Georg: (von Economo and Koskinas 1925)
  - Bailey Percival and von Bonin Gerhardt: (Bailey and Bonin 1951)
  - Sarkissov SA et al.: (Sarkissow et al. 1955)
- Myeloarchitectonics (Fig. 11.3)
  - Vogt Oskar and Vogt Cecile: (Vogt and Vogt 1919)
  - Flechsig Paul: (Flechsig 1920, 1927)

More recent approaches aim at producing multi-model maps of the brain by combining datasets derived from neuroimaging, receptor imaging by nuclear medicine techniques as well as receptor autoradiography using the human brain (Zilles et al. 2004; Zilles and Amunts 2009; Toga et al. 2006).

11.1.1.1 Cytoarchitectonics
(Fig. 11.2a–i)
- Delineation of cortical areas based on
  - Relative thickness of the cortex
  - Density of cortical neurons
  - Size
  - Shape
  - Arrangement
- Proponents:
  - Campbell Alfred (1905), 16 cortical areas (Campbell 1905)
  - Smith Grafton Elliot (1907), 50 subdivisions
  - Brodmann Korbinian (1909), 52 cortical areas, BA Brodmann areas (Brodmann 1909)

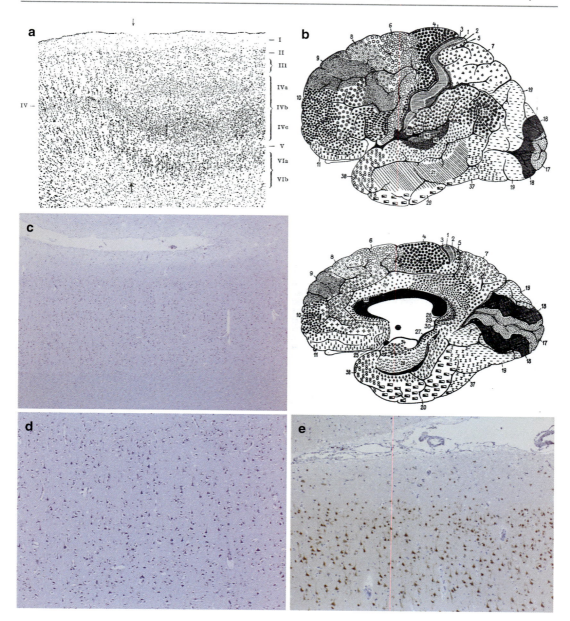

Fig. 11.2 Cytoarchitectonics: Layering of the striate area (**a**); parcellation of the brain into 55 areas (**b**) (**a, b**: Brodmann (1909)). Layering of the cerebral cortex as shown on cresyl violet-stained sections (**c, d**) and using an antibody against NeuN (**e, f**). "Give a name a face": Meynert, Campbell (**g**), Brodmann (**h**), von Economo and Koskinas (**i**) with kind permission from Catani and Thiebaut de Schotten (2012)

11.1 Cerebral Cortex

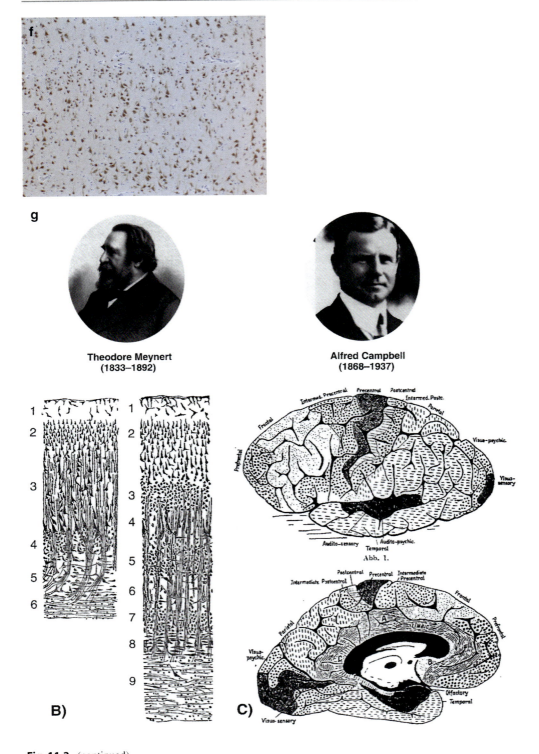

Fig. 11.2 (continued)

h

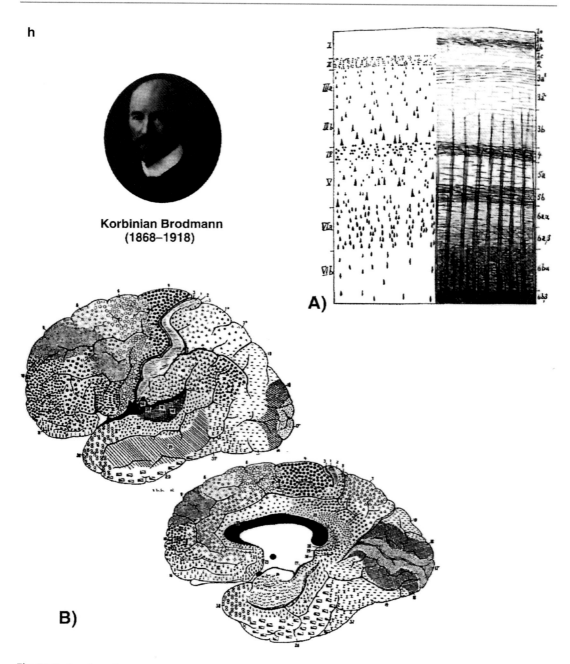

Fig. 11.2 (continued)

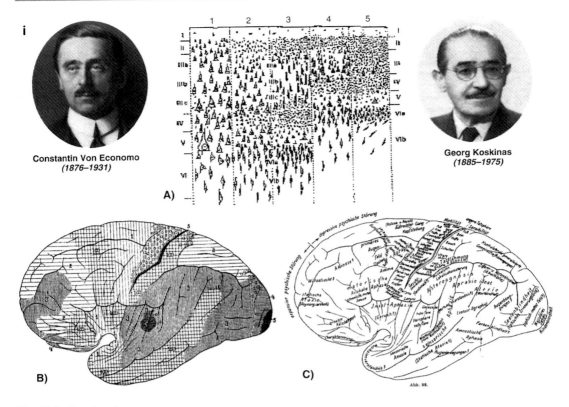

Fig. 11.2 (continued)

- Brodmann (Brodmann 1909)
  - described 55 distinct areas
  - the most frequently used cytoarchitectonic map of the human brain

A list of the most important Brodmann areas is provided in Table 11.1.

11.1.1.2 Myeloarchitectonics
(Fig. 11.3a–j)
- Describes the sequence in which myelinated fibers appear underneath the different parts of the cortex
- Proponents:
  - Flechsig 1920, 1927 (Flechsig 1920, 1927)
- Primordial fields:
  - stainable myelin before or at term
- Intermediate fields:
  - myelination takes place between 6 and 12-postnatal weeks
  - association areas
- Terminal fields:
  - myelinate after the 4th postnatal month
  - higher order association or integration areas

11.1.1.3 Pigmentarchitectonics
(Fig. 11.4a–d)
- Proponent:
  - Braak (1980)
- Distinguishes:
  - Granulous cores
  - Paragranulous belts
  - Magnopyramidal regions
  - Ganglionic cores
  - Paraganglionic belts

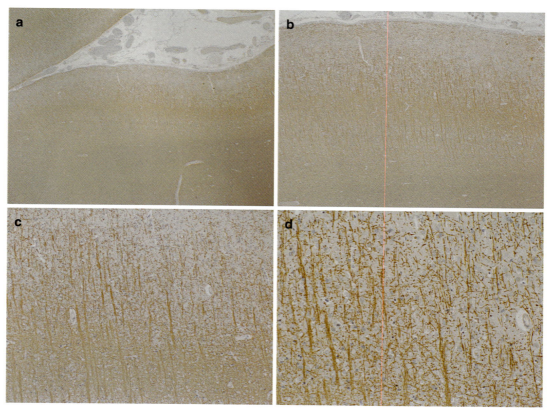

Fig. 11.3 Myeloarchitectonics: Myelin is immunohistochemically stained for myelin basic protein (MBP) in the striate area of the occipital lobe (**a–d**), examples of the variation between cortical areas (**e, f**). The four principal types of myeloarchitectonic layering: **a**: bistriate type, **b**: unistriate type, **c**: unitostriate type, **d**: striate type (**e**). Myeloarchitecture of some frontal areas after (Vogt and Vogt 1919). Comparison between cytoarchitectonic and myeloarchitectonic subdivisions of the cerebral cortex, with kind permission from (Palomero-Gallagher and Zilles 2017) (**g, h**). "Give a name a face": Flechsig (**i**), Cecile and Oskar Vogt (**j**) with kind permission from (Palomero-Gallagher and Zilles 2017)

11.1 Cerebral Cortex

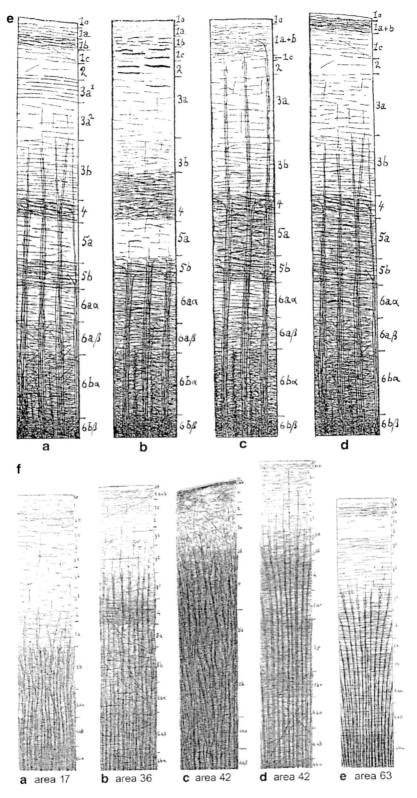

a area 17   b area 36   c area 42   d area 42   e area 63

Fig. 11.3 (continued)

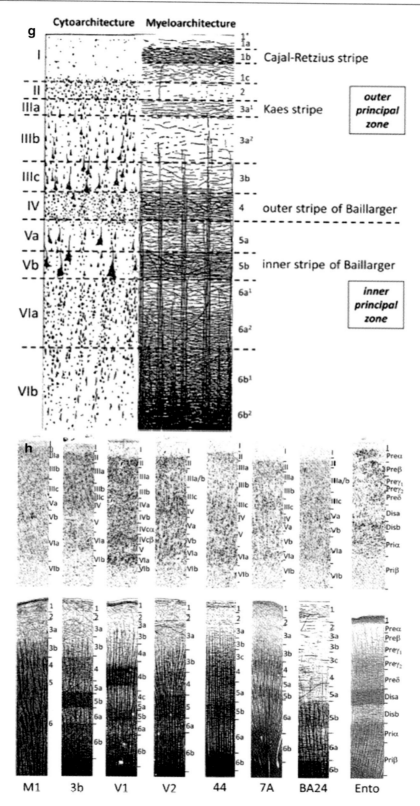

Fig. 11.3 (continued)

11.1 Cerebral Cortex

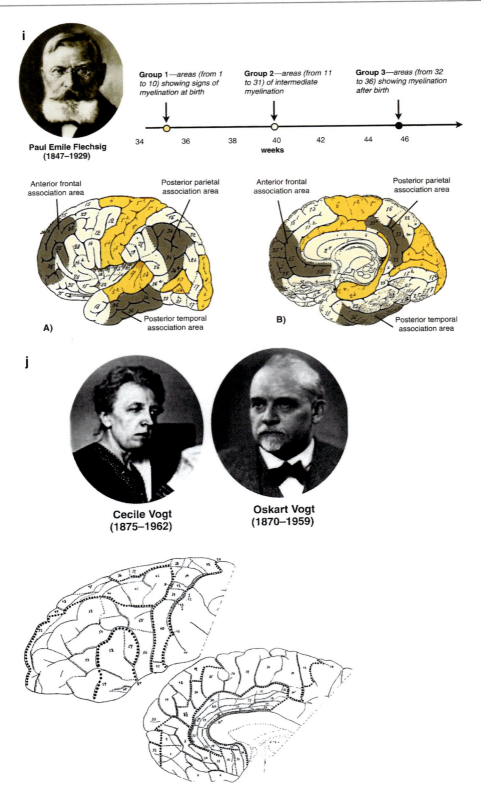

Fig. 11.3 (continued)

Table 11.1 The most important areas as described by Korbinian Brodmann (1909)

Cortical region	Brodmann area (BA)
Primary motor cortex	BA 4
Primary premotor cortex	BA 6
Frontal eye field	BA 8
Primary visual cortex	BA 17
Visual association cortex	BA 18, BA 19
Auditory cortex	BA 41, BA 42
Auditory association cortex	BA 22
Broca's speech area	BA 44
Sensory association cortex	BA 5, BA 7
Prefrontal cortex	BA 9, BA 10, BA 11, BA 12

A comparison of the nomenclature used in cytoarchitectonics, myeloarchitectonics, and pigmentarchitectonics to describe the various cortical layers is given in Table 11.2.

11.1.1.4 Angioarchitectonics
(Fig. 11.5a–c)
- Distribution of vessels to delineate brain regions (Pfeiffer 1928, 1930)

11.1.1.5 Chemoarchitectonics
- Uses for the delineation of brain regions the various amounts of enzymes present in different locations (Friede 1966a, b).
- Mapping of brain neurotransmitters, neuromodulators.

11.1.1.6 Dendrite Architectonics
- Recognizes the sequence in which the dendritic arbor of cortical pyramidal cells is established.
- Capricious silver impregnation techniques are required for staining.

11.1.1.7 Glia Architectonics
- Density of glial cells used to delineate brain regions

- Proponent:
  - Schlote (1959)

11.1.1.8 Receptor Architectonics
(Fig. 11.6a–f)
- Determining the varying density of transmitter receptors throughout the cortical depth.
- Receptor-dense and receptor-sparse layers.
- Do not correspond to the borders of layers in cyto- and myeloarchitectonics.
- Type- and region-specific layering pattern.
- Densities of transmitter receptors vary between areas of human cerebral cortex.
- Multi-receptor fingerprints segregate cortical layers.
- The densities of all examined receptor types together reach highest values in the supragranular stratum of all areas.
- The lowest values are found in the infragranular stratum.
- Multi-receptor fingerprints of entire areas and their layers segregate functional systems.
- Cortical types (primary sensory, motor, multimodal association) differ in their receptor fingerprints.
- Proponents:
  - (Palomero-Gallagher and Zilles 2017; Zilles and Palomero-Gallagher 2001; Amunts and Zilles 2015; Zilles et al. 2004)

11.1.1.9 In Vivo Architectonics
(Fig. 11.7)
- use of noninvasive structural imaging
- usefulness of cortical myelin maps (Van Essen and Glasser 2014)
  - as a way to identify cortical areas and functionally specialized regions in individuals and group averages
  - as a substrate for improved intersubject registration
  - as a basis for interspecies comparisons

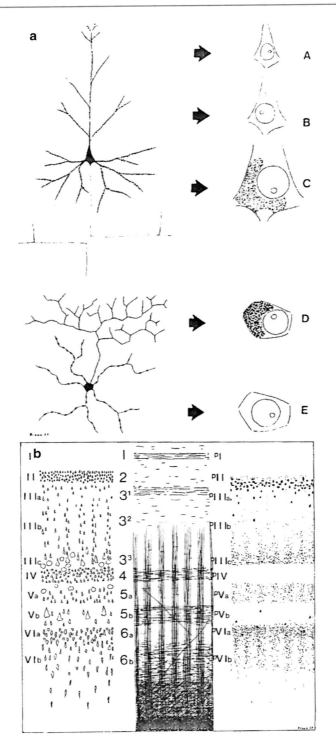

Fig. 11.4 Pigmentarchitectonics: Pyramidal neurons contain a loose distribution of finely grained pigment (A, B), a dense agglomeration of pigment is found in large pyramidal neurons of layers IIIc and Vb (C), stellate cells are either filled with coarse and intensely stained lipofuscin granules (D) or are devoid of pigment (E) (**a**), comparison between cytoarchitectonic, myeloarchitectonic, and pigmentarchitectonic maps (**b**), comparison between cytoarchitectonic, myeloarchitectonic, and pigmentarchitectonic maps for various brain regions (**c**), pigmentarchitectonic map of the frontal lobe (**d**). (Reproduced from Braak (1980) with kind permission by Springer Nature)

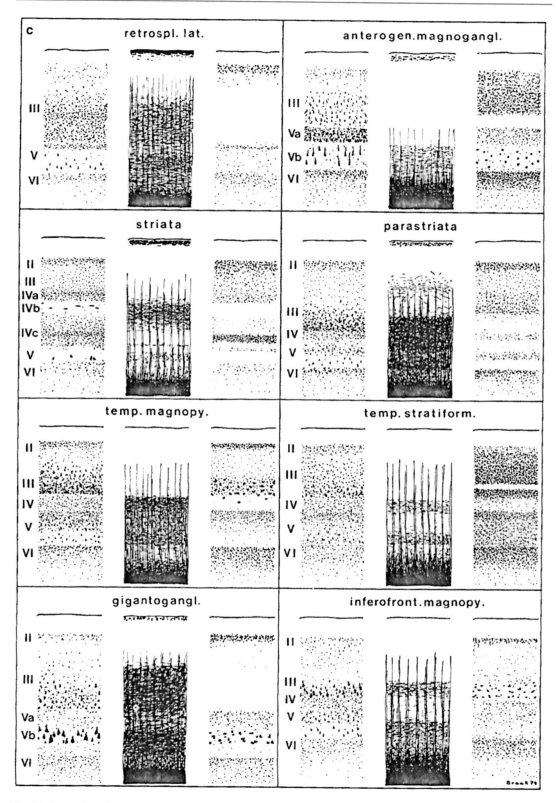

Fig. 11.4 (continued)

11.1 Cerebral Cortex

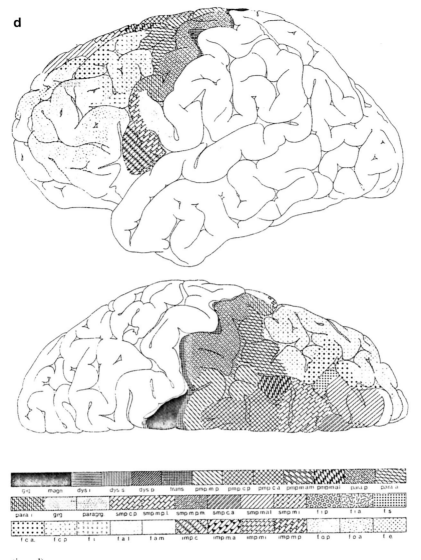

Fig. 11.4 (continued)

Table 11.2 Nomenclature used in cytoarchitectonics, myeloarchitectonics, and pigmentarchitectonics to describe the various cortical layers

Cytoarchitectonics	Myeloarchitectonics	Pigmentarchitectonics
Vogt and Vogt		
I. Molecular layer	1.. Zonal layer	P_I Molecular layer
II. Corpuscular layer	2 Dysfibrous layer	P_{II} Corpuscular layer
III Pyramidal layer	3. Suprastriate layer	P_{III} Pyramidal layer
IV. Granular layer	4. External stria	$Te(P_{IV})$ External tenia
V. Ganglionic layer	5a. Intrastriate layer	P_{Va} Ganglionic layer
	5b. Internal stria	$Ti(P_{Vb})$ Internal tenia
VI. Multiform layer	6. Substrate and limiting layers	P_{VI} Multiform layer

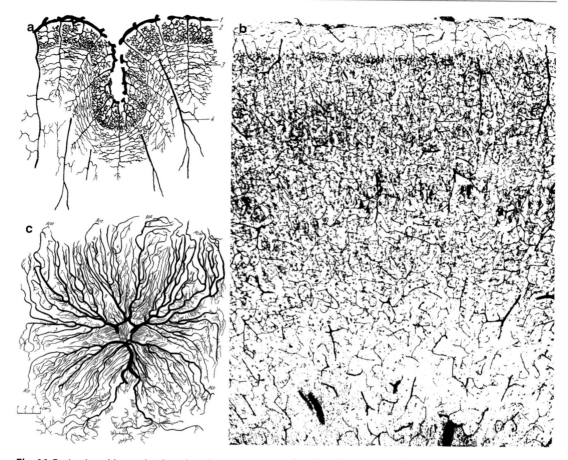

Fig. 11.5 Angioarchitectonics: based on the arrangement of arterial vascular supply (**a, b**) a parcellation of the cortex can be performed. (**a**) 1: arteries of the leptomeninges, 2: arteries applying the cerebral cortex, 3: arteries supplying the white matter, 4: long arteries supplying the white matter. The arterial architectonic map of man (**c**). (**a–c**) reproduced with kind permission from Sarkissow et al. (1955)

11.1.2 Layers and Networks of the Cerebral Cortex

11.1.2.1 General Aspects

The following six layers in the neocortex are defined in passing from the pial surface to the underlying white matter (Fig. 11.8a–c):

- **Layer I**: molecular layer
- **Layer II**: external granular layer
- **Layer III**: external pyramidal cell layer
- **Layer IV**: internal granular layer
- **Layer V**: internal pyramidal cell layer
- **Layer VI**: plexiform (multiform) layer

The six layers are characterized in the following way:

Layer I—Molecular layer
- Sparse population of cells.
- Contains:
  - cells with horizontal axons

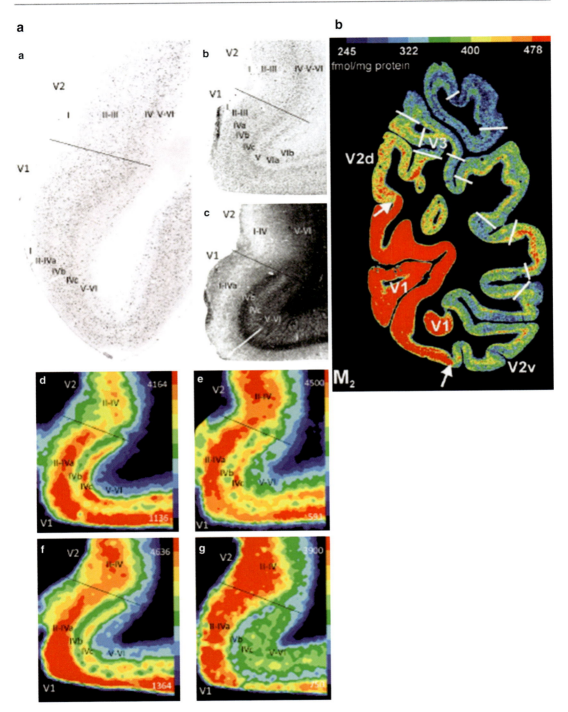

Fig. 11.6 Receptor architectonics: Correspondence of areal borders across different modalities (A) Allan brain atlas showing parvalbumin gene expression, (B) cell body-stained section, (C) myelin-stained section, (D) agonist-binding sites of GABA$_A$ receptor (E), antagonist-binding sites of the GABA$_A$ receptor (**a**) (Amunts and Zilles 2015); Coronal section showing the distribution pattern of the cholinergic muscarinic M2 receptor (**b**) (Zilles et al. 2004); receptor-, cyto-, and myeloarchitecture of the human primary motor cortex (M1, Brodmann area 4) (**c**), receptor-, cyto-, and myeloarchitecture of the human somatosensory cortex (S1, Brodmann area 3b) (**d**), laminar receptor profiles in the primary motor (M!) and somatosensory (S1) cortices (**e**), mean laminar receptor densities (**f**) (**c–f** reproduced with permission of Palomero-Gallagher and Zilles 2017)

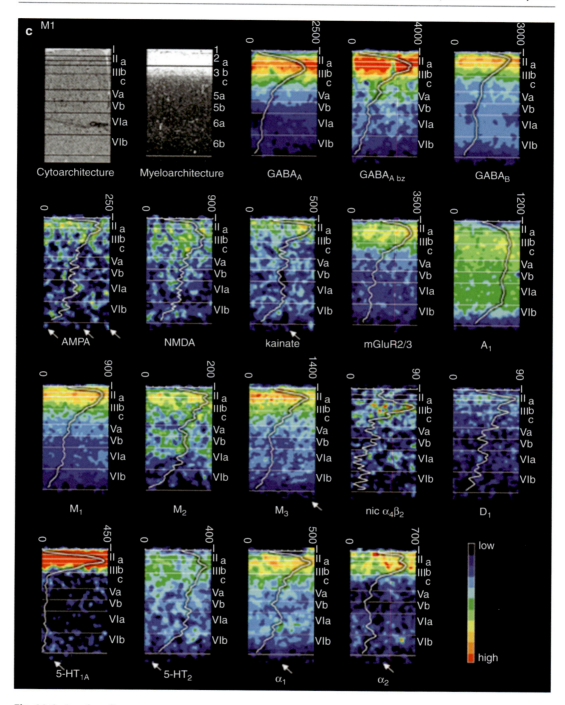

Fig. 11.6 (continued)

11.1 Cerebral Cortex

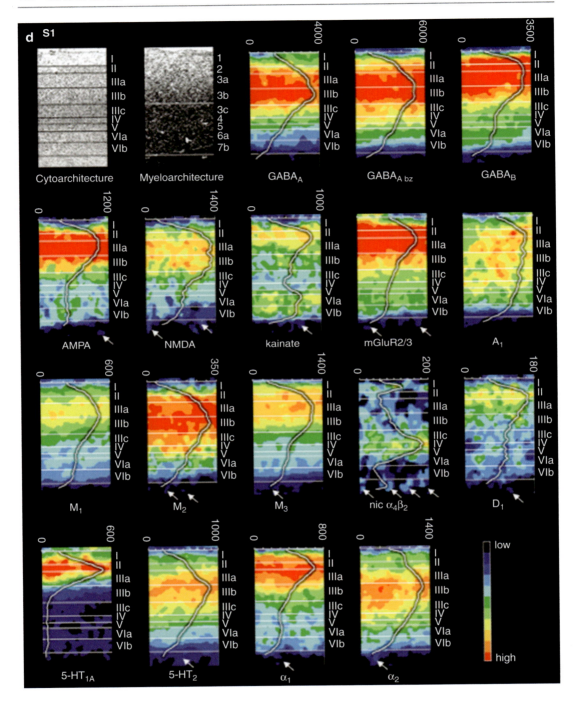

Fig. 11.6 (continued)

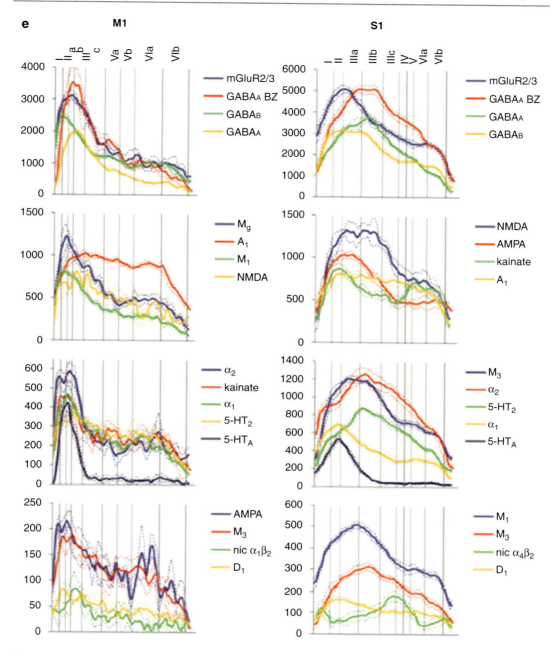

Fig. 11.6 (continued)

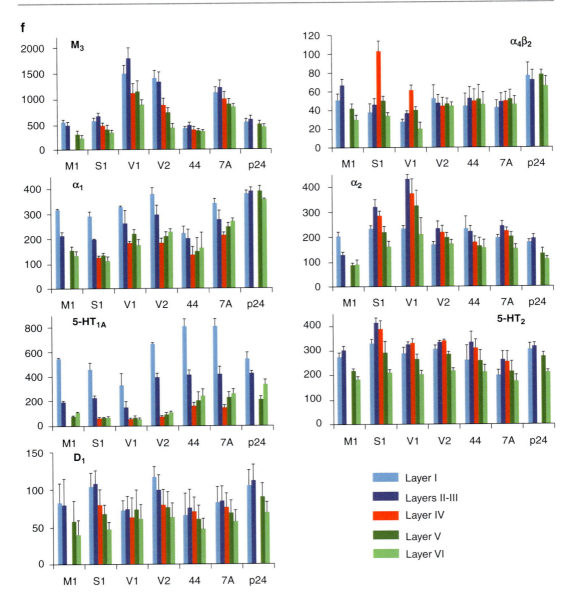

Fig. 11.6 (continued)

- Golgi type II cells
- terminal dendritic ramifications of the pyramidal and fusiform cells from the deeper layers
- axonal endings of stellate cells and of Martinotti cells
• These dendritic and axonal branches form a fairly dense tangential fiber plexus resulting in a large number of synaptic connections.

Layer II—External granular layer
• Consists of numerous closely packed small granule cells:
    - whose apical dendrites terminate in the molecular layer
    - whose axons descend to the deeper cortical layers
• This layer is poor in myelinated fibers.

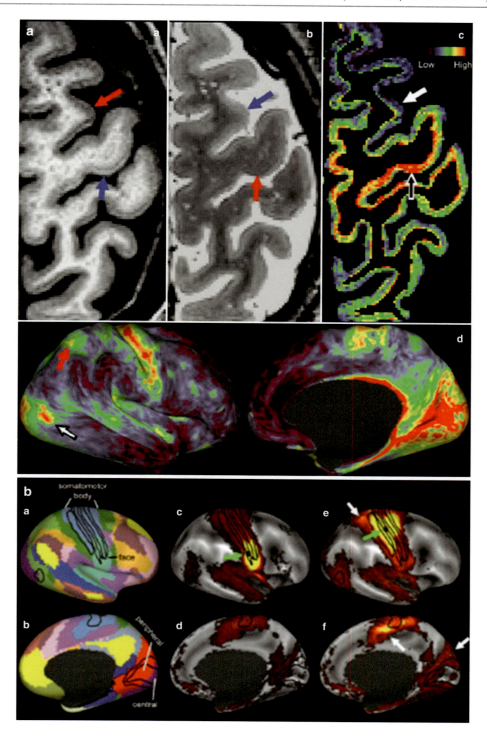

Fig. 11.7 In vivo architectonics: Myelin content estimated by taking the voxel-wise ratio of T1w (A) to T2w (B), and colorizing (C). (D) Myelin map on inflated right hemisphere of the same subject, including heavily myelinated hotspots centered on area MT+ (black/white arrow) and in the intraparietal sulcus (red arrow) (**a**). A, B. Functional network parcellation shows functional network boundaries that cut midway through architectonically defined somatosensory areas (panel A) and visual areas (panel B). C–F. Functional connectivity maps from the HCP Q1 unrelated 20 group average 20 for seeds within area 3b face representation (panels C, D) and upper body representation (panels E, F), including the arm and hand (**b**) reproduced with kind permission from Van Essen and Glasser (2014)

11.1 Cerebral Cortex

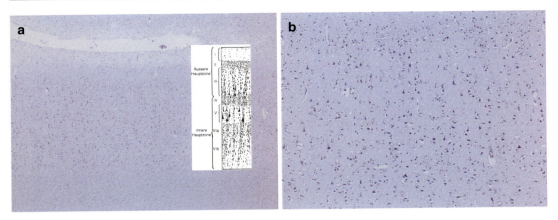

Fig. 11.8 Layers in cerebral cortex are best visualized using cresyl violet stain (Nissl stain (**a**, **b**))

Layer III—External pyramidal layer
- Comprising two sublayers of pyramidal neurons:
  - a superficial layer of medium cells
  - a deeper layer of large pyramidal cells
- Their apical dendrites abut in the molecular layer (layer I).
- Their axons enter the white matter as association or commissural fibers.
- Intermingled with the pyramidal neurons are granule and Martinotti cells.
- In the most superficial part of the layer, a number of horizontal myelinated fibers constitute the band of Kaes-Bechterew.

Layer IV—Internal granular layer
- Composed of
  - Closely packed stellate cells, many of which have short axons ramifying within the layer.
  - Other larger cells have descending axons that terminate in deeper layers, or may enter the white substance.
- The whole layer is permeated by a dense horizontal plexus of myelinated fibers, forming the external band of Baillarger.

Layer V—Internal pyramidal layer
- Consists of
  - medium- and large-size pyramidal neurons
  - intermingled with granule and Martinotti cells
- Apical dendrites of large pyramidal cells ascend to the molecular layer.

- Dendrites of small pyramidal cells ascend only to layer IV or may even arborize within this layer.
- Axons of these cells enter the white matter chiefly as projection fibers although a small number of callosal fibers are furnished by the smaller pyramidal cells.
- The horizontal fiber plexus in the deeper portion of this layer constitutes the internal band of Baillarger.

Layer VI—Multiform or fusiform layer
- Contains
  - Predominantly spindle-shaped fusiform cells whose long axes are perpendicular to the cortical surface. Like pyramidal neurons of layer V, the spindle cells vary in size.
  - The larger ones send dendrites into the molecular layer, while the dendrites of the smaller ones ascend only to layer IV, or arborize within the fusiform layer.
  - Small number of pyramidal cells and interneurons.
- The dendrites of many pyramidal and spindle cells from layers V and VI come into direct relation with the endings of sensory thalamocortical fibers, which ramify chiefly in the internal granular layer.
- Axons of the spindle cells enter the white substance mainly as projection fibers. Some of the short arcuate association fibers connecting adjacent convolutions are furnished by the deep stellate cells of layer VI (239).

- The multiform layer may be divided into an upper sublayer of densely packed large cells and a lower one of loosely arranged small cells.
- The whole layer is pervaded by fiber bundles which enter or leave the medullary substance.

Minicolumns
- Cortex also exhibits a vertical or radial arrangement of the cells, which gives the appearance of slender vertical cell columns extending the whole thickness of the cortex.
- These vertical columns are quite distinct in the parietal, occipital, and temporal lobes, but are practically absent in the frontal lobe.
- The columnar arrangement of cells in the cerebral cortex appears to be determined largely by the mode of termination of corticocortical afferents rather than specific sensory afferents.
- Corticocortical afferents are distributed throughout all layers of the cortex in columnar modules measuring 200–300 μm in diameter, while terminals of specific sensory afferents usually are restricted to layer IV.
- Columnar units of corticocortical afferents are all nearly the same size and have dimensions similar to physiologically identified columnar units in the specific sensory cortex.
- The arrangement into vertical cell columns is produced by the radial fibers of the cortex, just as the horizontal lamination is largely determined by the distribution of the tangential fibers.

Characterization of the cerebral cortex based on layer IV as:
- Granular cortex:
  - Clearly visible inner granular layer (layer IV)
  - Strongly developed layers II and IV
  - Receive afferents inputs
  - Primary sensory regions (visual, auditory, somatosensory cortex)
- Agranular cortex:
  - Absence of a visible inner granular layer (layer IV)
  - Contains large amount of pyramidal cells
  - Strongly developed pyramidal layers III and V
  - Give efferent impulses (motor cortex, frontal eye field)

The internal granular layer, which receives the main specific afferent projections and is best developed in the primary sensory areas, has been used to distinguish supragranular and infragranular layers:

- Supragranular layers: Layers I, II, III
- Granular layer: Layer IV
- Infragranular layers: Layers V and VI

The supragranular layers (I, II, and III)
- are the last to arise in brain development
- the most highly differentiated
- the most extensive in humans
- concerned mainly with associative cortical functions

The infragranular layers (V and VI)
- Well developed in all mammals.
- Give rise to subcortical projection fibers concerned with efferent mechanisms.
- Layers are not present in the archipallium or paleopallium.

Five fundamental types of isocortical structures were defined by von Economo and Koskinas (1925):
- Type 1: agranular motor cortex
- Type 2: frontal homotypical (frontal granular)
- Type 3: parietal homotypical
- Type 4: polar, e.g., BA 18
- Type 5: hypergranular or koniocortex

Flechsig distinguished (Flechsig 1920):
- Primordial fields:
  - stainable myelin before or at term
- Intermediate fields:
  - myelination takes place between 6 and 12-postnatal weeks
  - association areas
- Terminal fields:
  - Myelinate after the fourth postnatal month
  - Higher order association or integration areas

11.1 Cerebral Cortex

Heterotypic cortex
- Primary motor and sensory cortex.
- Has six identifiable definite layers.
- Layer IV has three sublayers.

Homotypic cortex
- Unimodal sensory and motor association and heteromodal or polymodal cortex.
- Has six identifiable, but relative obscure (not so definite), layers.
- Layer IV has no subdivision.

Functional subdivision of the cortex by Mesulam (2000)
- Primary sensory-motor
- Unimodal (modality-specific) association
- Heteromodal or higher order association areas
- Paralimbic
- Limbic

Functional cortical areas:
- Primary sensory-motor fields
  - receive projections from sensory relay nuclei in the thalamus
  - S1 (BA 3,1,2)
  - A1 (BA 41)
  - V1 (BA 17)
  - secondary sensory fields (S2 and BA 42 or A2)
- Unimodal (modality-specific) association fields
  - processing of:
  - somatosensory information (BA 5 and 7)
  - auditory information (BA 22)
  - visual information (BA 18 and 19)
- Heteromodal or higher order association areas
  - Receive information from several sensory modalities (parieto-occipital, limbic, prefrontal association areas)
- Modality-specific or unimodal motor cortex includes:
  - Lateral premotor cortex (lateral part of BA6)
  - Medial premotor area (supplementary motor area SMA, part of BA 6)
  - Frontal eye field (FEF)(BA 8)
- Primary motor cortex

Five large-scale neurocognitive networks (Mesulam 2000)
- Dorsal, parieto-frontal network for
  - Spatial orientation
- Limbic network for
  - Emotion and memory
- Perisylvian network for
  - Language
- Ventral, occipito-temporal network for
  - Face and object recognition
- Prefrontal network for
  - Executive function and comportment

The distribution of protein expression profiles according to specific layers in the cerebral cortex of rat is given in Table 11.3.

Based on embryonic origin the following interneurons are distinguished (Wamsley and Fishell 2017):
- Medial ganglionic eminence (MGE)
  - Parvalbumin (PV)
  - Somatostatin (SST)
- Caudal ganglionic eminence (CGE)
  - Vasoactive intestinal peptide (VIP)
  - Reelin (RELN)

Various features of different interneurons are given in Table 11.4.

A list of selected genes associated with interneurons in displayed in Table 11.5.

Table 11.3 Laminar distribution of protein expression profiles in the cerebral cortex of rat

Layer	Protein
I	• RELN (Reelin)
II–IV	• RASGFR2 (Ras protein-specific guanine nucleotide-releasing factor 2) • CUX1 (Cut-like homeobox 1) • POU3F2 (BRN2) (POU-class 3 homeobox 2) • NECAB1 (N-terminal EF-hand calcium-binding protein 1)
V	• PCP4 (Purkinje cell protein 4) • CNTC6
V and VI	• BCL11B (CTIP2) B-cell CLL/lymphoma 11B (zinc finger protein)
VI	• FOXP2 (Forkhead box P2) • TLE4 (Transducin-like enhancer of split 4)
VIb	• CTGF (Connective tissue growth factor)

Table 11.4 Various features of interneurons (Wamsley and Fishell 2017) reproduced with kind permission from Springer Nature

Cell type	Layers	Markers	Characteristics
Parvalbumin (PV)			
Basket	• Present in L2–6 • Highest density in L4 and L5	• Tachykinin 1 (TAC) • Cholecystokinin (CCK)	• Multipolar dendrites • Soma and proximal dendrites • Mainly target cortical pyramidal neurons and PV+ cortical interneurons • Intra- and interlaminar arbors • Intra- and intercolumnar arbors • Low input resistance • High firing frequency • Fast, strong, and depressing excitatory inputs and inhibitory output
Chandelier	• Mainly in L2–6	• Tachykinin 1 (TAC) • Cholecystokinin (CCK)	• Multipolar dendrites • Axonal initial segment • Mainly target cortical pyramidal neurons • Axonal arbor mainly local • Fast spiking pattern but slower than basket cells • Potentially depolarizing
Somatostatin (SST)			
Martinotti	• Present in L2–6 • Highest density in L5	• Calretinin (CR) • Neuronal nitric oxide synthase (nNOS) • Reelin (RELN) • Neuropeptide Y (NPY)	• Multipolar and bitufted dendrites • L1 axonal arbor plexus • Local axonal arbors • Translaminar and columnar axon • High input resistance • LTS adapting or burst firing
Non-Martinotti	• Present in L2–6 • Highest density in L5	• Calretinin (CR) • Neuronal nitric oxide synthase (nNOS) • Reelin (RELN) • Neuropeptide Y (NPY)	• Multipolar and bitufted dendrites • Local axonal arbors • L4 cells: PV+ cortical interneurons targeting preference • L5 cells: axon plexus in both L4 and L5 • Low input resistance • Potentially fast spiking
Vasoactive intestinal peptide (VIP)			

Bipolar	• Present in L2–3 and L5–6
	• Highest density in L2 and L3
		• Calretinin (CR)
		• ChAT
		• Cholecystokinin (CCK)
			• Vertical intralaminar dendrites
			• Soma and dendrite targeting
			• Intralaminar and columnar axon arbor
			• Cortical interneurons targeting (i.e., SST+ c cortical interneurons)
			• High input resistance
			• Many firing patterns:
			  – Irregular
			  – Bursting
			  – Adapting

Multipolar	• Present in L2–3 and L5–6 • Highest density in L2 and L3	• Calretinin (CR) • ChAT • Cholecystokinin (CCK)	• Vertical intralaminar dendrites
Reelin (RELN) (non-SST)			
Small Basket Cells (SBC)	• L1	• Neuronal nitric oxide synthase (nNOS) • Neuron-derived neurotrophic factor (NDNF) • Cholecystokinin (CCK)	• Multipolar dendrites • Narrow translaminar axon arbor • Cortical interneurons targeting

Table 11.4 (continued)

Cell type	Layers	Markers	Characteristics
Neurogliaform cell (NGFC)	• Present in L1–6	• Neuronal nitric oxide synthase (nNOS) • Neuron-derived neurotrophic factor (NDNF) • Cholecystokinin (CCK)	• Multipolar dendrites • Dense axon arbor plexus • Synaptic and volume transmission • High input resistance • Commonly LS firing • Electronically coupled to other cortical interneurons

Table 11.5 Genes associated with interneurons

HTR3A+ vasoactive intestinal peptide (VIP)–interneurons	Smad3	SMAD family member 3
	Ndnf Car4	Carbonic anhydrase 4
	Ndnf Cxcl14	C-X-C motif chemokine ligand 14
	Igtp	Interferon gamma-induced GTPase
Vasoactive intestinal peptide (VIP)+ interneurons	Vip Gpc3	Glypican-3
	Vip Chat	Choline O-acetyltransferase
	Vip Parm1	Prostate androgen-regulated mucin-like protein 1
	Vip Mybpc1	Myosin-binding protein C, slow type
	Vip Sncg	Synuclein gamma
	Sncg	Synuclein gamma
SST+ interneurons	Sst Chodl	Chondrolectin
	Sst Cdk6	Cyclin-dependent kinase 6
	Sst Cbln4	Cerebellin 4 precursor
	Sst Myh8	Myosin heavy chain 8
	Sst Tacstd2	Tumor-associated calcium signal transducer 2
	Sst Th	Tyrosine hydroxylase
PVALB+ interneurons	Pvalb Cpne5	Copine 5
	Pvalb Tpbg	Trophoblast glycoprotein
	Pvalb Obox3	Oocyte specific homeobox 3
	Pvalb Gpx3	Glutathione peroxidase 3
	Pvalb Rspo2	R-spondin 2
	Pvalb Wt1	Wilms tumor 1
	Pvalb Tacr3	Tachykinin receptor 3
L2/3 intratelencephalic (IT) neurons	L2 Ngb	Neuroglobin
	L2/3 Ptgs2	Prostaglandin-endoperoxide synthase 2
L4 neurons	L4 Arf5	ADP-ribosylation factor 5
	L4 Scnn1a	Sodium channel epithelial 1 alpha subunit
	L4 Ctxn3	Cortexin-3
L5a intratelencephalic (IT) neurons	L5a Hsd11b1	Hydroxysteroid 11-beta dehydrogenase 1
	L5a Tcerg1I	Transcription elongation regulator 1 like
	L5a Pde1c	Phosphodiesterase 1c
	L5a Batf3	Basic leucine zipper transcription factor, ATF-like 3
L6a intratelencephalic (IT) neurons	L6a Car12	Carbonic anhydrase 12
	L6a Syt17	Synaptotagmin 17
L5b pyramidal tract (PT) neurons	L5b Tph2	Tryptophan hydroxylase 2
	L5b Cdh13	Cadherin 13
L6a cortico-thalamic (CT) neurons	L6a Mgp	Matrix Gla protein
	L6a Sla	Src-like adaptor
New type of L5b cells	L5b Chrna6	Cholinergic receptor nicotinic alpha 6 subunit

(continued)

Table 11.5 (continued)

L6b sub-plate neurons	L6b Serpinb11	Serpin family B member 11
	L6b Rgs12	Regulator of G-protein signaling 12
Non-neuronal cells	Oligo Opalin	Oligodendrocyte-oligodendrocytic myelin paranodal and inner loop protein
	Oligo 96*Rik	Oligodendrocyte-RS2-interacting KH protein
	OPC Pdgfra	Oligodendrocyte-oligodendrocyte progenitor cell platelet-derived growth factor receptor alpha
	Astro Aqp4	Astrocyte-aquaporin 4
	SMC Myl9	Smooth muscle cell-myosin light chain 9
	Endo Xdh	Endothelial cell-xanthine dehydrogenase
	Micro Ctss	Microglia-cathepsin S

11.1.2.2 Frontal Lobe

Characterization

- Histological:
  - Granular
  - Dysgranular
  - Agranular
- Functional:
  - Primary motor cortex
  - Premotor
  - Prefrontal association cortices
  - Broca language region
  - Anterior cingulate region
  - Non-primary motor cortex

Precentral Gyrus
- Agranular
- Area 4
- Betz giant pyramidal cells (Fig. 11.9a–d)

11.1.2.3 Parietal Lobe

Characterization:
- Histological:
  - Granular
  - Agranular
- Functional:
  - Postcentral region
  - Parietal region
  - Superior parietal lobule
  - Inferior parietal lobule

11.1.2.4 Temporal Lobe

Characterization:
- Histological:
  - Granular
  - Agranular
- Functional:
  - Auditory cortex
  - Primary auditory cortex (Core region)
  - Secondary auditory cortex (Belt region)
  - Planum temporale
  - Inferotemporal zone

11.1.2.5 Occipital Lobe

Characterization:
- Histological:
  - Granular
  - Agranular
- Functional:
  - Primary visual cortex
  - Extrastriate visual cortex
    - V2, V3, VP, V3A, V4, V5/MT

Striate area (Fig. 11.10a–d)
- Area 17
- Prominent tripartite layer IV
  - sublayers IV A–C

11.2 Hippocampus

The hippocampus is bilaminar and consists of the following two major parts:

- Cornu ammonis (hippocampus proper)
- Dentate gyrus (fascia dentata)

One lamina is rolled up inside the other, resembling two interlocking, U-shaped laminae, one fitting into the other and separated from each other by the hippocampal sulcus.

11.2 Hippocampus

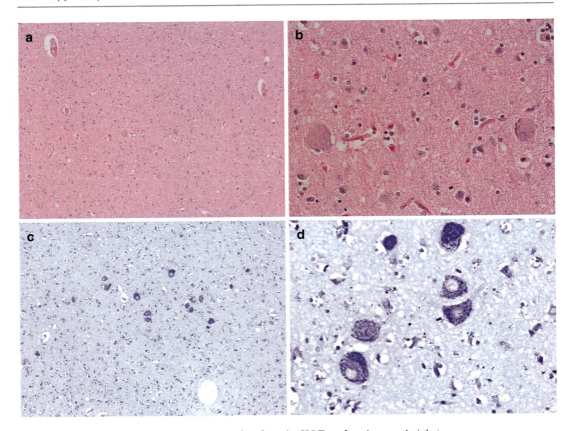

Fig. 11.9 Betz cells in the precentral gyrus (**a–d**; **a**, **b**: stain: H&E; **c**, **d**: stain: cresyl violet)

They are part of the allocortex or archeocortex.

The fine structural subdivision of these two major parts is given from outside to inside as follows (Fig. 11.11a–d):

- Cornu ammonis
  - Alveus
  - Stratum oriens
  - Stratum pyramidale with CA1, CA2, CA3, CA4 (Fig. 11.11b–f)
  - Stratum radiatum
  - Stratum lacunosum
  - Stratum moleculare
- Dentate gyrus (Fig. 11.11g, h)
  - Stratum moleculare
  - Stratum granulosum
  - Polymorphic layer

11.2.1 Cornu Ammonis (Hippocampus Proper)

Alveus
- Covers the intraventricular surface.
- Contains axons of the hippocampal and subicular neurons, which are the main efferent pathway of these structures.
- These fibers then enter the fimbria.
- The alveus also contains afferent fibers largely from the septum.

Stratum oriens
- The limits of the stratum oriens are poorly defined.
- It blends with the underlying stratum pyramidale.

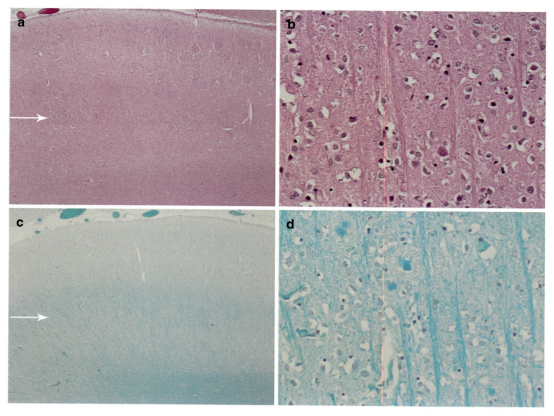

Fig. 11.10 Occipital cortex-striate area: the large tripartite layer IV is discernible (→) (**a**, **c**); nerve fiber bundles of the optic radiation are prominent (**b**, **d**). (**a**, **b**: stain: H&E; **c**, **d**: stain: LFB)

- It is composed of scattered nervous cells (basket cells) and is crossed by the axons of pyramidal neurons as they arrive at the alveus.

Stratum pyramidale
- Contains the pyramidal neurons.
  - A pyramidal soma is typically triangular.
  - Its base faces the alveus and its apex faces towards the vestigial hippocampal sulcus.
  - From its base, the axon traverses the stratum oriens to the alveus.
- Pyramidal neurons mainly project to the septal nucleus, but some are association fibers for the other pyramidal neurons and perhaps cross to the contralateral hippocampus. Such axons have Schaffer collaterals, which curve back into the stratum radiatum and reach other pyramidal neurons.
- At the apex of each pyramidal neuron is an apical dendrite which traverses the entire thickness of the cornu ammonis to reach the stratum molecular near the vestigial hippocampal sulcus.
- There are basal dendrites from the soma basal angles; some of these arborize in the stratum oriens.
- The soma is surrounded by a dense plexus of arborizations from basket cells with somata in the stratum oriens.
- Basket-type interneurons and stellate neurons are also scattered throughout the stratum pyramidale itself.

Stratum radiatum
- Consists mainly of apical dendrites from pyramidal neurons, the parallel arrangement of which gives this layer a striated appearance.
- Apical dendrites connect with Schaffer collaterals, fibers from septal nuclei, and commissural fibers.

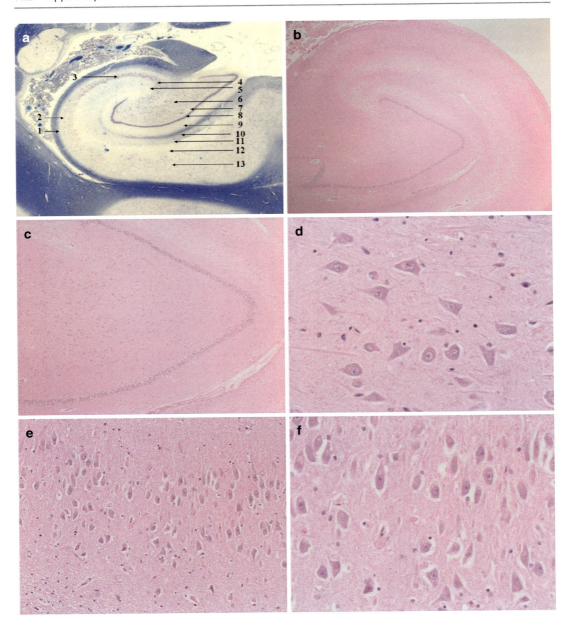

Fig. 11.11 Hippocampus: The hippocampus and its layers examined (**a**, **b**) (1) Alveus, (2) stratum oriens, (3) CA2-pyramidal layer, (4) CA3-pyramidal layer, (5) CA-stratum lucidum, (6)CA4-pyramidal layer, (7) dentate gyrus-polymorphic layer, (8) dentate gyrus-stratum granulare, (9) dentate gyrus-stratum moleculare, (10) CA-stratum moleculare, (11) CA-stratum lacunosum, (12) CA-stratum radiatum, and (13) CA1-pyramidal layer (**a**: stain: LFB, **b**: stain: H&E). CA4 (**c**, **d**), CA2 (**e**, **f**), dentate gyrus (**g**, **h**)

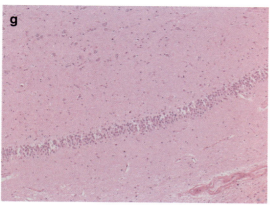
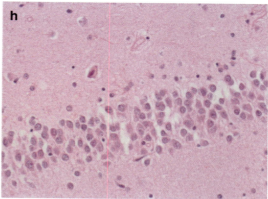

Fig. 11.11 (continued)

Stratum lacunosum
- Contains mainly numerous axonal fasciculi parallel to the surface of the cornu ammonis, formed mainly of perforant fibers and Schaffer collaterals

Stratum moleculare
- Adjoins the vestigial hippocampal sulcus.
- Blends with that of the gyrus dentatus.
- Contains few neurons (interneurons).
- Contains the original arborizations of apical dendrites of pyramidal neurons.
- By their prolongation, pyramidal neurons reach all layers of the cornu ammonis.

Regional Variations
- The cornu ammonis has been described as having four fields, named CA1–CA4 after Lorente de No (1934).

CA1
- Continues from the subiculum.
- Its pyramidal somata are typically triangular, generally small and scattered.
- The stratum pyramidale of human CA1 is large.
- Two sublayers have been distinguished in the stratum pyramidale of human CA1:
  - a stratum profundum, the former in contact with the stratum oriens, with few pyramidal neurons
  - a stratum superficiale, contains numerous ones

CA2
- composed of large, ovoid, densely packed somata
- making the stratum pyramidale dense and narrow, in sharp contrast to CA1

CA3
- Corresponds to the curve, or genu, of the cornu ammonis, where it enters the concavity of the gyrus dentatus.
- Its pyramidal somata are like those in CA2.
- Their density is less pronounced.
- A typical feature of CA3 is the presence of fine, non-myelinated fibers, the mossy fibers, which arise from the dentate gyrus. These fibers surround the pyramidal somata and are also compressed between the strata radiatum and pyramidale, thus forming a supplementary layer, the stratum lucidum that is characteristic of CA3.

CA4
- Is situated within the concavity of the dentate gyrus, which distinguishes it from CA3.
- Somata in this field are ovoid, large, few in number, and scattered among intertwined large and mossy myelinated fibers characteristic of CA4.
- It is now often admitted that CA4 is functionally assimilated to CA3.

Another division of the cornu ammonis into five sectors (H1–H5) by Rose (1927):

- H1 corresponds to CA1 but also extends into the adjacent subiculum.
- H2 and H3 correspond to CA2 and CA3, respectively.
- H4 and H5 correspond to CA4, slightly overlapping into CA3.

A subdivision into three fields by Vogt and Vogt (1937)

- H1 for CA1
- H2 for CA2 and CA3
- H3 for CA4

Based on its *sensitivity to hypoxia* in different fields in the cornu ammonis, the following designation is used:

- CA1 is said to be a "vulnerable sector," or Sommer sector (Sommer 1880).
- CA3 is called a "resistant sector," or Spielmeyer sector (Spielmeyer 1927).
- CA4 being a sector of medium vulnerability, or Bratz sector (Bratz 1899).

11.2.2 Gyrus Dentatus (Fascia Dentata, Gyrus Involutus)

The gyrus dentatus is
- A narrow, dorsally concave lamina.
- Its concavity envelopes the CA4 segment of the cornu ammonis.
- Separated from CA1–CA3 by the hippocampal sulcus.
- The cornu ammonis and the gyrus dentatus are thus fused together, separated only by the vestigial hippocampal sulcus.

The three layers of the allocortex are plainly visible, that is
- Stratum moleculare
- Stratum granulosum
- Polymorphic layer

The *stratum granulosum*
- The main layer contains somata of granular neurons, which are small and round but densely packed, making the layer easy to distinguish.
- Their axons are "mossy" and traverse the polymorphic layer to CA4 and CA3.
- A single dendrite escapes from the basal pole of each granular soma and extends into the stratum moleculare.

The *stratum moleculare*
- Is thick and separated from the stratum moleculare of the cornu ammonis by the vestigial hippocampal sulcus.
- Its external two thirds near the hippocampal sulcus receive fibers from the perforant pathway.
- Whereas the inner third, in contact with the stratum granulosum, is occupied by commissural and septal fibers.
- There are few interneurons.

The *polymorphic layer* (or plexiform layer)
- Unites granular layer to CA4.
- Is crossed by axons of granular neurons.
- There are few interneurons.

The *area dentate* comprises:
- gyrus dentatus (fascia dentata)
- CA4

Other names used for CA4 include:
- the end folium
- the end blade
- the hilus of fascia dentata

The hippocampus is prolonged by the *subiculum*
- Forms part of the parahippocampal gyrus.
- The end of the stratum radiatum of CA1 is considered to mark the division between the cornu ammonis and the subiculum.

The subiculum itself is divided into several segments:
- the *prosubiculum*, which continues CA1 (and whose existence is not accepted by all)
- the *subiculum proper*, partly hidden by the gyrus dentatus

- the *presubiculum*, whose small, superficial pyramidal neurons are packed in clusters, making it characteristically maculate
- the *parasubiculum*, which passes around the margin of the parahippocampal gyrus to the entorhinal area on the medial aspect of the gyrus

11.2.3 Entorhinal Cortex

- The *entorhinal area* (Brodmann's area 28) is itself poorly demarcated.
- Its presence in the uncus and anterior end of the parahippocampal gyrus is generally accepted.
- Posterior extension along the parahippocampal gyrus is uncertain.
- Most distinctive feature:
  - islands of darkly stained modified pyramidal and stellate cells that make up layer II.

11.2.4 Nucleus Basalis Meynert (Fig. 11.12a, b)

- A group of large neurons in the substantia innominata of the basal forebrain
- Has wide projections to the neocortex
- Is rich in acetylcholine and choline acetyltransferase

- The nucleus basalis is
  - inferior to the globus pallidus and within an area known as the substantia innominate
  - immediately inferior to the anterior commissure
  - superior and lateral to the anterior portion of the hypothalamus
- Subsectors:
  - anterior nbM
  - intermediate nbM
  - posterior nbM

11.3 Amygdala (Fig. 11.13a, b)

The amygdala belongs to the limbic lobe
- The cortical and medial nuclei are olfactory centers.
- The basal, lateral, and central nuclei have limbic functions.

Nuclei of the amygdala
- Corticomedial nuclear group (superficial nuclei)
  - Anterior amygdaloid area
  - Cortical amygdaloid nucleus
  - Medial amygdaloid nucleus
  - Nucleus of the lateral olfactory tract
  - Periamygdaloid cortex

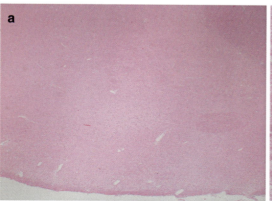
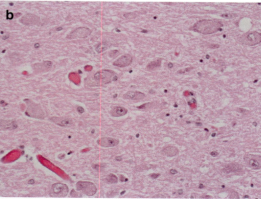

Fig. 11.12 Nucleus basalis Meynert (**a**, **b**). The basal nucleus Meynert is located beneath the anterior commissure (CA) → (**a**) and composed of large neurons (**b**)

11.5 Basal Ganglia

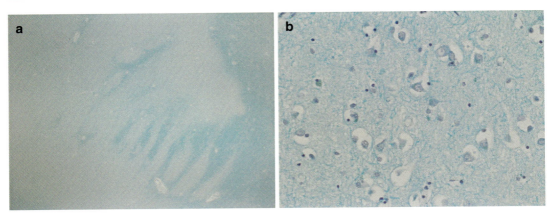

Fig. 11.13 Amygdala: a rough subdivision of the amygdala is seen on LFB-stained sections (**a**), neurons and glial cells (**b**)

- Central nuclear group
  - Central amygdaloid nucleus
  - Interstitial (intercalated) amygdaloid nuclei
- Basolateral nuclear group (deep nuclei)
  - Basolateral (basal) amygdaloid nucleus
  - Basomedial (accessory basal) amygdaloid nucleus
  - Lateral amygdaloid nucleus
- Transition areas
  - Amygdaloclaustral transition area
  - Amygdalohippocampal transition area
  - Amygdalopiriform transition area
  - Amygdalostriatal transition area

11.4 White Matter (Fig. 11.14a–f)

The white matter is made up of
- Myelinated nerve fibers
- Non-myelinated nerve fibers
- Astrocytes
- Oligodendrocytes
- Microglia
- Vessels

11.5 Basal Ganglia
(Figs. 11.15a–h and 11.16a, b)

11.5.1 Caudate Nucleus and Putamen

- Are cytologically identical
- Composed of many neurons without lamination
- Small cells outnumber large cells 20–60:1

Spiny neurons
- Most numerous
- Round to oval medium-sized cell
- Multiple primary dendrites covered with spines
- Long axons
- Spiny neuron type I
- Spiny neuron type II
- GABA-ergic
- Coexpress substance P, encephalin, dynorphin, neurotensin

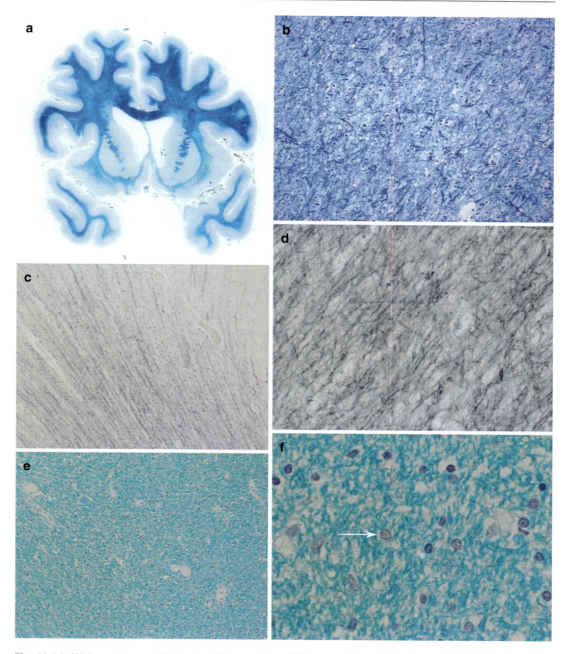

Fig. 11.14 White matter: myelin is stained blue on this bi-hemispheric section (**a**) and at higher magnification (**b**). Myelin can also be visualized in black using the Weigert myelin stain for the cerebral cortex (**c**) and deep white matter (**d**). The cellular elements of the white matter include astrocytes (→) and oligodendrocytes (∗) (**e**, **f**)

Aspiny neurons
- Short exons
- Absence or rarity of spines on dendrites
- Two types

- Giant aspiny interneurons
    - Elongated cell bodies
    - Few stout dendrites
    - Extensively branched axon
    - Cholinergic

11.5 Basal Ganglia

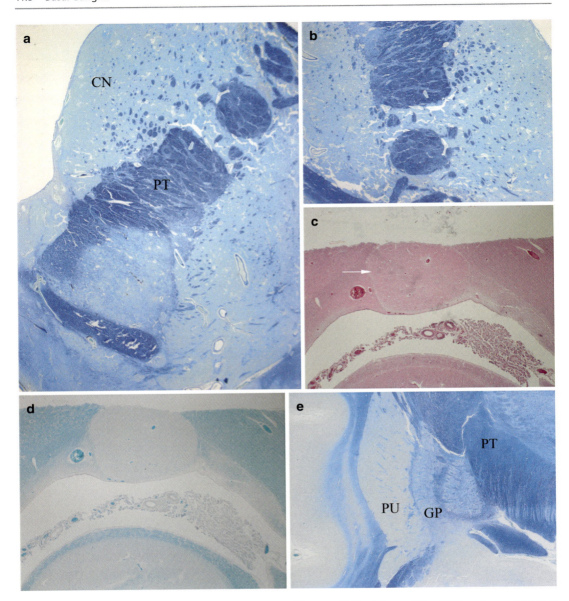

Fig. 11.15 Basal ganglia: The caudate nucleus and the pyramidal tract are discernible on LFB-stained sections (**a**, **b**). The tail of the caudate nucleus (→) located on the roof of the inferior horn of the lateral ventricle (**c**, **d**). Putamen (PU), globus pallidus (GP), and pyramidal tract (PT) are seen (**e**). Globus pallidus with its internal (GPi) and external segment (GPe) (**f**). Neurons and glial cells in the globus pallidus (**g**, **h**)

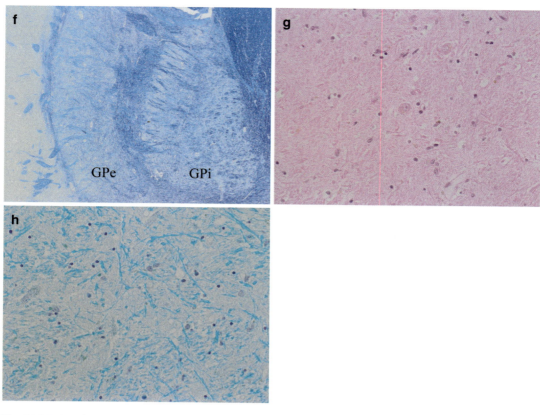

Fig. 11.15 (continued)

- Medium-sized interneurons
  - GABA-type
    - Round cell body
    - Curved dendrites
    - Short axon
    - GABA-ergic with parvalbumin
  - Somatostatin-type
    - Spheroid cell body
    - Few straight dendrites
    - Relatively short axon
    - Somatostatin and neuropeptide Y

11.5.2 Globus Pallidus (Fig. 11.15e–h)

- Neurons
  - Large ovoid to polygonal cells
  - Relatively smooth dendrites
  - Rich plexus of afferent fibers investing the long dendrites
  - Axons with few collaterals
  - GABA-ergic
- Bundles of myelinated fibers traversing the globus pallidus

11.5.2.1 Nucleus Accumbens

It is divided into two structures:
- the nucleus accumbens core
- the nucleus accumbens shell

Shell-Cell types:
- Neurons in the nucleus accumbens are mostly medium spiny neurons (MSNs).
- Containing mainly D1-type (i.e., DRD1 and DRD5) or D2-type (i.e., DRD2, DRD3, and DRD4) dopamine receptors.
- A subpopulation of MSNs contain both D1-type and D2-type receptors, with approximately 40% of striatal MSNs expressing both DRD1 and DRD2 mRNA.

11.6 Diencephalon

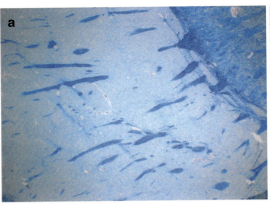 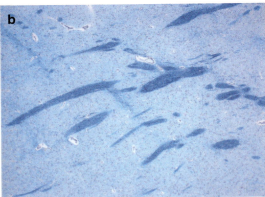

Fig. 11.16 Basal ganglia—Putamen: Bundles of nerve fibers crossing the putamen (**a**, **b**)

- These mixed-type NAcc MSNs with both D1-type and D2-type receptors are mostly confined to the NAcc shell.
- The neurons in the shell, as compared to the core, have a lower density of dendritic spines, less terminal segments, and less branch segments than those in the core.
- The shell neurons project to the subcommissural part of the ventral pallidum as well as the ventral tegmental area and to extensive areas in the hypothalamus and extended amygdala.

Core-Cell types:
- Made up mainly of medium spiny neurons containing mainly D1-type or D2-type dopamine receptors.
- The neurons in the core, as compared to the neurons in the shell, have
  - increased density of dendritic spines
  - increased branch segments
  - increased terminal segments.
- From the core, the neurons project to other subcortical areas such as the globus pallidus and the substantia nigra. GABA is one of the main neurotransmitters in the NAcc, and GABA receptors are also abundant.

11.6 Diencephalon

11.6.1 Thalamus

The microscopic analysis reveals that the thalamus is subdivided into the following nuclei, some of which might already be discerned at the macroscopic level (Fig. 11.17a–d):

- anterior nuclear group
- medial nuclear group
- ventrolateral nuclear group
- lateral geniculate body
- medial geniculate body
- reticular nucleus
- intralaminar nuclei

Some of the above-mentioned nuclei can be further subdivided as follows:

- Medial nuclear group
- Mediodorsal group: MD
- Ventrolateral nuclear group
  – Ventral anterior: VA
  – Ventral lateral: VL
  – Ventral posterior: VP
    o Ventral posterolateral: VPL
    o Ventral posteromedial: VPM
    o Lateral dorsal: LD
    o Lateral posterior: LP
    o Pulvinar: P

The ventral group is formed by:
- VA
- VL
- VP

The lateral group is formed by:
- LD
- LP
- Pulvinar P

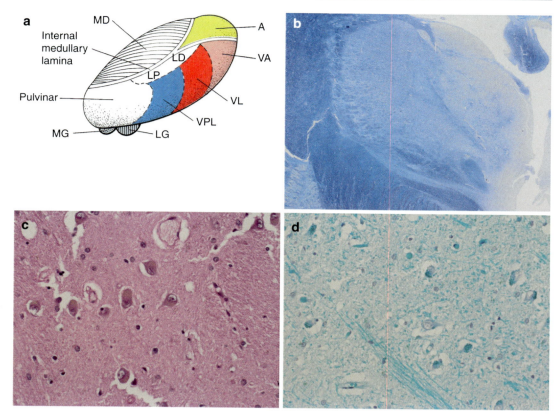

Fig. 11.17 Thalamus: The various thalamic nuclei (reproduced from Heimer (1983) with kind permission by Springer Nature (**a**) (*A* anterior nucleus, *VA* ventral anterior, *VL* ventral lateral, *VPL* ventral posterior lateral, *MD* medial dorsal; *MG* medial geniculate body, *LG* lateral geniculate body). The thalamus displaying a few nuclei on an LFB-stained section (**b**). Roughly the anterior nuclear group (AV) and the ventrolateral nuclear group (Va) are discernible. Neurons of the thalamus (**c, d**; **c**: stain H&E, **d** stain: LFB)

11.6.2 Hypothalamus (Fig. 11.18)

The hypothalamus is divided into:
- Medial hypothalamic region
  - Contains the majority of nuclei
- Lateral hypothalamic region
  - Contains the major fiber tracts

The medial hypothalamic region is subdivided into:
- Supraoptic region
  - Supraoptic nucleus
  - Suprachiasmatic nucleus
  - Paraventricular nucleus
- Tuberal region
  - Ventromedial nucleus
  - Dorsomedial nucleus
  - Infundubular nucleus
- Mammillary region
  - Mammillary body
  - Posterior nucleus

11.7 Mesencephalon

The following parts of the mesencephalon are distinguished as follows (Fig. 11.19):
- Caudal midbrain
  - Inferior colliculi
  - Parabigeminal area
  - Trochlear nerve (N.IV)
  - Tegmental and interpeduncular nuclei
- Rostral midbrain
  - Superior colliculi
  - Pretectal region

11.7 Mesencephalon

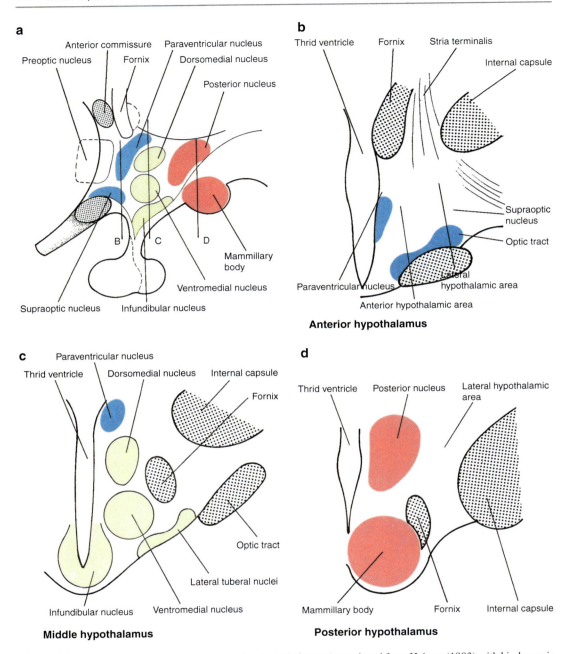

Fig. 11.18 Hypothalamus: The various nuclei of the hypothalamus (reproduced from Heimer (1983) with kind permission by Springer Nature)

- Posterior commissure
- Oculomotor nerve
- Midbrain tegmentum
  - Red nucleus (Nucleus ruber)
  - Reticular formation
- Substantia nigra
- Crus cerebri

11.7.1 Substantia Nigra
(Fig. 11.20a–d)

The substantia nigra is divided into:
- pars compacta (SNc)
  - dorsal tier
  - ventral tier

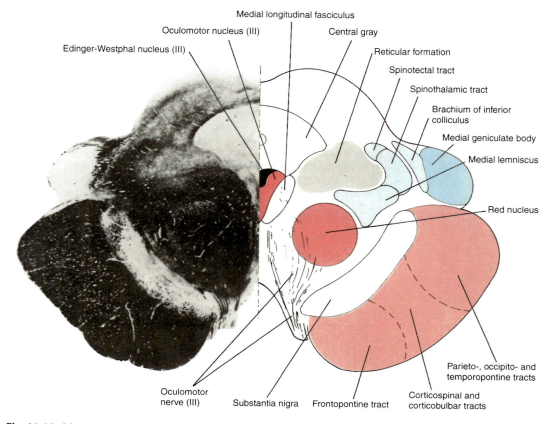

Fig. 11.19 Mesencephalon: Schematic drawing of the pons and its nuclei and tracts (reproduced from Heimer (1983) with kind permission by Springer Nature)

- pars reticulata (SNr)
- pars lateralis (SNl)

Pars compacta
- cell-rich zone
- numerous densely packed neurons
- neurons contain melanin pigment

Pars reticulata
- cell-poor zone
- neurons enmeshed in a dense striato-nigral fiber network

Pars lateralis
- most fibrous region
- contains fibers and neurons

11.7.2 Nucleus Ruber (Fig. 11.21a–d)

- round structure of 7–8 mm in diameter
- with reddish colored appearance (due to high iron content)
- lies between the periaqueductal gray and the substantia nigra
- is lined posteriorly by the reticular formation
- subdivided into:
  - magnocellular part: contains large neurons
  - parvocellular part: contains small neurons and makes up the largest portion of the nucleus

11.7 Mesencephalon

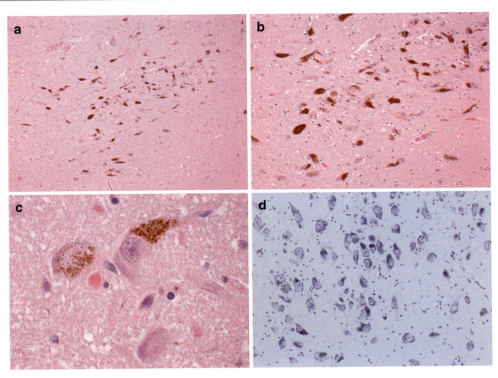

Fig. 11.20 Substantia nigra: Pigmented neurons in the substantia nigra (**a–d**, **a–c**: stain: H&E, **d**: stain: cresyl violet)

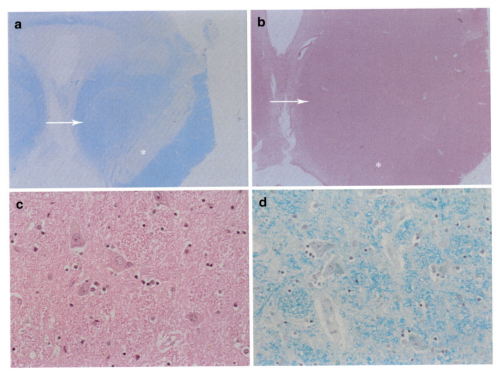

Fig. 11.21 Nc ruber: Low magnification to visualize the close proximity of the nucleus ruber (→) to the substantia nigra (∗) (**a, b**; **a**: LFB; **b**: H&E). The neurons of the nucleus ruber (**c, d**; **c**: H&E; **d**: LFB)

11.8 Pons

The following parts of the pons are distinguished (Fig. 11.22a–i):
- caudal pons
  - dorsal portion
  - ventral pons
- vestibulocochlear nerve (N. VIII)
  - cochlear nuclei
  - auditory fiber systems
  - labyrinthal nuclei
  - vestibular fiber systems
- facial nerve (N. VII)
- abducens nerve (N. VI)

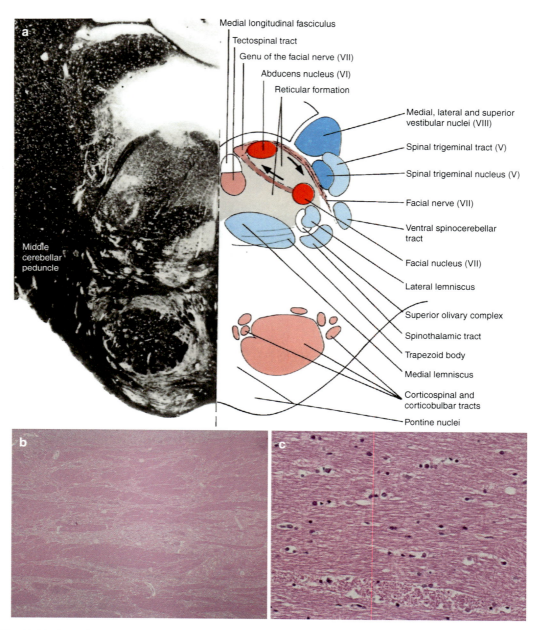

Fig. 11.22 Pons: Schematic drawing of the pons and its nuclei and tracts (reproduced from Heimer (1983) with kind permission by Springer Nature). (**a**). Transverse fiber systems (**b–e**; **b**, **c**: stain: H&E; **d**, **e**: stain: LFB); pontine nuclei (**f–i**; **f**, **g**: stain: H&E; **h**, **i**: stain: LFB)

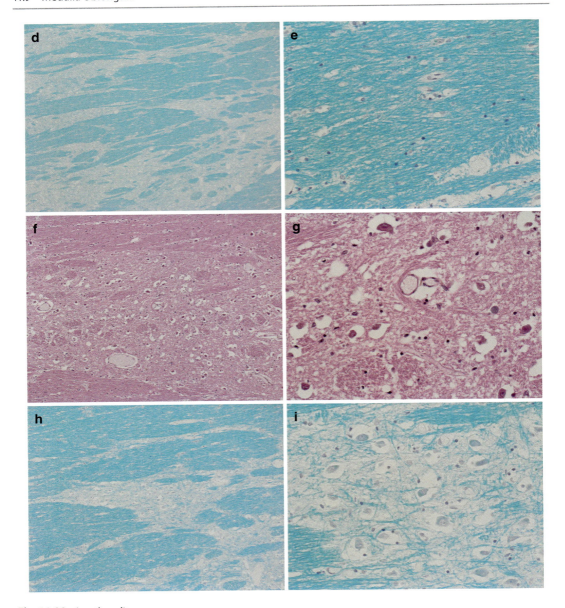

Fig. 11.22 (continued)

- trigeminal nerve (N.V)
- rostral pons-isthmus level
  - tegmentum
  - superior cerebellar peduncle
  - parabrachial nuclei
  - locus coeruleus
  - raphe nuclei
- reticular formation

Locus coeruleus (Fig. 11.23a–d)
- Bluish gray area rostral to the facial colliculus in the area of the sulcus limitans.
- cells contain melanin pigment.
- Gives rise to noradrenergic pathways.

11.9 Medulla Oblongata

The following parts of the medulla oblongata are distinguished (Fig. 11.24):
- spinomedullary transition with the following structures:
  - corticospinal decussation
  - posterior column nuclei

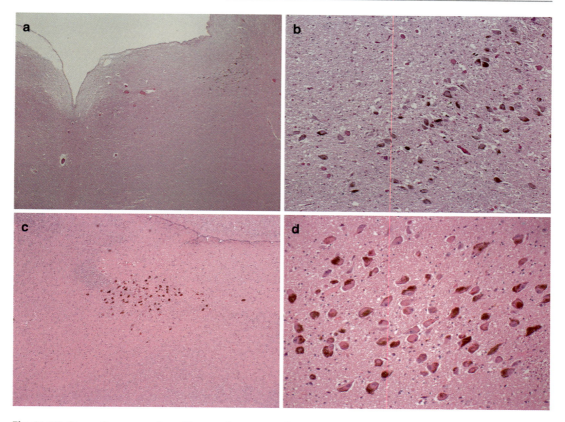

Fig. 11.23 Pons—Locus coeruleus: Pigmented neurons make up the locus coeruleus (**a–d**)

- decussation of the medial lemniscus
- spinal trigeminal complex
- area postrema
• inferior olivary complex
• medullary reticular formation
• ascending and descending tracts
• inferior cerebellar peduncle
• cranial nerves of the medulla
    - Hypoglossal nerve (N. XII)
    - Spinal accessory nerve (N. XI)
    - Vagus nerve (N. X)
    - Glossopharyngeal nerve (N. IX)
• Corticobulbar fibers
• Medullary-pontine junction

11.9.1 Area Postrema

It belongs to the circumventricular organs and consists of:
• Astroblast-like cells
• Arterioles
• Sinusoids
• Apolar or unipolar neurons

11.9.2 Pyramis (Fig. 11.25a–d)

• Cone-shaped eminence
• Contains the corticospinal tract

11.10 Cerebellum

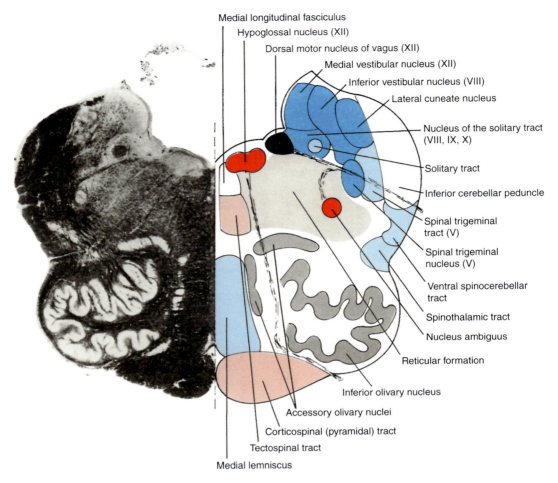

Fig. 11.24 Medulla oblongata: Schematic drawing of the medulla oblongata and its nuclei and tracts (reproduced from Heimer (1983) with kind permission by Springer Nature)

11.9.3 Inferior Olivary Complex
(Fig. 11.26a–d)

The inferior olivary complex consists of the following nuclei:
- Principal inferior olivary nucleus
- Medial accessory olivary nucleus
- Dorsal accessory olivary nucleus

The nuclei are made up of
- Small, round, or pear-shaped cells
- Numerous short branching dendrites

11.10 Cerebellum

The cerebellum is composed of:
- cerebellar cortex
- cerebellar white matter
- cerebellar nuclei embedded in the white matter

The major cell types of the cerebellar cortex include:
- Granular cells
- Golgi cells

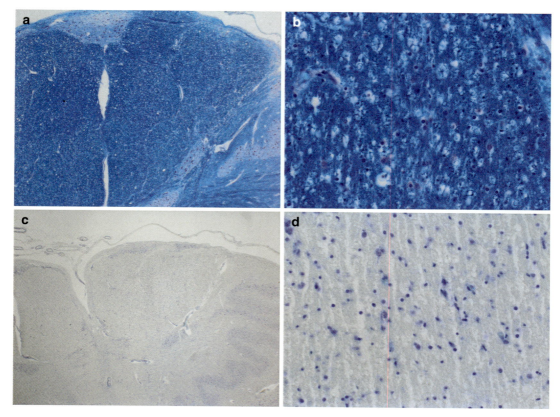

Fig. 11.25 Medulla oblongata—Pyramis: The myelinated fibers of the corticospinal tract make up the pyramis (**a**, **b**; stain: LFB), glial cells are seen on a cresyl violet-stained section (**c**, **d**)

- Purkinje cells
- Basket cells
- Stellate cells

The cerebellar cortex is composed of the following three layers from outwards to inwards (Fig. 11.27a–c):

- Layer 1: molecular layer
- Layer 2: Purkinje cell layer
- Layer 3: granular cell layer

Layer 1: Molecular layer (Fig. 11.27d, e)
- made up of stellate cells and basket cells
- dendritic arborizations of Purkinje cells and Golgi cells
- abundance of tightly packed granular cell axons, i.e., parallel fibers which run parallel to the direction of the folia

Layer 2: Purkinje cell layer (Fig. 11.27e–h)
- formed by a sheet of large Purkinje cells
- rich branching

11.10 Cerebellum

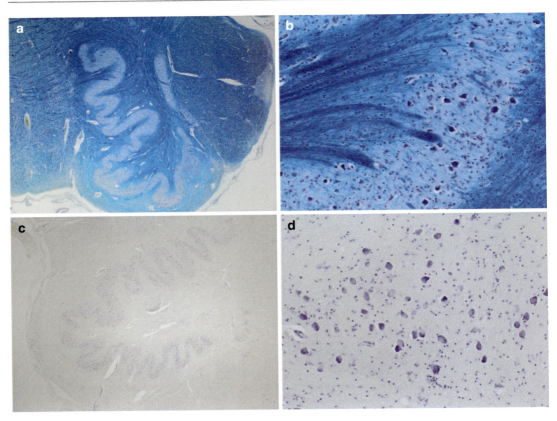

Fig. 11.26 Medulla oblongata-inferior olivary nucleus: The dentated structure of the nucleus is best seen on LFB-stained section (**a, b**) as well as on cresyl violet-stained sections (Nissl stain) (**c, d**)

- flattened dendritic tree extends throughout the molecular layer in a plane perpendicular to the longitudinal axis of the folium

Layer 3: Granular cell layer (Fig. 11.27i, j)
- granular cells, i.e., relay neurons
- limited number of large interneurons

- Golgi cells with large dendritic trees extending in all directions of the molecular layer

The cerebellar nuclei encompass:
- dentate nucleus (Fig. 11.28a–d)
- emboliform nucleus
- fusiform nucleus

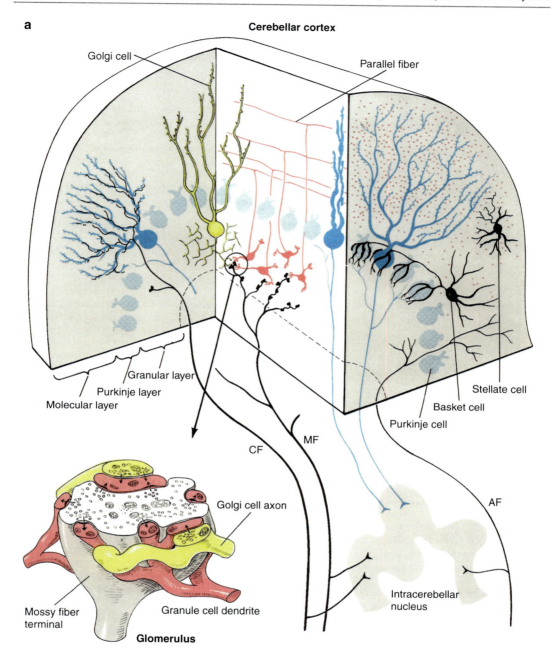

Fig. 11.27 Cerebellum: Schematic drawings of the layers of the cerebellar cortex (**a**, reproduced from Heimer (1983) with kind permission by Springer Nature); (**b**) with kind permission from Arslan (2015). The three layers (I, II, III) and the white matter (WM) (**c, d**), the granular cell layer (**e**), Purkinje cells (**f–i**), binucleated Purkinje cell (**h**), arborizations of the Purkinje cells in the molecular layer (**j**)

11.10 Cerebellum

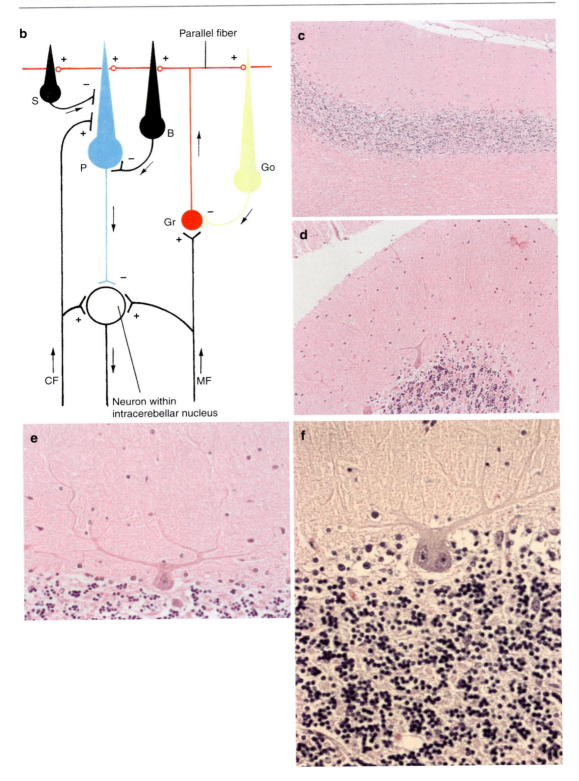

Fig. 11.27 (continued)

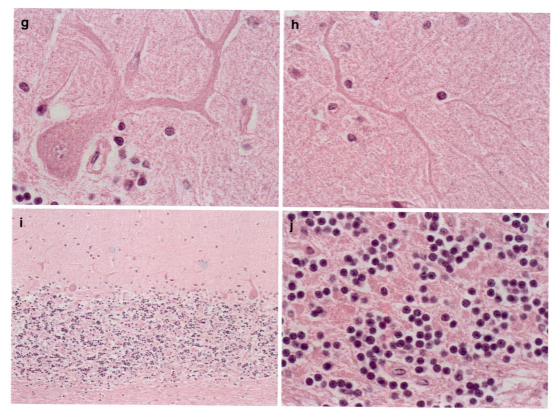

Fig. 11.27 (continued)

11.11 Spinal Cord

The spinal cord is made up of gray matter surrounded by white matter. On horizontal sections, the gray matter displays an H-like shape or the shape of a butterfly. The gray matter of the spinal cord is a symmetrical structure connected by the central gray commissure. In the middle of the central gray commissure, the central canal can easily be discerned. The gray matter is composed of longitudinally arranged columns and laminae whereas the white matter contains longitudinally arranged fiber systems.

A first rough subdivision of the gray matter for orientation purposes is given as follows and is shown in Fig. 11.29a–c:

- dorsal horn
- ventral horn
- lateral horn

The following nuclei are contained in the dorsal horn:

- posteromarginal nucleus
- substantia gelantinosa
- nucleus propius (principal sensory nucleus)

At the level of C8–L3, the dorsal nucleus of Clarke (Clarke's column) is found.

The dorsal horn contains in the above-mentioned structures relais-stations where primary sensory fibers terminate and synapse with

11.11 Spinal Cord

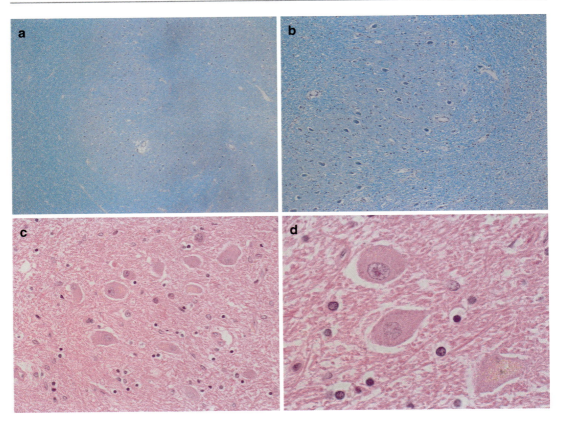

Fig. 11.28 Cerebellar dentate nucleus: The dentated structure of the nucleus is best seen on LFB-stained sections (**a**, **b**); the neurons of the dentate nucleus (**c**, **d**)

other fiber systems in order to integrate and modulate sensory information, to transmit information to higher centers (thalamus, cerebellum, brain stem), and to form reflex arcs.

The ventral horn contains the medial motor column and the lateral motor column. The medial motor extends throughout the total length of the spinal cord. The lateral motor columns are present in the cervical enlargement C5–T1 and in the lumbosacral enlargement L1–S3. The ventral horn contains the neuronal perikarya of those neurons that innervate striated muscle, i.e., the motorneurons (Fig. 11.29d).

The lateral column is made up of the intermediolateral cell column and the intermediomedial cell column. It contains preganglionic sympathetic neurons and is only visible at the level of T1–L3. The intermediomedial cell column contains neurons which are associated with visceral motor reflexes.

Another subdivision of the gray matter was proposed by Rexed. The subdivision does not consider the grouping of neurons into columns or nuclei but an organization into 10 laminae. The organization of the gray matter of the spinal cord into the laminae after Rexed is displayed in Fig. 11.29e. The correspondence of the Rexed laminae with the classical nuclei and columns is given in Table 11.6.

The central canal runs longitudinally through the length of the entire spinal cord

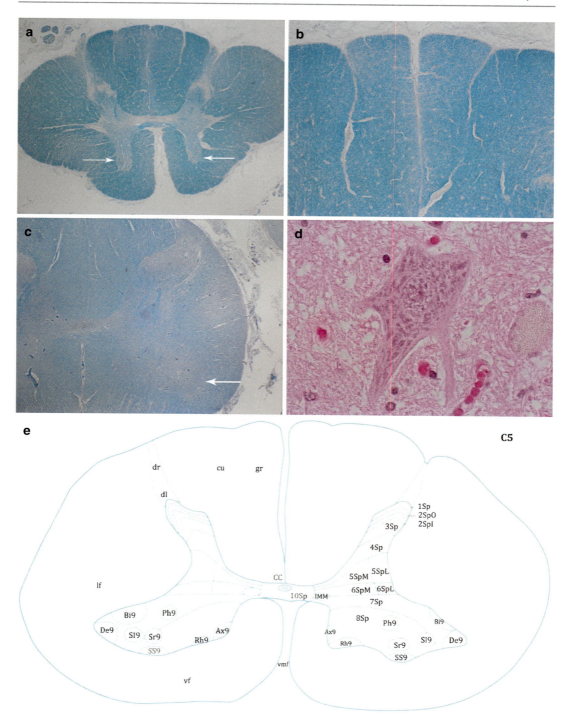

Fig. 11.29 Spinal cord: The gray matter appears bright on this LFB-stained section, the white matter stains blue (**a**), the posterior columns (**b**), anterior horn is seen → (**c**), motor neuron located in the anterior horn (**d**), central canal (**f**, **g**); (stain: LFB). Rexed laminae in C5 human spinal cord segment (**e**) (reproduced from Sengul and Watson (2012) with kind permission by Elsevier)

11.12 Ventricular System

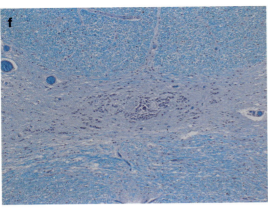
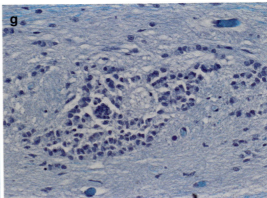

Fig. 11.29 (continued)

(Fig. 11.29f, g). It is space filled with cerebrospinal fluid. The central canal is continuous with the ventricular system of the brain. At the level of the obex, the fourth ventricle narrows to become the central canal of the spinal cord. The central canal helps to transport nutrients to the spinal cord as well as protect it by cushioning the impact of a force when the spine is affected. The central canal represents the adult remainder of the central cavity of the neural tube. The central canal is lined by ependymal cells.

11.12 Ventricular System

11.12.1 Ventricular Lining
(Fig. 11.30a, b)

- lined by a single layer of ependymal cells
- cuboidal cells
- numerous microvilli on the ventricular side
- Electron microscopic features include:
    - small slender mitochondria
    - vesicles or ergastoplasm
    - smooth endoplasmic reticulum
    - Golgi complex
    - compact bundles of intermediate filaments
- Tela choroidea: point of attachment formed of pia mater and ependymal cells
    - in the third, fourth, and lateral ventricles

Table 11.6 Rexed laminae

Rexed laminae		
Lamina I	Posteromarginal nucleus	
Lamina II	Substantia gelatinosa	
Lamina III	Nucleus proprius	
Lamina IV	Nucleus proprius	Dorsal horn
Lamina V	Base of dorsal horn medial complex	
Lamina VI	Base of dorsal horn lateral complex	
Lamina VII	Dorsal column of Clarke	
Lamina VIII	Intermediolateral column Intermediomedial column	Lateral horn
Lamina IX	Lateral and medial motor columns	Ventral horn
Lamina X	Central gray commissure	Central gray commissure

11.12.2 Choroid Plexus (Fig. 11.31a–f)

- villous structure
- single layer of cuboidal epithelium
    - rest on a basal lamina
- basal infoldings on the choroidal stroma
- apical microvilli in contact with CSF
- extensive capillary network
- connective tissue stroma

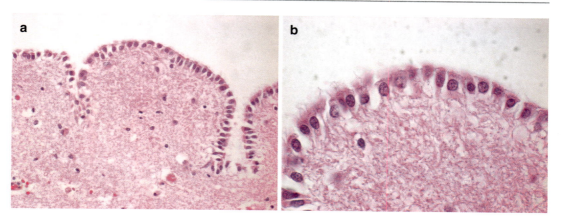

Fig. 11.30 Ventricular lining: made up of a single layer of ependymal cuboidal cells with numerous microvilli on the ventricular side (**a, b**)

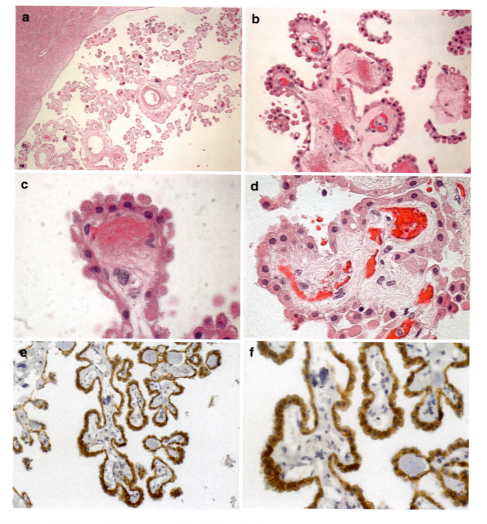

Fig. 11.31 Choroid plexus: villous structure formed by a single layer of cuboidal epithelium resting on a basal lamina (**a–d**). Immunophenotype: positive for pancytokeratin AE1/AE3 (**e, f**)

Selected References

Amunts K, Zilles K (2015) Architectonic mapping of the human brain beyond Brodmann. Neuron 88(6):1086–1107. https://doi.org/10.1016/j.neuron.2015.12.001

Arslan OE (2015) Neuroanatomical basis of clinical neurology, 2nd edn. CRC, Boca Raton, FL

Bailey P, Bonin VG (1951) The isocortex of man. University of Illinois Press, Champaign, IL

Braak H (1980) Architectonics of the human telencephalic cortex. Springer, Berlin

Bratz E (1899) Ammonshornbefunde der Epileptischen. Arch Psychiatr Nervenkr 31:820–836

Brodmann K (1909) Vergleichende Lokalisationslehre der Großhirnrinde in ihren Prinzipien dargestellt auf Grund des Zellenbaues. Verlag von Johann Ambrosius Barth, Leipzig

Campbell AW (1905) Histological studies on the localisation of cerebral function. Cambridge University Press, Cambridge

Catani M, Thiebaut de Schotten M (2012) Atlas of human brain connections. Oxford University Press, Oxford

Cusick CG, Seltzer B, Cola M, Griggs E (1995) Chemoarchitectonics and corticocortical terminations within the superior temporal sulcus of the rhesus monkey: evidence for subdivisions of superior temporal polysensory cortex. J Comp Neurol 360(3):513–535. https://doi.org/10.1002/cne.903600312

Fingelkurts AA, Fingelkurts AA (2008) Brain-mind operational architectonics imaging: technical and methodological aspects. Open Neuroimag J 2:73–93. https://doi.org/10.2174/1874440000802010073

Fingelkurts AA, Fingelkurts AA, Neves CF (2009) Brain and mind operational architectonics and man-made "machine" consciousness. Cogn Process 10(2):105–111. https://doi.org/10.1007/s10339-008-0234-y

Flechsig P (1920) Anatomie des menschlichen Gehirns und Rückenmarks auf myelogenetischer Grundlage. Thieme, Stuttgart

Flechsig P (1927) Meine myelogenetische Hirnlehre. Mit biographischer Einführung. Springer, Berlin

Friede RL (1960) A comparative study of cytoarchitectonics and chemoarchitectonics of the cerebral cortex of the guinea pig. Z Zellforsch Mikrosk Anat 52:482–493

Friede RL (1966a) The histochemical architecture of the Ammon's horn as related to its selective vulnerability. Acta Neuropathol 6(1):1–13

Friede RL (1966b) Topographic brain chemistry. Academic Press, Cambridge, MA

Heimer L (1983) The human brain and spinal cord: functional neuroanatomy and dissection guide. Springer, Berlin

Hubel DH, Wiesel TN (1977) Ferrier lecture. functional architecture of macaque monkey visual cortex. Proc R Soc Lond Ser B Biol Sci 198(1130):1–59

Jacobowitz DM, Kresse A, Skofitsch G (2004) Galanin in the brain: chemoarchitectonics and brain cartography—a historical review. Peptides 25(3):433–464. https://doi.org/10.1016/j.peptides.2004.02.015

Kusunoki T (1969) The chemoarchitectonics of the avian brain. J Hirnforsch 11(6):477–497

Lorente de No R (1934) Studies on the structure of the cerebral cortex. II. Continuation of the study of the Ammonic system. J Psychol Neurol 46:13–177

Matelli M, Luppino G (2004) Architectonics of the primates cortex: usefulness and limits. Cortex 40(1):209–210

Mesulam MM (2000) Behavioral neuroanatomy. large. scale networks, association cortex, frontal syndromes, the limbic system, and hemispheric specializations. In: Mesulam MM (ed) Principles of behavioral and cognitive neurology, 2nd edn. Oxford University Press, Oxford, pp 1–120

Mesulam MM, Geula C (1994) Chemoarchitectonics of axonal and perikaryal acetylcholinesterase along information processing systems of the human cerebral cortex. Brain Res Bull 33(2):137–153

Mesulam MM, Rosen AD, Mufson EJ (1984) Regional variations in cortical cholinergic innervation: chemoarchitectonics of acetylcholinesterase-containing fibers in the macaque brain. Brain Res 311(2):245–258

Ohm TG, Heilmann R, Braak H (1989) The human oral raphe system. Architectonics and neuronal types in pigment-Nissl preparations. Anat Embryol 180(1):37–43

Palomero-Gallagher N, Zilles K (2017) Cortical layers: cyto-, myelo-, receptor- and synaptic architecture in human cortical areas. NeuroImage https://doi.org/10.1016/j.neuroimage.2017.08.035

Pessacq TP (1988) Some considerations on the synaptic architectonics of the cerebral cortex. Morphol Embryol 34(1):9–11

Pfeiffer RA (1928) Die Angioarchitektonik der Großhirnrinde. Springer, Berlin

Pfeiffer RA (1930) Grundlegende Untersuchungen für die Angioarchitektonik des menschlichen Gehirns. Springer, Berlin

Roper WG (2016) Architectonics of male amygdala. Med Hypotheses 96:73–74. https://doi.org/10.1016/j.mehy.2016.09.026

Rose M (1927) Allocortex bei Tier und Mensch. Die sogenannte Riechrinde beim Menschen und beim Affen. J Psychol Neurol 34:261–401

Sarkissow SA, Filimonoff IN, Kononowa EP, Preobrachenskaja IS, Kukuew LA (1955) Atlas of the cytoarchitectonics of the human cerebral cortex. Medgiz, Leningrad

Schlote W (1959) On glia architectonics of the human cerebral cortex in the Nissl picture. Arch Psychiatr Nervenkr Z Gesamte Neurol Psychiatr 199:573–595

Sengul G, Watson C (2012) Spinal cord: regional anatomy, cytoarchitecture and chemoarchitecture. In: Mai JK, Paxinos G (eds) The human nervous system, 3rd edn. Elsevier, Amsterdam, pp 186–232

Smith GE (1907) A new topographical survey of the human cerebral cortex, being an account of the distribution of the anatomically distinct cortical areas and their relationship to the cerebral sulci. J Anat Physiol 41(Pt 4):237–254

Smith CU (1992) A century of cortical architectonics. J Hist Neurosci 1(3):201–218. https://doi.org/10.1080/09647049209525533

Sommer W (1880) Erkrankung des Ammonshorns als aetiologisches Moment der Epilepsie. Arch Psychiatr Nervenkr 10:631–675

Spielmeyer W (1927) Die Pathogenese des epileptischen Krampfes. Z Dtsch Ges Neurol Psychiatr 109:501–520

Toga AW, Thompson PM, Mori S, Amunts K, Zilles K (2006) Towards multimodal atlases of the human brain. Nat Rev Neurosci 7(12):952–966. https://doi.org/10.1038/nrn2012

Van Essen DC, Glasser MF (2014) In vivo architectonics: a cortico-centric perspective. Neuroimage 93(Pt 2):157–164. https://doi.org/10.1016/j.neuroimage.2013.04.095

Van Essen DC, Anderson CH, Felleman DJ (1992) Information processing in the primate visual system: an integrated systems perspective. Science 255(5043):419–423

Vogt C, Vogt O (1919) Allgemeinere Ergebnisse unserer Hirnforschung. J Psychol Neurol 25:279–468

Vogt C, Vogt O (1937) Sitz und Wesen der Krankheiten im Lichte der topistischen Hirnforschung und des Varierens der Tiere. Teil 1. Barth, Leipzig

von Economo C, Koskinas GN (1925) Die Cytoarchitektonik der Hirnrinde des erwachsenen Menschen. Springer, Berlin

Wamsley B, Fishell G (2017) Genetic and activity-dependent mechanisms underlying interneuron diversity. Nat Rev Neurosci 18(5):299–309. https://doi.org/10.1038/nrn.2017.30

Zilles K, Amunts K (2009) Receptor mapping: architecture of the human cerebral cortex. Curr Opin Neurol 22(4):331–339. https://doi.org/10.1097/WCO.0b013e32832d95db

Zilles K, Amunts K (2010) Centenary of Brodmann's map—conception and fate. Nat Rev Neurosci 11(2):139–145. https://doi.org/10.1038/nrn2776

Zilles K, Palomero-Gallagher N (2001) Cyto-, myelo-, and receptor architectonics of the human parietal cortex. Neuroimage 14(1 Pt 2):S8–S20. https://doi.org/10.1006/nimg.2001.0823

Zilles K, Palomero-Gallagher N, Grefkes C, Scheperjans F, Boy C, Amunts K, Schleicher A (2002) Architectonics of the human cerebral cortex and transmitter receptor fingerprints: reconciling functional neuroanatomy and neurochemistry. Eur Neuropsychopharmacol 12(6):587–599

Zilles K, Palomero-Gallagher N, Schleicher A (2004) Transmitter receptors and functional anatomy of the cerebral cortex. J Anat 205(6):417–432. https://doi.org/10.1111/j.0021-8782.2004.00357.x

Zykin PA, Moiseenko IA, Tkachenko LA, Nasyrov RA, Tsvetkov EA, Krasnoshchekova EI (2018) Peculiarities of cyto- and chemoarchitectonics of human entorhinal cortex during the fetal period. Bull Exp Biol Med 164(4):497–501. https://doi.org/10.1007/s10517-018-4020-2

Functional Systems

12.1 Introduction

Functional systems are composed of several morphological regions or structures involved in the coordination and execution of the same function.

The following main categories of functional systems can be defined:
- Sensory system
- Motor system
- Brain stem and cranial nerves
- Autonomic system
- Cerebral cortex and limbic system
- Hypothalamus and hypophyseal system

A further subdivision of the above-mentioned functional systems is given in Table 12.1.

Circuit:
- Neurons never function in isolation; they are organized into ensembles or circuits that process specific kinds of information (Purves et al. 2012).
- Some characteristic features:
  - The synaptic connections that define a circuit are typically made in a dense tangle of dendrites, axons terminals, and glial cell processes that together constitute neuropil.
  - The direction of information flow in any particular circuit is essential for understanding its function.
  - Neural circuits are both anatomical and functional entities.

Microcircuit:
- The way that nerve cells (and associated cells such as glia) are organized to carry out specific operations within a region of the nervous system (Shepherd and Grillner 2010).

12.2 Sensory System: Visual System

The following structures are involved (Figs. 12.1a–d and 12.2a–h):
- retina
- optic nerve, optic chiasm, optic tract
- lateral geniculate body
- optic radiation = geniculate calcarine tract
- primary visual cortex

The processing of the visual information is done in the following ways:
- The retina constitutes an evaginated part of the forebrain and thus, is part of the brain.

Table 12.1 A further subdivision of the main categories of functional systems

Sensory systems	• Visual system • Auditory system • Vestibular system • Olfactory system • Taste • Somatosensory system
Motor systems	• Peripheral motor neuron • Central motor system • Basal ganglionic system • Cerebellar system
Brain stem and cranial nerves	• Reticular formation • Cranial nerves
Autonomic system	• Peripheral autonomic system • Central autonomic system
Cerebral cortex and limbic system	• Cerebral cortex • Limbic system • Amygdalar system • Thalamic system • Hippocampal system
Hypothalamus and hypophyseal system	• Hypothalamus • Pituitary gland

- The retina is composed of rods and cones which function as visual receptors.
  - The rods are concerned with light and allow us to see in dim light.
  - The cones are responsible for color vision and allow us to see sharp images.
  - The fovea centralis of the retina contains only cones and represents the area of the highest visual acuity.
- Besides rods and cones, the retina also contains bipolar neurons and interneurons, i.e., the horizontal and the amacrine cells.
- Visual information is received by the receptors and transduced to the bipolar cells. The transduction of the information is modulated by the horizontal and the amacrine cells. The information is transmitted from the bipolar cells to the ganglion cells which send their axons to the optic disc.
- These axons are contained in the optic nerve, which, some cm posterior, forms the optic chiasm.
- In the optic chiasm, the fibers of the nasal half of the retina cross the contralateral side, whereas the fibers from the temporal half of the retina do not cross.
- All fibers then continue their course as the optic tract.
- The majority of the axons from the optic tract terminate in the lateral geniculate body (LGB).
  - The LGB is made up of six layers.
  - Layering reflects the fiber input from both eyes and the various retinal cells.
  - CGL is the first place where the fibers synapse.
- Some fibers terminate in the pretectal region and are involved in the control of eye movement and in the pupillary light reflex (see later).
- Other fibers terminate in the superior colliculus.
- The fibers continue their route as the optic radiation.

The optic radiation terminates predominantly in Brodmann area 17, i.e., primary visual cortex. A subdivision of the occipital lobe and the visual areas is given in Fig. 12.3 and Table 12.2.

Afferent and efferent fiber systems of Brodmann area 17 are listed in Table 12.3.

Evidence for two different streams in the dorsal visual system (see also Sect. 12.13):
- a *dorso-dorsal (d-d) stream* to area V6 and areas V6A and MIP of the SPL
  - The dorsal stream (or "where pathway") is involved with processing the object's spatial location relative to the viewer and with speech repetition.
  - Provide information for the control of action.
  - The **dorsal stream** is proposed to be involved in the guidance of actions and recognizing where objects are in space. Also known as the parietal stream, the "where" stream, or the "how" stream, this pathway stretches from the primary visual cortex (V1) in the occipital lobe forward into the parietal lobe. It is interconnected with the parallel ventral stream (the "what" stream) which runs downward from V1 into the temporal lobe.

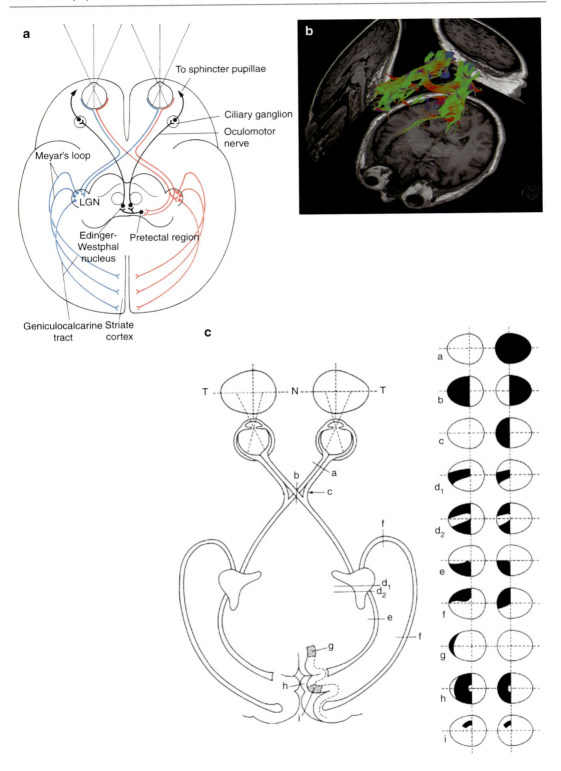

Fig. 12.1 Visual system: Scheme illustrating the visual system (**a**) (reproduced from Heimer (1983) with kind permission by Springer Nature). Reconstruction of the visual system based of DTI (**b**). Lesions associated with the visual system and pertinent dysfunctions (**c**) (reproduced from ten Donkelaar (2011) with kind permission by Springer Nature)

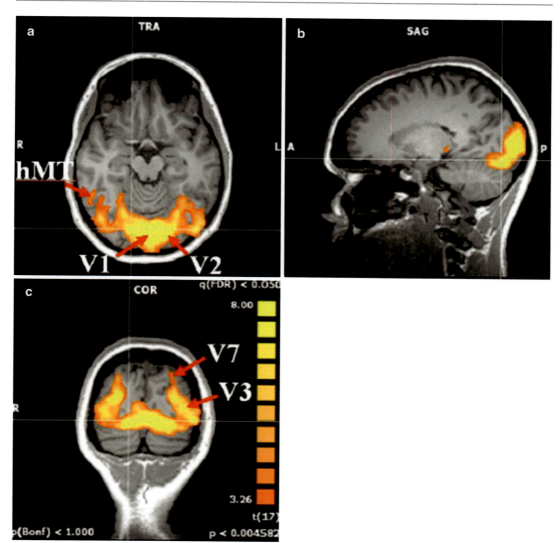

Fig. 12.2 Visual system shown by fMRI (**a**–**h**). Primary visual cortex V1, V2 (**a**, **b**), V3, V7 (**c**), summary of the brain regions involved in the processing of visual information (**d**), ventral and dorsal stream regions including the superior frontal gyrus (**e**), superior parietal lobe (**f**), precentral gyrus (**g**), and lateral geniculate body (**h**)

12.2 Sensory System: Visual System

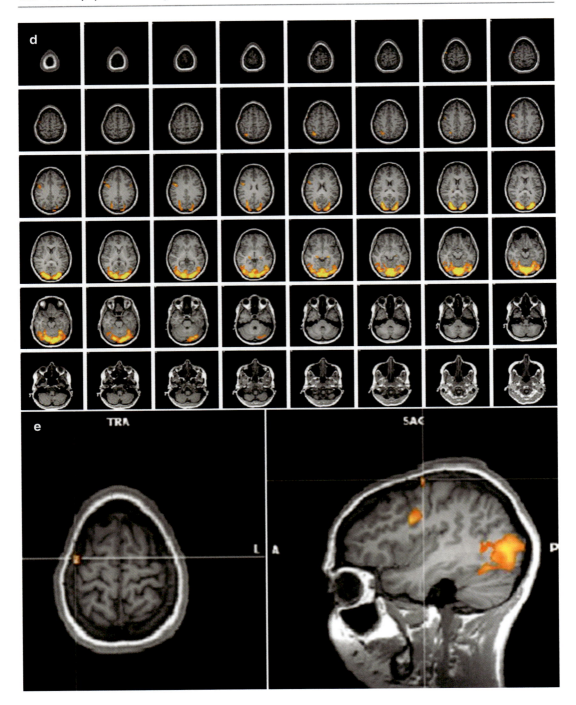

Fig. 12.2 (continued)

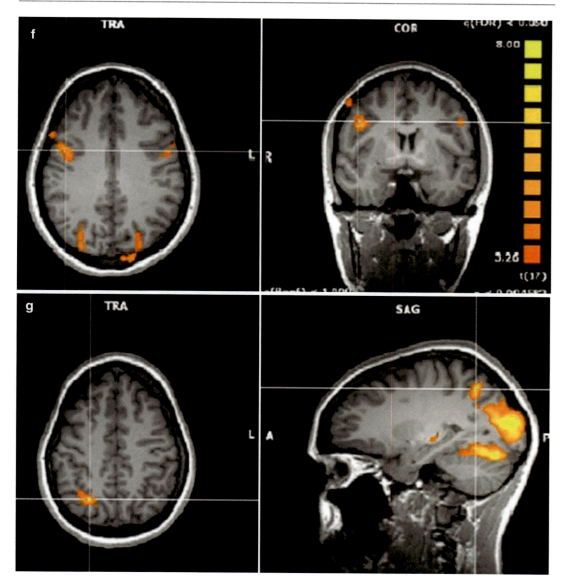

Fig. 12.2 (continued)

12.2 Sensory System: Visual System

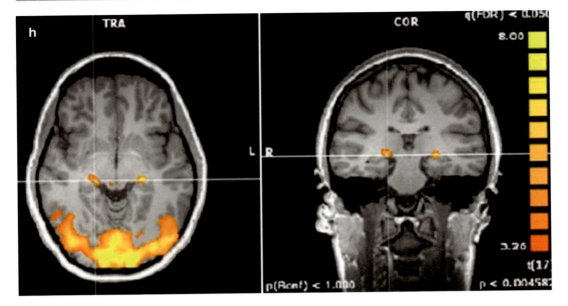

Fig. 12.2 (continued)

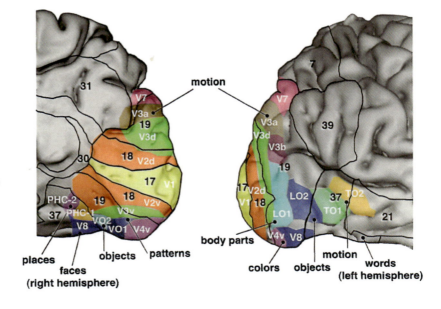

Fig. 12.3 Visual system: Parcellation of the occipital lobe into Brodmann areas 17, 18, 19 (cytoarchitectonics), and retinotopic areas (V1, V2v, V2d, etc.) based on functional imaging studies (reproduced from Catani and Thiebaut de Schotten (2012) with kind permission by Oxford University Press)

Table 12.2 Subdivisions of the occipital lobe and the visual areas

Area		Function
V1	Primary visual cortex	• Processing information about static and moving objects • Excellent in pattern recognition
V2	Secondary visual cortex Prestriate cortex	• Orientation • Spatial frequency • Color • Storage of object recognition memory • Conversion of short-term object memories into long-term memories
V3	Third visual complex	• Analysis of the form of stimuli
V3A		• Analysis of the form of stimuli
VP		• Analysis of the form of stimuli
V4	Extrastriate visual cortex	• Exhibits long-term plasticity • Encodes stimulus salience • Gated by signals coming from the frontal eye fields • Shows changes in the spatial profile of its receptive fields with attention
V5	Middle temporal visual cortex	• Motion perception and eye movements
V6	Dorsomedial area	• Sharp selectivity for the orientation of visual contours • Preference for long, uninterrupted lines covering large parts of the visual field

Table 12.3 Afferent and efferent fibers of Brodmann area 17

Cortical layer	Origin of afferent fibers	Terminal of efferent fibers
I	• Cortex • Lateral geniculate body • Pulvinar • Ventral tegmental area	• –
II-III	• Lateral geniculate body	• Ipsi- and contralateral cortex
IVA	• Lateral geniculate body • Cortex	• –
IVB	• Cortex	• Cortex
IVC	• Lateral geniculate body • Cortex • Raphe • Locus coeruleus	• –
V	• –	• Cortex • Pulvinar • Cranial colliculus • Pontine nuclei
VI	• Cortex • Claustrum • Pulvinar	• Claustrum • Lateral geniculate body

- The dorsal "action" stream transforms incoming visual information to the requisite egocentric (head-centered) coordinate system for skilled motor planning.
- Damage to the d-d stream leads to optic ataxia.
• a *ventro-dorsal (v-d) stream* to area MT and the visual areas of the IPL
  - The ventral stream (also known as the "what pathway") is involved with object and visual identification and recognition.
- Provide information for the control of action.
- May also play a crucial role in space perception and action understanding.
- According to their data, the ventral "perceptual" stream computes a detailed map of the world from visual input, which can then be used for cognitive operations.
- The **ventral stream** is associated with object recognition and form representation. Also described as the "what" stream, it has strong connections to the medial temporal lobe (which stores long-term memories), the limbic system (which controls emotions), and the dorsal stream (which deals with object locations and motion).

12.3 Motor System: Central Motor System

Regions involved in motor activity include (Figs. 12.4a, b and 12.5a–h):
- Pyramidal system
- Extrapyramidal system
- Cerebellum
- Lower motor neuron

Pyramidal system includes the following components:
- Corticospinal tract
- Corticobulbar tract

Extrapyramidal system includes the following components:
- Extrapyramidal areas
- Basal ganglia
- Afferents to the basal ganglia
- Cortical-striatal-pallidal-thalamocortical circuits
- Multisynaptic descending pathways

12.3.1 Corticospinal Tract

Coordinates precise movements of the upper and lower extremities
- precentral gyrus (Brodmann area 4)
  - somatotopical arrangement
  - 1.000.000.000 fibers
    - 30% from layer V of the primary motor cortex
    - 30% from the premotor cortex
    - 40% from the sensory parietal lobe
- Corona radiata
- Posterior limb of the internal capsule
- Cerebral peduncle of the midbrain
- Pyramidal tract in the pons
- Pyramis on the ventral aspect of the medulla oblongata
- Decussation of the pyramids (Decussation pyramis)
  - 90% of the fibers cross to the contralateral side
- Lateral corticospinal tract in the lateral funiculus of the spinal cord
- Uncrossed fibers run in the ventral funiculus as the anterior corticospinal tract

Upper motor neuron:
- Neuron from precentral gyrus synapsing with the lower motor neurons

Lower motor neuron:
- Located in the nuclei of the medial and lateral ventral gray matter (anterior horn)

12.4 Motor System: Basal Ganglionic System

Striatum: Caudate nucleus–putamen (Fig. 12.6a–f)
- Afferent connections
  - Cortico-striatal projections
  - Thalamo-striatal projections
  - Nigrostriatal projections
  - From raphe nuclei
  - Amygdalo-striatal projections
- Efferent connections
  - Striato-pallidal projections
  - Striato-nigral projections

Globus pallidus
- Afferent connections
  - Striato-pallidal projections
  - Subthalamo-pallidal projections
- Efferent connections
  - Ansa lenticularis
  - Lenticular fasciculus
  - Thalamic fasciculus
  - Pallido-thalamic projections
  - Pallido-habenular projections
  - Pallido-nigral projections
  - Pallido-tegmental projections
  - Subthalamic fasciculus

12.5 Sensory System: Somatosensory System

Sensory information from the peripheral receptors is carried via sensory paths to all parts of the CNS.

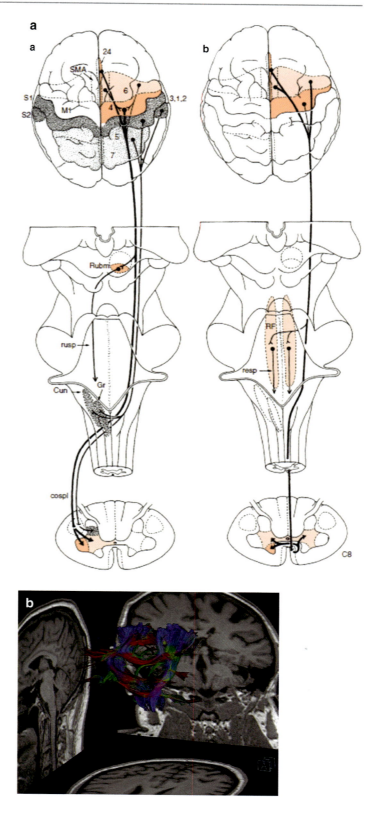

Fig. 12.4 Motor system: schematic drawing showing the various sites of origin of the lateral (**a**) and the anterior (**b**) corticospinal tracts. Abbreviations: *Cun* cuneate nucleus, *Gr* gracile nucleus, *cospa cospl* anterior and lateral corticospinal tracts, *M1* primary motor cortex, *resp* reticulospinal fibers, *RF* reticular formation, *Rubm* magnocellular part of red nucleus, *rusp* rubrospinal tract, *SMA* supplementary motor area, *S1*, *S2* primary and secondary somatosensory cortices, *1–24* Brodmann areas (**a**) (reproduced from ten Donkelaar (2011) with kind permission by Springer Nature). Visualization of the motor system using DTI (**b**)

12.5 Sensory System: Somatosensory System

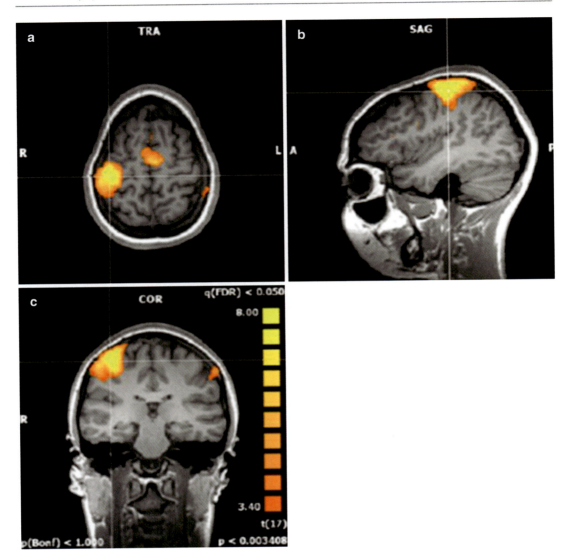

Fig. 12.5 Motor system: activation of the right precentral gyrus after movement of the left finger (**a–c**) as shown by fMRI. Summary of the brain regions involved in the processing of visual information (**d**). The motor information is further processed in the supplementary motor area (SMA) (**e**), frontal premotor cortex (**f**), inferior frontal gyrus (**g**), and cerebellum (**h**)

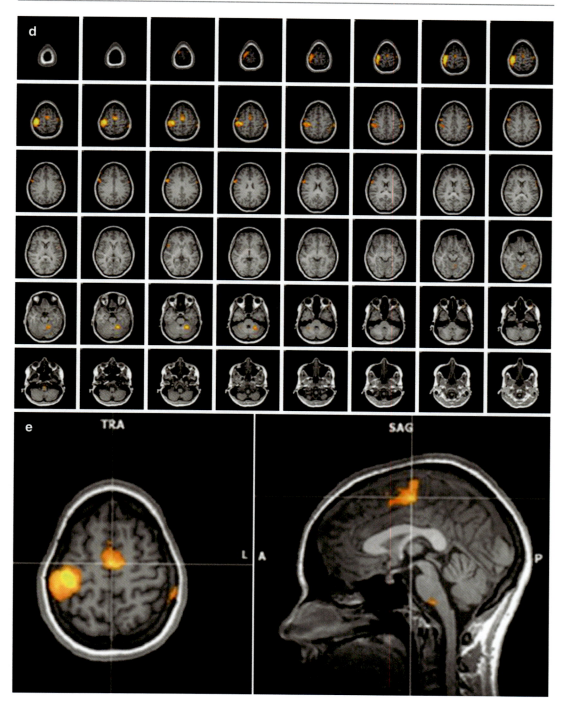

Fig. 12.5 (continued)

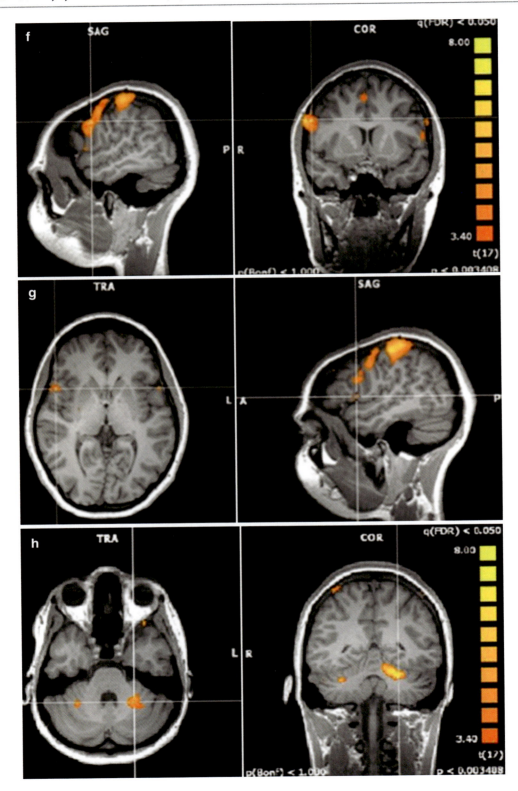

Fig. 12.5 (continued)

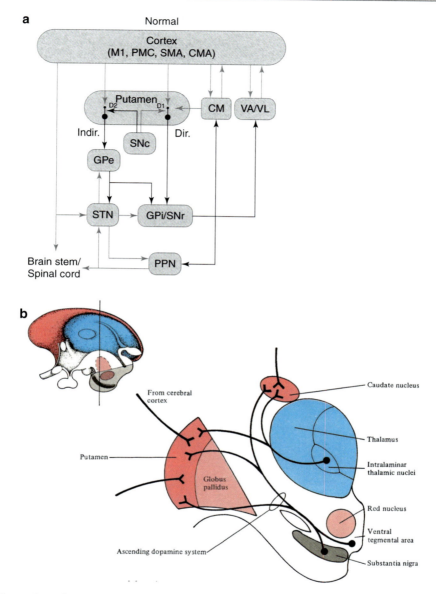

Fig. 12.6 Connections of the basal ganglia-thalamocortical motor circuit. Black arrows indicate inhibitory connections; gray arrows indicate excitatory connections. Abbreviations: *CM* centromedian nucleus of thalamus, *CMA* cingulate motor area, *Dir.* direct pathway, *D1, D2* dopamine receptor subtypes, *GPe* external segment of the globus pallidus, *GPi* internal segment of the globus pallidus, *Indir.* indirect pathway, *M1* primary motor cortex, *Pf* parafascicular nucleus of the thalamus, *PMC* premotor cortex, *PPN* pedunculopontine nucleus, *SMA* supplementary motor area, *SNc* substantia nigra pars compacta, *SNr* substantia nigra pars reticulate, *STN* subthalamic nucleus, *VA* ventral anterior nucleus of thalamus, *VL* ventrolateral nucleus of thalamus (**a**) (reproduced from Galvan and Wichmann (2008) with kind permission by Elsevier), afferent connections (**b**), striato-pallido-thalamic loop (**c**), nigral connections (**d**), pallido-subthalamic-pallidal loop (**e**), basal ganglia and the descending pathways (**f**) (**b–f**: reproduced from Heimer (1983) with kind permission by Springer Nature)

12.5 Sensory System: Somatosensory System

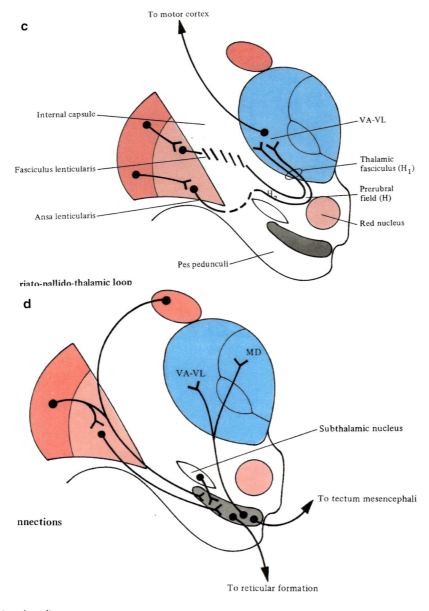

Fig. 12.6 (continued)

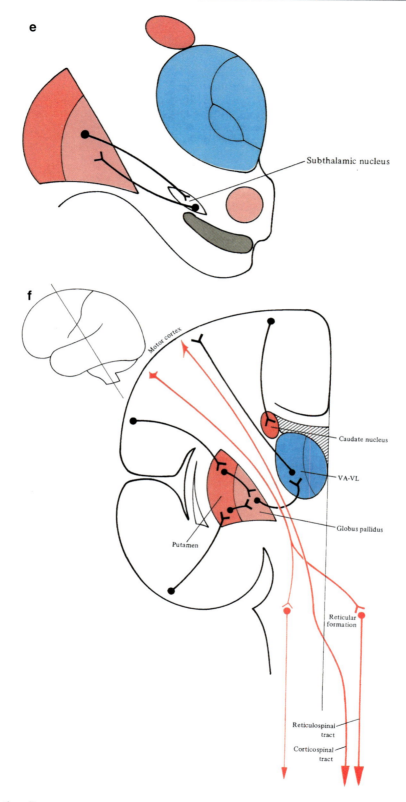

Fig. 12.6 (continued)

Sensory pathways are classified by function as follows (Fig. 12.7a, b):
- Somatic afferent pathways
  - pain, temperature, touch, pressure, vibration, proprioception
  - visual, auditory, vestibular
- Visceral afferent pathways
  - viscera, walls of vessels, olfactory, and gustatory
- Somatic efferent pathways
  - striated muscle
- Visceral efferent pathways
  - non-striated muscle, cardiac muscle, exocrine glands

Two major components:
- Spinothalamic system
  - lateral spinothalamic tract (LST)
    ○ pain, temperature sensation
  - anterior (ventral) spinothalamic tract
    ○ touch and pressure sensation
- Spino-reticulo-thalamic tract
  - visceral pain
- Ventral trigemino-thalamic tract
  - superficial pain, thermal discrimination
- Fasciculus gracilis, fasciculus cuneatus
  - tactile discrimination, pressure, proprioception, vibration from the body
- Dorsal columns-medial lemniscus system

12.6 Cerebral Cortex

The cerebral cortex is made up of six layers (for details, see Chap. 11).

An elementary cortical microcircuit centered on pyramidal neurons is composed of (Fig. 12.8a, b):

- Afferent fiber systems
- Intrinsic connections
- Classes of interneurons

Afferent fiber systems
- Extrinsic afferent fibers from
  - thalamus
  - ipsilateral or contralateral cortical areas
  - synapse with
    ○ dendritic spines
    ○ dendritic shafts of all spiny neurons (lesser extent)
    ○ dendrites of many smooth interneurons
- Nonspecific fibers from
  - monoaminergic systems of the brain stem
  - cholinergic systems of basal forebrain
  - synapse on
    • distal and proximal dendrites of spiny and non-spiny neurons

Intrinsic connections
- axon collaterals of pyramidal cells
  - asymmetric synapses with
    ○ somata and dendrites of interneurons
    ○ dendritic spines
    ○ dendritic shafts of other pyramidal cells
- interneurons
  - synapse with
    ○ somata and dendrites of other interneurons
    ○ all regions of pyramidal neurons
- spiny stellate cells
  - synapse with dendritic spines of other spiny neurons

Classes of interneurons
- based on the preferred postsynaptic region of the pyramidal neuron
- Axo-dendritic cells
  - axons form synapses with dendrites
- Axo-somatodendritic cells
  - axons form multiple synapses with dendrites and somata
- Axo-axonic or chandelier cells
  - axons synapse only with the axon initial segment

A definite elemental microcircuit of the human neocortex cannot yet be drawn (DeFilipe and Jones 2010). Sources of variation include:

- Vertical dimension
  - significant variation of the layers and sublayers
- Horizontal dimension
  - variation in the organization of periodic groups of synaptically associated cells receiving inputs from or projecting to a particular part of the brain

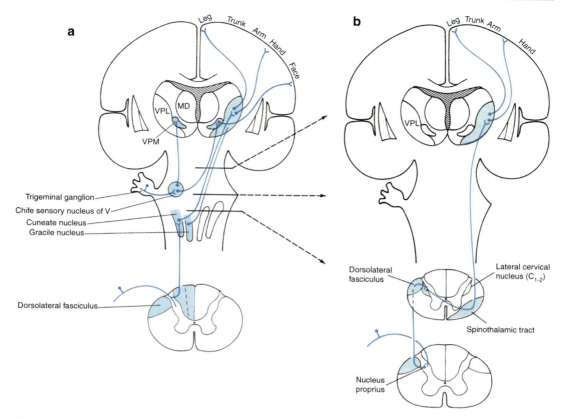

Fig. 12.7 Sensory system: pathways for tactile, vibratory, and proprioceptive impulses (**a**), the spinocervicothalamic pathway for touch and pressure (**b**). (**a, b**: reproduced from Heimer (1983) with kind permission by Springer Nature)

- Morphology
- Neurochemical characteristics

12.7 Limbic System

The limbic system is composed of the following structures (Fig. 12.9a):
- Olfactory system
- Septal area (ventral part of the subcallosal area)
- Mammillary bodies
- Anterior nuclear group of the thalamus
- Hippocampal formation
- Amygdaloid complex
- Cingulate gyrus
- Cortical limbic association areas (anterior temporal, cingulate, insular, orbital, frontal, and parahippocampal)

Cyclic limbic pathway (Fig. 12.9b, c)
- Starts in the mammillary body.
- The mammillothalamic tract projects impulses to the anterior nuclei of the thalamus.
- Thalamocingulate fibers project from the anterior nuclear thalamic group to the cingulate gyrus.
- The cingulum proceeds to the parahippocampal gyrus.
- Short association fibers connect the gyrus with the hippocampal formation and amygdala.
- The fornix arises in the hippocampal formation, passes beneath the corpus callosum, and terminates in the septal area.

Descending limbic pathways include:
- Habenulopeduncular tract
- Dorsal longitudinal fasciculus

12.7 Limbic System

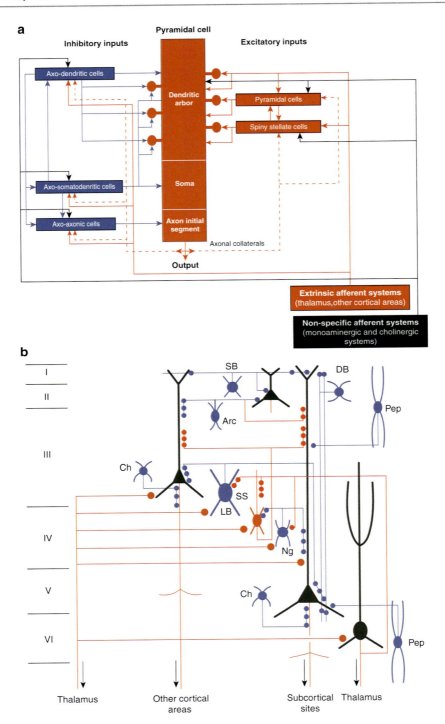

Fig. 12.8 Connections in the cerebral cortex: Basic cortical microcircuit (**a**). Circuit based on thalamic afferent fibers (**b**). Abbreviations: *Arc* neuron with arciform axon, *Ch* chandelier cells, *DB* double bouquet cell, *LB* large basket cell, *Ng* neurogliaform, *Pep* peptidergic neuron, *SS* stellate cell (reproduced from DeFilipe and Jones (2010) with kind permission by Oxford University Press). Simplified schematic representation of the neocortical microcircuitry. Red color indicates excitatory neurons, dendrites, and axons; blue color indicates inhibitory neurons, dendrites, and axons (reproduced from Markram (2010) with kind permission by Oxford University Press)

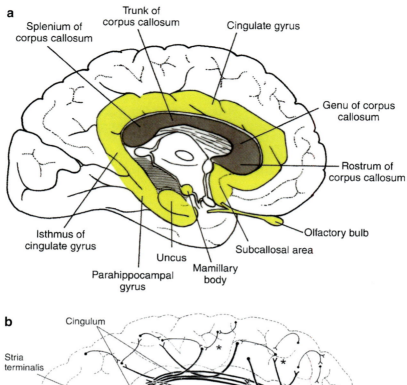

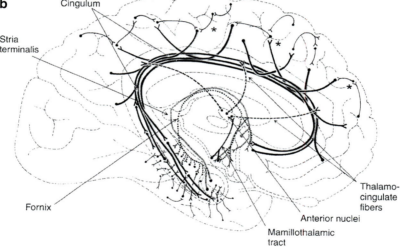

Fig. 12.9 Limbic system. Limbic areas (shown in yellow) on the medial surface of the hemisphere (**a**), connections of the limbic areas (**b**) (**a, b** reproduced from Augustine (2017) with kind permission by Wiley-Blackwell). Limbic system as originally proposed by Papez in 1937 (**a**) and in vivo tractographic reconstruction (**b**), diagram showing the limbic connections based on McLean's 1952 proposal for a unitary model (**c** reproduced from Catani and Thiebaut de Schotten (2012) with kind permission by Oxford University Press)

12.8 Hippocampal System

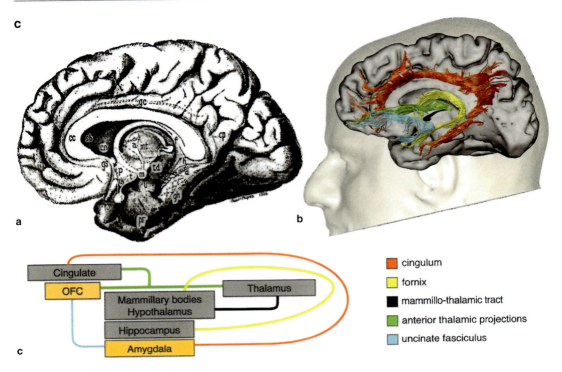

Fig. 12.9 (continued)

- Mammillotegmental tract
- Tegmentospinal tract

12.8 Hippocampal System

The hippocampus is a highly organized structure (Fig. 12.10a, b).

The intrahippocampal circuitries are divided into the following two pathways:
- Polysynaptic pathway (Fig. 12.10c)
  - links all parts of the hippocampus by a long neuronal chain
- Direct pathway (Fig. 12.10d)
  - directly reaches the output neurons of the hippocampus

12.8.1 Polysynaptic Intrahippocampal Pathway

- Composed of a long neuronal chain made up of
  - Entorhinal area
  - Dentate gyrus
  - CA3
  - CA1
  - Subiculum
- Entorhinal area
  - The *perforant path* arises from layer II of the *entorhinal cortex*.
  - The perforant path "perforates" the subiculum, traverses the vestigial hippocampal sulcus to reach the stratum moleculare of the dentate gyrus.
  - The fibers synapse on dendrites of granular cells in the external two thirds of the molecular layer.
  - The perforant path is composed of glutaminergic fibers; thus, it has an excitatory action on the dentate gyrus.
- Dentate gyrus
  - The next relay station is the *dentate gyrus*.
  - The axons of granular neurons, i.e., the mossy fibers, are glutaminergic and have a large content of zinc.
  - These fibers traverse the polymorphic layer and stimulate the dendrites of CA4 and especially those of CA3.

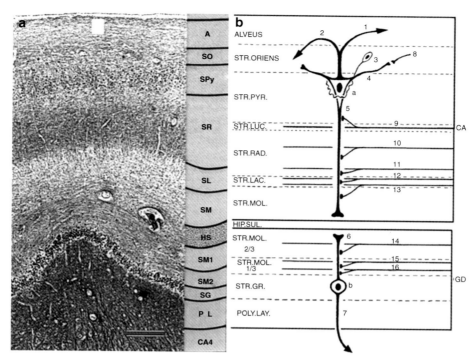

Fig. 12.10 Hippocampal connections (reproduced from Duvernoy et al. (2013) with kind permission by Springer Nature). Structure of the hippocampus (**a**). Cornu ammonis (CA): *A* alveus, *SO* stratum oriens, *Spy* stratum pyramidale, *SR* stratum radiatum, *SL* stratum lacunosum, *SM* stratum moleculare, *HS* vestigial hippocampal sulcus. Dentate gyrus (GD): *SM1* stratum moleculare, external two thirds, *SM2* stratum moleculare, inner third, *SG* stratum granulosum, *PL* polymorphic layer, *CA4* field of the cornu ammonis. Principal connections of pyramidal (**a**) and granular (**b**) neurons (**b**). *CA* cornu ammonis, *GD* gyrus dentatus. Layers of the cornu ammonis: alveus, stratum oriens (*STR. ORIENS*), stratum pyramidale (*STR. PYR.*), stratum lucidum (*STR. LUC.*), stratum radiatum (*STR. RAD.*), stratum lacunosum (*STR. LAC.*), stratum moleculare (*STR. MOL.*), vestigial hippocampal sulcus (*HIP. SUL.*). Layers of the gyrus dentatus: stratum moleculare, external two thirds (*STR. MOL. 2/3*), stratum moleculare, inner third (*STR. MOL. 1/3*), stratum granulosum (*STR. GR.*), polymorphic layer (*POLY. LAY.*). *1* axon of a pyramidal neuron, *2* Schaffer collateral, *3* basket cell, *4* basal dendrite, *5* apical dendrite, *6* apical dendrite of a granular neuron, *7* axon (mossy fiber) of a granular neuron, *8* connections of a basal dendrite of a pyramidal neuron with other pyramidal neurons and with septal and commissural fibers, *9* mossy fibers (stratum lucidum into CA3), *10* septal and commissural fibers, *11*, *12* Schaffer collaterals, *13*, *14* perforant path, *15* commissural fibers, *16* septal fibers. Polysynaptic intrahippocampal pathway (**c**-right). *A*–*E* are parts of the neural chain forming the polysynaptic intrahippocampal pathway. Cornu ammonis: *1* alveus, *2* stratum pyramidale, *3* Schaffer collaterals, *4* axons of pyramidal neurons (mainly to septal nuclei), *5* strata lacunosum and radiatum, *6* stratum moleculare, *7* vestigial hippocampal sulcus. Gyrus dentatus (GD): *8* stratum moleculare, *9* stratum granulosum. *CA1*, *CA3* fields of the cornu ammonis, *SUB* subiculum. *ENT* (Layer II of the entorhinal area) is the origin of this chain; its large pyramidal neurons are grouped in clusters, giving a granular aspect at the entorhinal surface. Cortical connections of the polysynaptic intrahippocampal pathway (**c**-left). Hippocampal outputs fibers to the cortex: arising from the hippocampus (*1*), fibers successively reach the body (*2*) and column (*3*) of fornix (*3 ¢*, anterior commissure), the mammillary body (*4*), and then, via the mammillothalamic tract (*5*), the anterior thalamic nucleus (*6*); some fibers reach this nucleus directly (*6 ¢*); from the anterior thalamic nucleus, the main cortical projections are the posterior cingulate (*area 23*) and retrosplenial (*areas 29*, *30*) cortices; some fibers may project to the anterior cingulate cortex (*area 24*). Input fibers from the cortex to hippocampus: the posterior parietal association cortex (*7*) in relation to the superior visual system (*8*) projects via the parahippocampal gyrus (*9*) to the entorhinal area (*10*); *10 ¢* perforant fibers. Direct intrahippocampal pathway (**d**-right). The entorhinal area (*ENT*) (layer III) projects directly (*1*) onto CA1 pyramidal neurons, which innervate (*2*) the subiculum (*SUB*). Subicular axons project back to the deep layers of the entorhinal cortex (*3*). The neurons of these layers send axons to the association cortex (*4*). The direct pathway receives inputs through the perirhinal cortex (*5*). *6* layer II of the entorhinal cortex. Cortical connections of the direct intrahippocampal pathway (**d**-left). *1* intrahippocampal circuitry. Hippocampal outputs fibers to the cortex: from the deep layers of the entorhinal cortex (*2*), fibers reach the inferior temporal association cortex (*3*), the temporal pole (*4*), and the prefrontal cortex (*5*). Input fibers from the cortex to hippocampus: the main origin of these fibers is the inferior temporal association cortex (*area 37*) in relation to the inferior visual system (*6*), reaching the entorhinal cortex through the perirhinal cortex (*areas 35*, *36*)

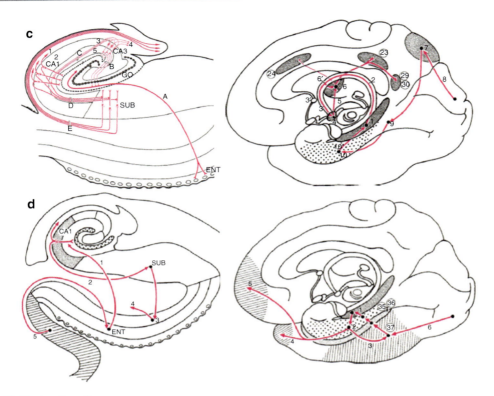

Fig. 12.10 (continued)

- CA3, CA4, CA1
  - The axons of CA3 and CA4 emit the Schaffer collaterals, which reach the apical dendrites of CA1 in the strata radiatum and lacunosum.
  - They enter the alveus and then the fimbria.
  - They represent the main output of the hippocampus by way of the *alveus* and then the fimbria.
  - By entering the alveus, the axons of CA1 produce collaterals which reach the subiculum.
- Subiculum
  - The *subiculum* therefore emits the definitive response, by fibers constituting the major part of the alveus and then the fimbria. The neurons of the subiculum are glutaminergic, as are those of the preceding parts of the polysynaptic chain.

Hippocampal Output to the Cortex
- The principal outputs follow the fimbria, the crus and body of the fornix, and the columns of the fornix, also known as the postcommissural fornix (behind the anterior commissure).
- The nervous impulses then reach the anterior thalamic nucleus, either directly or via the mammillary bodies, extending from there into the mammillothalamic tract.
- Other thalamic nuclei, such as the intralaminar nuclei, and the hypothalamus may possibly be reached.
- From the thalamus, impulses reach the posterior cingulated cortex (area 23) and the retrosplenial cortex (areas 29 and 30).

Input from the Cortex
- The fibers originate in a large cortical area which include many sites where the sensory informations converge such as posterior parietal association cortex (area 7) and the neighboring temporal and occipital cortices (areas 40, 39, and 22).
- The posterior parietal association cortex sends fibers to the entorhinal area through the parahippocampal gyrus. The main function attributed to

the posterior parietal association cortex, related to the superior visual system, is perception of the position of an object in space.
- This spatial perception is thought to then be memorized through the polysynaptic pathway, and the episodic memory and the memory of facts in relation to each other apparently also depend on this system.

12.8.2 Direct Intrahippocampal Pathway

The direct intrahippocampal pathway
- Fibers reach directly CA1 and the hippocampal outputs directly without following the polysynaptic chain.
- The origin of the direct pathway is found in layer III of the entorhinal cortex.
- From this layer, fibers directly reach the pyramidal neurons of CA1 by a different pathway from that of the perforant path.
- The CA1 neurons project onto the subiculum, the axons of which return to the deep layers of the entorhinal area.

Hippocampal Output to the Cortex
The output of the direct pathway to the cortex
- inferior temporal association cortex
- the temporal pole
- the prefrontal cortex

Input from the Cortex
- Inferior temporal association cortex (areas 37, 20), which reaches the entorhinal area through the perirhinal cortex (areas 35, 36)

12.8.3 Regulatory Circuits

- Numerous circuits may regulate the main principal pathways
  - internal regulatory circuits, entirely within the hippocampus
  - external regulatory circuits, which involve extrahippocampal structures

12.8.3.1 Internal Regulatory Circuits
- *Basket Neurons*
  - Are the basic elements in these circuits.
  - Occur in the cornu ammonis and gyrus dentatus.
  - Are largely situated in the stratum oriens but are also scattered in other layers
  - Receive impulses from pyramidal neurons.
  - Their axons return to numerous neurons, forming basket arborization around their cell bodies.
  - Their fibers are GABA-ergic.
  - Inhibit pyramidal neurons.
  - May influence granular neurons or pyramidal neurons.
  - Stimulated at first by collaterals of mossy fibers, basket neurons inhibit granular neurons by retroaction.
- *Neurotransmitters*
  - Interneurons produce neurotransmitters other than GABA.
  - The cornu ammonis and gyrus dentatus contain neurons producing:
    ○ substance P, vasoactive intestinal polypeptide (VIP), cholecystokinin (CCK), somatostatin, corticotropin-releasing factor (CRF), and neuropeptide Y.
  - Granular neurons from the gyrus dentatus may produce enkephalins and dynorphins.
  - All these neurons intervene in local inhibitory or excitatory circuits.
- *Pyramidal Neurons*
  - Pyramidal neurons might influence each other.
  - Collaterals of their axons connect with basal dendrites of other pyramidal neurons.

12.8.3.2 External Regulatory Circuits
The external regulatory circuits involve

- the septal nuclei
- the contralateral hippocampus by commissural fibers, neuromediators of extrahippocampal origin

- certain areas of cerebral cortex
- *Septal Nuclei*
  - Axons of hippocampal subicular pyramidal neurons are the origin of these circuits.
  - The fibers reach via the fimbria and the precommissural fornix the lateral septal nucleus; impulses then reach the important cholinergic centers, i.e., medial septal nucleus and the nucleus of the vertical limb of the diagonal band.
  - From these nuclei, cholinergic and GABAergic fibers project back to the hippocampus by the precommissural fornix and fimbria.
  - Septal cholinergic fibers end on granular neurons in the dentate gyrus and pyramidal neurons in the cornu ammonis.
  - The septum may control a special hippocampal activity, i.e., the rhythmic slow-wave activity or theta rhythm thought to be localized in the dentate gyrus and CA1.
- *Commissural Fibers*
  - The two hippocampi are joined via the fornix by commissural fibers.
  - The dorsal hippocampal commissure *in humans* connects mesiotemporal and particularly left and right entorhinal areas.
- *Neuromediators*
  - Numerous endings of nerve fibers of extrahippocampal origin liberate neuromediators:
    ○ Cholinergic septal fibers.
    ○ Terminals of monoaminergic pathways.
    ○ Noradrenergic fibers arising from the locus coeruleus and belonging to the dorsal noradrenergic bundle reach the hippocampus via the fornix but also via the longitudinal striae.
    ○ Serotoninergic fibers from the nuclei of the raphe reach the hippocampus via the longitudinal striae.
    ○ Dopaminergic projections.
    ○ Many neuropeptidergic terminals have been found in the hippocampus, such as vasopressin, somatostatin, substance P, neuropeptide Y, and a-melanocyte-stimulating hormone.

- *Cortical Regulation*
  - Direct connections exist between the neocortex and the hippocampus and include:
    ○ Direct projections from the cingulate gyrus to the hippocampus
    ○ Direct afferents from temporal and prefrontal lobes

12.9 Amygdalar System

Reciprocal connections with (Fig. 12.11a–c):
- Thalamus
- Basal ganglia
- Hypothalamus
- Temporal cortex
- Septal area
- Preoptic area

The afferent and efferent fiber systems of the amygdala are listed in Tables 12.4 and 12.5.

12.10 Cerebellum

The cerebellar cortex is made up of three layers (see Chap. 11) (Fig. 12.12a–c).

Afferent cerebellar connections include:
- Spinocerebellar tracts
- Vestibulocerebellar tracts
- Reticulocerebellar fibers
- Pontocerebellar fibers
- Olivocerebellar fibers
- Aminergic fibers from the raphe nuclei

Efferent cerebellar connections
- Cerebrovestibular fibers
- Cerebelloreticular fibers
- Cerebellorubral fibers
- Cerebellothalamic fibers

The major afferent fiber systems are:
- Mossy fibers from
  - spinal cord
  - vestibular system
  - reticular formation
  - pontine nuclei

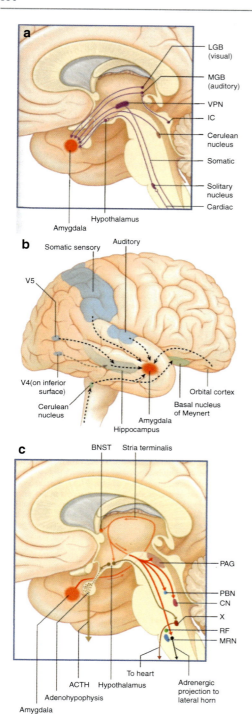

Table 12.4 Afferents to the amygdala

Nature	Cortical and subcortical source
Tactile	• Parietal lobe • Ventral posterior nucleus of the thalamus
Auditory	• Superior temporal gyrus • Medial geniculate body
Visual	• Occipital cortex • Lateral geniculate body
Olfactory	• Piriform lobe
Mnemonic	• Hippocampus/entorhinal cortex
Cardiac	• Insula • Hypothalamus
Nociceptive	• Midbrain reticular formation
Cognitive	• Orbital cortex
Attention-related	• Basal nucleus of Meynert • Nucleus coeruleus

- Climbing fibers from
  - inferior olivary nucleus
- Aminergic fibers from
  - raphe nucleus
  - locus coeruleus

Intrinsic microcircuit
- Afferent fiber abut on Purkinje cells.
- Purkinje cell axons project to intracerebellar nuclei.
- Efferent cerebellar fiber tracts originate in the intracerebellar nuclei.
- Climbing fibers
  - Make multiple and powerful contacts directly with proximal dendritic branches of a limited number of Purkinje cells.
- Mossy fibers
  - influence indirectly a large number of Purkinje cells by:
    ○ extensively branching in the white matter and granular layer
    ○ establishing synaptic contacts with the dendrites of several granule cells in complex synapses called glomeruli
  - Glomeruli
    ○ Contain a central mossy fiber terminal and boutons of the Golgi cell axons.
    ○ Synapse with the granule cells.
  - Axons of granule cells project to the molecular layer.
    ○ They bifurcate in a T-shaped manner forming the parallel fibers

Fig. 12.11 Amygdala: Subcortical afferents to the lateral nucleus of amygdala (**a**), cortical afferents to the lateral nucleus of amygdala (**b**), efferents from the central nucleus of amygdala via the stria terminalis (**c**) (reproduced from Fitzgerald et al. (2012) with kind permission by Elsevier)

12.12 Hypothalamus and Hypophyseal System

Table 12.5 Efferents from the central nucleus of the amygdala

Target nucleus/pathway	Function/effect
Periaqueductal gray matter to medulla/raphespinal tract	Antinociception
Periaqueductal gray matter to medullary reticulospinal tract	Freezing
Nucleus coeruleus	Arousal
Norepinephrine medullary neurons (projection to lateral horn)	Tachycardia/hypertension
Hypothalamus/dorsal nucleus of vagus (to heart)	Bradycardia/fainting
Hypothalamus (liberation of corticotropin-releasing hormone)	Stress hormone secretion
Parabrachial nucleus (to medullary respiratory nuclei)	Hyperventilation

- Parallel fibers
    - Run for several millimeters along the longitudinal extent of a folium.
- Aminergic fibers
    - contain biogenic amines
    - widespread distribution in the cerebellar cortex
    - are of two types:
        - serotoninergic axons from the raphe nuclei
        - noradrenergic axons from the locus coeruleus

12.11 Thalamic System

The thalamus (Fig. 12.13):
- identifies information (auditory, visual, tactile, and gustatory) that is transmitted to the brain
- analyses these information
- directs the sensory and motor information to the different locations in the brain
- → major integrator and relay of sensory information to the cortex
- regulates consciousness, sleep, and alertness

The afferent and efferent fiber systems of the thalamus are depicted in Table 12.6.

12.12 Hypothalamus and Hypophyseal System

The hypothalamus is made up of a magnitude of small nuclei (Fig. 12.14a).

The hypothalamus receives *afferent connections* from (Fig. 12.14b, c):
- olfactory and septal areas
    - medial forebrain bundle
    - smell
    - basic emotional drives
- hippocampus
    - learning and memory
    - fornix: connection between hippocampus and mammillary bodies
- amygdala
    - complex behavior
    - stria terminalis
- midbrain tegmentum (reticular formation)
    - autonomic functions
    - medial forebrain bundle
    - raphe nucleus: serotonin-containing fibers
    - locus coeruleus: norepinephrine-containing fibers
- dorsomedial and midline thalamic nuclei
    - emotional states
    - autonomic functions
    - thalamohypothalamic tract

The hypothalamus as a major output pathway from the limbic system sends *efferent connections* to (Fig. 12.14b, c):

- olfactory and septal areas
    - smell
    - emotional drives
- anterior thalamic nucleus
    - emotional states
    - memory
    - mammillothalamic tract
- preganglionic autonomic neurons of the brain stem and spinal cord

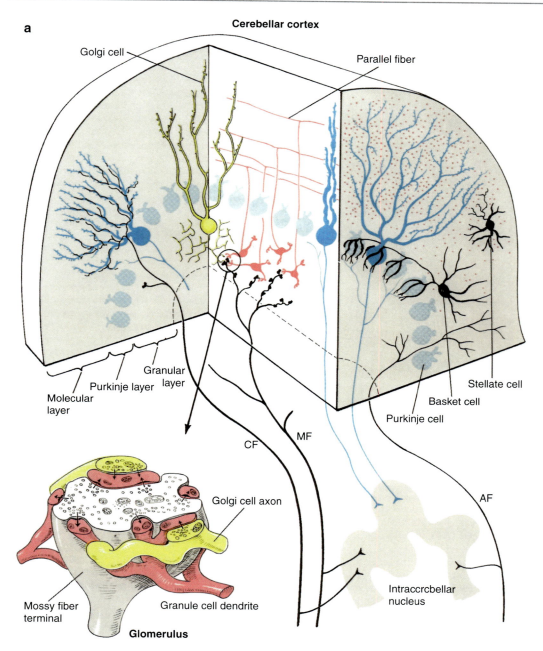

Fig. 12.12 Cerebellum. General organization of the cerebellar cortex (**a**) (reproduced from Heimer (1983) with kind permission by Springer Nature). Purkinje cells in blue, granule cells in red, Golgi cell in yellow, basket and stellate cells in black: *CF* climbing fibers, *MF* mossy fibers, *AF* aminergic fiber. Basic circuitry in the cerebellum (**b**) (reproduced from Heimer (1983) with kind permission by Springer Nature). Connections of the cerebellum (**c**) (reproduced from Heimer (1983) with kind permission by Springer Nature). Left side: climbing fiber input from the inferior olive to the Purkinje cells and the projections from the Purkinje cells to the intracerebellar nuclei. Right side: mossy fiber systems from the spinal cord, vestibular apparatus, and cerebral cortex. *P* pontocerebellum, *S* spinocerebellum, *V* vestibulocerebellum

12.12 Hypothalamus and Hypophyseal System

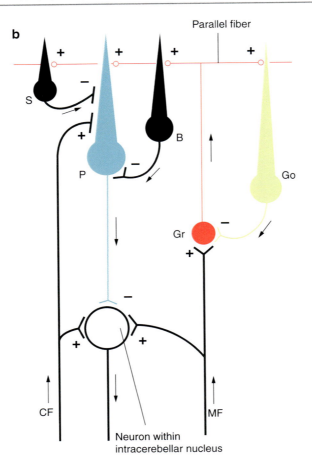

Fig. 12.12 (continued)

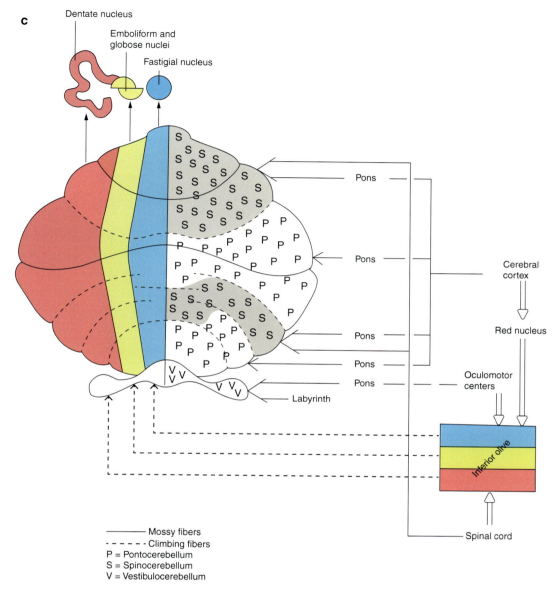

Fig. 12.12 (continued)

- autonomic functions
- dorsal longitudinal fasciculus: dorsal nucleus of vagus, intermediolateral cell column (spinal cord)
• posterior pituitary gland
  - paraventricular nuclei, supraoptic nuclei: supraoptic hypophyseal tract
• anterior pituitary gland
  - axoplasmic transport in the tuberoinfundibular tract

Functions of the hypothalamus include:
• Autonomic functions
  - Cardiovascular regulation
  - Regulation of body temperature
  - Regulation of water balance
  - Regulation of food intake
• Endocrine functions
  - Regulation of water balance
  - Regulation of reproductive functions
• Emotional behavior

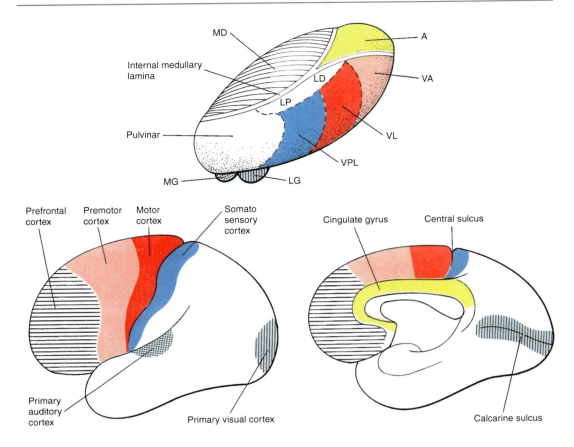

Fig. 12.13 Thalamic connections. Thalamocortical circuits. *A* Anterior nucleus, *VA* ventral anterior nucleus, *VL* ventral lateral nucleus, *VPL* ventral posterior nucleus, *LD* lateral dorsal nucleus, *LP* lateral-posterior nucleus, *MD* midline nucleus, *MG* Medical geniculate body, *LG* lateral geniculate body (reproduced from Heimer (1983) with kind permission by Springer Nature)

Clinical manifestations of hypothalamic lesions include:

- Disturbances of water balance
  - Diabetes insipidus
  - Syndrome of inappropriate secretion of antidiuretic hormone (SIADH)
- Disturbances of temperature regulation
- Obesity
- Hypogonadotropic hypogonadism
- Disturbances of emotional behavior

Neuronal circuit of emotional processing

- Dorsolateral prefrontal cortex
  - appraisal regulation
- Orbitofrontal cortex
- Anterior cingulate cortex
- Temporal pole

12.13 Two-stream Hypothesis

The **two-stream hypothesis** is a widely accepted and influential model of the neural processing for:

- vision
- hearing

12.13.1 Visual System: Two-Stream Hypothesis

As visual information exits the occipital lobe, and as sound leaves the phonological network, it follows two main pathways, or "streams" (Fig. 12.15a–c).

Table 12.6 Afferent and efferent connections of the various thalamic nuclei and their associated function

Nucleus	Afferent connection	Efferent connection	Function
Anterior nucleus	• Hypothalamus	• Cingulate gyrus	• Affective and emotional states • Memory
Ventral anterior and ventral lateral nuclei	• Basal ganglia • Cerebellum	• Motor cortex • Premotor cortex	• Relay motor information from basal ganglia and cerebellum to cortex
Ventral posterior nucleus	• Medial lemniscal tracts • Spinothalamic tracts • Trigeminal nerve	• Primary sensory cortex	• Affective and emotional states • Memory
Centromedian nucleus	• Cerebral cortex • Globus pallidus	• Caudate nucleus • Putamen	• Extrapyramidal motor system
Reticular nucleus	• Collateral branches of thalamocortical and corticothalamic fibers	• Other thalamic nuclei	• Modulates influence that thalamus exerts on cortex
Midline nucleus	• Brain stem reticular formation	• Limbic structures	• Unknown
Lateral dorsal nucleus	• Hippocampal formation	• Cingulate gyrus	• Affective and emotional states
Lateral-posterior nucleus	• Unknown	• Somatosensory association cortex	• Sensory processing
Pulvinar thalami	• Axons of neurons in the superior colliculus • Sensory association areas in the parietal, temporal, and occipital lobes	• Sensory association areas in the parietal, temporal, and occipital lobes	• Sensory processing
Dorsomedial nucleus	• Olfactory cortex • Amygdala • Hypothalamus	• Prefrontal cortex	• Affective and emotional states • Memory
Lateral geniculate body	• Retinal ganglion cells	• Primary visual cortex	• Visual processing
Medial geniculate body	• Axons of neurons in the inferior colliculus	• Primary auditory cortex	• Auditory processing

- The ventral stream–ventral perceptual stream (also known as the "what pathway")
  - is involved with object and visual identification and recognition
  - computes a detailed map of the world from visual input, which can then be used for cognitive operations (Goodale and Milner 1992)
- The dorsal stream–dorsal action stream (or, "where pathway")
  - is involved with processing the object's spatial location relative to the viewer and with speech repetition
  - transforms incoming visual information to the requisite egocentric (head-centered) coordinate system for skilled motor planning (Goodale and Milner 1992)

The model also posits that
- Visual perception
  - encodes spatial properties of objects, such as size and location, relative to other objects in the visual field; in other words, it utilizes relative metrics and scene-based frames of reference (Aglioti et al. 1995)
- Visual action planning and coordination
  - uses absolute metrics determined via egocentric frames of reference, computing the actual properties of objects relative to the observer (Aglioti et al. 1995)

A similar dual-process model of vision was proposed by Norman (2002) (Table 12.7).

Details are given elsewhere (McIntosh and Schenk 2009; Goodale 2011; Milner 2017; Milner and Goodale 2008; Fukushima and Ojima 2016;

12.13 Two-stream Hypothesis

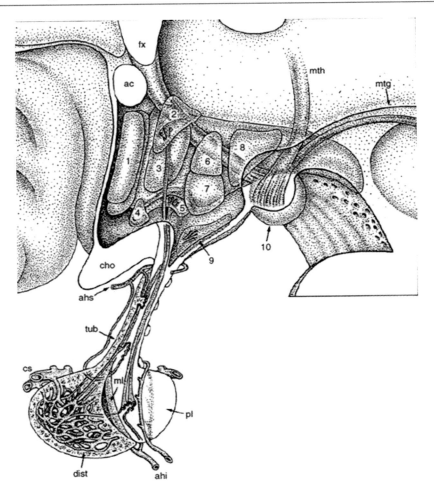

Fig. 12.14 Hypothalamic-Hypophyseal system. Schematic drawing of the hypothalamic region (reproduced from ten Donkelaar (2011) with kind permission by Springer Nature). *ac* anterior commissure, *ahi, ahs* inferior and superior hypophyseal arteries, *cho* chiasma opticum, *cs* cavernous sinus, *dist* distal part of anterior pituitary lobe, *fx* fornix, *ml* middle pituitary lobe, *mtg* mammillotegmental tract, *mth* mammillothalamic tract, *pl* posterior pituitary lobe, *tub* tuberal part of anterior pituitary lobe. (1) preoptic nucleus, (2) paraventricular nucleus, (3) anterior nucleus, (4) suprachiasmatic nucleus, (5) supraoptic nucleus, (6) dorsomedial nucleus, (7) ventromedial nucleus, (8) posterior nucleus, (9) arcuate or infundibular nucleus, (10) corpus mammillare, afferent connections (**b**), and efferent connections (**c**)

Murata et al. 2016; Reddy and Kanwisher 2006; Wilson and Wilkinson 2015; Atkinson 2017; Grinter et al. 2010; Milner 2012; Perry and Fallah 2014; Sakreida et al. 2016; Zaehle et al. 2008)

12.13.2 Ventral Stream

- Is associated with object recognition and form representation.
- Also described as the "what" stream.
- It has strong connections to
    - the medial temporal lobe (which stores long-term memories)
    - the limbic system (which controls emotions)
    - the dorsal stream (which deals with object locations and motion)
- Gets its main input from
    - The parvocellular (as opposed to magnocellular) layer of the lateral geniculate nucleus of the thalamus.
    - These neurons project to V1 sublayers 4Cβ, 4A, 3B, and 2/3a, successively.
- From there, the ventral pathway goes through V2 and V4 to areas of the inferior temporal lobe: PIT (posterior inferotemporal), CIT

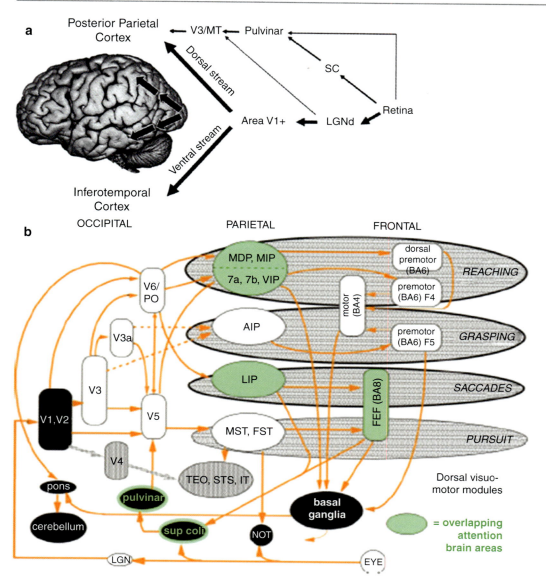

Fig. 12.15 Visual system: Dorsal and Ventral streams. Schematic view of the dorsal and ventral streams (**a**) (with permission from Goodale (2011)). Detailed diagrams of the dorsal stream (**b**) and ventral stream (**c**) (with permission from Atkinson (2017))

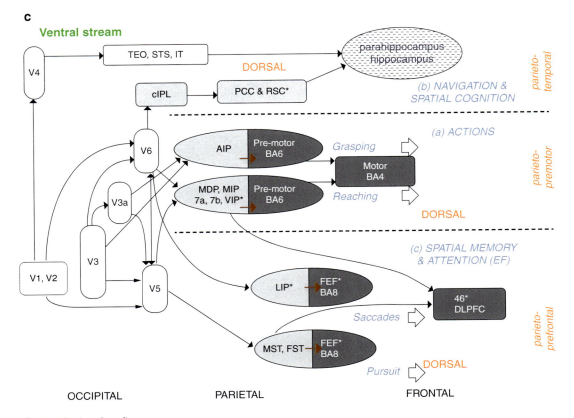

Fig. 12.15 (continued)

Table 12.7 Eight main differences between the two systems consistent with other two-system models

Factor	Ventral system	Dorsal system
Function	Recognition/identification	Visually guided behavior
Sensitivity	High spatial frequencies—details	High temporal frequencies—motion
Memory	Long-term stored representations	Only very short-term storage
Speed	Relatively slow	Relatively fast
Consciousness	Typically high	Typically low
Frame of reference	Allocentric or object-centered	Egocentric or viewer-centered
Visual input	Mainly foveal or parafoveal	Across retina
Monocular vision	Generally reasonably small effects	Often large effects, e.g., motion parallax

(central inferotemporal), and AIT (anterior inferotemporal).

- Each visual area contains a full representation of visual space. That is, it contains neurons whose receptive fields together represent the entire visual field. Visual information enters the ventral stream through the primary visual cortex and travels through the rest of the areas in sequence.

- Moving along the stream from V1 to AIT, receptive fields increase their size, latency, and the complexity of their tuning.
- All the areas in the ventral stream are influenced by extraretinal factors in addition to the nature of the stimulus in their receptive field. These factors include attention, working memory, and stimulus salience. Thus, the ventral stream does not merely provide a descrip-

tion of the elements in the visual world—it also plays a crucial role in judging the significance of these elements.

Damage to the ventral stream
- can cause inability to recognize faces or interpret facial expression

12.13.3 Dorsal Stream

- Is proposed involved in the guidance of actions and recognizing where objects are in space in spatial awareness and guidance of actions (e.g., reaching).
- It contains a detailed map of the visual field, and is also good at detecting and analyzing movements.
- Also known as the parietal stream, the "where" stream, or the "how" stream.
- Commences with purely visual functions in the occipital lobe before gradually transferring to spatial awareness at its termination in the parietal lobe.
- Pathway stretches from the primary visual cortex (V1) in the occipital lobe forward into the parietal lobe.
- The posterior parietal cortex is essential for "the perception and interpretation of spatial relationships, accurate body image, and the learning of tasks involving coordination of the body in space".
- It contains individually functioning lobules. The lateral intraparietal sulcus (LIP) contains neurons that produce enhanced activation when attention is moved onto the stimulus or the animal saccades towards a visual stimulus, and the ventral intraparietal sulcus (VIP) where visual and somatosensory information are integrated.
- It is interconnected with the parallel ventral stream (the "what" stream) which runs downward from V1 into the temporal lobe.

Damage to the posterior parietal cortex causes a number of spatial disorders including:
- Simultanagnosia:
  - The patient can only describe single objects without the ability to perceive it as a component of a set of details or objects in a context (as in a scenario, e.g., the forest for the trees).
- Optic ataxia:
  - The patient can't use visuospatial information to guide arm movements.
- Hemispatial neglect:
  - The patient is unaware of the contralesional half of space (i.e., they are unaware of things in their left field of view and focus only on objects in the right field of view; or appear unaware of things in one field of view when they perceive them in the other). For example, a person with this disorder may draw a clock, and then label it from 12, 1, 2, ..., 6, but then stop and consider their drawing complete.
- Akinetopsia:
  - inability to perceive motion
- Apraxia:
  - inability to produce discretionary or volitional movement in the absence of muscular disorders

12.14 The Connectome

A connectome is (Seung 2012) (Fig. 12.16a–e):
- the totality of connections between neurons in a nervous system
- all of the connections
- the wiring diagram of the brain

Connectional neuroanatomy delineates the origin, course, and termination of connecting pathways (Catani and Thiebaut de Schotten 2012).

The functional implications for the interpretation of the connectome are:
- Minds differ because connectomes differ.
- Personality and IQ might be explained by the connectome.
- Memories are encoded in your connectome.
- Your connectome changes throughout life.
- We shape our own connectomes.
- Neuronal activity changes the connectome.
- Curing mental disorders is about repairing connectomes.

12.14 The Connectome

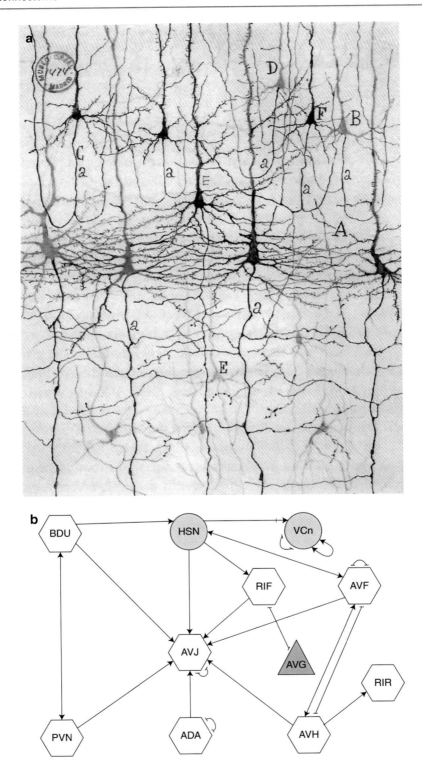

Fig. 12.16 A world of brain connections: Neuronal connections of the cerebral cortex as illustrated by Cajal (**a**), "reduced" connectome of *C. elegans* (**b**), visual connectome of the rhesus monkey (**c**), connectome of *C. elegans* (**d**), the connectome of the first author of this book (**e**). (**a–d**: with permission from Seung (2012))

c

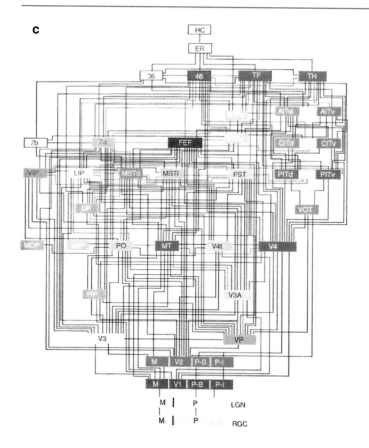

d

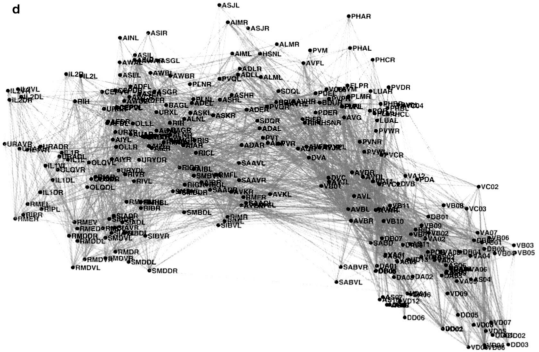

Fig. 12.16 (continued)

12.15 Rich-Club Organization

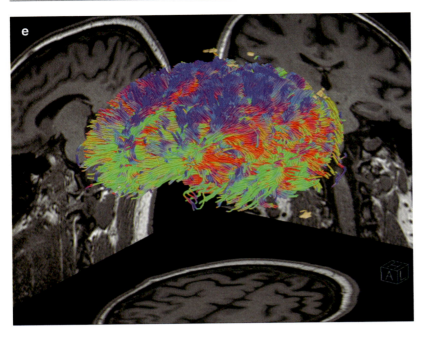

Fig. 12.16 (continued)

Minds differ because of genomes. You are more than your genes. You are your connectome (Seung 2012).

Neurons
- reconnect by creating and eliminating synapses
- rewire by growing and retracting branches (dendritic tree)

Changes of the connectome occur by
- reweighting
- reconnection
- rewiring
- regeneration

Connectionism
- Attempt to explain how regions of the brain actually work.
- A brain region is not an elementary unit but a complex network composed of a large number of neurons.

The connectome defines the pathways along which neural activity can flow; we might regard it as the streambed of consciousness.

Connectopathies
- abnormal patterns of neural connection
- might underlie mental disorders

Currently, the most prominent attempt along these lines is the Human Connectome Project (http://www.neuroscienceblueprint.nih.gov/connectome/). This project aims to derive a complete map of all major connections between brain areas by measuring dMRI as well as functional connectivity and genetic data in more than 1000 individuals (twin pairs and their siblings from 300 families). Besides deriving a connectivity map—the human connectome—the measured data of structural and functional connectivity will be shared to stimulate research in the emerging field of human connectomics as well as providing the basis for future studies of abnormal brain circuits in neurological and psychiatric disorders (Sporns 2011, 2012).

12.15 Rich-Club Organization

The name "rich-club" originates from the observation that, in social networks, certain (often wealthy) people have a high number of connections, and are also very strongly connected with each other. The "rich-club" is a pattern of organization established in healthy human brains (Fig. 12.17a, b).

The brain is a complex network of interlinked regions. Structural connections are not uniform but are organized across the brain in a non-homogeneous fashion. A number of highly connected and highly central neocortical hub regions exist which play a role in global information integration between different parts of the network. A set of brain regions, known as a "**rich-club**," provides for intramodular connectivity and is thought to play a central role in maintaining network integ-

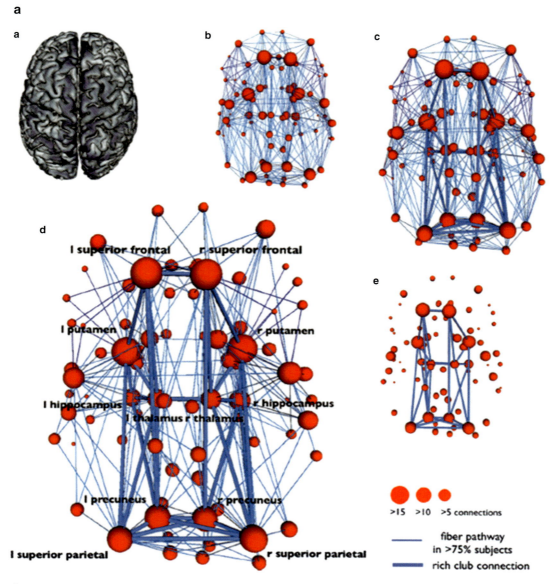

Fig. 12.17 Rich-club organization: Rich-club regions and connections (**a**) (with permission from van den Heuvel and Sporns (2011): anatomical perspective (**a**), group-averaged connectome (**b**), group connectome with rich-club connections marked in dark blue (**c**), connections between rich-club region (dark blue) and connections from rich-club nodes to the other brain regions of the brain network (light blue) (**d**), rich-club connections (**e**). Applications of disturbed connectomes in control as compared to patients with ASD (autism spectrum disorder) and ADHD (attention-deficit hyperactivity disorders) (with permission from Ray et al. (2014))

12.15 Rich-Club Organization

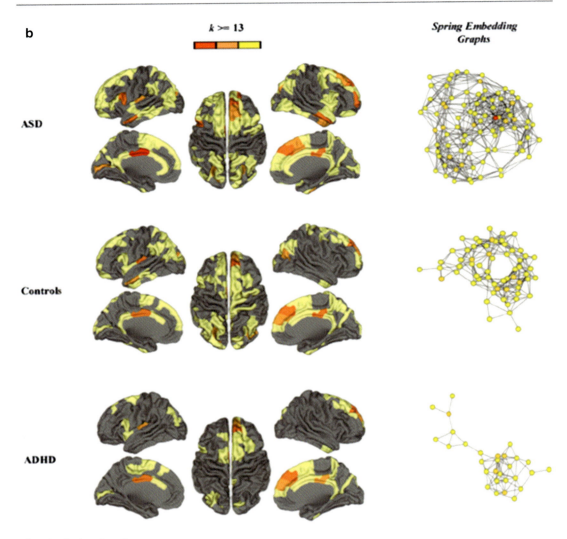

Fig. 12.17 (continued)

rity (van den Heuvel et al. 2012). Specific hub ("rich-club") brain regions are more highly connected to each other, forming a selective network with higher connectivity than other brain regions (van den Heuvel and Sporns 2011). Such topological centrality of the rich-club network supports integrative processing and adaptive behaviors (Senden et al. 2014). Consistent with this, the degree of structural rich-club connectivity predicts general cognitive performance in healthy older adults (Fig. 12.17a, b) (Baggio et al. 2015).

Rich-club regions in the brain have a high number of connections and, critically, are also more connected with each other than would be expected by chance. The latter feature effectively implies a redundancy of connections that link segregated modules. Taken together, modularity and rich-club organization characterizes a relatively sparse but, nevertheless, efficient connectivity structure at both local and global levels (Markov et al. 2013). Disturbances of their structural and functional connectivity profile are associated with neuropathology.

The "rich-club" phenomenon in networks is present when the hubs of a network tend to be more densely connected among themselves than nodes of a lower degree. Strongly interconnected bi-hemispheric hub regions include the precuneus, superior frontal and superior parietal cortex, subcortical hippocampus, putamen, insula, and thalamus (van den Heuvel and Sporns 2011; van den Heuvel et al. 2013).

Disturbances in rich-club organization are reported to occur in schizophrenia, psychosis, patients with generalized tonic-clonic seizures, migraine sufferers, brain ischemia protein interaction network, brain aging, autism spectrum disorders and attention-deficit/hyperactivity disorder, Alzheimer disease (Fig. 12.17a, b) (Alawieh et al. 2015; Baggio et al. 2015; Ball et al. 2014; Beggs et al. 2016; Collin et al. 2014; Daianu et al. 2013; Forcellini et al. 2018; Grayson et al. 2014; Li et al. 2017; Li et al. 2016; Nigam et al. 2016; Ray et al. 2014; Senden et al. 2014; van den Heuvel and Sporns 2011; van den Heuvel et al. 2013; Zhao et al. 2017)

Selected References

Aglioti S, DeSouza JF, Goodale MA (1995) Size-contrast illusions deceive the eye but not the hand. Curr Biol 5(6):679–685
Alawieh A, Sabra Z, Sabra M, Tomlinson S, Zaraket FA (2015) A Rich-Club Organization in brain ischemia protein interaction network. Sci Rep 5:13513. https://doi.org/10.1007/s00429-015-1096-6
Atkinson J (2017) The Davida Teller Award Lecture, 2016: Visual Brain Development: a review of "Dorsal Stream Vulnerability"-motion, mathematics, amblyopia, actions, and attention. J Vis 17(3):26. https://doi.org/10.1167/17.3.26
Augustine JR (2017) Human neuroanatomy, 2nd edn. Wiley Blackwell, Hoboken, NJ
Baggio HC, Segura B, Junque C, de Reus MA, Sala-Llonch R, Van den Heuvel MP (2015) Rich Club Organization and cognitive performance in healthy older participants. J Cogn Neurosci 27(9):1801–1810. https://doi.org/10.1162/jocn_a_00821
Ball G, Aljabar P, Zebari S, Tusor N, Arichi T, Merchant N, Robinson EC, Ogundipe E, Rueckert D, Edwards AD, Counsell SJ (2014) Rich-club organization of the newborn human brain. Proc Natl Acad Sci U S A 111(20):7456–7461. https://doi.org/10.1073/pnas.1324118111
Beggs JM, Scheinost D, Kwon SH, Shen X, Lacadie C, Schneider KC, Dai F, Ment LR, Constable RT (2016) Preterm birth alters neonatal, functional rich club organization. J Neurosci 221(6):3211–3222. https://doi.org/10.1007/s00429-015-1096-6
Catani M, Thiebaut de Schotten M (2012) Atlas of human brain connections. Oxford University Press, Oxford
Collin G, Sporns O, Mandl RC, van den Heuvel MP (2014) Structural and functional aspects relating to cost and benefit of rich club organization in the human cerebral cortex. Cereb Cortex 24(9):2258–2267. https://doi.org/10.1093/cercor/bht064
Daianu M, Dennis EL, Jahanshad N, Nir TM, Toga AW, Jack CR Jr, Weiner MW, Thompson PM (2013) Alzheimer's disease disrupts Rich Club Organization in brain connectivity networks. Proc IEEE Int Symp Biomed Imaging 2013:266–269. https://doi.org/10.1109/isbi.2013.6556463
DeFilipe J, Jones EG (2010) Neocortical microcircuits. In: Shepard GM, Grillner S (eds) Handbook of brain microcircuits. Oxford University Press, Oxford, pp 5–14
Duvernoy H, Cattin F, Risold PY (2013) The human hippocampus. functional anatomy, vascularization and serial sections with MRI, 4th edn. Springer, Berlin
Fitzgerald MJT, Gruener G, Mtui E (2012) Clinical neuroanatomy and neuroscience, 6th edn. Elsevier Saunders, Philadelphia, PA
Forcellini G, O'Donoghue S, Kenney J, McInerney S, Scanlon C, Nabulsi L, McPhilemy G, Kilmartin L, O'Hora D, Hallahan B, Cannon DM, McDonald C (2018) Structural connectivity and rich-club organization in recent onset psychosis. Schizophr Res 192:477–478. https://doi.org/10.1016/j.schres.2017.05.018
Fukushima M, Ojima H (2016) Information processing in the auditory ventral stream. Brain Nerve 68(11):1371–1378. https://doi.org/10.11477/mf.1416200600
Galvan A, Wichmann T (2008) Pathophysiology of parkinsonism. Clin Neurophysiol 119(7):1459–1474. https://doi.org/10.1016/j.clinph.2008.03.017
Goodale MA (2011) Transforming vision into action. Vision Res 51(13):1567–1587. https://doi.org/10.1016/j.visres.2010.07.027
Goodale MA, Milner AD (1992) Separate visual pathways for perception and action. Trends Neurosci 15(1):20–25
Grayson DS, Ray S, Carpenter S, Iyer S, Dias TG, Stevens C, Nigg JT, Fair DA (2014) Structural and functional rich club organization of the brain in children and adults. PLoS One 9(2):e88297. https://doi.org/10.1371/journal.pone.0088297
Grinter EJ, Maybery MT, Badcock DR (2010) Vision in developmental disorders: is there a dorsal stream deficit? Brain Res Bull 82(3-4):147–160. https://doi.org/10.1016/j.brainresbull.2010.02.016
Heimer L (1983) The human brain and spinal cord: functional neuroanatomy and dissection guide. Springer, Berlin
Li R, Liao W, Li Y, Yu Y, Zhang Z, Lu G, Chen H (2016) Disrupted structural and functional rich club organization of the brain connectome in patients with generalized tonic-clonic seizure. Hum Brain Mapp 37(12):4487–4499. https://doi.org/10.1002/hbm.23323
Li K, Liu L, Yin Q, Dun W, Xu X, Liu J, Zhang M (2017) Abnormal rich club organization and impaired correlation between structural and functional

connectivity in migraine sufferers. Brain Imaging Behav 11(2):526–540. https://doi.org/10.1007/s11682-016-9533-6

Markov NT, Ercsey-Ravasz M, Van Essen DC, Knoblauch K, Toroczkai Z, Kennedy H (2013) Cortical high-density counterstream architectures. Science 342(6158):1238406. https://doi.org/10.1126/science.1238406

Markram H (2010) Microcircuitry of the neocortex. In: Shepard GM, Grillner S (eds) Handbook of brain microcircuits. Oxford University Press, Oxford, pp 22–30

McIntosh RD, Schenk T (2009) Two visual streams for perception and action: current trends. Neuropsychologia 47(6):1391–1396. https://doi.org/10.1016/j.neuropsychologia.2009.02.009

Milner AD (2012) Is visual processing in the dorsal stream accessible to consciousness? Proc Biol Sci 279(1737):2289–2298. https://doi.org/10.1098/rspb.2011.2663

Milner AD (2017) How do the two visual streams interact with each other? Exp Brain Res 235(5):1297–1308. https://doi.org/10.1007/s00221-017-4917-4

Milner AD, Goodale MA (2008) Two visual systems reviewed. Neuropsychologia 46(3):774–785. https://doi.org/10.1016/j.neuropsychologia.2007.10.005

Murata A, Wen W, Asama H (2016) The body and objects represented in the ventral stream of the parieto-premotor network. Neurosci Res 104:4–15. https://doi.org/10.1016/j.neures.2015.10.010

Nigam S, Shimono M, Ito S, Yeh FC, Timme N, Myroshnychenko M, Lapish CC, Tosi Z, Hottowy P, Smith WC, Masmanidis SC, Litke AM, Sporns O (2016) Rich-Club Organization in effective connectivity among cortical neurons. J Neurosci 36(3):670–684. https://doi.org/10.1523/jneurosci.2177-15.2016

Norman J (2002) Two visual systems and two theories of perception: an attempt to reconcile the constructivist and ecological approaches. Behav Brain Sci 25(1):73–96. discussion 96-144

Perry CJ, Fallah M (2014) Feature integration and object representations along the dorsal stream visual hierarchy. Front Comput Neurosci 8:84. https://doi.org/10.3389/fncom.2014.00084

Purves D, Augustine GL, Hall WC, LaMantia AS, White LE (2012) Neuroscience, 5th edn. Sinauer Associates, Sunderland, MA

Ray S, Miller M, Karalunas S, Robertson C, Grayson DS, Cary RP, Hawkey E, Painter JG, Kriz D, Fombonne E, Nigg JT, Fair DA (2014) Structural and functional connectivity of the human brain in autism spectrum disorders and attention-deficit/hyperactivity disorder: a Rich Club-Organization study. Hum Brain Mapp 35(12):6032–6048. https://doi.org/10.1002/hbm.22603

Reddy L, Kanwisher N (2006) Coding of visual objects in the ventral stream. Curr Opin Neurobiol 16(4):408–414. https://doi.org/10.1016/j.conb.2006.06.004

Sakreida K, Effnert I, Thill S, Menz MM, Jirak D, Eickhoff CR, Ziemke T, Eickhoff SB, Borghi AM, Binkofski F (2016) Affordance processing in segregated parieto-frontal dorsal stream sub-pathways. Neurosci Biobehav Rev 69:89–112. https://doi.org/10.1016/j.neubiorev.2016.07.032

Senden M, Deco G, de Reus MA, Goebel R, van den Heuvel MP (2014) Rich club organization supports a diverse set of functional network configurations. Neuroimage 96:174–182. https://doi.org/10.1016/j.neuroimage.2014.03.066

Seung S (2012) Connectome. How the brain's wiring makes us who we are. Houghton Mifflin Harcourt, Boston, MA

Shepherd GM, Grillner S (2010) Handbook of brain microcircuits. Oxford University Press, Oxford

Sporns O (2011) Networks of the brain. MIT, Cambridge, MA

Sporns O (2012) Discovering the human connectome. MIT, Cambridge, MA

ten Donkelaar HJ (2011) Clinical neuroanatomy. Brain circuitry and its disorders. Springer, Berlin

van den Heuvel MP, Sporns O (2011) Rich-club organization of the human connectome. J Neurosci 31(44):15775–15786. https://doi.org/10.1523/jneurosci.3539-11.2011

van den Heuvel MP, Kahn RS, Goni J, Sporns O (2012) High-cost, high-capacity backbone for global brain communication. Proc Natl Acad Sci U S A 109(28):11372–11377. https://doi.org/10.1073/pnas.1203593109

van den Heuvel MP, Sporns O, Collin G, Scheewe T, Mandl RC, Cahn W, Goni J, Hulshoff Pol HE, Kahn RS (2013) Abnormal rich club organization and functional brain dynamics in schizophrenia. JAMA Psychiat 70(8):783–792. https://doi.org/10.1001/jamapsychiatry.2013.1328

Wilson HR, Wilkinson F (2015) From orientations to objects: configural processing in the ventral stream. J Vis 15(7):4. https://doi.org/10.1167/15.7.4

Zaehle T, Geiser E, Alter K, Jancke L, Meyer M (2008) Segmental processing in the human auditory dorsal stream. Brain Res 1220:179–190. https://doi.org/10.1016/j.brainres.2007.11.013

Zhao X, Tian L, Yan J, Yue W, Yan H, Zhang D (2017) Abnormal Rich-Club Organization associated with compromised cognitive function in patients with schizophrenia and their unaffected parents. Neurosci Bull 33(4):445–454. https://doi.org/10.1007/s12264-017-0151-0

Neurotransmitter Systems

The transmission of information between neurons is done using chemical substances, i.e., the neurotransmitters. Transmission also occurs between neurons and glial cells (i.e., astrocytes) (see tripartite synapse).

A substance is defined as a neurotransmitter if the following criteria are fulfilled:
- Presence in nerve terminals
- Release from electrically stimulated neurons
- Presence of a mechanism for terminating the action of the released substance
- The application to target neurons mimics the action
- Existence of specific receptors

The following aspects are applicable:
- There exist excitatory transmitters as well as inhibitory transmitters.
- The effect of the neurotransmitter depends also on the receptor with which it reacts.
- Excitatory and inhibitory receptors may exist for the same transmitter.
- In many neurons, more than one neurotransmitter is present.
- Synaptic transmission is rapid in onset and termination with a maximal duration of 30 ms.
- Binding to postsynaptic receptors leads to:
  - opening of ionic channels
  - activation of longer lasting intraneuronal processes (second messenger, e.g., cyclic AMP, signal transduction)

The steps in the process of synaptic transmission can be described as follows:
- Transport down the axon.
- Electrically excitable membrane of the axon.
- Organelles and enzymes present in nerve terminal responsible for
  - synthesis
  - storage
  - release of transmitter.
- Synaptic vesicle.
- Process of active reuptake.
- Enzymes in the extracellular space for catabolizing excess transmitter released from nerve terminal.
- Enzymes in the glial cells (astrocytes) for catabolizing excess transmitter released from nerve terminal.
- Postsynaptic receptor triggers the response.
- Organelles in the postsynaptic cell respond to the receptor trigger.

- Interaction between genetic expression of postsynaptic cells and cytoplasmic organelles.

A subdivision of transmitters into categories is provided in Table 13.1.

The family of neuropeptides is very large as shown in Table 13.2.

Based on their function, the transmitters can be grouped into:
- Mainly *excitatory* neurotransmitters include:
  - Glutamic acid
  - Aspartic acid
- Mainly *inhibitory* neurotransmitters include:
  - GABA
  - Glycine

Widely projecting systems
- Monoamines
  - Catecholamines
    - Dopamine
    - Norepinephrine
    - Epinephrine
  - Indoleamine
    - Serotonin
  - Histamine
- Acetylcholine
- Neuropeptides
  - Orexins

Neuromodulators
- Influence the process of transmission by affecting
  - the amount of transmitter released
  - the time course of transmitter release
  - regulating sensitivity of the receptors
- Liberated by
  - neurons
  - glial cells
  - ependymal
  - neurosecretory cells
  - gland cells

Table 13.1 Subdivision of transmitters into categories

Group	Transmitter
Acetylcholine	• Acetylcholine
Catecholamines	• Dopamine • Noradrenaline • Adrenaline • Serotonin • Histamine
Amino acids	• γ-aminobutyric acid (GABA) • Glutamate • Aspartate • Glycine • Taurine
Neuropeptides	• see Table 13.2
Gut-brain peptides	• Substance P • Vasoactive intestinal peptide • Cholecystokinin • Neurotensin
Hypophysiotropic peptides	• Corticotropin-releasing factor • Luteinizing hormone-releasing hormone • Somatostatin • Thyrotropin-releasing hormone
Neurohypophyseal peptides	• Vasopressin • Oxytocin
Proopiomelanocortin derivatives	• Corticotropin • Melanocyte-stimulating hormone • ß-endorphin
Enkephalins and dynorphins	• Encephalin • Dynorphin
Angiotensin II	• Angiotensin II
Gas	• Nitric oxide (NO) • Carbon monoxide
Neurotrophic factors	• Neurotrophins • GDNF family • CNTF • Ephrins • EGF family • VEGF • Interleukins • TGF family • Chemokines
Endogenous cannabinoids	
Purines	

Table 13.2 The families of neuropeptides

Calcitonin family	• Calcitonin • Calcitonin gene-related peptide
Hypothalamic (neurohypophyseal) hormones	• Vasopressin • Oxytocin
Hypothalamic releasing and inhibitory hormones (Hypophysiotropic peptides)	• Corticotropin-releasing factor (CRF or CRH) • Gonadotropin-releasing hormone (GnRH) • Growth hormone-releasing hormone (GHRH) • Somatostatin • Thyrotropin-releasing hormone (TRH)
Neuropeptide Y family	• Neuropeptide Y (NPY) • Neuropeptide YY (PYY) • Pancreatic polypeptide (PP)
Opioid peptides	• ß-endorphin • Dynorphin peptides • Leu-enkephalin • Met-enkephalin
Pituitary hormones	• Adrenocorticotropic hormone (ACTH) • α-Melanocyte-stimulating hormone (α-MSH) • Growth hormone (GH) • Follicle-stimulating hormone (FSH) • Luteinizing hormone (LH)
Tachykinins	• Neurokinin A • Neurokinin B • Neuropeptide K • Substance P
VIP-glucagon family	• Glucagon • Glucagon-like peptide 1 (GLP-1) • Pituitary adenylate cyclase-activating peptide (PACAP) • Vasoactive intestinal polypeptide (VIP)
Some other peptides	• Agouti-related peptide (ARP) • Bradykinin • Cholecystokinin • Cocaine- and amphetamine-regulated transcript (CART) • Galanin • Ghrelin • Melanin-concentrating hormone (MCH) • Neurotensin • Orexins (or hypocretins) • Orphanin FQ

- effect lasts longer than that of conventional neurotransmitter
- change the capacity of their target cells
- no sharp distinction between neuromodulator and neurotransmitter

Neurotransmitter transporters (Table 13.3)
- Are a class of membrane transport proteins.
- Span the cellular membranes of neurons.
- Carry neurotransmitters across these membranes and to direct their further transport to specific intracellular locations.
- Use electrochemical gradients that exist across cell membranes to carry out their work.
- Serve to remove neurotransmitters from the synaptic cleft and prevent their action or bring it to an end.

Table 13.3 Neurotransmitter transporters, modified after Nestler et al. (2015)

Amine/GABA Family Transporters (SLC6A Genes)	Transmitter	Localization
GAT-1	GABA	Neurons (presynaptic and postsynaptic); glia
GAT-2	GABA	Glia
GAT-3 (GAT-4)	GABA	Glia
BGT-1	GABA	Glia
GlyT1	Glycine	Neurons and glia
GlyT2	Glycine	Neurons
DAT	Dopamine	Dopaminergic neurons
SERT	Serotonin	Serotonergic neurons
NET	Norepinephrine	Noradrenergic and adrenergic neurons
Glutamate Family Transporters (SLC1A Genes)	**Transmitter**	**Localization**
EAAT1 (GLAST1)	Glutamate	Astrocytes
EAAT2 (GLT-1)	Glutamate	Astrocytes
EAAT3 (EAAC1)	Glutamate	Neurons
EAAT4	Glutamate	Purkinje cells
EAAT5	Glutamate	Retina
Choline Transporter	**Transmitter**	**Localization**
CHT (SLC5A7)	Choline	Retina
Vesicular Transporters	**Transmitter**	**Localization**
VGAT-3 (SLC32A genes)	GABA; glycine	Synaptic vesicles
VMAT1 (SLC18A1)	Monoamines	Non-neuronal vesicles
VMAT2 (SLC18A2)	Monoamines	Synaptic vesicles; dense core vesicles
VAChT (SLC18A3)	Acetylcholine	Synaptic vesicles
VGluT1-3 (SLC17A members)	Glutamate	Synaptic vesicles
VNuT (SLC17A9 gene)	ATP	Synaptic vesicles

- Transporters can work in reverse, transporting neurotransmitters into the synapse, allowing these neurotransmitters to bind to their receptors and exert their effect: "nonvesicular release."

Vesicular transporters
- Move neurotransmitters into synaptic vesicles.
- Regulate the concentrations of substances within the vesicles.
- Rely on a proton gradient created by the hydrolysis of adenosine triphosphate (ATP) in order to carry out their work:
  - v-ATPase hydrolyzes ATP, causing protons to be pumped into the synaptic vesicles and creating a proton gradient.
- The efflux of protons from the vesicle provides the energy to bring the neurotransmitter into the vesicle.

The visualization of receptors represents one application field in nuclear medicine. The frequently investigated transmitter systems with their receptors are given in Table 13.4. In other investigations, opioid, adenosine, and cholinergic receptors are investigated; however, there is no direct clinical application ensuing.

Table 13.4 The visualization of transmitter receptors is widely used in nuclear medicine and includes the following transmitter receptors

Transmitter	Receptor type	Application
Dopamine	• DAT • D2	• Parkinson disease • Atypical Parkinson syndrome
Serotonin	• HT5 1A	• Depression
Somatostatin	• SSR 2,3,5 (mainly 2)	• GEP-NET • Sympatho-adrenal system tumors • Medullary thyroid carcinoma • Merkel cell carcinoma • Small cell lung cancer • Pituitary adenoma • Meningioma
GABA	• A	• Neuronal integrity (epilepsy)

13.1 Acetylcholine

ACh was the first identified neurotransmitter
- Choline acetyltransferase (ChAT) synthesizes Ach by transferring an acetyl group from acetyl coenzyme A to choline.
- Acetylcholinesterase (AChE) degrades (hydrolyzes) Ach into acetate and choline.
- ChAT used for immunhistochemical staining.

ACh-positive structures and systems (Fig. 13.1a, b):
- Skeletal motoneurons in brain stem and spinal cord
- Preganglionic autonomic neurons in brain stem and spinal cord
- Auditory receptor cells in the organ of Corti
- Rhombencephalic medial reticular formation
- Lateral tegmental area of the rostral rhombencephalon (→dorsal tegmental pathway)
- Basal forebrain neurons extending from the septal region rostrally to the subthalamic nucleus:
  - Ch1 group: medial septal nucleus (10% cholinergic neurons)
  - Ch2 group: vertical limb of the nucleus of the diagonal band of Broca (70% cholinergic neurons)
  - Ch3 group: horizontal limb of the nucleus of the diagonal band of Broca (1% cholinergic neurons)
  - Ch4 group: nucleus basalis Meynert (90% cholinergic neurons)
  - Ch5 group: lateral rhombencephalic tegmental area
  - Ch6 group: adjacent sector of the central gray

Cholinergic pathways are given in Table 13.5.

Physiological and behavioral processes include:
- Memory
- Affective behavior
- Arousal
- Cortical responsiveness to sensory input
- Emotional states
- Learning
- Memory

Acetylcholine receptors:
- Muscarinic receptors (Table 13.6)
  - GPCR superfamily
- Nicotinic receptors
  - ligand-gated ion channel superfamily

Nicotinic receptors
- localization
  - neuromuscular junction
  - autonomic ganglia

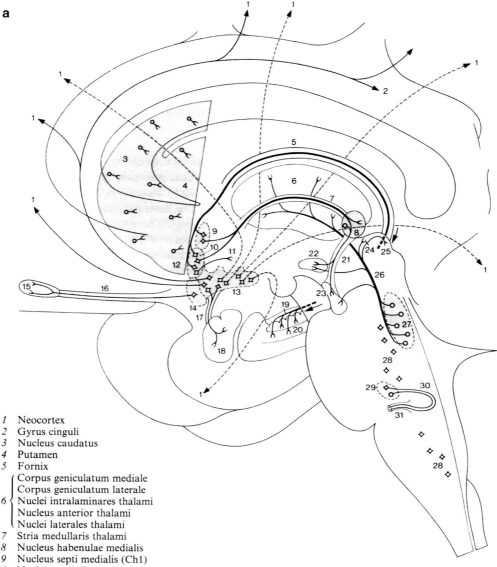

1 Neocortex
2 Gyrus cinguli
3 Nucleus caudatus
4 Putamen
5 Fornix
6 {Corpus geniculatum mediale
Corpus geniculatum laterale
Nuclei intralaminares thalami
Nucleus anterior thalami
Nuclei laterales thalami
7 Stria medullaris thalami
8 Nucleus habenulae medialis
9 Nucleus septi medialis (Ch1)
10 Nucleus gyri diagonalis, pars dorsalis (Ch2)
11 Area lateralis hypothalami
12 Nucleus accumbens
13 Nucleus basalis of Meynert (Ch4)
14 Nucleus gyri diagonalis, pars ventralis (Ch3)
15 Bulbus olfactorius
16 Tractus olfactorius
17 Fibrae amygdalofugales ventrales
18 Nucleus basalis amygdalae
19 Fimbria hippocampi
20 Hippocampus
21 Tractus habenulointerpeduncularis
22 Area tegmentalis ventralis
23 Nucleus interpeduncularis
24 Area pretectalis
25 Colliculus superior
26 Fasciculus tegmentalis dorsalis (Shute and Lewis)
27 Area tegmentalis dorsolateralis (including nuclei parabrachiales) plus adjacent central grey (Ch5+Ch6)
28 Formatio reticularis medialis
29 Nuclei periolivares
30 Fasciculus olivocochlearis (Rasmussen)
31 Nervus vestibulocochlearis

Fig. 13.1 Cholinergic projections (**a**) (reproduced from Nieuwenhuys (1985) with kind permission by Springer Nature). Cholinergic synapse (**b**) (reproduced from Iversen et al. (2009) with kind permission by Oxford University Press)

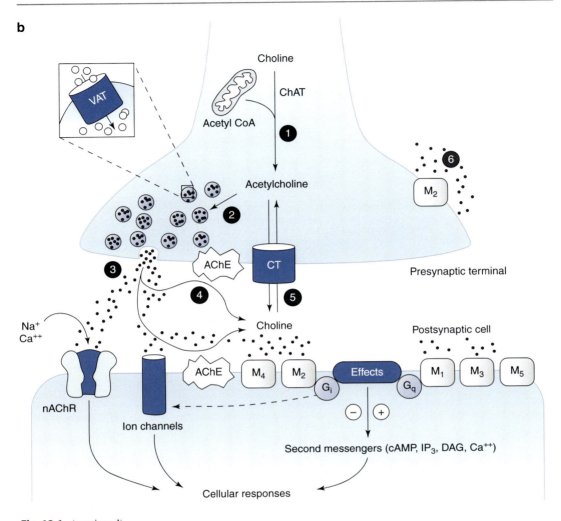

Fig. 13.1 (continued)

Table 13.5 Cholinergic projections

Cholinergic cell groups	Pathway	Termination
Ch1, Ch2, Ch3	Stria medullaris	Base of midbrain • Interpeduncular nucleus • Area tegmentalis Medial habenular nucleus
Ch1, Ch2	Fornix	Hippocampus
Ch2		Lateral hypothalamus
Ch3		Olfactory bulb
Ch4 (antero-lateral portion)	Ventral amygdalofugal	Amygdala
Ch4		Neocortex

Table 13.6 Muscarinic cholinergic receptors, modified after Nestler et al. (2015)

Receptor	G-protein	Localization	Function
M_1	$G_{q/11}$	• Cortex • Hippocampus • Striatum	• mediate some of the effects of Ach on learning and memory • mediate cholinergic signaling in extrapyramidal motor circuits and in response to rewards
M_2	$G_{i/o}$	• Basal forebrain • Thalamus	• autoreceptors to control Ach synthesis and release
M_3	$G_{q/11}$	• Cortex • Hippocampus • Thalamus	• mediate some of the effects of Ach on learning and memory
M_4	$G_{i/o}$	• Cortex • Striatum • Hippocampus	• mediate some of the effects of Ach on learning and memory • mediate cholinergic signaling in extrapyramidal motor circuits and in response to rewards
M_5	$G_{q/11}$	• Substantia nigra	

- adrenal medulla
- CNS
• function
  - rapid influx of NA^+ and Ca^+ and subsequent cellular depolarization
  - rapid desensitization
• Subunits
  - α-subunits ($α_2 - α_9$)
  - ß subunits ($ß_2 - ß_4$)
• Roles
  - arousal
  - attention
  - memory

13.2 Catecholamines Monoamines

The biogenic amines include:
• Catecholamines
  - Dopamine
  - Noradrenaline (norepinephrine)
  - Adrenaline (epinephrine)
• Indolamine
  - Serotonin (5-hydroxytryptamine)

Biosynthesis of catecholamines is as follows:
• L-amino acid tyrosine converted by tyrosine hydroxylase (TH) into L-dihydroxyphenylalanine (DOPA)
• DOPA converted by L-aromatic amino acid decarboxylase (AADC) into dopamine (DA)
• Dopamine converted by dopamine-ß-hydroxylase (DBH) into norepinephrine (NE)
• Noradrenaline converted by phenylethanolamine-N-methyl-transferase (PNMT) into adrenaline

Based on the transmitter synthesized, the following cell groups have been identified:
• A1–A15: dopaminergic and noradrenergic
• B1–B9: serotoninergic
• C1–C2: adrenergic

13.2.1 Dopamine

Biosynthesis of dopamine is as follows:
• L-amino acid tyrosine is converted by tyrosine hydroxylase (TH) into L-dihydroxyphenylalanine (DOPA).
• DOPA is converted by aromatic amino acid decarboxylase (AADC) into dopamine.

Dopamine synthesizing neurons are located in (Fig. 13.2a–e):
• Mesencephalon (A8, A9, A10)
  - A8: area tegmentalis lateralis
  - A9: substantia nigra, pars compacta
  - A10: ventral tegmental area
• Diencephalon (A11, A12, A13, A14)
  - A11: caudal hypothalamus
  - A12: infundibular nucleus

13.2 Catecholamines Monoamines

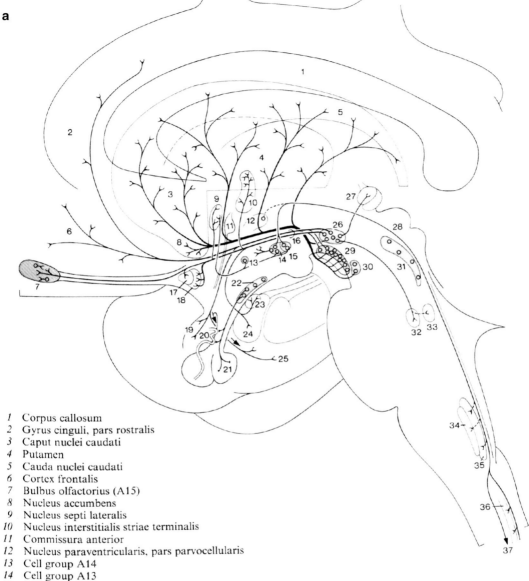

1. Corpus callosum
2. Gyrus cinguli, pars rostralis
3. Caput nuclei caudati
4. Putamen
5. Cauda nuclei caudati
6. Cortex frontalis
7. Bulbus olfactorius (A15)
8. Nucleus accumbens
9. Nucleus septi lateralis
10. Nucleus interstitialis striae terminalis
11. Commissura anterior
12. Nucleus paraventricularis, pars parvocellularis
13. Cell group A14
14. Cell group A13
15. Cell group A11
16. Fasciculus telencephalicus medialis
17. Nucleus olfactorius anterior
18. Substantia perforata anterior
19. Cortex praepiriformis
20. Eminentia mediana
21. Lobus posterior hypophyseos
22. Nucleus infundibularis (A12)
23. Nucleus centralis amygdalae
24. Nucleus basalis amygdalae
25. Cortex entorhinalis
26. Area tegmentalis ventralis (A10)
27. Nucleus habenulae lateralis
28. Fasciculus longitudinalis dorsalis
29. Substantia nigra, pars compacta (A9)
30. Area tegmentalis lateralis (A8)
31. Nucleus raphes dorsalis
32. Locus coeruleus
33. Nucleus parabrachialis lateralis
34. Nucleus dorsalis nervi vagi
35. Nucleus solitarius
36. Substantia gelatinosa
37. Nucleus intermediolateralis

Fig. 13.2 Dopaminergic projections (**a**) (reproduced from Nieuwenhuys (1985) with kind permission by Springer Nature) central dopaminergic synapse (**b**) (reproduced from Iversen et al. (2009) with kind permission by Oxford University Press), basal ganglia are visualized with DOPA (**c**), D2 postsynaptic receptor with fallypride (**d**), dopamine transporter with FP-CIT (*N*-3-fluoropropyl-2-beta-carboxymethoxy-3-beta-(4-iodophenyl) nortropane) (**e**)

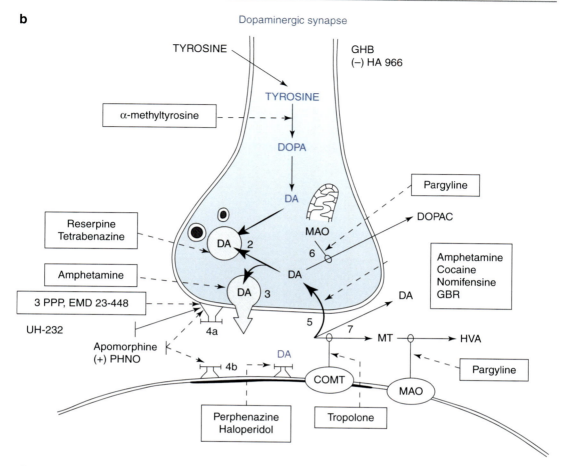

Fig. 13.2 (continued)

13.2 Catecholamines Monoamines

Fig. 13.2 (continued)

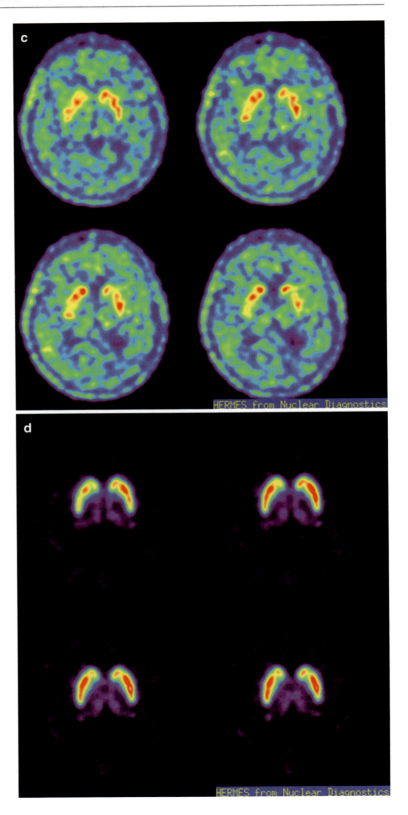

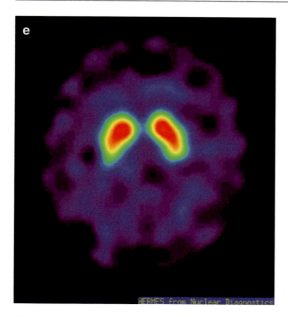

Fig. 13.2 (continued)

- A13: zona incerta
- A14: periventricular zone of the rostral hypothalamus
- Telencephalon (A15)
  - A15. Olfactory bulb

Dopaminergic ascending projections:
- Nigrostriatal system (origin A9)
- Mesolimbic system (origin A10)
- Mesotelencephalic system
  - Meso-striatal projection
    - (origin A8, A9, A10)
    - Terminals: A10: nucleus accumbens, A8: ventral putamen)
    - Regulates complex behavior
    - Determines the ability of the organism to cope with available exteroceptive sensory information in various ways
  - Mesolimbic projection
    - Origin A10
    - Terminals: telencephalon, i.e., bulbus olfactorius, anterior olfactory nucleus, olfactory tubercle, lateral septal nucleus, bed nucleus of the stria terminalis, amygdala
    - Enhanced locomotor activity
  - Meso-cortical projection
    - Origin: A10
    - Terminals: limbic system (i.e., medial part of the frontal lobe, prepiriform and piriform cortices, anterior cingulate cortex)

Four efferent systems originating from A11-A14 dopaminergic cell groups:
- Tuberoinfundibular dopaminergic projection
  - Origin: a12
  - Terminals: median eminence
- Incerto-hypothalamic dopaminergic projection
  - Origin: A11 and A13
  - Terminals: dorsal and rostral hypothalamic regions
- Diencephalon-septal dopaminergic projection
  - Origin: A11, A13, A14
  - Terminals: lateral septal nucleus
- Dopaminergic hypothalamo-spinal projection
  - Origin: A11
  - Terminals: ipsilateral half of the spinal cord

The various dopaminergic receptors and their respective area of anatomical localization are listed in Table 13.7.

Reuptake into nerve terminals via neurotransmitter-specific transporters

- Catabolized by monoamine oxidase (MAO)
- intracellular and extracellular forms

Table 13.7 Dopamine receptors, modified after Nestler et al. (2015)

Receptor	G-protein coupling	Areas of localization
D_1	GS	• Neostriatum • Cerebral cortex • Olfactory tubercle • Nucleus accumbens
D_2	G1/0	• Neostriatum • Olfactory tubercle • Nucleus accumbens
D_3	G1/0	• Nucleus accumbens • Islands of Calleja
D_4	G1/0	• Midbrain • Amygdala
D_5	GS	• Hippocampus • Hypothalamus

13.2 Catecholamines Monoamines

- two major forms:
  MAO$_A$ expressed in noradrenergic neurons, dopaminergic neurons
  MAO$_B$ expressed in serotonergic and histaminergic neurons
- Metabolized by catechol-O-methyltransferase (COMT)

Functional aspects include:
- promotes cognitive control of behavior in the prefrontal cortex
- working memory

Involvement in the following diseases:
- Attention-deficit hyperactivity disorder (ADHD)
- Addiction
- Impulse control disorders
- Schizophrenia
- Parkinson disease

13.2.2 Noradrenaline

Biosynthesis of noradrenaline is as follows:
- L-amino acid tyrosine is converted by tyrosine hydroxylase(TH)intoL-dihydroxyphenylalanine (DOPA).
- DOPA is converted by aromatic amino acid decarboxylase (AADC) into dopamine.
- Dopamine is converted by dopamine-ß-hydroxylase (DBH) into noradrenaline.

Noradrenaline-synthesizing neurons are located in (Fig. 13.3a–c):
- Pontine regions, locus coeruleus
- Medullary tegmental regions
- A1, A2: lower part of the medulla oblongata
- A1: around the nucleus of the lateral funiculus
- A2: nucleus solitaries, the dorsal vagal nucleus, intervening area (noradrenergic dorsal medullary group)
- A3: in rat: inferior olivary nucleus
- A4: superior cerebellar peduncle
- A5: pontine tegmentum
- A6: locus coeruleus
- A7: rostral pontine part of the lateral reticular formation

Efferents of the most important noradrenergic center, i.e., locus coeruleus:
- Dorsal noradrenergic bundle (dorsal tegmental bundle)
  - Origin: A6
  - Terminals:
    o Mesencephalon: central gray substance, dorsal raphe nucleus, superior and inferior colliculi, interpeduncular nucleus
    o Diencephalic: internal lamina of the thalamus, thalamus, epithalamus, hypothalamus
    o Telencephalic: amygdala, olfactory tubercle, anterior olfactory nucleus, olfactory bulb, nucleus of the diagonal band, medial septal nucleus, bed nucleus of the stria terminalis, hippocampal formation, entire neocortex
- Dorsal periventricular pathway
  - Origin: A6
  - Terminals.
    o Hypothalamus
    o Caudal limb of the dorsal periventricular pathway: dorsal vagus nucleus
    o Caudal limb of the dorsal periventricular bundle: lateral funiculus of the spinal cord

Functional aspects:
- regulator of the sleep-wake cycle
- regulator of levels of arousal
- attention and vigilance
- anxiety
- regulation of the cerebral microcirculation
- control of heart rate and blood pressure
- part of an alarm system (threatening stimuli)-survival-related behaviors
- stress dampening functions
- continuously monitors the environment for important stimuli and prepares the organism to cope with emergency situations

Ventral noradrenergic pathway
- Origin: A2, A1, A5, A7
- Terminals: mesencephalon (ventrolateral part of the substantia grisea centralis), diencephalon (hypothalamus), telencephalon (preoptic area, bed nucleus of the stria terminalis)

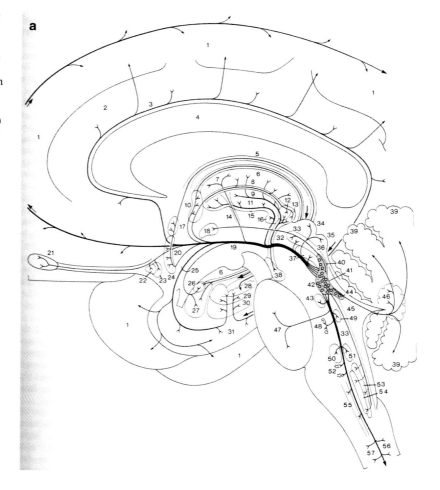

Fig. 13.3 Noradrenergic projection from the locus coeruleus (**a**) and from the remaining cell groups (**b**) (reproduced from Nieuwenhuys (1985) with kind permission by Springer Nature) noradrenergic synapse (**c**) (reproduced from Iversen et al. (2009) with kind permission by Oxford University Press)

Fig. 13.3 (continued)

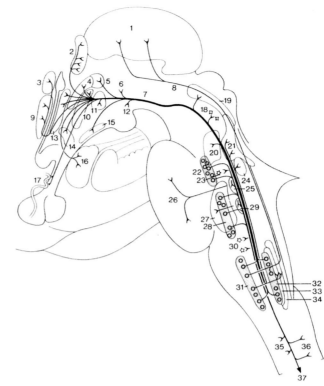

1. Thalamus, periventricular region
2. Nucleus interstitialis striae terminalis
3. Nucleus septi lateralis
4. Nucleus paraventricularis, pars magnocellularis
5. Nucleus paraventricularis, pars parvocellularis
6. Area lateralis hypothalami
7. Fasciculus telencephalicus medialis
8. Fasciculus longitudinalis dorsalis
9. Nucleus gyri diagonalis
10. Nucleus anterior hypothalami
11. Nucleus dorsomedialis
12. Area caudalis hypothalami
13. Nucleus praeopticus medialis
14. Nucleus supraopticus
15. Nucleus infundibularis
16. Corpus amygdaloideum
17. Eminentia mediana
18. Formatio reticularis mesencephali
19. Griseum centrale mesencephali
20. Nucleus centralis superior
21. Locus coeruleus
22. Cell group A7
23. Formatio reticularis metencephali
24. Nuclei parabrachiales
25. Nucleus motorius nervi trigemini
26. Nuclei pontis
27. Nucleus raphes magnus
28. Cell group A5
29. Nucleus nervi facialis
30. Formatio reticularis myelencephali
31. Cell group A1
32. Cell group A2
33. Nucleus dorsalis nervi vagi
34. Nucleus solitarius
35. Substantia grisea centralis
36. Substantia gelatinosa
37. Nucleus intermediolateralis

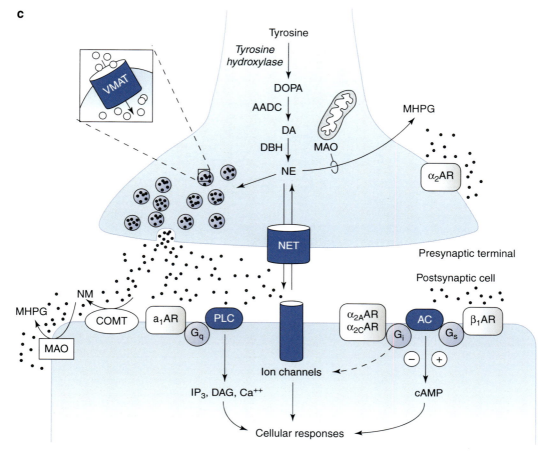

Fig. 13.3 (continued)

13.2.3 Monoamines: Adrenaline

Biosynthesis of adrenaline is as follows:
- L-amino acid tyrosine converted by tyrosine hydroxylase (TH) into L-dihydroxyphenylalanine (DOPA)
- DOPA converted by aromatic amino acid decarboxylase (AADC) into dopamine
- Dopamine converted by dopamine-ß-hydroxylase (DBH) into noradrenaline
- Noradrenaline converted by phenylethanolamine-N-methyl-transferase (PNMT) into adrenaline

Adrenaline-synthesizing neurons, visualized by the presence of PNMT, are located in:
- Caudal rhombencephalon
- C1: ventrolateral myelencephalon between the inferior olivary complex and the nucleus funiculi lateralis
- C2: adjacent to the nucleus solitaries
- C3: between the dorsal raphe region and hypoglossal nerve
- Terminals: thalamic midline nuclei, dorsomedial and paraventricular hypothalamic nuclei, ventral part of the periaqueductal gray, locus coeruleus, nucleus solitaries, nucleus dorsalis of the vagal nerve, nucleus intermediolateralis in the spinal cord

Functional aspects include:
- Oxytocin and vasopressin secretion
- Influence on food intake
- Regulation of blood pressure and respiration

13.2 Catecholamines Monoamines

Table 13.8 Adrenergic receptor family, modified after Nestler et al. (2015)

Receptor	G-protein coupling	Areas of localization
α_{1A}	$G_{q/11}$	• Cortex • Hippocampus
α_{1B}	$G_{q/11}$	• Cortex • Brain stem
α_{1D}	$G_{q/11}$	
α_{2A}	$G_{i/o}$	• Cortex • Brain stem • Midbrain • Spinal cord
α_{2B}	$G_{i/o}$	• Diencephalon
α_{2C}	$G_{i/o}$	• Basal ganglia • Cortex • Cerebellum • Hippocampus
β_1	G_S	• Olfactory nucleus • Cortex • Cerebellar nuclei • Brain stem nuclei • Spinal cord
β_2	G_S	• Olfactory bulb • Piriform cortex • Hippocampus • Cerebellar cortex
β_3	$G_S/G_{i/o}$	

A list of adrenergic receptors and their anatomical localization is provided in Table 13.8.

13.2.4 Monoamines: Serotonin

The biosynthesis of serotonin is as follows:
- Tryptophan is converted by tryptophan hydroxylase (TPH) into 5-hydroxytryptophan.
- 5-hydroxytryptophan is converted by aromatic amino acid decarboxylase (AADC) into serotonin.

DA is
- synthesized in the cytoplasm
- packaged in storage vesicles by the vesicular monoamine transporter protein (VMAT)

Serotonin-containing neurons are located in the median and paramedian parts of (Fig. 13.4a, b):
- Mesencephalon
- Pons
- Medulla oblongata

Fig. 13.4 Serotoninergic projections (**a**) (reproduced from Nieuwenhuys (1985) with kind permission by Springer Nature), serotoninergic synapse (**b**) (reproduced from Iversen et al. (2009) with kind permission by Springer Nature)

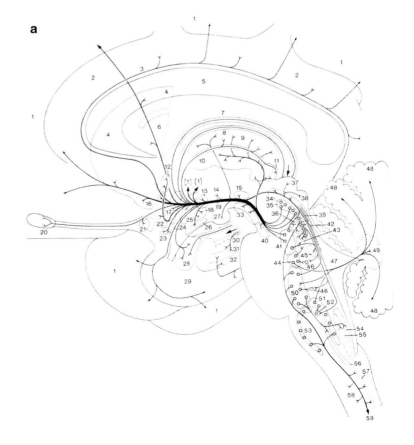

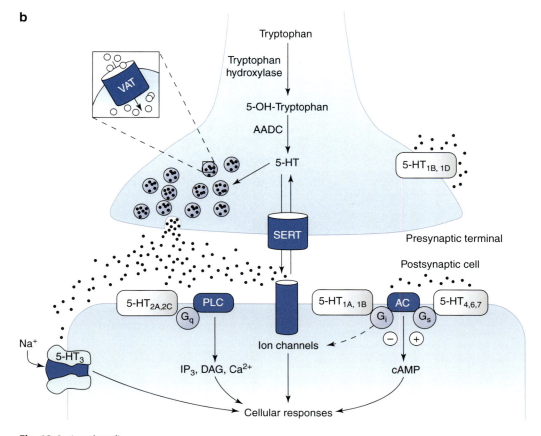

Fig. 13.4 (continued)

They are mainly, but not exclusively, confined to the nuclei of the raphe. On the other hand, not all nuclei of the raphe are serotoninergic and express dopamine, noradrenaline, GABA, etc.

The serotoninergic neuronal groups are defined as follows:
- B1: ventral part of the medulla oblongata, nucleus raphe pallidus
- B2: more distal position, nucleus raphe obscurus
- B3: between medulla oblongata and pons, nucleus raphe magnus
- B4: difficult to delineate, dorsal to the nucleus prepositus hypoglossi
- B5: nucleus raphe pontis
- B6: nucleus centralis superior
- B7: nucleus raphe dorsalis
- B8: nucleus centralis superior

The following serotoninergic projections are distinguished:
- Ventral ascending pathway
- Dorsal ascending pathway
- Projections to rhombencephalic centers
- Cerebellar pathways
- Bulbospinal pathways
- Supra-ependymal plexus

The origin and termination of following serotoninergic projections are given as follows:
- Ventral ascending pathway
  - Origin: B6-B8

- Terminal: lateral hypothalamus, interpeduncular nucleus, substantia nigra; ansa peduncularis–ventral amygdalofugal pathway: amygdala, striatum, external capsule, lateral and caudal parts of the neocortex; medioventral fibers: preoptic and hypothalamic centers
- Further split-up of the pathway to terminate in: periventricular regions of the thalamus, amygdala, dentate gyrus, medial and lateral septal nuclei, neocortex, hippocampus, olfactory bulb
- Dorsal ascending pathway
  - Origin: B7, B6, B8
  - Terminals: hypothalamic area, joins the ventral pathway
- Projections to rhombencephalic centers
  - Origin: B7
  - Terminals: e.g., nucleus solitarius, locus coeruleus
- Cerebellar pathways
  - Origin: all raphe nuclei
  - Terminals: cerebellar cortex and central nuclei
- Bulbospinal pathways
  - Origin: B1-B3
  - Terminals: dorsal and ventral horns of the spinal cord
- Supra-ependymal plexus
  - Origin: B6-B8
  - Terminals: supra-ependymal plexus throughout the ventricular system

Possible functions
- Neuron-vascular contacts
- Endocrine-neural transducer cells
- Regulation of blood flow
- Central control of cardiovascular function
- Regulation of sleep
- Inhibitory influence on the locus coeruleus and substantia nigra
- Transmission of nociceptive messages
- Sleep
- Arousal
- Attention
- Processing of sensory information
- Emotion and mood regulation

Serotoninergic receptors and their anatomical localization are listed in Table 13.9.

Table 13.9 Serotonin receptors, modified after Nestler et al. (2015)

Receptor	G-protein	Localization
$5HT_{1A}$	$G_{i/o}$	• Hippocampus • Septum • Amygdala • Dorsal raphe • Cortex
$5HT_{1B}$	$G_{i/o}$	• Substantia nigra • Basal ganglia
$5HT_{1D}$	$G_{i/o}$	• Substantia nigra • Striatum • Nucleus accumbens • Hippocampus
$5HT_{1E}$	$G_{i/o}$	
$5HT_{1F}$	$G_{i/o}$	• Dorsal raphe • Hippocampus • Cortex
$5HT_{2A}$	$G_{q/11}$	• Cortex • Olfactory tubercle • Claustrum
$5HT_{2B}$	$G_{q/11}$	• Not located in the brain
$5HT_{2C}$	$G_{q/11}$	• Basal ganglia • Choroid plexus • Substantia nigra
$5HT_3$	Ligand-gated channel	• Spinal cord • Cortex • Hippocampus • Brain stem nuclei
$5HT_4$	G_S	• Hippocampus • Nucleus accumbens • Striatum • Substantia nigra
$5HT_{5A}$	G_S	• Cortex • Hippocampus • Cerebellum
$5HT_6$	G_S	• Striatum • Olfactory tubercle • Cortex • Hippocampus
$5HT_7$	G_S	• Hypothalamus • Thalamus • Cortex • Suprachiasmatic nucleus

13.3 Amino Acids

Amino acid transmitters are the major transmitters in the mammalian central nervous system.

Amino acid transmitters are divided into two major groups:
- Excitatory amino acid transmitters
  - Glutamate (Glu)
  - Aspartate (Asp)
  - Cysteate
  - Homocysteate
- Inhibitory amino acid transmitters
  - γ-aminobutyric acid (GABA)
  - Glycine (Gly)
  - Taurine
  - ß-alanine

13.3.1 γ-Aminobutyric Acid (GABA)

Most important inhibitory transmitter in the central nervous system

The biosynthesis of GABA is as follows:
- GABA shunt
  - precursors: glucose, pyruvate
  - conversion of α-ketoglutarate into glutamate by α-oxoglutarate transaminase (GABA transaminase GABA-T)
- Glutamate is decarboxylated by glutamic acid decarboxylase (GAD) to form GABA.

Release and reuptake
- removed from the synaptic cleft by several types of plasma membrane GAB transporters
- returned to GABAergic nerve terminals
- uptake by glial cells
- metabolized into succinic semialdehyde by GABA-T in the presence of α-ketoglutarate
- back conversion of GABA to glutamic acid and transferred back to neuron

Distribution of GABA-ergic neurons (Fig. 13.5a–c):
- Local circuit neurons
- Interneurons of the spinal cord
- Purkinje cells of the cerebellum
- Nucleus raphes dorsalis
- Superior colliculus
- Nucleus reticularis thalami
- Extrapyramidal motor system (caudate nucleus, putamen, globus pallidus, nucleus accumbens, substantia nigra
- Hypothalamus
- Septum and nucleus of the diagonal Band of Broca
- Olfactory bulb (granule cells, periglomerular cells)
- Hippocampal region
- Neocortex

GABA plays a role in:
- Epilepsy
- Huntington disease
- Tardive dyskinesia
- Alcoholism
- Addiction
- Sleep disorders
- Autoantibodies against GAD in stiff-person syndrome

GABA receptors (Table 13.10):
- ionotropic receptor
  - $GABA_A$
  - $GABA_C$
- metabotropic receptor
  - $GABA_B$

13.3 Amino Acids

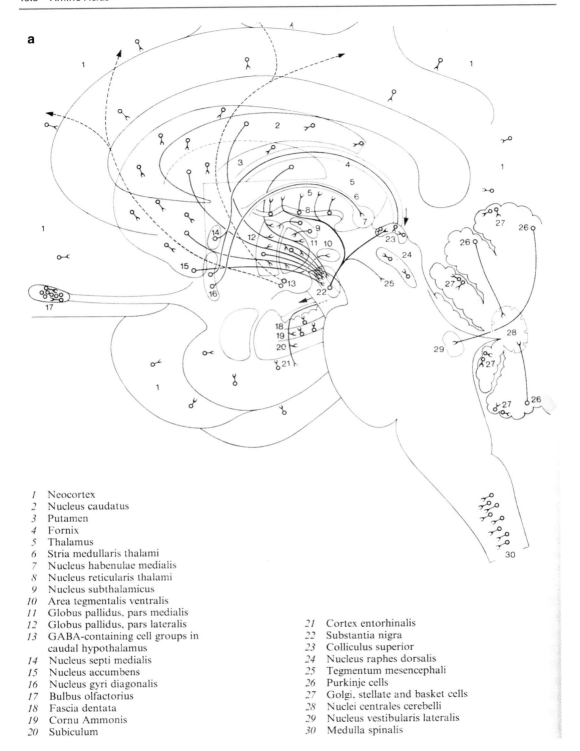

1. Neocortex
2. Nucleus caudatus
3. Putamen
4. Fornix
5. Thalamus
6. Stria medullaris thalami
7. Nucleus habenulae medialis
8. Nucleus reticularis thalami
9. Nucleus subthalamicus
10. Area tegmentalis ventralis
11. Globus pallidus, pars medialis
12. Globus pallidus, pars lateralis
13. GABA-containing cell groups in caudal hypothalamus
14. Nucleus septi medialis
15. Nucleus accumbens
16. Nucleus gyri diagonalis
17. Bulbus olfactorius
18. Fascia dentata
19. Cornu Ammonis
20. Subiculum
21. Cortex entorhinalis
22. Substantia nigra
23. Colliculus superior
24. Nucleus raphes dorsalis
25. Tegmentum mesencephali
26. Purkinje cells
27. Golgi, stellate and basket cells
28. Nuclei centrales cerebelli
29. Nucleus vestibularis lateralis
30. Medulla spinalis

Fig. 13.5 GABA-ergic projection (**a**) (reproduced from Nieuwenhuys (1985) with kind permission by Springer Nature), GABA-ergic synapse (**b**) (reproduced from Iversen et al. (2009) with kind permission by Oxford University Press), $GABA_A$ receptor visualization with Flumazenil (**c**)

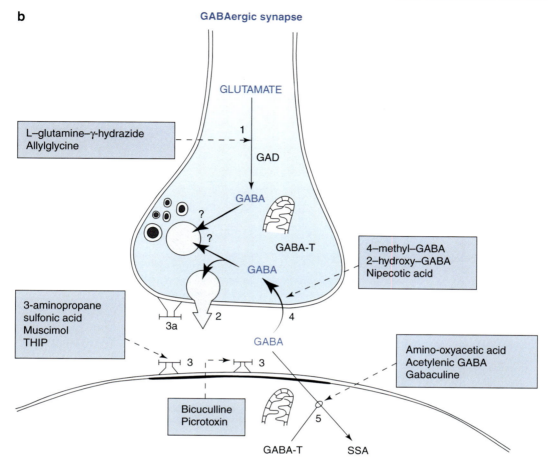

Fig. 13.5 (continued)

13.3 Amino Acids

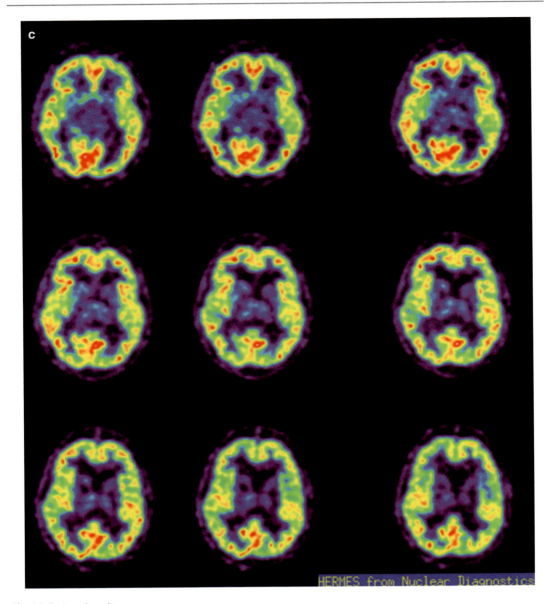

Fig. 13.5 (continued)

Table 13.10 GABA receptors, modified after Nestler et al. (2015)

	Gene families
Ionotropic GABA$_A$ receptor	• α1–α6 • ß1–ß3 • γ1–γ2 • δ • ρ1–ρ3 • ε • π
Metabotropic GABA$_B$ receptor	• GABA$_B$R$_{1a}$ • GABA$_B$R$_{1b}$ • GABA$_B$R$_2$

13.3.2 Glutamic Acid (Glu)

Major excitatory neurotransmitter

Synthesis and metabolism:
- synthesized in nerve terminals
  - from glucose via Krebs cycle
  - from glutamine (Gln) synthesized in glial cells
  - transported into nerve terminals
  - converted by glutaminase into Glut

- after release
  - Glut taken up by glial cells
  - in glial cells conversion into glutamine by glutamine synthetase
  - Gln transported out of glial by system N1 (SN1)
- uptake of Gln by neurons
  - back conversion into glutamate by glutaminase

Glut transporters
- EAAT1 (glutamate-aspartate transporter GLAST1)
- EAAT2 (glutamate transporter-1 GLT-1)
- EAAT3 (excitatory amino acid carrier-1 EAAC1)
- EAAT4
- EAAT5
- EAAT1 and EAAT2
  - expressed in glial cells
  - responsible for the majority of glutamate reuptake

Neuroanatomical localization of glutamatergic structures (Fig. 13.6a, b):
- Neocortical pyramidal cells
- GLUT-ergic corticofugal projections:
  - corticostriatal
  - corticothalamic
  - corticotectal
  - corticonigral
  - corticopontine
- GLUT-ergic pathways of the hippocampus:
  - perforant path
  - fibers from the cornu ammonis
  - fibers from the subiculum
- Other GLUT-ergic brain regions:
  - olfactory bulb
  - cerebellar cortex
  - auditory nerve
  - large, myelinated, non-nociceptive primary afferent fibers

Glutamate receptors (Table 13.11):
- Ionotropic receptors
  - ligand-gated ion channel
  - α-amino-3-hydroxy-5-methyl-4-isoxazole propionic acid (AMPA) receptor
  - kainate receptor
  - N-methyl-D-aspartate (NMDA) receptor
- Metabotropic receptors
  - G-protein-coupled
  - 8 subtypes

Ionotropic ligand-gated ion channel
AMPA receptor
- Mediate majority of synaptic excitatory transmission
- Coassembled from subunits GluA1-GluA4
- Region-specific expression in the brain
- Exist in *flip* and *flop* forms
- Some AMPA receptors are permeable to Ca^{2+}.
- Number of GluA2-lacking AMPA receptors is subject to dynamic regulation.
  - →mechanism of neural and behavioral plasticity

Kainate receptors
- cation-selective ligand-gated channels
- on presynaptic terminals of excitatory and inhibitory synapses
  - can facilitate or depress transmitter release
- on postsynaptic neurons
  - generate slow, small, but functionally important, postsynaptic potentials
- play a role in the development of temporal lobe epilepsy
- alleles of GluK2 linked to Huntington disease

NMDA receptor
- highly permeable to calcium
- voltage-dependent
- → calcium entry only if the cell is depolarized
- trigger synaptic plasticity
- when overactivated → trigger excitotoxicity

Metabotropic receptors
- G-protein-coupled receptors
- presynaptic terminal
  - → inhibit neurotransmitter release
- postsynaptic membrane
  - → complex modulatory effects through specific signal transduction cascades
  - → excitatory or inhibitory effects

13.3 Amino Acids

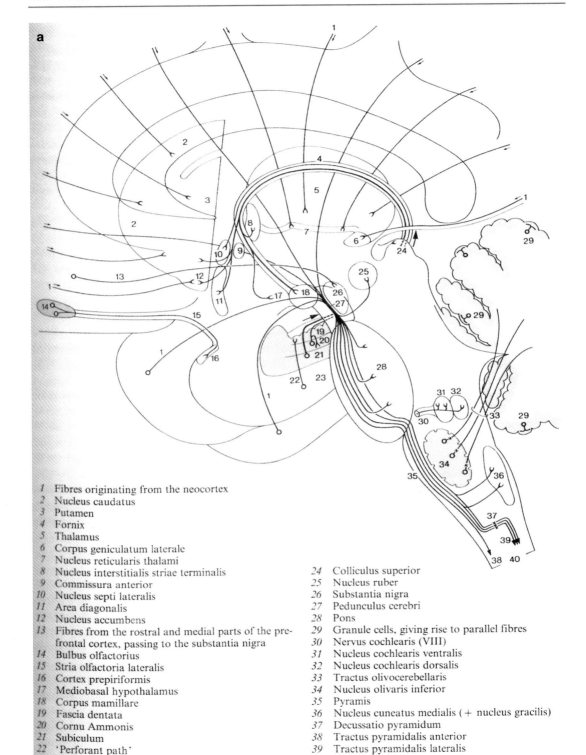

1. Fibres originating from the neocortex
2. Nucleus caudatus
3. Putamen
4. Fornix
5. Thalamus
6. Corpus geniculatum laterale
7. Nucleus reticularis thalami
8. Nucleus interstitialis striae terminalis
9. Commissura anterior
10. Nucleus septi lateralis
11. Area diagonalis
12. Nucleus accumbens
13. Fibres from the rostral and medial parts of the prefrontal cortex, passing to the substantia nigra
14. Bulbus olfactorius
15. Stria olfactoria lateralis
16. Cortex prepiriformis
17. Mediobasal hypothalamus
18. Corpus mamillare
19. Fascia dentata
20. Cornu Ammonis
21. Subiculum
22. 'Perforant path'
23. Gyrus parahippocampalis
24. Colliculus superior
25. Nucleus ruber
26. Substantia nigra
27. Pedunculus cerebri
28. Pons
29. Granule cells, giving rise to parallel fibres
30. Nervus cochlearis (VIII)
31. Nucleus cochlearis ventralis
32. Nucleus cochlearis dorsalis
33. Tractus olivocerebellaris
34. Nucleus olivaris inferior
35. Pyramis
36. Nucleus cuneatus medialis (+ nucleus gracilis)
37. Decussatio pyramidum
38. Tractus pyramidalis anterior
39. Tractus pyramidalis lateralis
40. Medulla spinalis

Fig. 13.6 Glutamatergic projections (**a**) (reproduced from Nieuwenhuys (1985) with kind permission by Springer Nature), glutamatergic synapse (**b**) (reproduced from Iversen et al. (2009) with kind permission by Oxford University Press)

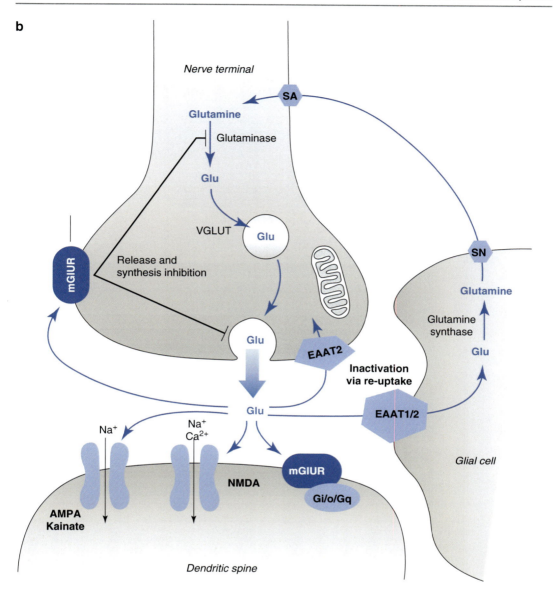

Fig. 13.6 (continued)

Table 13.11 Glutamate receptors modified after Nestler et al. (2015)

	Functional class	Gene families	Agonists	Antagonists
Ionotropic	AMPA	• GluA 1–4	• Glutamate • AMPA	• CNQX • NBQX
	Kainate	• GluK 1–5	• Glutamate • Kainate • ATPA • Domoic acid	• CNQX
	NMDA	• GluN1 • GluN2A-D • GluN3A	• Glutamate • Aspartate • NMDA	• Phencyclidine • Ketamine
Metabotropic	Group I	• mGlu1,5	• 1S, 3R-ACPD • DHPG	• AIDA
	Group II	• mGlu2,3	• 1S, 3R-ACPD • DCG-IV • PCCG-4	• EGLU
	Group II	• mGlu4, 6–8	• L-AP4 • 1S, 3R-ACPD	• MAP4

Selected References

Alsharafi WA, Luo Z, Long X, Xie Y, Xiao B (2017) MicroRNA in glutamate receptor-dependent neurological diseases. Clin Sci 131(14):1591–1604. https://doi.org/10.1042/cs20170964

Ashok AH, Marques TR, Jauhar S, Nour MM, Goodwin GM, Young AH, Howes OD (2017) The dopamine hypothesis of bipolar affective disorder: the state of the art and implications for treatment. Mol Psychiatry 22(5):666–679. https://doi.org/10.1038/mp.2017.16

Bai W, Zhou YG (2017) Homeostasis of the intraparenchymal-blood glutamate concentration gradient: maintenance, imbalance, and regulation. Front Mol Neurosci 10:400. https://doi.org/10.3389/fnmol.2017.00400

Belujon P, Grace AA (2017) Dopamine system dysregulation in major depressive disorders. Neural Plast 20(12):1036–1046. https://doi.org/10.1093/ijnp/pyx056

Bertrand D, Terry AV Jr (2018) The wonderland of neuronal nicotinic acetylcholine receptors. Biochem Pharmacol 151:214–225. https://doi.org/10.1016/j.bcp.2017.12.008

Blows WT (2000) Neurotransmitters of the brain: serotonin, noradrenaline (norepinephrine), and dopamine. J Neurosci Nurs 32(4):234–238

Bouzat C, Sine SM (2018) Nicotinic acetylcholine receptors at the single-channel level. Br J Pharmacol 175(11):1789–1804. https://doi.org/10.1111/bph.13770

Brooks DJ (2016) Molecular imaging of dopamine transporters. Ageing Res Rev 30:114–121. https://doi.org/10.1016/j.arr.2015.12.009

Brunello N, Blier P, Judd LL, Mendlewicz J, Nelson CJ, Souery D, Zohar J, Racagni G (2003) Noradrenaline in mood and anxiety disorders: basic and clinical studies. Int Clin Psychopharmacol 18(4):191–202. https://doi.org/10.1097/01.yic.0000073880.93678.68

Cameron JD, Chaput JP, Sjodin AM, Goldfield GS (2017) Brain on fire: incentive salience, hedonic hot spots, dopamine, obesity, and other hunger games. Annu Rev Nutr 37:183–205. https://doi.org/10.1146/annurev-nutr-071816-064855

Canavier CC, Evans RC, Oster AM, Pissadaki EK, Drion G, Kuznetsov AS, Gutkin BS (2016) Implications of cellular models of dopamine neurons for disease. J Neurophysiol 116(6):2815–2830. https://doi.org/10.1152/jn.00530.2016

Chen W, Nong Z, Li Y, Huang J, Chen C, Huang L (2017) Role of dopamine signaling in drug addiction. Curr Top Med Chem 17(21):2440–2455. https://doi.org/10.2174/1568026617666170504100642

Clevenger SS, Malhotra D, Dang J, Vanle B, IsHak WW (2018) The role of selective serotonin reuptake inhibitors in preventing relapse of major depressive disorder. Therapeut Adv Psychopharmacol 8(1):49–58. https://doi.org/10.1177/2045125317737264

Cohen EJ, Quarta E, Fulgenzi G, Minciacchi D (2015) Acetylcholine, GABA and neuronal networks: a working hypothesis for compensations in the dystrophic brain. Brain Res Bull 110:1–13. https://doi.org/10.1016/j.brainresbull.2014.10.004

Commons KG (2016) Ascending serotonin neuron diversity under two umbrellas. Brain Struct Funct 221(7):3347–3360. https://doi.org/10.1007/s00429-015-1176-7

Correa AMB, Guimaraes JDS, Dos Santos EAE, Kushmerick C (2017) Control of neuronal excitability by Group I metabotropic glutamate receptors. Biophys Rev 9(5):835–845. https://doi.org/10.1007/s12551-017-0301-7

Cryer PE (1993) Adrenaline: a physiological metabolic regulatory hormone in humans? Int J Obes Relat Metab Disord 17(Suppl 3):S43–S46. discussion S68

Danbolt NC, Furness DN, Zhou Y (2016) Neuronal vs glial glutamate uptake: resolving the conundrum. Neurochem Int 98:29–45. https://doi.org/10.1016/j.neuint.2016.05.009

Dani JA (2015) Neuronal nicotinic acetylcholine receptor structure and function and response to nicotine. Int Rev Neurobiol 124:3–19. https://doi.org/10.1016/bs.irn.2015.07.001

De Felice LJ (2016) A current view of serotonin transporters. F1000Res 5. https://doi.org/10.12688/f1000research.8384.1

de Kloet SF, Mansvelder HD, De Vries TJ (2015) Cholinergic modulation of dopamine pathways through nicotinic acetylcholine receptors. Biochem Pharmacol 97(4):425–438. https://doi.org/10.1016/j.bcp.2015.07.014

Deneris E, Gaspar P (2018) Serotonin neuron development: shaping molecular and structural identities. Wiley Interdiscip Rev Dev Biol 7(1). https://doi.org/10.1002/wdev.301

Diana A, Pillai R, Bongioanni P, O'Keeffe AG, Miller RG, Moore DH (2017) Gamma aminobutyric acid (GABA) modulators for amyotrophic lateral sclerosis/motor neuron disease. Cochrane Database Syst Rev 1:Cd006049. https://doi.org/10.1002/14651858.CD006049.pub2

Elam M, Grassi G (2000) Adrenaline and hypertension: new evidence for a guilty verdict? J Hypertens 18(6):675–677

Esler M, Alvarenga M, Pier C, Richards J, El-Osta A, Barton D, Haikerwal D, Kaye D, Schlaich M, Guo L, Jennings G, Socratous F, Lambert G (2006) The neuronal noradrenaline transporter, anxiety and cardiovascular disease. J Psychopharmacol 20(4 Suppl):60–66. https://doi.org/10.1177/1359786806066055

Faure P, Tolu S, Valverde S, Naude J (2014) Role of nicotinic acetylcholine receptors in regulating dopamine neuron activity. Neuroscience 282:86–100. https://doi.org/10.1016/j.neuroscience.2014.05.040

Ferraguti F (2018) Metabotropic glutamate receptors as targets for novel anxiolytics. Curr Opin Pharmacol 38:37–42. https://doi.org/10.1016/j.coph.2018.02.004

Ferrari A, Rustichelli C, Baraldi C (2017) Glutamate receptor antagonists with the potential for migraine treatment. Expert Opin Investig Drugs 26(12):1321–1330. https://doi.org/10.1080/13543784.2017.1395411

Fillenz M, Lowry JP, Boutelle MG, Fray AE (1999) The role of astrocytes and noradrenaline in neuronal glucose metabolism. Acta Physiol Scand 167(4):275–284. https://doi.org/10.1046/j.1365-201x.1999.00578.x

Fischer AG, Ullsperger M (2017) An update on the role of serotonin and its interplay with dopamine for reward. Front Hum Neurosci 11:484. https://doi.org/10.3389/fnhum.2017.00484

Fitzgerald PJ (2009) Is elevated noradrenaline an aetiological factor in a number of diseases? Auton Autacoid Pharmacol 29(4):143–156. https://doi.org/10.1111/j.1474-8665.2009.00442.x

Garcia-Sainz JA (1995) Adrenaline and its receptors: one hundred years of research. Arch Med Res 26(3):205–212

Ghasemi M, Hadipour-Niktarash A (2015) Pathologic role of neuronal nicotinic acetylcholine receptors in epileptic disorders: implication for pharmacological interventions. Rev Neurosci 26(2):199–223. https://doi.org/10.1515/revneuro-2014-0044

Gilsbach R, Hein L (2008) Presynaptic metabotropic receptors for acetylcholine and adrenaline/noradrenaline. Handb Exp Pharmacol 184:261–288. https://doi.org/10.1007/978-3-540-74805-2_9

Gingrich JA, Malm H, Ansorge MS, Brown A, Sourander A, Suri D, Teixeira CM, Caffrey Cagliostro MK, Mahadevia D, Weissman MM (2017) New insights into how serotonin selective reuptake inhibitors shape the developing brain. Birth Defects Res 109(12):924–932. https://doi.org/10.1002/bdr2.1085

Gottesmann C (2008) Noradrenaline involvement in basic and higher integrated REM sleep processes. Prog Neurobiol 85(3):237–272. https://doi.org/10.1016/j.pneurobio.2008.04.002

Grasing K (2016) A threshold model for opposing actions of acetylcholine on reward behavior: molecular mechanisms and implications for treatment of substance abuse disorders. Behav Brain Res 312:148–162. https://doi.org/10.1016/j.bbr.2016.06.022

Gurevich EV, Gainetdinov RR, Gurevich VV (2016) G protein-coupled receptor kinases as regulators of dopamine receptor functions. Pharmacol Res 111:1–16. https://doi.org/10.1016/j.phrs.2016.05.010

Hadzic M, Jack A, Wahle P (2017) Ionotropic glutamate receptors: which ones, when, and where in the mammalian neocortex. J Comp Neurol 525(4):976–1033. https://doi.org/10.1002/cne.24103

Haga T (2013) Molecular properties of muscarinic acetylcholine receptors. Proc Jpn Acad Ser B Phys Biol Sci 89(6):226–256

Hirasawa H, Contini M, Raviola E (2015) Extrasynaptic release of GABA and dopamine by retinal dopaminergic neurons. Philos Trans R Soc Lond B Biol Sci 370(1672). https://doi.org/10.1098/rstb.2014.0186

Holgate JY, Bartlett SE (2015) Early life stress, nicotinic acetylcholine receptors and alcohol use disorders. Brain Sci 5(3):258–274. https://doi.org/10.3390/brainsci5030258

Holly EN, Miczek KA (2016) Ventral tegmental area dopamine revisited: effects of acute and repeated stress. Psychopharmacology (Berl) 233(2):163–186. https://doi.org/10.1007/s00213-015-4151-3

Hoops D, Flores C (2017) Making dopamine connections in adolescence. Trends Neurosci 40(12):709–719. https://doi.org/10.1016/j.tins.2017.09.004

Houwing DJ, Buwalda B, van der Zee EA, de Boer SF, Olivier JDA (2017) The serotonin transporter and early life stress: translational perspectives. Front Cell Neurosci 11:117. https://doi.org/10.3389/fncel.2017.00117

Ito S (2016) GABA and glycine in the developing brain. J Physiol Sci 66(5):375–379. https://doi.org/10.1007/s12576-016-0442-7

Iversen LL, Iversen SD, Bloom FE, Roth RH (2009) Introduction to neuropsychopharmacology. Oxford University Press, Oxford

Jembrek MJ, Vlainic J (2015) GABA receptors: pharmacological potential and pitfalls. Curr Pharm Des 21(34):4943–4959

Kaasinen V, Vahlberg T (2017) Striatal dopamine in Parkinson disease: A meta-analysis of imaging studies. Ann Neurol 82(6):873–882. https://doi.org/10.1002/ana.25103

Khazipov R, Valeeva G, Khalilov I (2015) Depolarizing GABA and developmental epilepsies. CNS Neurosci Ther 21(2):83–91. https://doi.org/10.1111/cns.12353

Kobayashi K, Yasoshima Y (2001) The central noradrenaline system and memory consolidation. Neuroscientist 7(5):371–376. https://doi.org/10.1177/107385840100700506

Koenig MK, Hodgeman R, Riviello JJ, Chung W, Bain J, Chiriboga CA, Ichikawa K, Osaka H, Tsuji M, Gibson KM, Bonnen PE, Pearl PL (2017) Phenotype of GABA-transaminase deficiency. Neurology 88(20):1919–1924. https://doi.org/10.1212/wnl.0000000000003936

Korshunov KS, Blakemore LJ, Trombley PQ (2017) Dopamine: a modulator of circadian rhythms in the central nervous system. Front Cell Neurosci 11:91. https://doi.org/10.3389/fncel.2017.00091

Kraus C, Castren E, Kasper S, Lanzenberger R (2017) Serotonin and neuroplasticity—links between molecular, functional and structural pathophysiology in depression. Neurosci Biobehav Rev 77:317–326. https://doi.org/10.1016/j.neubiorev.2017.03.007

Kruse AC, Kobilka BK, Gautam D, Sexton PM, Christopoulos A, Wess J (2014) Muscarinic acetylcholine receptors: novel opportunities for drug development. Nat Rev Drug Discov 13(7):549–560. https://doi.org/10.1038/nrd4295

Kubista H, Boehm S (2006) Molecular mechanisms underlying the modulation of exocytotic noradrenaline release via presynaptic receptors. Pharmacol Ther 112(1):213–242. https://doi.org/10.1016/j.pharmthera.2006.04.005

Lauder JM (2016) Serotonin as a differentiation signal. Dev Neurosci 38(4):239–240. https://doi.org/10.1159/000448373

Lee JH, Lee S, Kim JH (2016) Amygdala circuits for fear memory: a key role for dopamine regulation. Neuroscientist. https://doi.org/10.1177/1073858416679936

Leresche N, Lambert RC (2018) GABA receptors and T-type Ca(2+) channels crosstalk in thalamic networks. Neuropharmacology 136(Pt A):37–45. https://doi.org/10.1002/dneu.22536

Liu J, Wang LN, Ma X, Ji X (2016) Gamma aminobutyric acid (GABA) receptor agonists for acute stroke. Cochrane Database Syst Rev 10:Cd009622. https://doi.org/10.1002/14651858.CD009622.pub4

Liu B, Liu J, Wang M, Zhang Y, Li L (2017) From serotonin to neuroplasticity: evolvement of theories for maor depressive disorder. Front Cell Neurosci 11:305. https://doi.org/10.3389/fncel.2017.00305

Lombardo S, Maskos U (2015) Role of the nicotinic acetylcholine receptor in Alzheimer's disease pathology and treatment. Neuropharmacology 96(Pt B):255–262. https://doi.org/10.1016/j.neuropharm.2014.11.018

Lorenz-Guertin JM, Jacob TC (2018) GABA type a receptor trafficking and the architecture of synaptic inhibition. Dev Neurobiol 78(3):238–270. https://doi.org/10.1002/dneu.22536

Luhmann HJ, Fukuda A, Kilb W (2015) Control of cortical neuronal migration by glutamate and GABA. Front Cell Neurosci 9:4. https://doi.org/10.3389/fncel.2015.00004

Marazziti D (2017) Understanding the role of serotonin in psychiatric diseases. F1000 Res 6:180. https://doi.org/10.12688/f1000research.10094.1

Mayer ML (2017) The challenge of interpreting glutamate-receptor ion-channel structures. Biophys J 113(10):2143–2151. https://doi.org/10.1016/j.bpj.2017.07.028

McQuail JA, Frazier CJ, Bizon JL (2015) Molecular aspects of age-related cognitive decline: the role of GABA signaling. Trends Mol Med 21(7):450–460. https://doi.org/10.1016/j.molmed.2015.05.002

Melroy-Greif WE, Stitzel JA, Ehringer MA (2016) Nicotinic acetylcholine receptors: upregulation, age-related effects and associations with drug use. Genes Brain Behav 15(1):89–107. https://doi.org/10.1111/gbb.12251

Meneses A (2015) Serotonin, neural markers, and memory. Front Pharmacol 6:143. https://doi.org/10.3389/fphar.2015.00143

Momiyama T, Nishijo T (2017) Dopamine and serotonin-induced modulation of GABAergic and glutamatergic transmission in the striatum and basal forebrain. Front Neuroanat 11:42. https://doi.org/10.3389/fnana.2017.00042

Nestler EJ, Hyman SE, Holtzman DM, Malenka RC (2015) Molecular neuropsychopharmacology. A foundation for clinical neuroscience. McGraw Hill, New York

Nieuwenhuys R (1985) Chemoarchitecture of the brain. Springer, Berlin

O'Donovan SM, Sullivan CR, McCullumsmith RE (2017) The role of glutamate transporters in the pathophysiology of neuropsychiatric disorders. NPJ Schizophr 3(1):32. https://doi.org/10.1038/s41537-017-0037-1

Oda A, Tanaka H (2014) Activities of nicotinic acetylcholine receptors modulate neurotransmission and synaptic architecture. Neural Regen Res 9(24):2128–2131. https://doi.org/10.4103/1673-5374.147943

Pagano G, Niccolini F, Fusar-Poli P, Politis M (2017) Serotonin transporter in Parkinson's disease: a meta-analysis of positron emission tomography studies. Ann Neurol 81(2):171–180. https://doi.org/10.1002/ana.24859

Palacios JM (2016) Serotonin receptors in brain revisited. Brain Res 1645:46–49. https://doi.org/10.1016/j.brainres.2015.12.042

Papke RL (2014) Merging old and new perspectives on nicotinic acetylcholine receptors. Biochem Pharmacol 89(1):1–11. https://doi.org/10.1016/j.bcp.2014.01.029

Perrier JF (2016) Modulation of motoneuron activity by serotonin. Danish Med J 63(2)

Plaitakis A, Kalef-Ezra E, Kotzamani D, Zaganas I, Spanaki C (2017) The glutamate dehydrogenase pathway and its roles in cell and tissue biology in health and disease. Biology 6(1):E11. https://doi.org/10.3390/biology6010011

Prieto GA (2017) Abnormalities of dopamine D3 receptor signaling in the diseased brain. J Central Nerv Syst Dis 9:1179573517726335. https://doi.org/10.1177/1179573517726335

Puig MV, Gener T (2015) Serotonin modulation of prefronto-hippocampal rhythms in health and disease. ACS Chem Nerosci 6(7):1017–1025. https://doi.org/10.1021/cn500350e

Qian F, Tang FR (2016) Metabotropic glutamate receptors and interacting proteins in epileptogenesis. Curr Neuropharmacol 14(5):551–562

Ribeiro FM, Vieira LB, Pires RG, Olmo RP, Ferguson SS (2017) Metabotropic glutamate receptors and neurodegenerative diseases. Pharmacol Res 115:179–191. https://doi.org/10.1016/j.phrs.2016.11.013

Rimmele TS, Rosenberg PA (2016) GLT-1: the elusive presynaptic glutamate transporter. Neurochem Int 98:19–28. https://doi.org/10.1016/j.neuint.2016.04.010

Rizzi G, Tan KR (2017) Dopamine and Acetylcholine, a circuit point of view in Parkinson's disease. Front Neural Circuits 11:110. https://doi.org/10.3389/fncir.2017.00110

Rose CR, Felix L, Zeug A, Dietrich D, Reiner A, Henneberger C (2017) Astroglial glutamate signaling and uptake in the hippocampus. Front Mol Neurosci 10:451. https://doi.org/10.3389/fnmol.2017.00451

Rowley NM, Madsen KK, Schousboe A, Steve White H (2012) Glutamate and GABA synthesis, release, transport and metabolism as targets for seizure control. Neurochem Int 61(4):546–558. https://doi.org/10.1016/j.neuint.2012.02.013

Ryczko D, Dubuc R (2017) Dopamine and the brainstem locomotor networks: from lamprey to human. Am J Med Genet B Neuropsychiatr Genet 11:295. https://doi.org/10.3389/fnins.2017.00295

Sadigh-Eteghad S, Majdi A, Mahmoudi J, Golzari SE, Talebi M (2016) Astrocytic and microglial nicotinic acetylcholine receptors: an overlooked issue in Alzheimer's disease. J Neural Transm 123(12):1359–1367. https://doi.org/10.1007/s00702-016-1580-z

Salatino-Oliveira A, Rohde LA, Hutz MH (2018) The dopamine transporter role in psychiatric phenotypes. Am J Med Genet B Neuropsychiatr Genet 177(2):211–231. https://doi.org/10.1177/1179573517726335

Salminen A, Jouhten P, Sarajarvi T, Haapasalo A, Hiltunen M (2016) Hypoxia and GABA shunt activation in the pathogenesis of Alzheimer's disease. Neurochem Int 92:13–24. https://doi.org/10.1016/j.neuint.2015.11.005

Schmidt KT, Weinshenker D (2014) Adrenaline rush: the role of adrenergic receptors in stimulant-induced behaviors. Mol Pharmacol 85(4):640–650. https://doi.org/10.1124/mol.113.090118

Schousboe A (2019) Metabolic signaling in the brain and the role of astrocytes in control of glutamate and GABA neurotransmission. Neurosci Lett 689:11–13. https://doi.org/10.1016/j.neulet.2018.01.038

Scimemi A (2014) Structure, function, and plasticity of GABA transporters. Front Cell Neurosci 8:161. https://doi.org/10.3389/fncel.2014.00161

Sigel E, Steinmann ME (2012) Structure, function, and modulation of GABA(A) receptors. J Biol Chem 287(48):40224–40231. https://doi.org/10.1074/jbc.R112.386664

Smythies J (2005) Section IV. The adrenaline system. Int Rev Neurobiol 64:213–215. https://doi.org/10.1016/s0074-7742(05)64004-4

Song NN, Huang Y, Yu X, Lang B, Ding YQ, Zhang L (2017) Divergent roles of central serotonin in adult hippocampal neurogenesis. Front Cell Neurosci 11:185. https://doi.org/10.3389/fncel.2017.00185

Spencer S, Scofield M, Kalivas PW (2016) The good and bad news about glutamate in drug addiction. J Psychopharmacol 30(11):1095–1098. https://doi.org/10.1177/0269881116655248

Spitzer S, Volbracht K, Lundgaard I, Karadottir RT (2016) Glutamate signalling: a multifaceted modulator of oligodendrocyte lineage cells in health and disease. Neuropharmacology 110(Pt B):574–585. https://doi.org/10.1016/j.neuropharm.2016.06.014

Strobel C, Hunt S, Sullivan R, Sun J, Sah P (2014) Emotional regulation of pain: the role of noradrenaline in the amygdala. Sci China Life Sci 57(4):384–390. https://doi.org/10.1007/s11427-014-4638-x

Szeitz A, Bandiera SM (2018) Analysis and measurement of serotonin. Biomed Chromatogr 32(1). https://doi.org/10.1002/bmc.4135

Terbeck S, Savulescu J, Chesterman LP, Cowen PJ (2016) Noradrenaline effects on social behaviour, intergroup relations, and moral decisions. Neurosci Biobehav Rev 66:54–60. https://doi.org/10.1016/j.neubiorev.2016.03.031

Tessier CJG, Emlaw JR, Cao ZQ, Perez-Areales FJ, Salameh JJ, Prinston JE, McNulty MS, daCosta CJB (2017) Back to the future: rational maps for exploring acetylcholine receptor space and time. Biochim Biophys Acta 1865(11 Pt B):1522–1528. https://doi.org/10.1016/j.bbapap.2017.08.006

Tritsch NX, Granger AJ, Sabatini BL (2016) Mechanisms and functions of GABA co-release. Nat Rev Neurosci 17(3):139–145. https://doi.org/10.1038/nrn.2015.21

van Galen KA, Ter Horst KW, Booij J, la Fleur SE, Serlie MJ (2018) The role of central dopamine and serotonin in human obesity: lessons learned from molecular neuroimaging studies. Metab Clin Exp 85:325–339. https://doi.org/10.1016/j.metabol.2017.09.007

Verberne AJ, Korim WS, Sabetghadam A, Llewellyn-Smith IJ (2016) Adrenaline: insights into its metabolic roles in hypoglycaemia and diabetes. Br J Pharmacol 173(9):1425–1437. https://doi.org/10.1111/bph.13458

Vishnoi S, Raisuddin S, Parvez S (2016) Glutamate excitotoxicity and oxidative stress in epilepsy: modulatory role of melatonin. J Environ Pathol Toxicol Oncol 35(4):365–374. https://doi.org/10.1615/JEnvironPatholToxicolOncol.2016016399

Vizi ES, Elenkov IJ (2002) Nonsynaptic noradrenaline release in neuro-immune responses. Acta Biol Hung 53(1-2):229–244. https://doi.org/10.1556/ABiol.53.2002.1-2.21

Volkow ND, Wise RA, Baler R (2017) The dopamine motive system: implications for drug and food addiction. Ann Neurol 18(12):741–752. https://doi.org/10.1038/nrn.2017.130

Walker MC, van der Donk WA (2016) The many roles of glutamate in metabolism. J Ind Microbiol Biotechnol 43(2-3):419–430. https://doi.org/10.1007/s10295-015-1665-y

Wang R, Reddy PH (2017) Role of glutamate and NMDA receptors in Alzheimer's disease. J Alzheimers Dis 57(4):1041–1048. https://doi.org/10.3233/jad-160763

Warren N, O'Gorman C, Lehn A, Siskind D (2017) Dopamine dysregulation syndrome in Parkinson's disease: a systematic review of published cases. J Neurol Neurosurg Psychiatry 88(12):1060–1064. https://doi.org/10.1136/jnnp-2017-315985

Wirth A, Holst K, Ponimaskin E (2017) How serotonin receptors regulate morphogenic signalling in neurons. Prog Neurobiol 151:35–56. https://doi.org/10.1016/j.pneurobio.2016.03.007

Wu C, Sun D (2015) GABA receptors in brain development, function, and injury. Metab Brain Dis 30(2):367–379. https://doi.org/10.1007/s11011-014-9560-1

Wu ZS, Cheng H, Jiang Y, Melcher K, Xu HE (2015) Ion channels gated by acetylcholine and serotonin: structures, biology, and drug discovery. Acta Pharmacol Sin 36(8):895–907. https://doi.org/10.1038/aps.2015.66

Yamamoto K, Hornykiewicz O (2004) Proposal for a noradrenaline hypothesis of schizophrenia. Prog Neuropsychopharmacol Biol Psychiatry 28(5):913–922. https://doi.org/10.1016/j.pnpbp.2004.05.033

Yamasaki M, Takeuchi T (2017) Locus coeruleus and dopamine-dependent memory consolidation. Neural Plast 2017:8602690. https://doi.org/10.1155/2017/8602690

Yoon BE, Lee CJ (2014) GABA as a rising gliotransmitter. Front Neural Circuits 8:141. https://doi.org/10.3389/fncir.2014.00141

Yoon BE, Woo J, Lee CJ (2012) Astrocytes as GABAergic and GABA-ceptive cells. Neurochem Res 37(11):2474–2479. https://doi.org/10.1007/s11064-012-0808-z

Yu XX, Fernandez HH (2017) Dopamine agonist withdrawal syndrome: a comprehensive review. J Neurol Sci 374:53–55. https://doi.org/10.1016/j.jns.2016.12.070

Yuan S, Zhang ZW, Li ZL (2017) Cell death-autophagy loop and glutamate-glutamine cycle in amyotrophic lateral sclerosis. Biophys Rev 10:231. https://doi.org/10.3389/fnmol.2017.00231

Zenko D, Hislop JN (2018) Regulation and trafficking of muscarinic acetylcholine receptors. Neuropharmacology 136(Pt C):374–382. https://doi.org/10.1016/j.neuropharm.2017.11.017

Zhao Y (2016) The oncogenic functions of nicotinic acetylcholine receptors. J Oncol 2016:9650481. https://doi.org/10.1155/2016/9650481

Zhou Y, Danbolt NC (2013) GABA and glutamate transporters in brain. Front Endocrinol 4:165. https://doi.org/10.3389/fendo.2013.00165

Localization of Brain Function   14

Localization of brain function has since the early times been a very tedious task. The information provided in the following chapter mainly falls into the field of cognitive neuroscience, behavioral neurology, and clinical neuroanatomy.

Historically, localization of brain function could only be done while studying the autopsied brain by exactly describing in which brain region a lesion was encountered and correlating the morphological with the functional lesion. In addition, experimentally produced lesions in specific brain regions were performed in animals, and the functional outcome studied.

The pioneering work of Wilder Penfield, a neurosurgeon at the Montreal Neurological Institute, laid the ground for intraoperative stimulation of the cortical surface and watching, for example, movement in parts of the limb while stimulating the motor cortex. These electrical stimulation paradigms are still utilized for delineating eloquent regions (e.g., speech) during awake surgeries for tumor removal aiming at removing as much of the tumor as possible without causing a major functional lesion.

The following armamentarium is at the disposal of the researcher to elucidate topographical aspects of brain function:

- Connectional methods
  - Diffusion tensor imaging (DTI)
- Correlational methods
  - Magnetic resonance imaging (MRI)
  - Functional magnetic resonance imaging (fMRI)
  - Voxel-based morphometry
  - Positron emission tomography (PET)
  - Magnetoencephalography
  - Microelectrodes
  - Microdialysis
  - Voltammetry
  - Electroencephalography
- Lesion models
  - Traumatic brain injuries
  - Stroke
  - Tumor
- Stimulation methods
  - Transcranial magnetic stimulation (TMS)
  - Repetitive transcranial magnetic stimulation (rTMS)
  - Transcranial direct current stimulation (tDCS)

Theories of brain function include the following models (Catani and Thiebaut de Schotten 2012) (Fig. 14.1):

- Holistic
- Localizationist
- Associationist

Holistic models
- All regions as mutually interconnected through a network of homogeneously distributed association fibers.

- Normal functioning:
  - Cognitive functions are the result of the simultaneous activity of all regions acting as a whole through the association pathways.
- Dysfunction
  - In case of damage to one area, the network allows the redistribution of the lost function to undamaged brain regions.
- It follows that for holistic approaches function cannot be localized, the symptoms resulting from the loss of a "quantity" of cerebral cortex rather than a localized area.

Localizationist models
- Give little importance to interregional connections.
- Normal functioning:
  - Each function is carried out by discrete independent regions.
- Dysfunction:
  - Damage (black) results in the complete functional loss of the lesioned area.
- Hence, localization of symptoms corresponds to localization of functions.

Associationist models
- Consider the brain as organized in parallel distributed networks around cortical epicenters.
- Normal functioning:
  - Primary sensory and motor functions are localized but higher cognitive functions are distributed within large-scale networks.
- Dysfunction:
  - A cortical lesion causes functional loss of the damaged area (black) and partial dysfunction of those regions connected to the lesioned area (yellow).

Functions attributed to the major four lobes are shown in Table 14.1.

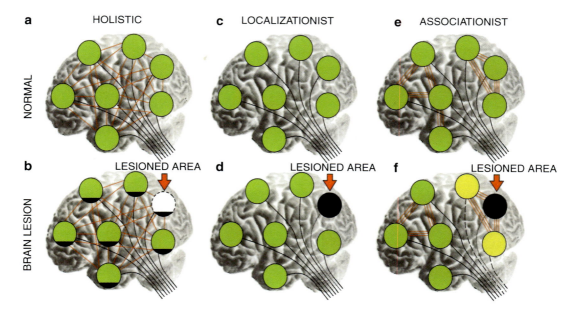

Fig. 14.1 Theories of brain function based on the holistic (**a, b**), localizationist (**c, d**), and associationist models (**e, f**) (reprinted from Catani and Thiebaut de Schotten (2012) with kind permission by Oxford University Press)

14.1 Frontal Cortex

Table 14.1 The traditional brain–behavior relationships are given as follows (modified from Anderson et al. (2013))

Frontal	Temporal	Parietal	Occipital
• Motor planning • Voluntary movement • Language (fluency) • Motor prosody • Motivation • Working memory • Executive function • Comportment	• Audition • Auditory association • Language (comprehension) • Sensory prosody • Visual recognition • Declarative memory • Emotional generation • Olfaction	• Somatosensation • Somatosensory association • Cross-modal sensory association • Visuospatial function • Praxicon • Derivative language functions (reading, writing, calculation)	• Vision • Visual perception

14.1 Frontal Cortex

14.1.1 Primary Motor Cortex

- Brodmann area 4
- Represents the contralateral half of the body, inverted
- Function:
  - Execution of movement
- Deficit:
  - Spastic paralysis
  - Face area
    - Dysarthria
    - Dysphagia
  - Hand area
    - Contralateral weakness, clumsiness, spasticity
  - Leg area
    - Contralateral weakness
    - Gait apraxia
    - Urinary incontinence

14.1.2 Supplementary Motor Area

- Brodmann area 6 on the medial surface
- Predominantly represents the contralateral side of the face rostrally and the legs caudally
- Function:
  - Movement planning or programming
- Deficits:
  - Spastic paralysis
  - Normal or increased tone
  - Reduction of spontaneous or voluntary contralateral movement
  - Automatic motor activity relatively unaffected
  - Hemineglect or apraxia
  - Mute/Speech deficits

14.1.3 Premotor Cortex

- Brodmann area 6
- Represents predominantly the contralateral side
- Function:
  - Movement planning or programming
- Deficits:
  - Impairment of movement execution in absence of paralysis (apraxia)
  - Middle frontal gyrus (F2)
    - Impaired contralateral saccades
    - Pure agraphia (dominant hemisphere)
    - Contralateral weakness of shoulder and hip muscles plus limb-kinetic apraxia
    - Hemiakinesia
  - Inferior frontal gyrus (F3)
    - Motor aphasia (dominant hemisphere)
    - Motor aprosodia (non-dominant hemisphere)

14.1.4 Prefrontal Cortex (Frontal Association Cortex)

- Brodmann areas 9, 10, 11, 12
- Areas of the frontal pole
- Function:
  - Affective aspects of motor behavior
  - Personality
  - Judgment
  - Foresight
  - Intellectual and emotional aspects of behavior
  - Executive function
- Deficit:
  - Impairment of
    - Personality
    - Judgment

- Foresight
- Intellect
- Emotions

14.1.5 Frontal Pole: Orbitofrontal Area

- Blunted affect (apathetic, indifferent)
- Impaired appreciation of social nuances
- Impaired conflict resolution
- Impaired emotion regulation (changes in affect, euphoria, emotional instability)
- Impaired ability to multitask
- Impaired goal-directed behavior
- Impotence
- Facetiousness ("Witzelsucht" or moria)
- Environmental dependency syndrome
- Speech apraxia
- Inability to plan and execute multistepped processes
- Abulia (poverty of thought, action, and emotion), apathy, and deficiency of motivated behavior

14.1.6 Mesial Aspect: Cingulate Gyrus

- Akinesia (bilateral akinetic mutism)
- Perseveration
- Hand and foot grasp
- "Salutatory" seizures
- Alien hand sign
- Transcortical motor aphasia (dominant hemisphere)
- Difficulty with initiating contralateral arm movements
- Bilateral ideomotor apraxia

Anosognosia

- The term is used to indicate a general lack of awareness of one's disease or disorder.
- Superior frontal gyrus.

The supplementary cortical motor area for coordination of locomotion is located in the superior frontal gyrus, while that for the line of sight and head rotation is located in the middle frontal gyrus. Broca's speech area is localized mainly in the triangular part and partly in the opercular part of the inferior frontal gyrus. Lesions in this region lead to Broca's aphasia, i.e., expressive aphasia. This type of aphasia is characterized by decreased speech fluency with poor articulation as well as by phonetic paraphasias and agrammatism.

A summary of clinical signs and lesion localization in the frontal lobe are given in Table 14.2.

Table 14.2 Summary of clinical signs and lesions in the frontal lobe

Symptoms	Lesion site
Disturbance of motor Function	
Loss of movements	Area 4
Loss of strength	Areas 4, 6, dorsolateral
Poor movement programming	Premotor, dorsolateral
Poor voluntary eye gaze	Frontal eye fields
Poor corollary discharge	Premotor, dorsolateral
Broca's aphasia	Area 44
Loss of divergent thinking	
Reduced spontaneity	Orbital
Poor strategy formation	Dorsolateral
Poor frequency estimate	Dorsolateral
Environment control and behavior	
Poor response inhibition	Prefrontal
Impaired associate learning	Dorsolateral
Risk taking and rule breaking	Prefrontal
Gambling	Orbital
Self-regulatory disorder	Orbital
Poor temporal memory	
Poor working memory	Dorsolateral
Poor delayed response	Dorsolateral
Other symptoms	
Impaired social behavior	Orbital, dorsolateral
Altered sexual behavior	Orbital
Impaired olfactory discrimination	Orbital
Disorders associated with damage to the facial area	Face

14.2 Parietal Cortex

14.2.1 Primary Somatosensory Cortex

- Brodmann areas 3, 1, and 2
- Contralateral half of the body, inverted

- Function:
  - Tactile representation of the body
- Deficit
  - Impairment of discriminative sensation

14.2.2 Secondary Somatosensory Cortex

- Superior lip of posterior limb of lateral fissure
- Function:
  - Less discriminative aspects of sensation
- Deficit:
  - Non-ascribed

14.2.3 Somatosensory Association Area

- Brodmann areas 5 and 7
- Function:
  - Relates new sensory experiences to old
  - Generating conscious constructs of objects in the world → associated with language use
  - Object location in space (BA 7)
  - Object location in relation to own body (BA 7)
  - Visuomotor coordination (BA 7)
- Deficit:
  - Impairment in understanding of significance of sensory information

14.2.4 Postcentral Gyrus

- is recognized to be the primary somatosensory cortex.
- is somatotopically organized.
- All pieces of information from superficial and deep receptors are processed in this brain region.
- Deficits:
  - Simple somatosensory disturbances
    - Contralateral sensory loss (object recognition > position sense > pain and temperature touch)
    - Tactile extinction
    - Contralateral pain, paresthesia

14.2.5 Superior and Inferior Parietal Lobules

- Neuronal information concerned with the understanding and interpretation of sensory signals is processed.
- Thus, in both lobules secondary cortical regions concerned with the processing of superficial and deep sensations as well as orientation are localized.
- Deficits:
  - Dominant hemisphere
    - Parietal apraxia
    - Finger agnosia
    - Acalculia
    - Right-left disorientation
    - Literal alexia (supramarginal gyrus)
    - Conduction aphasia
  - Non-dominant hemisphere
    - Anosognosia
    - Autotopagnosia
    - Spatial disorientation
    - Hemispatial neglect
    - Constructional apraxia
    - Dressing apraxia
    - Loss of topographical memory
    - Allesthesia
    - Hemiasomatognosia
    - Asymbolia for pain

14.2.6 Supramarginal and Angular Gyri

- The secondary centers of the optic speech region.
- The centers for writing and reading are localized.
- Lesions may result in receptive/Wernicke's aphasia (supramarginal gyrus).

Table 14.3 Summary of clinical signs and lesions in the parietal lobe (PF, PE, PG von Ecomono)

Symptom	Lesion site
Disorders of tactile function	Brodmann areas 1, 2, 3
Tactile agnosia	Area PE
Defects in eye movement	Areas PE, PF
Misreaching	Area PE
Manipulation of objects	Areas PF, PG
Apraxia	Areas PF, PG, left
Constructional apraxia	Area PG
Acalculia	Areas PG, STS
Impaired cross-modal matching	Areas PG, STS
Contralateral neglect	Area PG right
Impaired object recognition	Area PG right
Disorders of body image	Area PE
Right-left confusion	Areas PF, PG
Disorders of spatial ability	Areas PE, PG
Disorders of drawing	Area PG

14.2.7 Angular Gyrus

- visual-auditory integration
- understanding visually perceived words
- lesions result in disruption of receptive language abilities

14.2.8 Mesial Aspect: Cuneus

- transcortical sensory aphasia
- attentional disorder

A summary of clinical signs and lesion localization in the parietal lobe is found in Table 14.3.

14.3 Occipital Cortex

14.3.1 Primary Visual Cortex
(Fig. 14.2)

- posterior pole of the occipital lobe, and abuts on the calcarine fissure of the medial surface
- Brodmann area 17
- Function:
  - Processing of visual information
- Deficit:
  - Homonymous hemianopsia with macular sparing
  - Simple visual hallucinations

14.3.2 Visual Association Cortex
(Fig. 14.2)

- Brodmann areas 18 and 19
- Function:
  - Relates new visual representations to old
  - Depth perception
- Deficit:
  - Visual field deficits
  - Visual agnosia
  - Complex visual hallucinations

14.3.3 Mesial Aspect

- Visual field deficits
- Visual agnosia
- Visual hallucinations
- Alexia without agraphia
- Visual anosognosia, Anton syndrome

14.3 Occipital Cortex

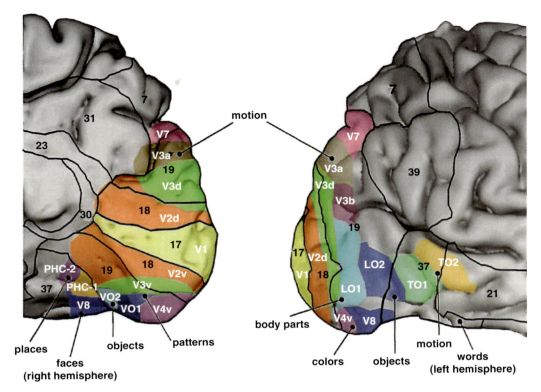

Fig. 14.2 Cytoarchitectonic, retinotopic, and functionally specialized areas of the medial and lateral surface of the human occipital cortex (reprinted from Catani and Thiebaut de Schotten (2012) with kind permission by Oxford University Press)

14.3.4 Lateral Aspect

- Alexia with agraphia
- Impaired optokinetic nystagmus
- Impaired ipsilateral scanning
- Palinopsia
- Visual allesthesia

A summary of clinical signs and lesion localization in the occipital lobe is displayed in Tables 14.4 and 14.5.

Table 14.4 Summary of clinical signs and lesions in the occipital lobe (Kolb and Whishaw, 2015)

Loss of function	Lesion site
Monocular blindness	Destruction of the retina Destruction of the optic nerve of one eye
Bitemporal hemianopia	Medial region of the optic chiasm severing the crossing fibers
Right nasal hemianopia	Lateral chiasm
Homonymous hemianopia	Complete section of the optic tract Lateral geniculate body V1 area
Quadrant anopia	Visual cortex lesions
Macular sparing	Sparing of the central, or macular, region of the visual field

Table 14.5 Summary of clinical signs and lesions in visual regions beyond the occipital lobe (Kolb and Whishaw, 2015)

Region	Proposed function
Ventral Stream Regions	
LO—Lateral occipital	Object analysis
FFA—Fusiform face area	Face analysis
EBA—Extrastriate body area	Body analysis
FBA—Fusiform body area	Body analysis
STS— Superior temporal sulcus	Analysis of biological motion
STSp—Superior temporal sulcus (posterior)	Moving-body analysis
PPA—Parahippocampal place area	Analysis of landmarks
Dorsal stream Regions	
LIP—Lateral intraparietal sulcus	Voluntary eye movement
AIP—Anterior intraparietal sulcus	Object-directed grasping
VIP—Ventral intraparietal sulcus	Visuomotor guidance
PRR—Parietal reach region	Visually guided reach
cIPS—Intraparietal sulcus	Object-directed action

14.4 Temporal Cortex

14.4.1 Primary Auditory Cortex

- Brodmann area 41 and 42
- Heschl transverse convolutions, superior temporal gyrus
- Function
  - Auditory processing
- Deficit
  - Impairment in perception and sound direction

14.4.2 Auditory Association Cortex

- Brodmann area 22
- Superior temporal gyrus posterior part, floor of the lateral sulcus
- Function
  - Higher level processing of acoustic information
- Deficit
  - Wernicke's aphasia, which is characterized by phonetic and/or semantic paraphasias, neologisms, disturbed speech understanding, and restricted communicative abilities

14.4.3 Inferomedial Aspect (Amygdala and Hippocampus)

- Amnesia (impaired storage)
  - Greater for verbal information with left involvement
  - Greater for visuospatial material with right involvement

14.4.4 Anterior Tip (Including Amygdala; Bilateral Lesions)

- Klüver–Bucy syndrome
  - Visual agnosia
  - Oral-exploratory behavior
  - Tameness (amygdala)
  - Hypersexuality
  - Hypomotility
  - Hypermetamorphosis
  - Amnesia
  - Diminished emotional response/affect

14.4.5 Latero-inferior Aspect

- Dominant hemisphere
  - Transcortical sensory aphasia
  - Word selection anomia
  - Agitated delirium
- Non-dominant hemisphere
  - Impaired recognition of facial emotional expression

14.4.6 Latero-superior Aspect

- Dominant hemisphere
  - Pure word deafness
  - Sensory aphasia

- Non-dominant hemisphere
  - Sensory amusia
  - Sensory aprosodia
- Bilateral lesions
  - Auditory agnosia
  - Pure word deafness
- Contralateral superior quadrantanopia

14.4.7 Non-localizing

- Auditory hallucinations
- Complex visual hallucinations

14.4.8 With Epileptogenic Lesions

- Interictal manifestations
  - Deepening of emotions
  - Tendency to transcendentalize minutia (cosmic vision)
  - Concern with minor detail
  - Paranoid ideation
  - Hyposexuality
  - Abnormal religiosity
  - Left hemispheric foci
    - Ideational aberration
    - Paranoia
    - Sense of personal destiny
  - Right hemisphere foci
    - Emotional disturbances (sadness, elation)
    - Denial
- Ictal manifestations
  - Hallucinations of smell and taste (amygdala)
  - Visual delusions (déjà vu, jamais vu)
  - Experiential delusions (déjà vecu, jamais vecu)
  - Psychomotor seizures

A summary of clinical signs and lesion localization in the temporal lobe is shown in Table 14.6.

Table 14.6 Summary of clinical signs and lesions in the temporal lobe (Kolb and Whishaw, 2015)

Symptoms	Lesion site
Disturbances of auditory sensation	Areas 41, 42, 22
Disturbance of visual- and auditory-input selection	Areas TE, STS
Disorders of visual perception	Areas TE, STS, amygdala
Disorders of auditory perception	Areas 41, 42, 22
Disorders of music perception	Superior temporal gyrus
Impaired organization and categorization of material	Areas TE, STS
Poor contextual use	Area TE
Disturbances of language comprehension	Area 22 left
Poor long-term memory	Areas TE, TF, TH, 48
Changes in personality and affect	Area TE, amygdala
Changes in sexual activity	Amygdala

14.5 Language Areas

The following two principal areas in the dominant hemisphere are the anatomic substrate for language (Fig. 14.3a–e) (Table 14.7):

- Wernicke's area
- Broca's area

Wernicke's area
- Receptive language area
- Brodmann area 22
- Dorsal region of the superior temporal gyrus
- May involve the supramarginal and angular gyri of the inferior parietal lobule
- Reception and comprehension of written and spoken language

Broca's area
- Expressive language area
- Brodmann areas 44, 45

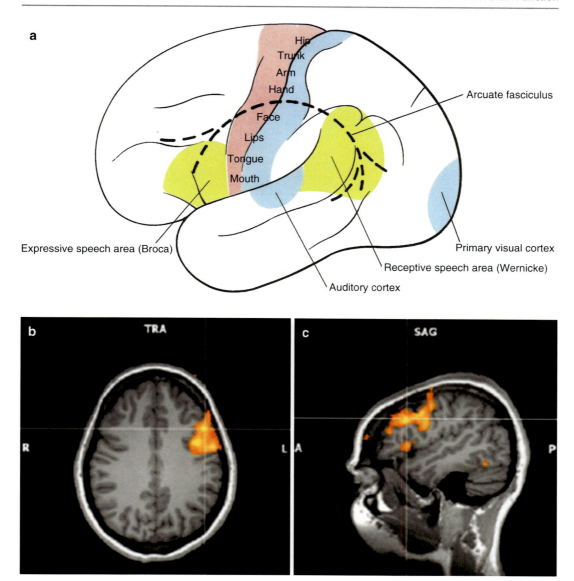

Fig. 14.3 The expressive and receptive speech areas are shown in yellow (reproduced from Heimer (1983) with kind permission by Springer Nature) (**a**) activation of the speech area as revealed by fMRI (**b–e**)

14.5 Language Areas

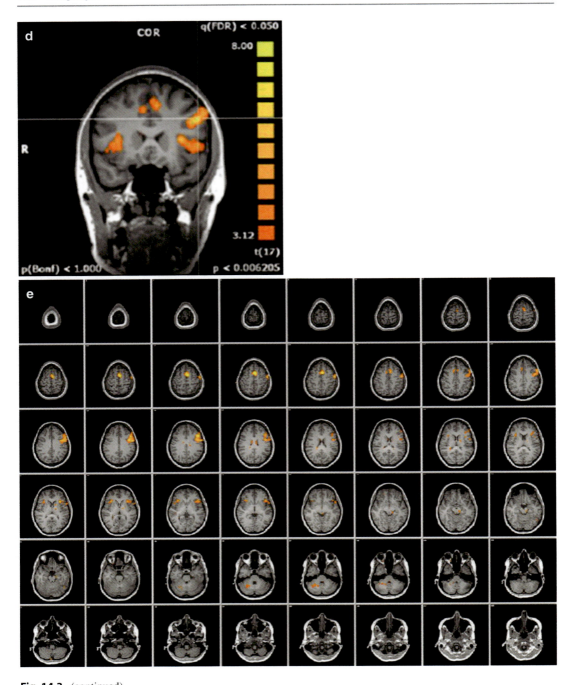

Fig. 14.3 (continued)

Table 14.7 Summary of various types of aphasia, lesion site, and outcome in fluency, comprehension, repetition, and naming

Type of Aphasia	Lesion location	Fluency	Comprehension	Repetition	Naming
Broca	Frontoparietal operculum	↓	Good	↓	↓
Wernicke	Infero-posterior perisylvian	Good	↓	↓	↓
Conduction	Posterior perisylvian	Good	Good	↓	↓
Transcortical motor	Frontal Striatum	↓	Good	Good	May be normal
Transcortical sensory	Parietal Temporal Thalamus	Good	↓	Good	Usually normal
Anomic	Depends on type of anomia	Good	Good	Good	↓
Global	Perisylvian	↓	↓	↓	↓

- Inferior frontal gyrus, pars opercularis, and triangularis
- Translates memory images of a word into the grammatical structure of a phrase

14.6 Cortical Syndromes

Right (non-dominant) hemisphere syndromes
- Constructional apraxia
  - Inability to draw or construct two- or three-dimensional objects
  - Disorder in learned movements
  - Parietal lobe
- Dressing apraxia
  - Inability to properly cloth, often leaving side of the body undressed
  - Parietal lobe
- Neglect and denial
  - Neglect: patient neglects half of the space contralateral to a lesion
  - Anosognosia: patient is unaware of the presence of an obvious disability
  - Denial: patient denies the presence of an obvious disability
  - Parietal and occipital lobes
- Color blindness
  - Inability to sort colors according the hue
  - Inferior occipito-temporal region

Dominant (Left) hemisphere syndromes
- Ideomotor apraxia
  - Inability to correctly imitate hand gestures or mime tool use of previously learned motor acts

- Visual agnosia
  - Inability to recognize objects visually
  - Bilateral visual association cortex or dominant occipital cortex and posterior corpus callosum
- Alexia without agraphia
  - The patient is unable to read but able to write.
  - Dominant occipital cortex and posterior corpus callosum.
- Gerstmann's syndrome
  - Defined by: dyscalculia, finger agnosia, left-finger disorientation, dysgraphia
  - Angular gyrus
- Color agnosia
  - Inability to name or point to colors in the presence of an intact ability to sort colors according to hue
  - Inferomedial occipital and temporal lobes

Bi-hemispheric syndromes
- Ideational apraxia
  - Defect of motor planning of a higher order
  - Bilateral lesion or diffuse cortical involvement
- Anton syndrome
  - Denial of blindness in a case of cortical blindness
  - Bilateral occipital lobe lesions

Aphasias
- Global aphasia
  - Disturbance in all aspects of language (comprehension, repetition, expression)
  - Wernicke's area and Broca's area

- Broca's aphasia
  - Non-fluent aphasia: agrammatic or telegraphic speech
- Wernicke's aphasia
  - Fluent aphasia: effortless spontaneous speech with many paraphasic errors
- Conduction aphasia
  - Fluent pattern of speech with significant word-finding difficulties and paraphasias
  - Supramarginal gyrus, arcuate fasciculus
- Transcortical sensory aphasia
  - Intact repetition but impaired comprehension
  - Borderzone between anterior and middle cerebral artery
- Transcortical motor aphasia
  - Intact repetition but impaired spontaneous speech
  - Borderzone between anterior and middle cerebral artery

14.7 Limbic System

The limbic system plays a major role in maintaining homeostasis by activating visceral effector mechanisms, by modulating the secretion of hypophyseal hormones, and by regulating sexual and reproductive behavior.

14.7.1 Hippocampus

- Recent memory
  - Retrieve material after an interval of minutes, hours, or days
  - Other involved regions include:
    - mammillary bodies
    - dorsomedial nucleus of the thalamus
- Modulation of emotions

14.7.2 Amygdala

Modulation of multiple functions:

- Olfaction
- Emotive behavior
  - Fear, anxiety, placidity, sexual activity
- Integration of autonomic visceral activity
  - Blood pressure, respiration, bowel, and bladder control

14.7.3 Stria Terminalis

- Autonomic response to fear, rage, and other emotions

14.7.4 Septal Nuclei

- Pleasure center of the brain

14.7.5 Cingulate Cortex

- Cortical regulation of basic autonomic functions
  - Respiration
  - Circulation
  - Digestion
- Behavior
- Emotional modulation of pain

14.8 Corpus Callosum

Lesions of the corpus callosum include:

- Lack of kinesthetic transfer
  - Inability to mimic position of the contralateral hand
  - Left hand apraxia
  - Left hand agraphia
  - Right hand constructional apraxia
  - Intermanual conflict (alien left hand)
- Perplexity trying to explain left-handed activity
- Double hemianopia
- Left hemiparalexia

Callosal disconnection syndromes are listed in Table 14.8.

Table 14.8 Callosal disconnection syndromes modified after Catani and Thiebaut de Schotten (2012)

Lesion site	Callosal syndromes	Description
Genu, anterior body	Alien hand syndrome "Diagnostic dyspraxia"	Involuntary intermanual conflict resulting in one hand (usually left) interfering with the correct execution of the movements of the other hand.
Body	Anarchic hand syndrome	Complex involuntary goal-directed movements of one hand (i.e., the anarchic hand) that the patient perceives as his own hand but with a will of its own.
Posterior body	Left hand tactile anomia and agnosia	Inability to name objects presented to the left hand. The inability to recognize objects after tactile presentation (i.e., tactile agnosia) has also been described.
Body-splenium	Left hand apraxia	Impaired ability to execute with the left hand goal-directed movements on imitation (when presented to the right hemifield) or under verbal command.
Body-splenium	Left hand agraphia	Failure to write the left hand.
Body-splenium	Hemispatial neglect	Failure to respond or reorient to novel or meaningful stimuli presented to one hemifield.
Isthmus-splenium	"Main étrangère"	A condition characterized by the patient's inability to recognize his left hand as his own when the hand is held in the other hand and is out of the visual field.
Isthmus-splenium	Dichotic listening suppression	When auditory stimuli are simultaneously presented to both ears, patients find easier to recognize verbal linguistic stimuli (e.g., words, digits) presented to the right ear and tend to ignore those presented to the left ear (left ear suppression).
Posterior body-splenium	Bilateral crossed optic ataxia	Specific visuomotor difficulty in reaching objects located contralaterally to the hand used.
Splenium	Deficits in binocular stereopsis and vergence eye movements	Reduced ability to perceive tridimensional objects and inability to produce appropriate convergent or divergent eye movements while fixating targets on the midsagittal plane.
Splenium	Optic aphasia	Failure to name objects presented visually, with preserved ability to name the same objects to definition
Splenium	Color anomia	Inability to name visually presented colors
Splenium	Alexia without agraphia (pure alexia)	Inability to read with preserved ability to write due to a disconnection between both occipital visual areas and the visual word form system.
Splenium	Left visual hemianomia and hemialexia	Inability to name objects (or read words) presented tachiscopically in the left half visual field. The right hemisphere maintains a normal capacity for visual recognition but has lost its access to the contralateral language regions.

14.9 Basal Ganglia

Table 14.9 Clinical manifestations of basal ganglia lesions

Dyskinesia (Hyperkinesia-Hypotonia syndrome)	• Chorea • Tardive dyskinesia • Orofacial dyskinesia • Abdominal dyskinesia • Ballismus • Akathisia • Athetosis • Dystonia • Torticollis • Paroxysmal dyskinesia • Myoclonus • Painful legs and moving toes • Restless legs syndrome and periodic limb movements of sleep • Tics • Tremor
Hypokinetic and bradykinetic disorders (Hypokinesia-Hypertonia syndrome)	• Parkinsonism • Stiff-person syndrome • Cortical-basal ganglionic degeneration • Progressive supranuclear palsy • Lewy body dementia • Multiple systems atrophy • Paraneoplastic movement disorders

14.9 Basal Ganglia

The function of the basal ganglia is complex and many aspects are not yet clearly understood. The main functions include (Table 14.9):

- regulation of motor function
- initiation and coordination of motor activities
- cognitive functioning

Ansa lenticularis:
- involved in motor function

Nucleus accumbens
- Shell
  - Cognitive processing of reward, including subjective "liking" reactions to certain pleasurable stimuli.
  - Motivational salience.
  - Positive reinforcement.
  - Mediate specific Pavlovian-instrumental transfer.
  - A "hedonic hotspot" or pleasure center which is responsible for the pleasurable or "liking" component of some intrinsic rewards.
  - D1-type medium spiny neurons in the Nacc shell mediate reward-related cognitive processes.
  - D2-type medium spiny neurons in the Nacc shell mediate aversion-related cognition.
  - Addictive drugs have a larger effect on dopamine release in the shell than in the core.
- Core
  - cognitive processing of motor function related to reward and reinforcement
  - encodes new motor programs which facilitate the acquisition of a given reward in the future
  - mediate general Pavlovian-instrumental transfer

Chorea
- Involuntary, arrhythmic movements of a forcible, rapid jerky type
  - Involves distal parts of extremities
  - Tongue movements, facial grimacing

Athetosis
- Slow, sinuous, involuntary movements
  - Extremities, face and tongue

Dystonia
- Slow, sustained, involuntary movements or postures
  - Large muscles of the trunk and limb girdle

Ballism
- Flinging and violent movements
  - Proximal extremities
  - Unilateral (hemiballism)

Parkinsonism
- Hypokinesia
  - Slowness of movement
- Rigidity
  - Resistance to passive movement
- Tremor
  - Rhythmic oscillation (4–6 Hz) between agonist and antagonist

14.10 Thalamus

Important functions of the organism are regulated by and coordinated in the thalamus (Tables 14.10 and 14.11). It is a relay station for afferent nerve fibers. The information carried by these fibers is filtered and processed in the thalamus and, subsequently, conducted to the cerebral cortex. Thus, the electrical activity of the cortex is regulated. Furthermore, the thalamus contains relay stations for nerve fibers from the basal ganglia and the cerebellum. It also fulfills some integrative functions of the motor system.

Clinical manifestations
- Sensory disturbances
  - Sensory loss and/or pain
  - Paresthesias
  - Ventral posterior nucleus
- Motor disturbances
  - Hemiataxia
  - Action tremor
  - Choreoathetosis
  - Ventral anterior and ventral lateral nuclei
- Disturbances of alertness
  - Intralaminar nuclei
  - Disconnection of
    - Ascending reticular activating system
- Disturbances of mood and affect
  - Apathy
  - Disinterest
  - Lack of initiative and drive
  - Anterior and dorsomedial nuclei
  - Disconnection between
    - Thalamus and limbic system
    - Thalamus and frontal cortex
- Disturbances of memory
  - Anterograde amnesia
  - Dorsomedial nucleus
- Visual disturbances
  - Contralateral hemianopsia
  - Lateral geniculate body
- Autonomic disturbances
  - Kleine–Levin syndrome
- Disturbances of complex sensorimotor functions
  - Motor neglect
  - Thalamic aphasia
  - Prosopoaffective agnosia
- Disturbances of executive function

Table 14.10 Functions of specific thalamic nuclei

Nucleus	Function
Anterior nucleus	• Affective and emotional states • Memory • Alertness
Ventral anterior and ventral lateral nuclei	• Relay motor information from basal ganglia and cerebellum to cortex
Ventral posterior nucleus	• Affective and emotional states • Memory • Touch, pain, temperature, itch, taste, arousal, body position
Centromedian nucleus	• Extrapyramidal motor system
Reticular nucleus	• Modulates influence that thalamus exerts on cortex
Midline nucleus	• Unknown
Lateral-dorsal nucleus	• Affective and emotional states
Lateral-posterior nucleus	• Sensory processing
Pulvinar thalami	• Sensory processing
Dorsomedial nucleus	• Affective and emotional states • Memory
Lateral geniculate body	• Visual processing
Medial geniculate body	• Auditory processing

Table 14.11 Thalamic regions associated with clinical dysfunctions

Thalamic region	Clinical function
Anterior thalamic region	• Language disturbances • Inattention • Akinesia • Amnesia • Attentional disturbances
Medial thalamic region	• Impairment of recent memory • Apathy • Agitation • Somnolence • Coma
Ventrolateral thalamic region	• Sensory loss • Paroxysmal pain • Hemiataxia • Postural abnormalities
Posterior thalamic region	• Hemianesthesia • Thalamic pain • Visual field defects • Attentional disorder

14.11 Hypothalamus

The hypothalamus regulates functions of metabolism, body temperature, sleep, and emotional behavior (Table 14.12).

Autonomic functions:
- Cardiovascular regulation
- Regulation of body temperature
- Regulation of water balance
- Regulation of food intake

Endocrine functions:
- Regulation of water balance
- Regulation of reproductive functions

Table 14.12 Lesions in various regions of the hypothalamus and the resulting dysfunctions

Hypothalamic region	Clinical finding
Anterior hypothalamus	• Hypothermia • Insomnia • Diabetes insipidus • Emaciation
Posterior hypothalamus	• Hypothermia • Poikilothermia • Hypersomnia, coma • Apathy • Ipsilateral Horner syndrome
Medial hypothalamus	• Hyperdipsia • Diabetes insipidus • Syndrome of inappropriate antidiuretic hormone • Secretion • Obesity • Amnesia • Rage • Dwarfism
Arcuate nucleus and infundibulum	• Hypopituitarism
Lateral hypothalamus	• Adipsia • Emaciation • Apathy
Pituitary gland	• Visual field defects • Headache • Decreased hormonal action • Dwarfism • Hypogonadism • Hypothyroidism • Glucocorticoid deficiency • Excessive hormonal secretion • Cushing syndrome • Gigantism (Child) • Acromegaly (Adult) • Hyperprolactinemia

Emotional behavior
- Physiological expression of emotional states
  - Lateral hypothalamus
    - Stimulation: rage and fear
    - Lesions: passive behavior
  - Ventromedial hypothalamus
    - Stimulation: placidity and tameness
    - Lesions: aggressiveness and rage

Clinical manifestations (Brazis et al. 2016)
- Disturbances of temperature regulation
  - Hypothermia
  - Hyperthermia
  - Poikilothermia
- Disturbances of alertness and sleep
  - Hypersomnia
  - Narcolepsy
  - Insomnia
  - Circadian abnormalities
- Autonomic disturbances
  - Cardiac
  - Pulmonary
  - Gastrointestinal
  - "Diencephalic epilepsy"
  - Anhidrosis
- Disturbances of water balance
  - Diabetes insipidus
  - Inappropriate secretion of antidiuretic hormone
  - Essential hypernatremia
  - Reset osmostat hyponatremia
  - Primary hyperdipsia
- Disturbances of caloric balance
  - Obesity
  - Emaciation
- Disturbances of reproductive functions
  - Hypogonadotropic hypogonadism
  - Nonpuerperal galactorrhea
  - Precocious puberty
  - Uncontrollable sexual behavior
- Disturbances of memory
- Disturbances of emotional behavior and affect
  - Rage and fear
  - Apathy and chronic fatigue
  - Depression
- Gelastic seizures
- Impaired visual acuity, field defects
- Diplopia, papillary changes
- Headache

14.12 Cerebellum

The cerebellum is functionally concerned with the coordination of locomotion, the control of muscle tone, and the regulation of equilibrium (Table 14.13).

Clinical signs of cerebellar disease are grouped into:

- Symptoms of cerebellar disease
  - Headache
  - Nausea and vomiting
  - Gait difficulties
  - Vertigo
- Signs of midline cerebellar disease
  - Gait difficulties
  - Truncal imbalance

Table 14.13 Functional deficits of cerebellar lesions based on location, modified after Catani and Thiebaut de Schotten (2012)

Localization	Function	Clinical manifestations
Anterior lobe and vermis	• Motor	• Gait ataxia • Limb ataxia • Dysarthric speech • Intention tremor • Hypotonia
Flocculo-nodular lobe	• Vestibular	• Vertigo • Nausea • Nystagmus • Gait ataxia
Posterior cerebellum	• Cognition	• Inattentiveness • Distractibility • Hyperactivity • Perseveration • Impulsiveness • Disinhibition • Difficulty shifting focus of attention • Reduced verbal fluency
Posterior cerebellum	• Thought • Personality • Social behavior	• Obsessional thinking • Compulsive and ritualistic behavior • Thought disorders and paranoid delusions • Oppositional behavior • Disinhibition • Passivity • Immaturity • Childishness • Difficulty with social interactions • Unawareness of social cues or boundaries • Overly gullible and trusting behavior
Flocculo-nodular lobe	• Emotion	• Lability • Incongruous feelings • Pathological laughing and crying • Anxiety • Agitation • Irritability • Anger • Aggression • Flattened affect • Emotional blunting • Apathy • Anhedonia • Depression

- Abnormal head posture
- Ocular motor dysfunction
• Signs of lateral (hemispheric) cerebellar disease
  - Hypotonia
  - Dysarthria
  - Limb ataxia
  - Intention tremor
  - Impaired check and excessive rebound
  - Oculomotor disorders

14.13 White Matter

Although white matter represents a large amount of brain tissue, its significance in the clinical setting has only been investigated in detail during the last decades (Tables 14.14, 14.15, 14.16, 14.17, and 14.18).

Table 14.14 Main white matter bundles and the resulting dysfunctions

Structure	Function/dysfunction
Superior longitudinal fasciculus	• SFL I: regulate motor behavior, conditional associative tasks • SFL II: perception of visual space, spatial attention regulate selection and retrieval of spatial information • SFL III: transfers somatosensory information (language articulation)
Arcuate fasciculus	• Interconnects Wernicke receptive language area with Broca's expressive language area • Conduction aphasia
Uncinate fasciculus	• Autonoetic self-awareness (right uncinate fasciculus) • Proficiency in auditory-verbal memory and declarative memory (left uncinate fasciculus) • Social anxiety, Alzheimer disease, bipolar disorder, depression
Anterior commissure	• Interhemispheric exchange of information • Between one anterior olfactory nucleus and the contralateral olfactory bulb

Table 14.15 Clinical presentations caused by lesions affecting the *perisylvian white matter*, modified after Catani and Thiebaut de Schotten (2012)

Tracts involved	Symptoms	Clinical presentation
Anterior and long segment	Broca's aphasia	• Non-fluent speech • Impaired repetition • Intact comprehension
Posterior and long segment	Wernicke's aphasia	• Impaired auditory comprehension and repetition • Fluent speech
Long segment	Conduction aphasia	• Repetition deficits • Paraphasias • Relatively intact comprehension and fluency
Anterior segment	Transcortical motor aphasia	• Impaired fluency • Intact repetition and comprehension
Posterior segment	Transcortical sensory	• Impaired comprehension • Intact fluency and repetition
Anterior, posterior, and long segments	Global aphasia	• Severe deficit in language comprehension, production, and repetition
Posterior segment	Pure alexia	• Acquired reading impairment often associated with color agnosia • Spontaneous writing and writing to dictation are preserved
Anterior segment, posterior segment	Dyslexia	• Developmental reading difficulties
Anterior segment	Dysgraphia	• Deficits in spontaneous writing and on dictation
Anterior, posterior, and long segments	Working memory deficits	• Impaired digit span

Table 14.15 (continued)

Tracts involved	Symptoms	Clinical presentation
Anterior and posterior segments	Apraxia	• Loss of the ability to perform voluntary skilled movements without sensorimotor deficits
Right hemisphere		
Anterior, posterior, and long segments SLF II	Unilateral spatial neglect	• Failure to respond or reorient to novel meaningful stimuli presented to the left hemispace
Anterior segment, long segment	Expressive amusia	• Inability to play a previously learned instrument • Loss of the ability to write musical annotations
Posterior segment, long segment	Receptive amusia	• Difficulties to recognize out-of-tune notes, familiar melodies, or read musical annotations
Anterior segment, long segment	Anterior affective-aprosodia	• Flatness of speech and loss of gestural abilities involving the face and limbs
Posterior segment, long segment	Posterior affective-aprosodia	• Inability to comprehend or repeat emotional gestures and discern speech intonation

Table 14.16 Clinical presentations caused by lesions affecting the early visual pathways matter, modified after Catani and Thiebaut de Schotten (2012)

Lesion location	Disorder	Disorder description
• Optic radiations • Calcarine cortex	• Visual field defects (scotoma, quadrantanopsia, hemianopsia)	• A partial of vision in a small region of the visual field (scotoma), a single quadrant (quadrantanopsia), or an entire hemifield (hemianopsia). • The visual deficit is always opposite to the lesion (e.g., left hemifield due to a right calcarine lesion). • A left or right upper quadrantanopsia is indicative of a lesion to the Flechsig-Meyer loop.
	• Cortical blindness	• Complete visual loss due to extensive bilateral occipital lesions. Some patients maintain the ability to consciously perceive and discriminate visual motion in their otherwise blind visual field when stimulated with fast motion (Riddoch phenomenon). Rarely the blind patient denies his visual deficit and gives confabulatory responses (Anton syndrome).
	• Aperceptive agnosia	• Inability to recognize, discriminate, or copy objects in a patient with otherwise normal visual ability. • Lesions are always close to the primary visual area or its connections to neighboring gyri.
	• Simple hallucinations (or phosphenes)	• Spontaneous of activity in the primary visual cortex due to local irritative pathology (e.g., epilepsy), or a distant hodological effect (e.g., de-afferentation caused by eye disease in Charles Bonnet syndrome).

14.13 White Matter

Table 14.17 Clinical presentations caused by lesions affecting the white matter of the ventral and dorsal visual pathways matter, modified after Catani and Thiebaut de Schotten (2012)

Lesion location	Disorder	Disorder description
• Ventral visual stream (specialized for objects, patterns, colors, faces, body parts, and words)	• Object agnosia • Achromatopsia • Prosopagnosia • Alexia	• Inability to recognize objects, colors, faces, and words due to de-afferentation or direct lesion of the specialized areas.
	• Object, color, face, text illusion/hallucination, visual functional hallucinations	• Hyperactivity of specialized cortex can cause visual of distorted objects (metamorphosias), faces (prosopmetamorphopsias), or text. Objects can appear larger (macropsia), smaller (micropsia), nearer (pelopsia), or further away (teleopsia). Seeing objects, colors, faces, or letters in the absence of a real visual stimulus can present spontaneously or sometimes can be triggered by a normal visual percept (functional hallucinations).
• Dorsal visual stream (specialized for motion, spatial coordinates, and depth)	• Akinetopsia	• Loss of motion vision following lesions of lateral occipital motion-specialized cortex. Lesions disconnection motion-specialized cortex and coordinate frames in the parietal lobe may present with "cinematographic vision," where moving objects appear as a series of static freeze frames at different spatial locations.
	• Illusions and hallucinations of object position and movement	• Increased perceptual activity within dorsal an lateral occipital and parietal cortex can manifest with distorted perception of multiple copies of the same object (polyopia), objects remaining fixed in retinal coordinates with eye movements (visual perseveration), or a pattern spreading from an object to it surrounds (illusory visual spread). Hallucinations typically involve moving objects (motion hallucination) and person or animals that pass sideways out of the visual field (passage hallucination).

Table 14.18 Clinical presentations caused by lesions affecting the white matter of extended visual pathways matter, modified after Catani and Thiebaut de Schotten (2012)

Lesion location	Disorder	Disorder description
• Perisylvian language and motor regions, limbic areas, frontal cortex (arcuate fasciculus, cingulum inferior fronto-occipital fasciculus, inferior longitudinal fasciculus, superior longitudinal fasciculus)	• Color and object anomia	• Disconnection of visual language areas results in specific deficits of color or object naming.
	• Visual amnesia	• Memory deficit for visually presented material due to a lesion of the inferior longitudinal fasciculus disconnecting visual areas and hippocampus.
	• Visual hypo-emotionality • Visual de-realization • Capgras syndrome • Fear recognition deficits	• These disconnection syndromes follow damage to the fibers of the inferior longitudinal and inferior fronto-occipital fasciculus connecting visual areas and anterior limbic structures (e.g., amygdala and orbitofrontal cortex). The patients report lack of emotional response to images (visual hypo-emotionality) or threatening situations (fear recognition deficits). Others complain of visual experiences being unreal (de-realization) or faces of known persons having been replaced by impostors (Capgras syndrome).

Table 14.18 (continued)

Lesion location	Disorder	Disorder description
	• Visual imagery deficits • Visual anoneria	• Inability to retrieve visual mental representations either during the day or while dreaming.
	• Hemispatial visual neglect	• Lesions of the inferior longitudinal fasciculus or inferior fronto-occipital fasciculus disconnecting visual areas and right frontoparietal visuospatial network manifesting with a failure to respond or reorient to novel or meaningful stimuli presented to the left hemispace.
	• Imitative an oculomotor apraxia • Utilization behavior • Optic apraxia	• Disconnection between motor and visual areas can result in the inability to imitate actions (imitative apraxia) or in the automatic use of objects placed within the field of view and reach (utilization behavior). Balint syndrome is a degenerative disorder characterized by simultagnosia, optic ataxia, and aculomotor apraxia.
	• Synaesthesia across sensory modalities • Reflex hallucinations	• A percept in one sensory modality evoking a parallel percept usually in a different sensory modality (e.g., seeing colored music) due to abnormal hyperconnectivity between distant sensory regions. Sometimes the percept triggers reflex hallucinations in a different modality (e.g., seeing a butterfly whenever the thumb is touched).
	• Flashbacks • Memory hallucinations • Phobias • Fregoli phenomenon	• A wide range of disorders related to hyperconnectivity between visual and limbic areas resulting in an excessive emotional response to visual perception or memories.

Selected References

Acciarresi M (2012) Agnosia, apraxia, callosal disconnection and other specific cognitive disorders. Front Neurol Neurosci 30:75–78. https://doi.org/10.1159/000333419

Acharya AB, Dulebohn SC (2018a) Aphasia, Broca. In: StatPearls. StatPearls Publishing LLC., Treasure Island

Acharya AB, Dulebohn SC (2018b) Aphasia, Wernicke. In: StatPearls. StatPearls Publishing, LLC., Treasure Island

Anderson CA, Arciniegas DB, Hall DA, Filley CM (2013) Behabioral neuroanatomy. In: Arciniegas DB, Anderson CA, Filley CM (eds) Behavioral neurology & neuropsychiatry. Cambridge University Press, Cambridge, pp 12–31

Bartolo A, Ham HS (2016) A cognitive overview of limb apraxia. Curr Neurol Neurosci Rep 16(8):75. https://doi.org/10.1007/s11910-016-0675-0

Boukrina O, Barrett AM (2017) Disruption of the ascending arousal system and cortical attention networks in post-stroke delirium and spatial neglect. Neurosci Biobehav Rev 83:1–10. https://doi.org/10.1016/j.neubiorev.2017.09.024

Brazis P, Masdeu JC, Biller J (2016) Localization in clinical neurology, 7th edn. Lippincott Williams & Wilkinson, Philadelphia

Cahana-Amitay D, Albert ML (2015) Neuroscience of aphasia recovery: the concept of neural multifunctionality. Curr Neurol Neurosci Rep 15(7):41. https://doi.org/10.1007/s11910-015-0568-7

Caro MA, Jimenez XF (2016) Mesiotemporal disconnection and hypoactivity in Kluver-Bucy syndrome: case series and literature review. J Clin Psychiatry 77(8):e982–e988. https://doi.org/10.4088/JCP.14r09497

Catani M, Thiebaut de Schotten M (2012) Atlas of human brain connections. Oxford University Press, Oxford

Corbetta M (2014) Hemispatial neglect: clinic, pathogenesis, and treatment. Semin Neurol 34(5):514–523. https://doi.org/10.1055/s-0034-1396005

Crinion JT, Leff AP (2015) Using functional imaging to understand therapeutic effects in poststroke aphasia. Curr Opin Neurol 28(4):330–337. https://doi.org/10.1097/wco.0000000000000217

de Freitas GR (2012) Aphasia and other language disorders. Front Neurol Neurosci 30:41–45. https://doi.org/10.1159/000333402

Ellis C, Urban S (2016) Age and aphasia: a review of presence, type, recovery and clinical outcomes. Top Stroke Rehabil 23(6):430–439. https://doi.org/10.1080/10749357.2016.1150412

Enderby P (2013) Disorders of communication: dysarthria. Handb Clin Neurol 110:273–281. https://doi.org/10.1016/b978-0-444-52901-5.00022-8

Selected References

Foundas AL (2013) Apraxia: neural mechanisms and functional recovery. Handb Clin Neurol 110:335–345. https://doi.org/10.1016/b978-0-444-52901-5.00028-9

Goldenberg G (2009) Apraxia and the parietal lobes. Neuropsychologia 47(6):1449–1459. https://doi.org/10.1016/j.neuropsychologia.2008.07.014

Gorno-Tempini ML, Hillis AE, Weintraub S, Kertesz A, Mendez M, Cappa SF, Ogar JM, Rohrer JD, Black S, Boeve BF, Manes F, Dronkers NF, Vandenberghe R, Rascovsky K, Patterson K, Miller BL, Knopman DS, Hodges JR, Mesulam MM, Grossman M (2011) Classification of primary progressive aphasia and its variants. Neurology 76(11):1006–1014. https://doi.org/10.1212/WNL.0b013e31821103e6

Gross RG, Grossman M (2008) Update on apraxia. Curr Neurol Neurosci Rep 8(6):490–496

Harris JM, Jones M (2014) Pathology in primary progressive aphasia syndromes. Curr Neurol Neurosci Rep 14(8):466. https://doi.org/10.1007/s11910-014-0466-4

Heilman KM (2014) Possible mechanisms of anosognosia of hemiplegia. Cortex 61:30–42. https://doi.org/10.1016/j.cortex.2014.06.007

Heimer L (1983) The human brain and spinal cord: functional neuroanatomy and dissection guide. Springer, Berlin

Hillis AE (2006) Neurobiology of unilateral spatial neglect. The Neuroscientist: a review journal bringing neurobiology. Fortschr Neurol Psychiatr 12(2):153–163. https://doi.org/10.1177/1073858405284257

Husain M (2008) Hemispatial neglect. Handb Clin Neurol 88:359–372. https://doi.org/10.1016/s0072-9752(07)88018-3

Jordan LC, Hillis AE (2006) Disorders of speech and language: aphasia, apraxia and dysarthria. Curr Opin Neurol 19(6):580–585. https://doi.org/10.1097/WCO.0b013e3280109260

Jung Y, Duffy JR, Josephs KA (2013) Primary progressive aphasia and apraxia of speech. Semin Neurol 33(4):342–347. https://doi.org/10.1055/s-0033-1359317

Karnath HO, Rorden C (2012) The anatomy of spatial neglect. Neuropsychologia 50(6):1010–1017. https://doi.org/10.1016/j.neuropsychologia.2011.06.027

Kertesz A, Harciarek M (2014) Primary progressive aphasia. Scand J Psychol 55(3):191–201. https://doi.org/10.1111/sjop.12105

Kolb B, Whishaw IQ (2015) Fundamentals of Neuropsychology. Worth Publishers, 7th edition

Li K, Malhotra PA (2015) Spatial neglect. Pract Neurol 15(5):333–339. https://doi.org/10.1136/practneurol-2015-001115

Lippe S, Gonin-Flambois C, Jambaque I (2013) The neuropsychology of the Kluver-Bucy syndrome in children. Handb Clin Neurol 112:1285–1288. https://doi.org/10.1016/b978-0-444-52910-7.00051-9

Marien P, van Dun K, Verhoeven J (2015) Cerebellum and apraxia. Cerebellum (London, England) 14(1):39–42. https://doi.org/10.1007/s12311-014-0620-1

Milner AD, McIntosh RD (2005) The neurological basis of visual neglect. Curr Opin Neurol 18(6):748–753

Park JE (2017) Apraxia: review and update. J Clin Neurol (Seoul, Korea) 13(4):317–324. https://doi.org/10.3988/jcn.2017.13.4.317

Petreska B, Adriani M, Blanke O, Billard AG (2007) Apraxia: a review. Prog Brain Res 164:61–83. https://doi.org/10.1016/s0079-6123(07)64004-7

Pia L, Neppi-Modona M, Ricci R, Berti A (2004) The anatomy of anosognosia for hemiplegia: a meta-analysis. Cortex 40(2):367–377

Prigatano GP (2009) Anosognosia: clinical and ethical considerations. Curr Opin Neurol 22(6):606–611. https://doi.org/10.1097/WCO.0b013e328332a1e7

Ptak R, Fellrath J (2013) Spatial neglect and the neural coding of attentional priority. Neurosci Biobehav Rev 37(4):705–722. https://doi.org/10.1016/j.neubiorev.2013.01.026

Radanovic M, Mansur LL (2017) Aphasia in vascular lesions of the basal ganglia: a comprehensive review. Brain Lang 173:20–32. https://doi.org/10.1016/j.bandl.2017.05.003

Rampello L, Rampello L, Patti F, Zappia M (2016) When the word doesn't come out: a synthetic overview of dysarthria. J Neurol Sci 369:354–360. https://doi.org/10.1016/j.jns.2016.08.048

Rode G, Fourtassi M, Pagliari C, Pisella L, Rossetti Y (2017) Complexity vs. unity in unilateral spatial neglect. Rev Neurol 173(7–8):440–450. https://doi.org/10.1016/j.neurol.2017.07.010

Rosen HJ (2011) Anosognosia in neurodegenerative disease. Neurocase 17(3):231–241. https://doi.org/10.1080/13554794.2010.522588

Spencer KA, Slocomb DL (2007) The neural basis of ataxic dysarthria. Cerebellum (London, England) 6(1):58–65. https://doi.org/10.1080/14734220601145459

Thiel A, Zumbansen A (2016) The pathophysiology of post-stroke aphasia: a network approach. Restor Neurol Neurosci 34(4):507–518. https://doi.org/10.3233/rnn-150632

Tippett DC (2015) Update in aphasia research. Curr Neurol Neurosci Rep 15(8):49. https://doi.org/10.1007/s11910-015-0573-x

Tippett DC, Hillis AE (2017) Where are aphasia theory and management "headed"? F1000Res 6. https://doi.org/10.12688/f1000research.11122.1

Turnbull OH, Fotopoulou A, Solms M (2014) Anosognosia as motivated unawareness: the 'defence' hypothesis revisited. Cortex 61:18–29. https://doi.org/10.1016/j.cortex.2014.10.008

Wilson RS, Sytsma J, Barnes LL, Boyle PA (2016) Anosognosia in dementia. Curr Neurol Neurosci Rep 16(9):77. https://doi.org/10.1007/s11910-016-0684-z

Ziegler W, Aichert I, Staiger A (2012) Apraxia of speech: concepts and controversies. J Speech Lang Hear Res 55(5):S1485–S1501. https://doi.org/10.1044/1092-4388(2012/12-0128

Part III

The Brain Diseases: Edema and Hydrocephalus

Brain Edema: Intracranial Pressure—Herniation

15.1 Definition

Increase in brain volume due to a localized or diffuse abnormal accumulation of water and sodium within the brain parenchyma. The term "brain edema" can interchangeably be used with the term "brain swelling."

Based on the pathogenesis, the following types of edema are distinguished:

- Vasogenic edema
- Cytotoxic edema
- Hydrocephalic or interstitial edema
- Osmotic edema

15.2 Epidemiology

Vasogenic edema
- Represents the most common form of edema
- Encountered in:
  - Brain tumors
  - Abscesses
  - Hemorrhage
  - Infarction
  - Contusion

Cytotoxic edema
- Encountered in:
  - Cerebral ischemia (focal or global)
  - Traumatic brain injury
  - Infections
  - Metabolic disorders

Hydrocephalic edema
- Non-communicating hydrocephalus

Osmotic edema
- Hypo-osmolar conditions
  - Improper administration of intravenous fluids leading to acute dilutional hyponatremia
  - Inappropriate antidiuretic hormone secretion
  - Excessive hemodialysis of uremic patients
  - Diabetic ketoacidosis

Age Incidence
- Any age

Sex Incidence
- No preference

15.3 Localization

Vasogenic edema
- white matter

15.4 General Imaging Findings

Edema: General or focal brain swelling with consecutive effacement of sulci and compression of ventricles and/or basal cisterns.

Herniation: Increased intracranial pressure leads to herniation of brain parenchyma from its normal location into an adjacent space.

CT non-contrast-enhanced (Figs. 15.1a, b, 15.2a, b, and 15.3)

- Effacement of sulci and compressed ventricles and/or basal cisterns
- Vasogenic edema: white matter predominantly affected
- Cytotoxic edema: pronounced in gray matter, loss of gray/white matter differentiation
- Complications of cerebral edema: herniation, infarction due to compressed vessels

CT contrast-enhanced
- Enhancement if blood–brain barrier breaks down

MRI-T2 (Figs. 15.4a and 15.5a)
- Edema hyperintense

MRI-FLAIR (Figs. 15.4b and 15.5b)
- Edema hyperintense

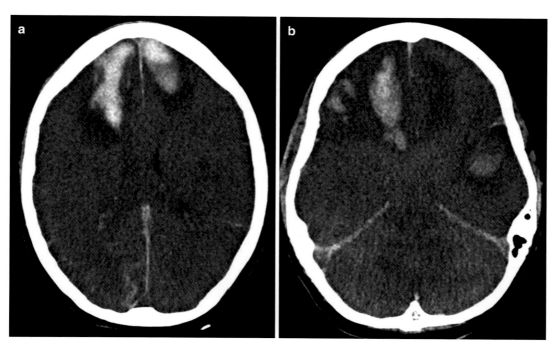

Fig. 15.1 General posttraumatic brain swelling (CT)—effacement of sulci and compressed ventricles (**a**), compressed basal cisterns (**b**)

15.4 General Imaging Findings

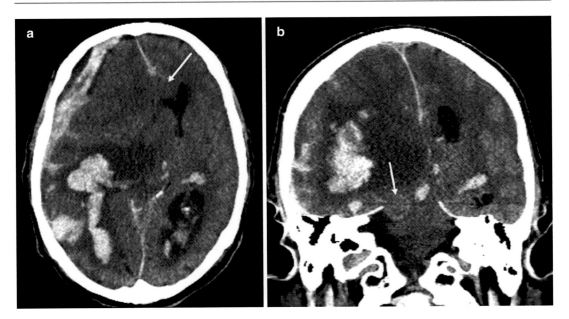

Fig. 15.2 Traumatic SDH and intracerebral hematomas with subfalcial (arrow) (**a**) and transtentorial (arrow) (**b**) herniation; CT axial (**a**) and coronal (**b**)

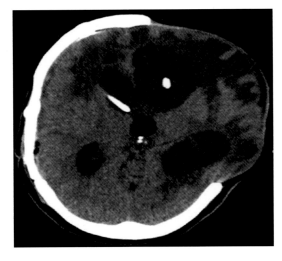

Fig. 15.3 Transcalvarial herniation (CT)

MRI-T1 (Figs. 15.4c and 15.5c)
- Edema hypointense

MRI-T1 contrast-enhanced (Figs. 15.4d, e and 15.5d)
- Impaired blood–brain barrier leads to enhancement

MRI-T2∗/SWI
- May detect associated hemorrhage

MR-Diffusion Imaging (Figs. 15.4f, g and 15.5e, f)
- DWI + ADC best imaging tool to differentiate between vasogenic and cytotoxic edema
- Vasogenic edema: no restricted diffusion, high signal in ADC

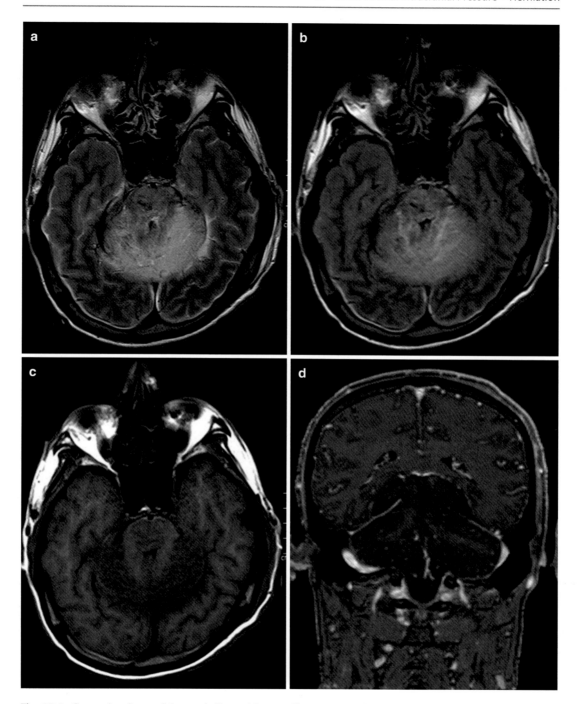

Fig. 15.4 Cytotoxic edema of the cerebellum with ascending transtentorial herniation; T2 (**a**), FLAIR (**b**), T1 (**c**), T1-contrast coronal (**d**) and sagittal (**e**), DWI (**f**) and ADC (**g**) demonstrate restricted diffusion

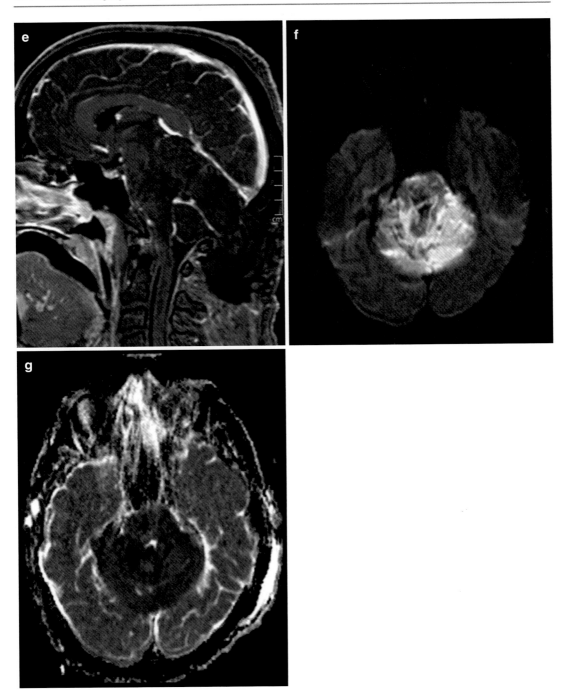

Fig. 15.4 (continued)

- Cytotoxic edema: restricted diffusion with decreased ADC

MRI-Perfusion
- Perfusion may be decreased due to increasing intracranial pressure

MR-Diffusion Tensor Imaging
- Decreased anisotropy

MR-Spectroscopy
- Low NAA values
- Increased choline values

Nuclear Medicine Imaging Findings (Fig. 15.6)
- There is usually no indication for nuclear medicine diagnostics.
- In brain tumors, the effect of brain edema on the gray matter can be seen as a distinct reduction of FDG uptake.
- Measuring intracranial pressure can be used in the diagnosis of brain death. Thus, after brain death, the intracranial pressure is elevated and if it reaches a level that exceeds that of blood pressure, no uptake of a CBF agent is seen.

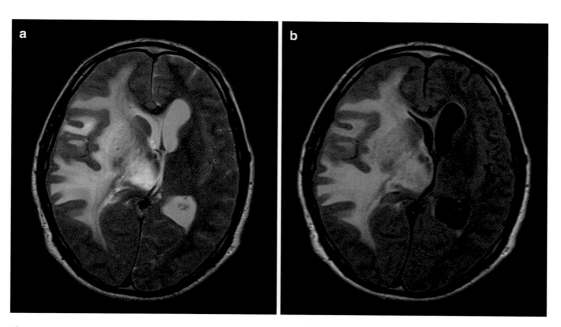

Fig. 15.5 Peritumoral vasogenic edema predominantly affecting white matter; T2 (**a**), FLAIR (**b**), T1 (**c**), enhancing tumor (glioblastoma multiforme) on T1-contrast (**d**), DWI (**e**) and ADC (**f**) without restricted diffusion

15.4 General Imaging Findings

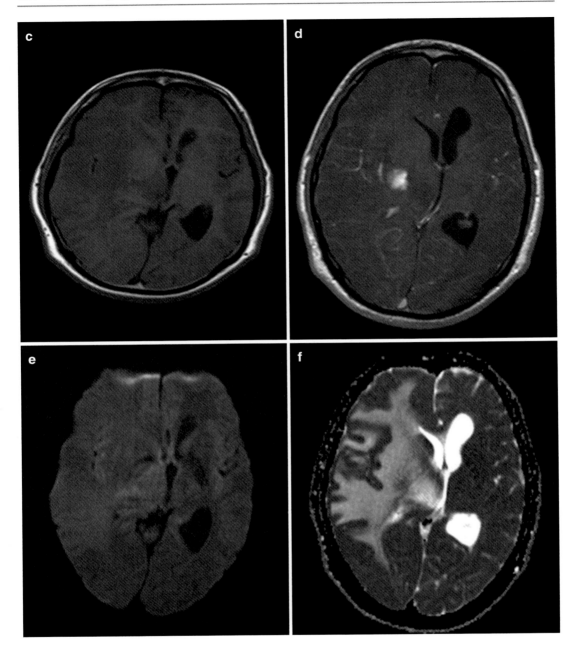

Fig. 15.5 (continued)

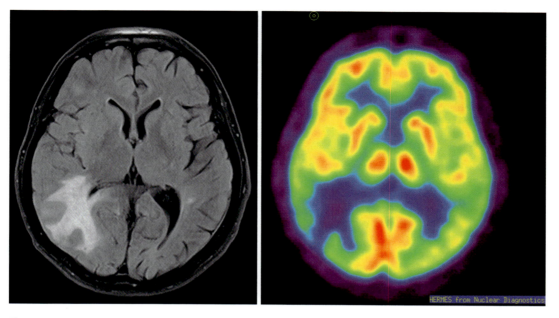

Fig. 15.6 Effect of brain edema in a patient with right temporal non-Hodgkin lymphoma and granulomatous inflammation. Co-registered MRI FLAIR and FDG-PET

15.5 Neuropathology Findings

Macroscopic Features (Figs. 15.7, 15.8, 15.9, 15.10, and 15.11)

The edematous brain shows:

- Softer consistency
- Larger size
- Heavier weight
- Flattened gyri
- Narrowed sulci
- Slit-like ventricles

In case of severe brain edema, the following signs of herniation can be observed:

- *Transtentorial herniation*: Tentorial (uncal or lateral transtentorial) herniation (Fig. 15.7)

– The most frequent and important herniation phenomenon.
– Increasing lesion above the cerebellar tentorium.
– Herniation of the hippocampal formation and uncus of the parahippocampal gyrus over the edge of the tentorium, i.e., "uncal herniation."
– Focal necrosis associated with hemorrhage can be found.
– If patient survives, local gliosis might develop.
– Increased herniation might lead to the compression of the posterior cerebral artery resulting in incomplete or complete infarction of the medial temporal lobe and/or the medial occipital lobe.
– Compression of the third cranial nerve is possible manifesting as pupillary constric-

15.5 Neuropathology Findings

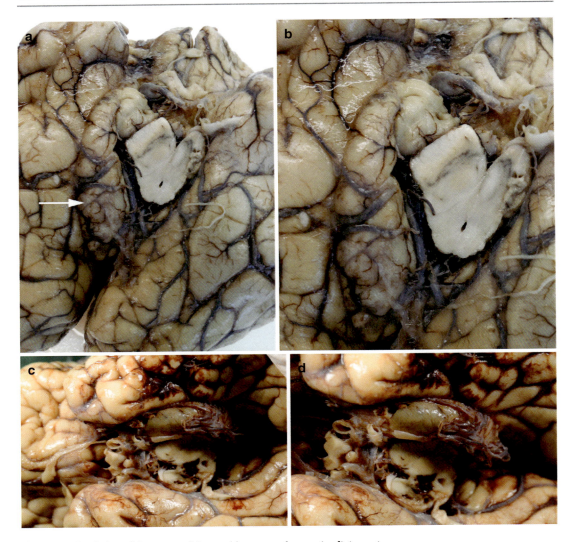

Fig. 15.7 Herniation of the uncus of the parahippocampal gyrus (**a–d**) (arrow)

tion (irritation of the parasympathetic fibers) or pupillary mydriasis (resulting from unopposed sympathetic stimulation).
- **Kernohan's notch**: notching of the brain stem produced by compression against the edge of the tentorium.
- Further downward movement of the midbrain leads to compression of the cerebral aqueduct with narrowing and occlusion leading to hydrocephalus of the third and lateral ventricles.
- **Duret hemorrhages** develop after the midbrain descends through the incisure stretching, shearing, and tearing the sharply angulated upper branches of the basilar artery.

- *Cerebellar tonsillar herniation:* Tonsillar herniation (foraminal impaction, cerebellar cone) (Fig. 15.8)
  - Cerebellar tonsils descend through the foramen magnum leading to a compression of the medulla oblongata with dysfunction of the vital centers of respiration and cardiac rhythmic control.
  - Due to a mass lesion in the posterior fossa, seldom due to a supratentorial mass lesion.
  - Histologically herniated cerebellar tissue shows early changes of infarction while the medulla oblongata shows edema and more advanced stages of tissue death.
- *Subfalcial herniation:* Supracallosal (subfalcine or cingulate) herniation (Fig. 15.9)
  - The medial surface of the hemisphere usually the cingulate gyrus or the supracingulate gyrus is pressed against the rigid midline falx cerebri and herniates under its edge.
  - Occurs in one-sided mass increase of the hemisphere.
  - Focal necrosis associated with hemorrhage can be found.
- *Subarachnoid cerebellar tissue emboli*
  - Herniated cerebellar tissue is shed into the subarachnoidal space through the pia.
  - Can be found as far down as the cauda equina.
  - Often encountered in patients with brain death.
- *Fungus cerebri* (Fig. 15.11)
  - Protrusion of the brain in a mushroom (fungus) way through a defect in the skull resulting from trauma or surgery (decompressive surgery for increased cerebral pressure)
  - Associated with fatal outcome
- *Anterior-to-middle fossa herniation*
  - Inferior aspects of the frontal lobe herniate over the edge of the sphenoid wing into the middle cranial fossa.
- *Upward transtentorial herniation*
  - Superior cerebellum and upper pons are forced through the incisure, compressing the midbrain.
  - Due to a mass lesion in the posterior fossa.
- *Spinal cord herniation*
  - Uncommon phenomenon
  - Movement of spinal cord tissue occurring after myelogram or lumbar puncture

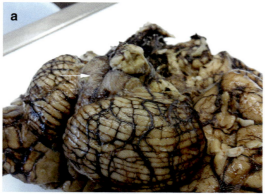
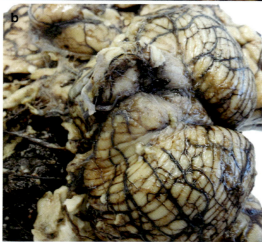
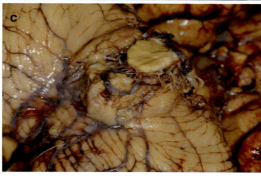

Fig. 15.8 Herniation of the cerebellar tonsils (**a–c**) (arrow)

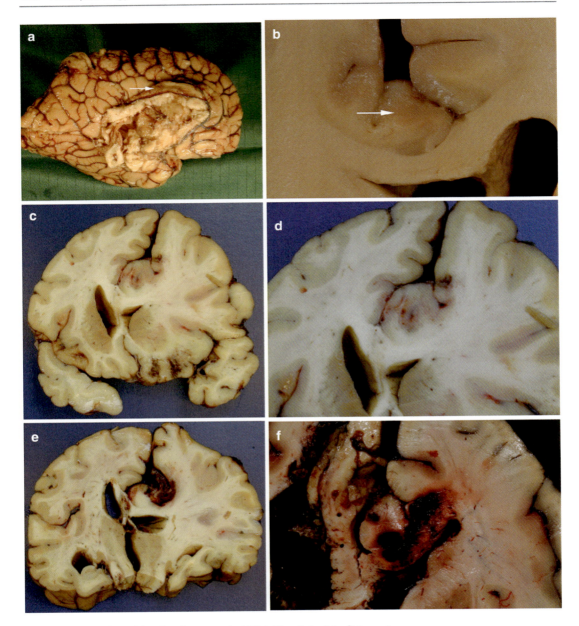

Fig. 15.9 Herniation of the cingulate gyrus (subfalcial herniation) (**a–f**) (arrow)

- Complication of spinal cord tumor, epidural metastatic tumor, or epidural hematoma
- Resulting in paralysis of the lower extremities and bowel and bladder dysfunction

Besides edema, all mass-increasing lesions, i.e., tumor, hemorrhage result in one or more of the above-described herniations.

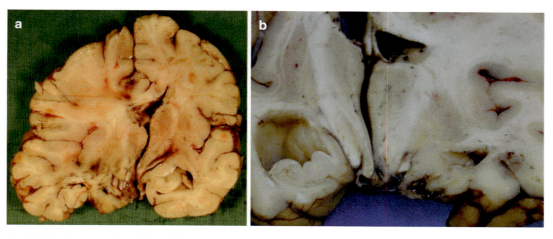

Fig. 15.10 Downward herniation of diencephalic brain regions (**a**, **b**)

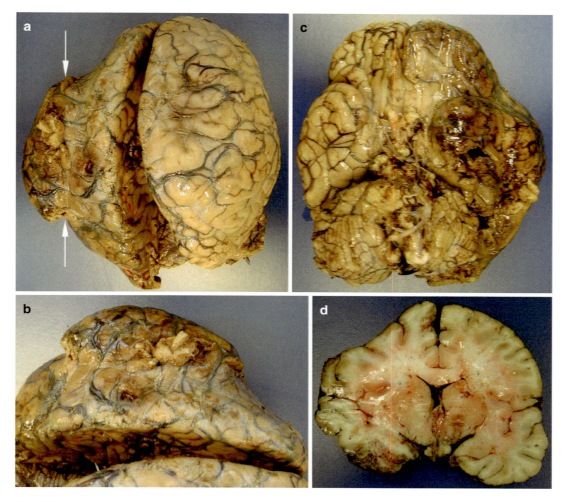

Fig. 15.11 Fungus cerebri (**a–h**)

15.5 Neuropathology Findings

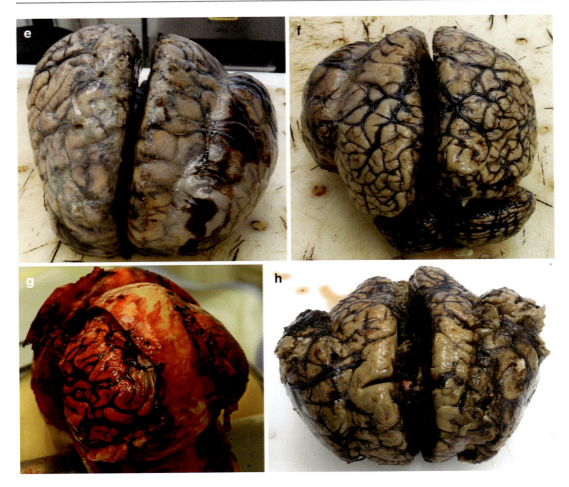

Fig. 15.11 (continued)

15.5.1 Microscopic Features
(Fig. 15.12)

Vasogenic edema (Fig. 15.12a–f)
- Increased permeability of the capillary endothelium
- Extravasation of fluid and plasma proteins (albumin being the major constituent)

Cytotoxic edema (Fig. 15.12a–f)
- Swelling of cellular elements, i.e., endothelia, glia, neurons
- Reduction of the extracellular space

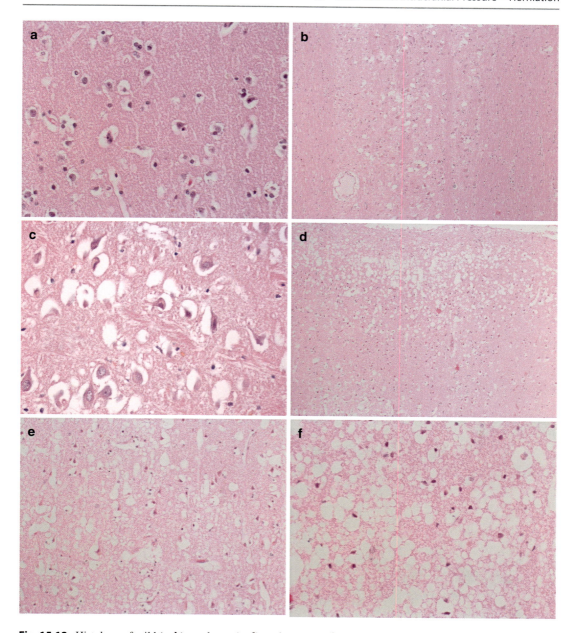

Fig. 15.12 Histology of mild (**a**, **b**), moderate (**c**, **d**), and severe (**e**, **f**) edematous tissue changes

15.5.2 Ultrastructural Features

Vasogenic edema
- Disruption of tight junctions
- Increased number of cytoplasmic vesicles in the endothelial cells

15.6 Molecular Neuropathology

Vasogenic edema
- Breakdown of the blood–brain barrier
- Expansion of the extracellular spaces
- Moves easily between the fibers of the white matter

Cytotoxic edema
- Results from pathological processes that damage cell membranes
- Constricts the extracellular spaces
- Constrains movement of fluid between cells

Injury cascade
- Depletion of energy and glutamate release into the extracellular space (cytotoxic).
- Opening of calcium channels on cell membranes.
- Entry of extracellular calcium into the brain.
- Accumulation of sodium within the cell creates an osmotic gradient that pulls water into the cell.
- Activation of intracellular cytotoxic processes leads to cell death.
  - Initiation of an inflammatory response by formation of immediate early genes and cytokines, chemokines
  - Activation of microglial cells
  - Release of free radicals and proteases

Mediators of brain edema
- Vaso-active agents,
  - i.e., arachidonic acid, bradykinin, complement-derived polypeptide C3a-desArg, glutamate, histamine, interleukins IL-1α, IL-1β, IL-2, leukotrienes, macrophage inflammatory proteins MIP-1, MIP-2, nitric oxide, oxygen-derived free radicals, phospholipase A2, platelet-activating factor, prostaglandins, purine nucleotides ATP, ADP, AMP, thrombin, and serotonin
- Aquaporins
- Matrix metalloproteinases
- Growth factors
  - Vascular endothelial growth factor A (VEGF-A)
  - Vascular endothelial growth factor B (VEGF-B)
- Angiopoietins

15.7 Treatment and Prognosis

Treatment
- Reduction of volume
  - blood volume (hyperventilation)
  - CSF volume (intraventricular drainage)
  - reduce production of CSF
- Osmotic treatment with mannitol
- Corticosteroids
  - in vasogenic edema
  - less effective in cytotoxic edema
  - contraindicated in edema secondary to stroke and hemorrhage
- Hypothermia
- Ventricular drainage
- Surgical cranial decompression (large craniectomy)

Biologic Behavior–Prognosis–Prognostic Factors
- Variable from full recovery to death
- Depends on etiology, duration, and treatment
  Comorbid disease states

Selected References

Adeva MM, Souto G, Donapetry C, Portals M, Rodriguez A, Lamas D (2012) Brain edema in diseases of different etiology. Neurochem Int 61(2):166–174. https://doi.org/10.1016/j.neuint.2012.05.007

Alexander AL, Lee JE, Lazar M, Field AS (2007) Diffusion tensor imaging of the brain. Neurotherapeutics 4(3):316–329. https://doi.org/10.1016/j.nurt.2007.05.011

Butterworth RF (2015) Pathogenesis of hepatic encephalopathy and brain edema in acute liver failure. J Clin Exp Hepatol 5(Suppl 1):S96–S103. https://doi.org/10.1016/j.jceh.2014.02.004

Filippidis AS, Kalani MY, Rekate HL (2012) Hydrocephalus and aquaporins: the role of aquaporin-4. Acta Neurochir Suppl 113:55–58. https://doi.org/10.1007/978-3-7091-0923-6_12

Ho ML, Rojas R, Eisenberg RL (2012) Cerebral edema. AJR Am J Roentgenol 199(3):W258–W273. https://doi.org/10.2214/ajr.11.8081

Jia SW, Liu XY, Wang SC, Wang YF (2016) Vasopressin hypersecretion-associated brain edema formation in ischemic stroke: underlying mechanisms. J Stroke

Cerebrovasc Dis 25(6):1289–1300. https://doi.org/10.1016/j.jstrokecerebrovasdis.2016.02.002

Kahle KT, Simard JM, Staley KJ, Nahed BV, Jones PS, Sun D (2009) Molecular mechanisms of ischemic cerebral edema: role of electroneutral ion transport. Physiology (Bethesda, Md) 24:257–265. https://doi.org/10.1152/physiol.00015.2009

Maegele M, Stuermer EK, Hoeffgen A, Uhlenkueken U, Mautes A, Schaefer N, Lippert-Gruener M, Schaefer U, Hoehn M (2015) Multimodal MR imaging of acute and subacute experimental traumatic brain injury: time course and correlation with cerebral energy metabolites. Acta Radiol Short Rep 4(1):2047981614555142. https://doi.org/10.1177/2047981614555142

Marmarou A (2007) A review of progress in understanding the pathophysiology and treatment of brain edema. Neurosurg Focus 22(5):E1

Michinaga S, Koyama Y (2015) Pathogenesis of brain edema and investigation into anti-edema drugs. Int J Mol Sci 16(5):9949–9975. https://doi.org/10.3390/ijms16059949

Na DG, Kim EY, Ryoo JW, Lee KH, Roh HG, Kim SS, Song IC, Chang KH (2005) CT sign of brain swelling without concomitant parenchymal hypoattenuation: comparison with diffusion- and perfusion-weighted MR imaging. Radiology 235(3):992–948. https://doi.org/10.1148/radiol.2353040571

Nag S, Manias JL, Stewart DJ (2009) Pathology and new players in the pathogenesis of brain edema. Acta Neuropathol 118(2):197–217. https://doi.org/10.1007/s00401-009-0541-0

Platten M, Wick W (2012) Blood-brain barrier and brain edema. Handb Clin Neurol 104:53–62. https://doi.org/10.1016/b978-0-444-52138-5.00005-0

Rama Rao KV, Jayakumar AR, Norenberg MD (2014) Brain edema in acute liver failure: mechanisms and concepts. Metab Brain Dis 29(4):927–936. https://doi.org/10.1007/s11011-014-9502-y

Roth P, Regli L, Tonder M, Weller M (2013) Tumor-associated edema in brain cancer patients: pathogenesis and management. Expert Rev Anticancer Ther 13(11):1319–1325. https://doi.org/10.1586/14737140.2013.852473

Stokum JA, Kurland DB, Gerzanich V, Simard JM (2015) Mechanisms of astrocyte-mediated cerebral edema. Neurochem Res 40(2):317–328. https://doi.org/10.1007/s11064-014-1374-3

Stokum JA, Gerzanich V, Simard JM (2016) Molecular pathophysiology of cerebral edema. J Cereb Blood Flow Metab 36(3):513–538. https://doi.org/10.1177/0271678x15617172

von Kummer R, Dzialowski I (2017) Imaging of cerebral ischemic edema and neuronal death. Neuroradiology 59(6):545–553. https://doi.org/10.1007/s00234-017-1847-6

Wang YF, Parpura V (2016) Central role of maladapted astrocytic plasticity in ischemic brain edema formation. Front Cell Neurosci 10:129. https://doi.org/10.3389/fncel.2016.00129

Winkler EA, Minter D, Yue JK, Manley GT (2016) Cerebral edema in traumatic brain injury: pathophysiology and prospective therapeutic targets. Neurosurg Clin N Am 27(4):473–488. https://doi.org/10.1016/j.nec.2016.05.008

Xi G, Keep RF, Hoff JT (2002) Pathophysiology of brain edema formation. Neurosurg Clin N Am 13(3):371–383

Hydrocephalus 16

The cerebrospinal fluid (CSF) is produced by the choroid plexus.

- CSF production amounts to 0.35 mL/min or 500 mL/24 h.
- The total CSF volume measures 150 mL.
- Renewal of CSF takes place 4–5 times per day.

16.1 Definition

Condition of the brain with altered circulation of the cerebrospinal fluid resulting in an expansion of the ventricular system.

The following types of hydrocephalus are distinguished:

- Non-communicating hydrocephalus
  - Aqueductal stenosis with hydrocephalus
- Communicating hydrocephalus
  - e.g., overproduction of CSF (choroid plexus papilloma)
  - impaired reabsorption of CSF
- Normal pressure hydrocephalus
  - Special form of communication hydrocephalus with normal intracranial pressure

16.2 Clinical Signs and Symptoms

- Aqueductal stenosis with hydrocephalus
  - Headache
  - Gait disturbance
  - Memory impairment
  - Urinary incontinence
- Communicating hydrocephalus
  - Headache
  - Frontal lobe dysfunction
  - Gait disorders
  - Urinary incontinence
  - Increased intracranial pressure
- Normal pressure hydrocephalus
  - Urinary incontinence
  - Gait disorder
  - Cognitive impairment

16.3 Epidemiology

Incidence
- Aqueductal stenosis with hydrocephalus
  - 0.2–0.8 children per 1000 live births
- Communicating hydrocephalus
  - 1–2 per 1000 persons
- Normal pressure hydrocephalus
  - 1 per 2000 persons
  - Elderly: 1 in 200 persons
  - Persons with dementia: 1 in 100 persons

Age Incidence
- Aqueductal stenosis with hydrocephalus
  - Infancy (shortly after birth)
  - Adulthood
- Communicating hydrocephalus
- Normal pressure hydrocephalus

Sex Incidence
- Communicating hydrocephalus
  - No gender difference
- Normal pressure hydrocephalus
  - No gender difference

Localization
- Ventricular system

16.4 General Imaging Findings

Ventriculomegaly with narrowed or normal outer CSF spaces, decompensation leads to transependymal edema

CT non-contrast-enhanced (Fig. 16.1a, b)
- Enlargement of lateral ventricles and third ventricle
- Narrowed outer CSF spaces and basal cisterns in obstructive hydrocephalus
- Normal sulci, enlarged basal cisterns, and Sylvian fissures in normal pressure hydrocephalus (NPH)
- Periventricular hypodensities in case of acute obstruction = transependymal edema
- Thinned corpus callosum
- Widened optic and infundibular recesses of third ventricle

CT contrast-enhanced
- In general no enhancement

MRI-T2 (Figs. 16.1c, g and 16.2a, g)
- Periventricular hyperintensities in case of transependymal edema
- Aqueductal flow void sign in communicating hydrocephalus, absent in aqueductal stenosis

MRI-FLAIR (Figs. 16.1d and 16.2b)
- Periventricular hyperintensities in case of transependymal edema

MRI-T1 (Figs. 16.1e and 16.2c)
- Enlarged third and lateral ventricles

MRI-T1 contrast-enhanced (Figs. 16.1f and 16.2d)
- Leptomeninges may enhance in obstructive hydrocephalus (vascular stasis).

MRI-CISS (Figs. 16.1h and 16.2h)
- Sequence to delineate ventricular system, may detect septa in aqueduct

MR-Spectroscopy
- NPH: elevated lactate values in lateral ventricles compared to other types of dementia

Nuclear Medicine Imaging Findings (Fig. 16.3)
- Historically normal pressure hydrocephalus was addressed by cisternography.
- Later on studies dealing with the assessment of luxury perfusion in hydrocephalus and differentiation between normal pressure hydrocephalus and Alzheimer disease with CBF-SPECT and FDG-PET were published.
- More recent studies showed an increase in global cerebral metabolic rate of glucose after surgery in idiopathic normal pressure hydrocephalus. A correlation between early metabolic changes and clinical symptoms (activities of daily living, cognition, and urinary incontinence) 1 week after surgery was described.
- CBF-SPECT showed significant differences in regional cerebral blood flow 2 weeks after surgery between shunt-effective and shunt-ineffective patients.
- 11C-raclopride-PET demonstrated significant postoperative upregulation of D2 receptors in the nucleus accumbens and dorsal putamen with a significant association with emotional and navigational improvement.

16.2 General Imaging Findings

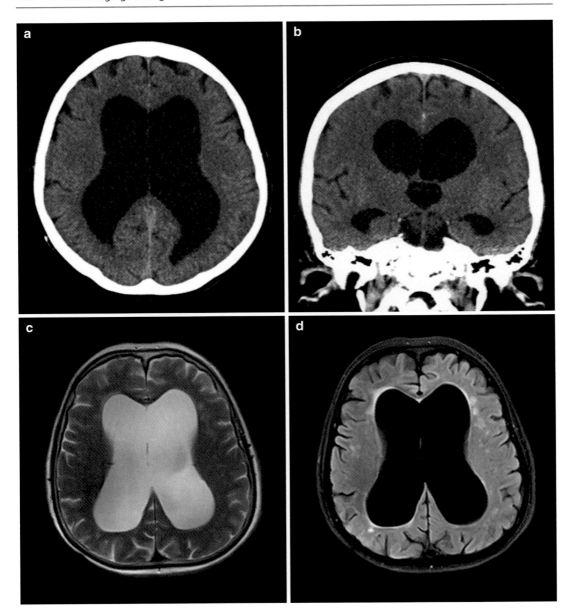

Fig. 16.1 Normal pressure hydrocephalus without transependymal edema, no aqueductal stenosis, aqueductal flow void sign on sagittal T2; CT non-contrast-enhanced axial (**a**) and coronary (**b**), T2 (**c**), FLAIR (**d**), T1 (**e**), T1 contrast (**f**), sagittal T2 (**g**), CISS (**h**)

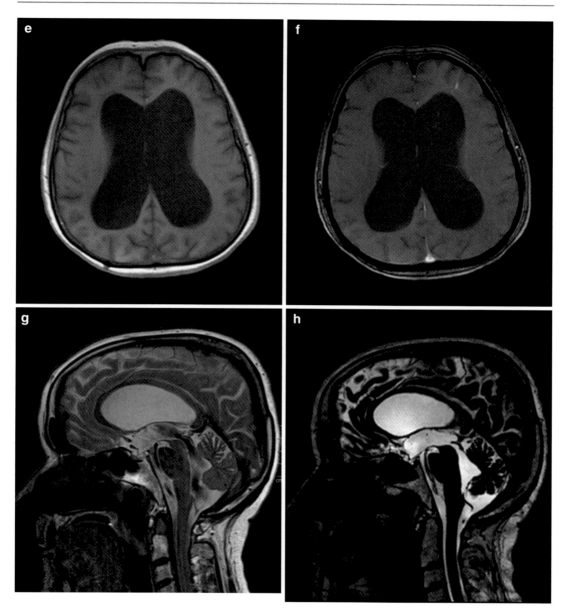

Fig. 16.1 (continued)

16.2 General Imaging Findings

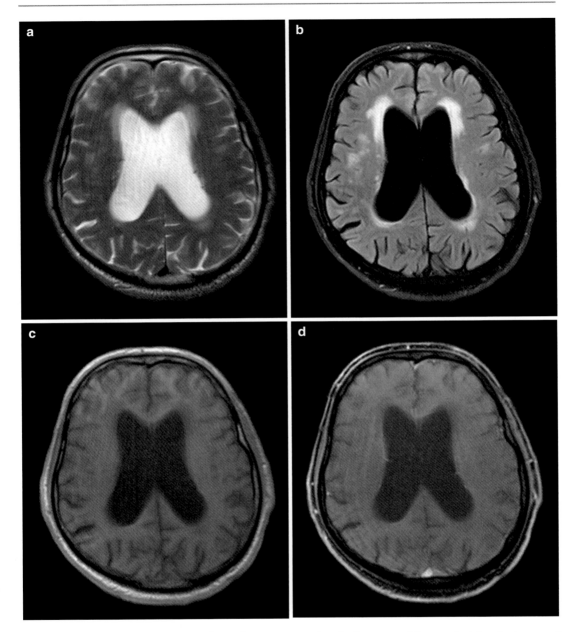

Fig. 16.2 Obstructive hydrocephalus with moderate transependymal edema caused by aqueductal web, absence of aqueductal flow void sign; T2 (**a**), FLAIR (**b**), T1 (**c**), T1 contrast (**d**), DWI (**e**), ADC (**f**), T2 sagittal (**g**), CISS (**h**)

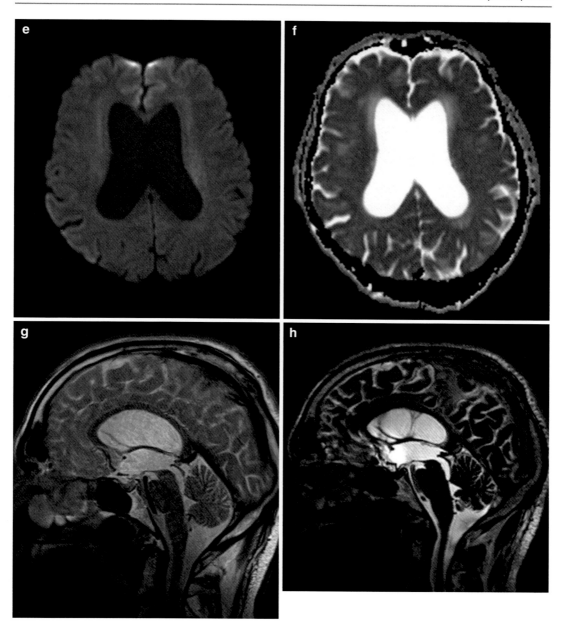

Fig. 16.2 (continued)

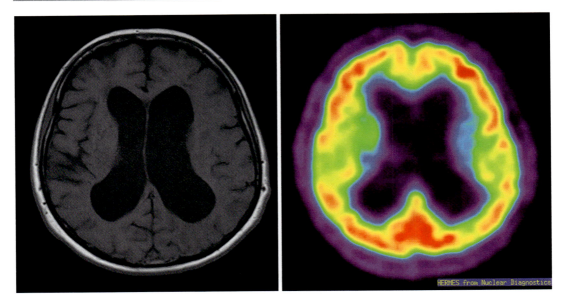

Fig. 16.3 Co-registered MRI and PET of a patient with hydrocephalus

16.5 Neuropathology Findings

Macroscopic Features (Figs. 16.4, 16.5, and 16.6)
- Enlargement of the ventricular system (Figs. 16.4, 16.5, and 16.6)
  - Aqueductal stenosis with hydrocephalus: lateral ventricles and third ventricle enlarged
  - Communicating hydrocephalus: enlarged ventricles with free communication with the lumbar subarachnoidal space
- Depends on degree of resistance to absorb and the distensibility of the ventricular system
  - Frontal and occipital lateral ventricles enlarge first
  - Temporal lateral ventricles and third ventricle
  - Least likely to dilate is the aqueduct of Sylvius
- Atrophy of corpus callosum
- Atrophy of fornix/fimbria
- Distortion of hypothalamus
- Rarely: cortical thinning

Microscopic Features
- Ependymal lining compromised or disrupted
- Ependymal granulations (in chronic high pressure)
- Subependymal gliosis
- Rarefied periventricular white matter with
  - Loss of oligodendrocytes
  - Gliosis
- Choroid plexus
  - Epithelial atrophy
  - Cytological changes
  - Stromal sclerosis
- Petechial hemorrhages
- Increased pinocytotic activity in capillary endothelium

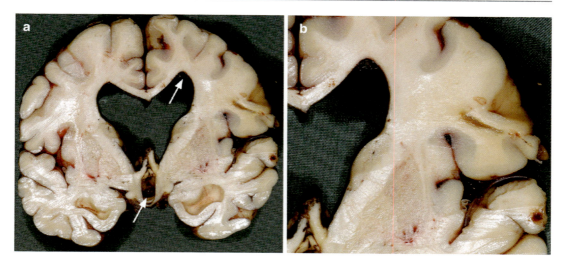

Fig. 16.4 Hydrocephalus with enlargement of the ventricular system, i.e., lateral ventricles and, third ventricle (arrow) (**a**) rounding of the upper roof (arrow) (**b**)

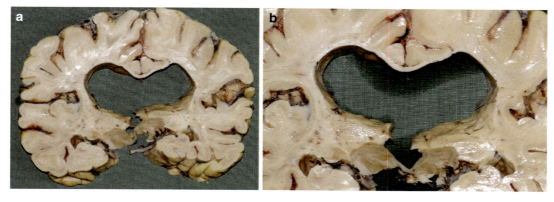

Fig. 16.5 Hydrocephalus with enlargement of the ventricular system, thinning of the corpus callosum, and atrophy of the basal ganglia and thalamus (**a, b**)

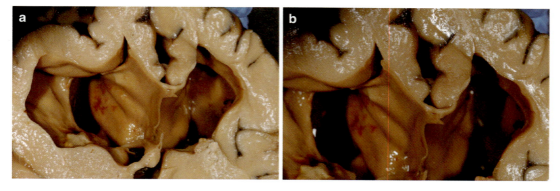

Fig. 16.6 Hydrocephalus in a child with massive atrophy of the corpus callosum and reduced volume of white matter (**a, b**)

16.6 Molecular Neuropathology

Congenital hydrocephalus
- In most cases not known
- Maternal infection (toxoplasmosis, cytomegalovirus, mumps, rubella, varicella)
- Nutritional disorders (hypovitaminosis A)
- Teratogenesis (radiation, lysergic acid diethylamide)
- Genetic factors (X-linked)

Aqueductal stenosis with hydrocephalus
- Aqueduct abnormalities
  - Congenital narrowing
  - Agenesis
  - Atresia
  - Gliosis
  - Forking
  - Membrane occlusion
- Midbrain tumors
- Perinatal intraventricular hemorrhage
- Meningitis
- Ventriculitis

Communicating hydrocephalus
- Blockage of the
  - flow of CSF in the subarachnoidal space over the convexities of the brain
  - resorption of CSF at the arachnoidal villi along the sagittal sinus
- Infection (meningitis, ventriculitis)
- Inflammation (neurosarcoidosis)
- Hemorrhage (intraventricular hemorrhage, aneurysmal subarachnoidal hemorrhage)

Normal pressure hydrocephalus
- Block in flow of CSF in the subarachnoidal spaces
- Failure to resorb CSF at the arachnoid villi
- Reduction of cerebral blood flow and oxidative metabolism
- Tearing and stretching of axons
- Activation of proteolytic calpains
- Elevated activity of nitric oxide synthase (NO) and NO production

16.7 Treatment and Prognosis

Treatment
- Aqueductal stenosis with hydrocephalus
  - Ventricular drainage using a shunt with an adjustable valve
- Communicating hydrocephalus
  - Ventriculo-peritoneal shunt
  - Ventriculostomy
- Normal pressure hydrocephalus
  - Ventriculo-peritoneal shunt

Biologic Behavior–Prognosis–Prognostic Factors
- Aqueductal stenosis with hydrocephalus
  - Complications due to shunt infection, overdrainage, subdural hematoma, subdural hygroma
- Communicating hydrocephalus
  - Dramatic improvement after shunting
- Normal pressure hydrocephalus
  - Improvement of gait in 63% after 3 months
  - Sustained improvement of cognition in 10% of patients after 5 years
  - Patients with NPH have higher risk of dying

Selected References

Bergsneider M, Miller C, Vespa PM, Hu X (2008) Surgical management of adult hydrocephalus. Neurosurgery 62(Suppl 2):643–659; discussion 659–660. https://doi.org/10.1227/01.neu.0000316269.82467.f7

Del Bigio MR (2010) Neuropathology and structural changes in hydrocephalus. Dev Disabil Res Rev 16(1):16–22. https://doi.org/10.1002/ddrr.94

Filippidis AS, Kalani MY, Rekate HL (2012) Hydrocephalus and aquaporins: the role of aquaporin-4. Acta Neurochir Suppl 113:55–58. https://doi.org/10.1007/978-3-7091-0923-6_12

Finney GR (2009) Normal pressure hydrocephalus. Int Rev Neurobiol 84:263–281. https://doi.org/10.1016/s0074-7742(09)00414-0

Hamilton MG (2009) Treatment of hydrocephalus in adults. Semin Pediatr Neurol 16(1):34–41. https://doi.org/10.1016/j.spen.2009.02.001

Kalani MY, Filippidis AS, Rekate HL (2012) Hydrocephalus and aquaporins: the role of aquaporin-1. Acta Neurochir Suppl 113:51–54. https://doi.org/10.1007/978-3-7091-0923-6_11

Kartal MG, Algin O (2014) Evaluation of hydrocephalus and other cerebrospinal fluid disorders with MRI: an update. Insights Imaging 5(4):531–541. https://doi.org/10.1007/s13244-014-0333-5

Kitagaki H, Mori E, Ishii K, Yamaji S, Hirono N, Imamura T (1998) CSF spaces in idiopathic normal pressure hydrocephalus: morphology and volumetry. AJNR Am J Neuroradiol 19(7):1277–1284

Kizu O, Yamada K, Nishimura T (2001) Proton chemical shift imaging in normal pressure hydrocephalus. AJNR Am J Neuroradiol 22(9):1659–1664

Oi S (2010) Hydrocephalus research update—controversies in definition and classification of hydrocephalus. Neurol Med Chir 50(9):859–869

Oi S (2011) Classification of hydrocephalus: critical analysis of classification categories and advantages of "multi-categorical hydrocephalus classification" (McHC). Childs Nerv Syst 27(10):1523–1533. https://doi.org/10.1007/s00381-011-1542-6

Penn RD, Linninger A (2009) The physics of hydrocephalus. Pediatr Neurosurg 45(3):161–174. https://doi.org/10.1159/000218198

Rosseau G (2011) Normal pressure hydrocephalus. Dis Mon 57(10):615–624. https://doi.org/10.1016/j.disamonth.2011.08.023

Schumacher DJ, Tien RD, Friedman H (1994) Gadolinium enhancement of the leptomeninges caused by hydrocephalus: a potential mimic of leptomeningeal metastasis. AJNR Am J Neuroradiol 15(4):639–641

Siraj S (2011) An overview of normal pressure hydrocephalus and its importance: how much do we really know? J Am Med Dir Assoc 12(1):19–21. https://doi.org/10.1016/j.jamda.2010.05.005

Stagno V, Navarrete EA, Mirone G, Esposito F (2013) Management of hydrocephalus around the world. World Neurosurg 79(2 Suppl):S23.e17–S23.e20. https://doi.org/10.1016/j.wneu.2012.02.004

Symss NP, Oi S (2013) Theories of cerebrospinal fluid dynamics and hydrocephalus: historical trend. J Neurosurg Pediatr 11(2):170–177. https://doi.org/10.3171/2012.3.peds0934

Virhammar J, Laurell K, Cesarini KG, Larsson EM (2014) Preoperative prognostic value of MRI findings in 108 patients with idiopathic normal pressure hydrocephalus. AJNR Am J Neuroradiol 35(12):2311–2318. https://doi.org/10.3174/ajnr.A4046

Part IV

The Brain Diseases: Vascular system

Vascular Disorders: Hypoxia

17.1 Introduction

Oxygen delivery and metabolism
- The adequacy of tissue oxygenation depends on
  - the rate of oxygen delivered to the tissues (oxygen delivery (DO_2))
  - the rate of oxygen consumed by the tissues (oxygen consumption or oxygen uptake (VO_2))
- *Oxygen delivery (DO_2)* is
  - the volume of oxygen delivered to the systemic vascular bed per minute
  - the product of cardiac output (CO) and arterial oxygen concentration (CaO_2): $DO_2 = CO \times CaO_2$
- *Oxygen uptake* is
  - The amount of oxygen that diffuses from capillaries to mitochondria.
  - Tissue oxygenation is adequate when tissues receive sufficient oxygen to meet their metabolic needs.
  - When tissues do not receive sufficient oxygen, cellular injury could potentially occur.
- Oxygen deprivation may cause tissue damage
  - directly if energy supplied to meet the tissue demands is insufficient
  - indirectly during the reperfusion of the tissue

- Factors affecting oxygen transport
  - limiting factors of O_2 uptake
    - convection
    - diffusion
  - specifically affected by several factors with a risk of O_2 uptake alteration include:
    - Blood flow
    - Blood oxygenation parameters: O_2 content, arterial O_2 partial pressure, hemoglobin oxygen affinity
    - Structural and functional characteristics of the microcirculatory network
- Factors affecting O_2 diffusion
  - Changes in arterial PO_2
  - Changes in hemoglobin O_2 affinity
  - Changes in the diffusing capacity of the microvascular network

Adequate oxygen (O_2) supply for gray matter: 6 mL/100 g/min

Hypoxia
- decreased oxygen
- leads to cell injury

Ischemia:
- Decreased blood flow
- Hypoxia plus lack of nutrients
- Accumulation of toxic cellular metabolites

Anoxia:
- total depletion in the level of oxygen, an extreme form of hypoxia

Brain death clinically defined as

- Irreversible coma
- Apnea
- Loss of all brain stem reflexes

Classification of hypoxia
- Hypoxic hypoxia
  - Blood oxygen tension below 40 mmHg
  - Occurs in:
    ○ In acute respiratory arrest
    ○ Chronic obstructive pulmonary disease
    ○ Alveolar hypoventilation
    ○ Near-drowning
    ○ Diminished oxygen concentration in the air
    ○ Weakness of respiratory muscles
    ○ Status epilepticus
- Anemic hypoxia
  - Oxygen-carrying hemoglobin falls to half its normal concentration
  - Occurs in:
    Severe blood loss
    Chronic anemia
- Histotoxic hypoxia
  - Caused by toxic substances including:
    Carbon monoxide
    Cyanide
    Sulfide
  - Prevention of oxygen utilization by neural tissue
- Ischemic/Stagnant hypoxia (cardiac arrest encephalopathy, transient global ischemia).
  - Blood falls below 18 mL/100 g tissue/min
  - Regional confined to arterial territory
  - Global generalized cerebral hypoperfusion
  - Occurs in:
    Cardiac arrest
    Cardiac arrhythmias
    Sudden hypotension from myocardial infarct
    Severe raise of intracranial pressure
- Non-perfused brain (respirator brain, permanent global ischemia).
- Different types of hypoxia are combined in certain clinical situations.

17.2 Clinical Signs

Clinical signs and symptoms
- Syncope
  - Momentary loss of consciousness
  - From transient global ischemia of a few seconds duration
- Hypoxic and ischemic encephalopathy
  - Mild to moderate continuous hypoxia
    ○ Symptoms include:
      - Headaches
      - Confusion
      - Memory and cognitive impairment
      - Seizures
      - Myoclonus
      - Motor and sensory deficits
  - Severe hypoxia (duration of 10 min)
    ○ Symptoms include:
      - Lethargy to deep coma
      - Seizures
      - Myoclonic jerks
      - Changes of muscle tone
- Pathologic reflexes

17.3 Epidemiology

Incidence
- Uncommon

Age Incidence
- Middle-aged persons
- Elderly persons

Sex Incidence
- Male:Female ratio: 1:1

Localization
- Regional confined to arterial territory
- Global generalized cerebral hypoperfusion

17.4 Neuroimaging Findings

General Imaging Findings
Global hypoxia (hypoxic-ischemic injury) presents with watershed zone infarcts in mild cases. Severe hypoxia results in infarcts of

17.4 Neuroimaging Findings

basal ganglia, cortex, thalami, hippocampi, and cerebellum.

CT non-contrast-enhanced (Figs. 17.1e and 17.2a)
- Diffuse edema
- Loss of gray-white matter differentiation
- Atrophy in chronic stage

CT contrast-enhanced
- Linear cortical enhancement in later series

MRI-T2/FLAIR (Figs. 17.1a, b and 17.2b, c, h, i)
- Hyperintensity of basal ganglia, cortex, hippocampi, cerebellum following DWI lesions

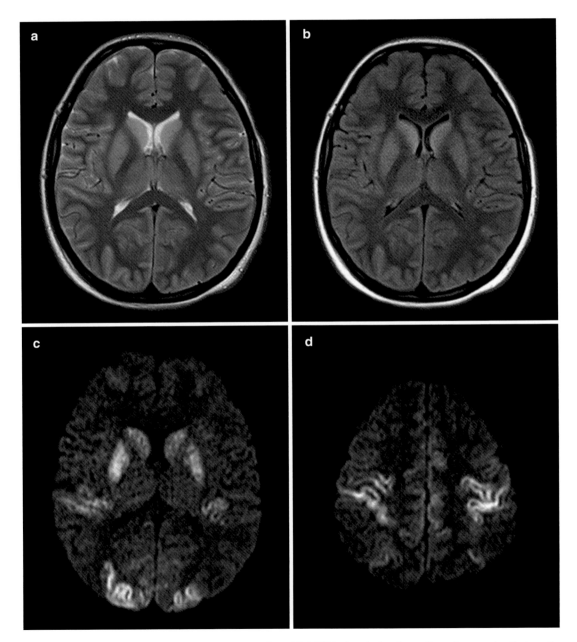

Fig. 17.1 MR 4 days after hypoxia, T2 (**a**), FLAIR (**b**), with DWI lesions in basal ganglia and cortex (**c, d**). Atrophy and gliosis after 2 months CT (**e**) and T2 (**f**)

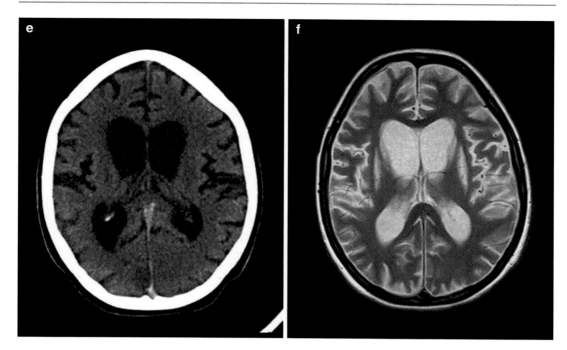

Fig. 17.1 (continued)

MRI-T1 (Fig. 17.2d, j)
- Cortical hyperintensities in late subacute/chronic stage represent cortical laminar necrosis.

MRI-T1 contrast-enhanced (Fig. 17.2e, k)
- Subacute gyriform enhancement

MR-Diffusion Imaging (Figs. 17.1c, d and 17.2f, g)
- Restricted diffusion due to cytotoxic edema in basal ganglia, cortex, hippocampi, thalami, and cerebellum.
- DWI hyperintensities pseudo-normalize by the end of the first week.

MRI-T2∗/SWI
- No hemorrhage or calcification

Nuclear Medicine Imaging Findings (Figs. 17.3, 17.4, and 17.5)
- CBF-SPECT demonstrates perfusion deficits and thereby damage caused by hypoxia.
- FDG-PET can demonstrate the reduced glucose uptake und utilization in impaired neuronal structures resulting in an overall reduced uptake of FDG.
- Flumazenil PET, which shows the distribution of $GABA_A$ receptors, can demonstrate the neuronal damage caused by hypoxia resulting in an overall reduced uptake of flumazenil.
- 15-O PET can demonstrate a reduced oxygen extraction fraction.
- Presynaptic and postsynaptic SPECT and PET studies can show a reduced tracer uptake, even with a reduction in caudate nucleus in presynaptic studies.

17.4 Neuroimaging Findings

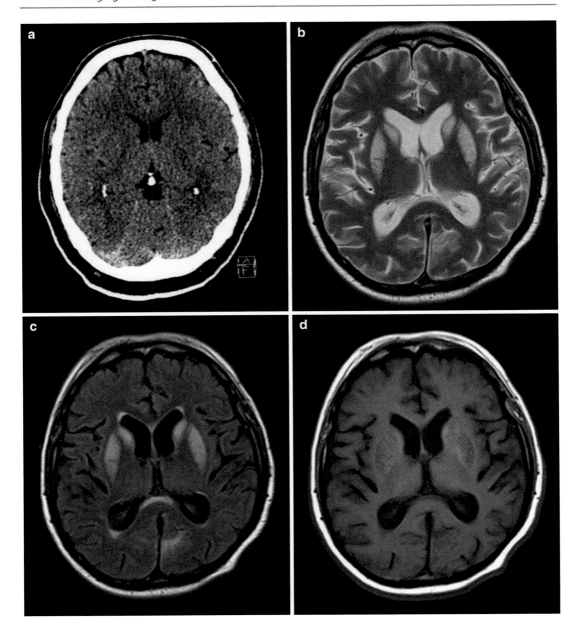

Fig. 17.2 CT 2 days after cardiac arrest (**a**) with loss of caudate head density, MR after 1 month with signal changes in basal ganglia in T2 (**b**), FLAIR (**c**), T1 (**d**), T1 contrast (**e**) and regressive DWI lesions (**f**), ADC (**g**). Cortical necrosis in T2 (**h**), FLAIR (**i**), T1 (**j**), and T1 contrast (**k**)

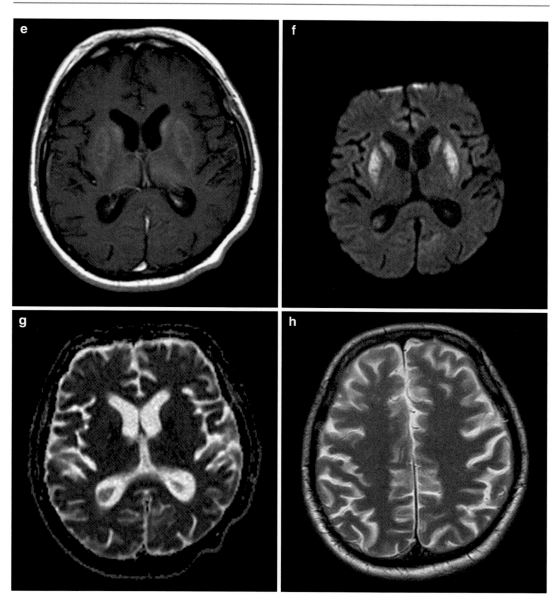

Fig. 17.2 (continued)

17.4 Neuroimaging Findings

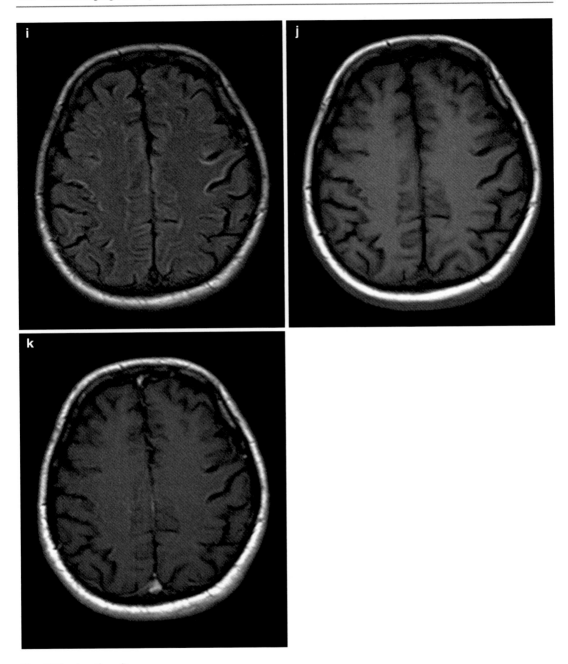

Fig. 17.2 (continued)

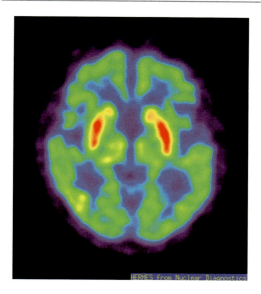

Fig. 17.3 FDG-PET of a patient with brain damage caused by hypoxia

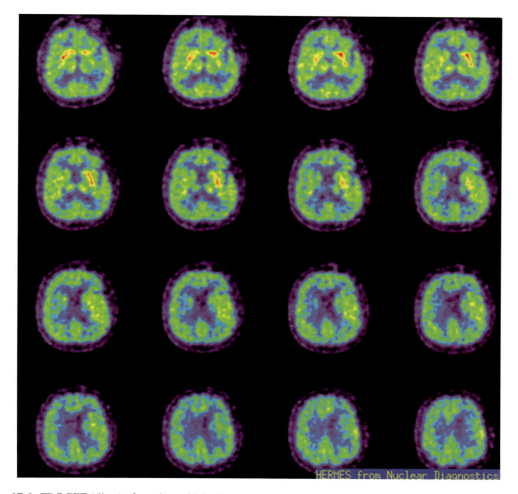

Fig. 17.4 FDG-PET (slices) of a patient with brain damage caused by hypoxia

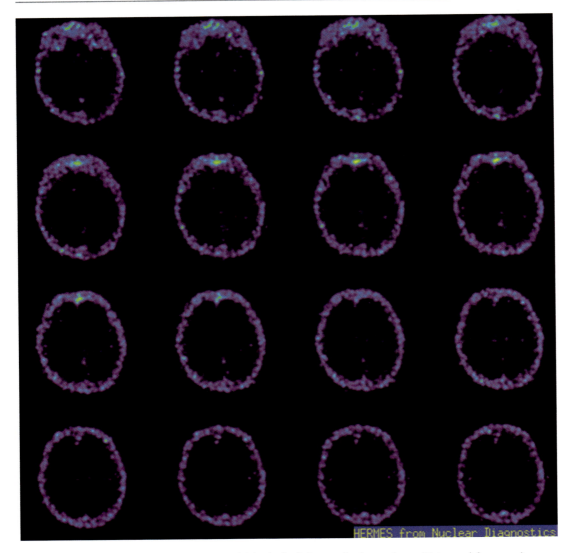

Fig. 17.5 Perfusion scintigraphy of a patient with brain death (no uptake due to elevated intracranial pressure)

17.5 Neuropathology Findings

Macroscopic Features
- Unremarkable
- Softening of the fixed brain tissue
- Severe form in apallic syndrome (Fig. 17.6a–h)
  - Atrophy of the cerebral gray matter

Microscopic Features (Fig. 17.7a–f)
- Neuronal necrosis:
  - Red neurons
  - Shrunken neuronal cell body
  - Bright eosinophilia of the perikaryon
  - Shrunken basophilic homogeneous nucleus
- Ghost neurons
  - Faintly stained perikaryon and nucleus
- Dark neurons
  - Condensed, darkly stained perikaryon
  - Corkscrew contournament of the apical dendrite
- Ferruginated neurons
  - Dead neurons become encrusted with calcium and iron salts.
- Enlargement of the perineuronal space

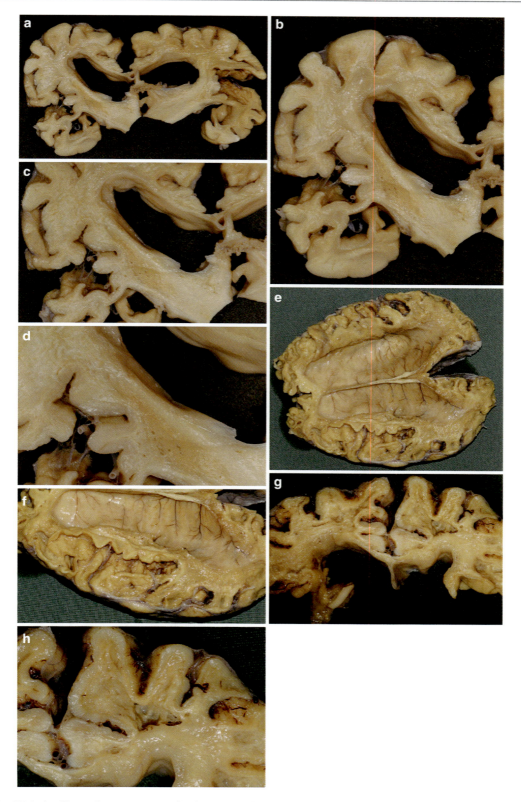

Fig. 17.6 Apallic syndrome: macroscopic changes seen in apallic syndrome consist of thinning of the cortical ribbon and enlargement of the ventricular system (**a–h**)

17.5 Neuropathology Findings

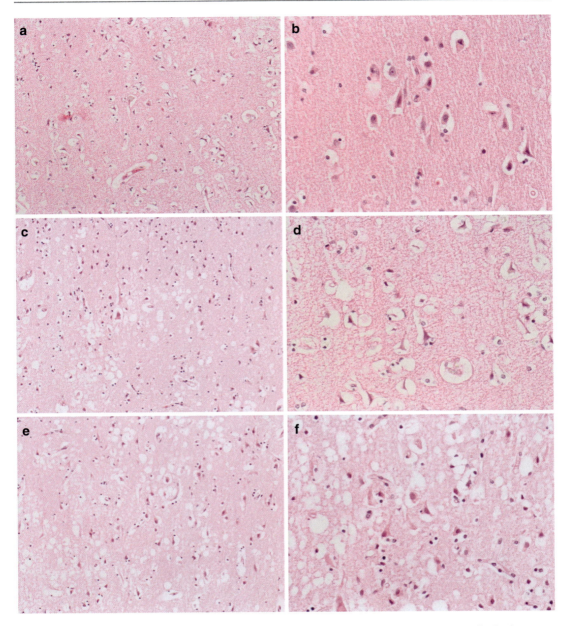

Fig. 17.7 Histological appearance of mild (**a**, **b**), moderate (**c**, **d**), and severe hypoxia (**e**, **f**). Red neurons (arrow) (**b**, **c**)

Table 17.1 Selective regional vulnerability determines the anatomic distribution of the lesions

Anatomic region	Affected cells
Hippocampus	Pyramidal neurons in CA1 sector (Sommer sector)
Neocortex	Neurons of layers III, V, and VI
Cerebellum	Purkinje cells
Thalamus	Anterior and dorsomedial nuclei
Basal ganglia	Spiny neurons

- Pale coloration of the tissue section
- Selective regional vulnerability (Table 17.1)
- Cortical laminar neuronal necrosis
  - Involves one or several cortical layers
  - Dense astrocytic fibrillary gliosis
- Cortical laminar pan-necrosis
  - Affects neurons, oligodendrocytes, astrocytes, myelin, and axons
  - Involves one or several cortical layers or the entire width of the cortex
  - Infarction:
    - Prominent endothelial swelling and proliferation
    - Macrophages, microglia, and blood monocytes
    - Astrocytic proliferation, gemistocytic astrocytes
- Hypoxic-ischemic leukoencephalopathy
  - Rare condition
  - Less severe but prolonged hypotension and cerebral hypoperfusion
  - Multiple small areas of myelin loss
  - Variable axonal changes
  - Absence of macrophages
  - Insignificant astrocytic reaction
- Respirator brain
  - Due to permanent non-perfusion
- Apallic syndrome (Figs. 17.8 and 17.9)
  - thinned cortical (cerebral and cerebellar) ribbon due to neuronal loss (Fig. 17.8a–j)
  - reactive astrogliosis (Fig. 17.9a–d)
  - reactive microgliosis (Fig. 17.9e–h)

Immunohistochemical Staining Characteristics
- GFAP for assessing astrocytic reaction
- HLA-DRII (Cr3/43) for assessing microglial reaction
- CD68

Differential Diagnosis
- Infectious process
- Demyelination

17.6 Molecular Neuropathology

- Decrease in oxygen
  - leads to a decreased production of ATP
  - leads to failure of NA/K$^+$ pump and Ca^{2+} pump
  - sodium enters the cell
  - causes cell swelling
- Entrance of Ca into the cells
  - activates endonucleases, proteases, phospholipases, and DNAses
  - leading to cell damage
- Switch to anaerobic respiration by the cell
  - accumulation of lactic acid
  - decreased cellular pH
  - causes disaggregation of ribosomes from endoplasmic reticulum

Pathogenesis of selective neuronal necrosis

- Excitotoxicity due to the excitatory neurotransmitter glutamate
  - Depolarizes the neuronal membrane
  - Excessive influx of sodium, chloride, water, and calcium
  - Swelling, metabolic dysfunction, disruption of the cellular membrane
- Molecular chaperone proteins
- Immediate early genes
- Ischemic "tolerance," repetitive cerebral ischemia

17.6 Molecular Neuropathology

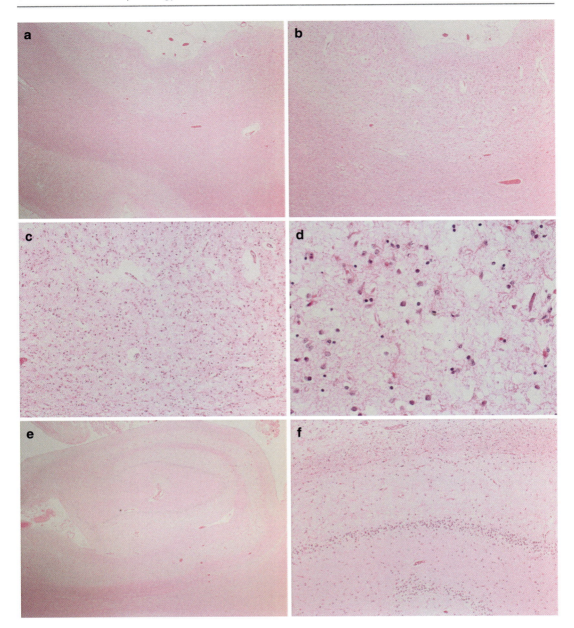

Fig. 17.8 Apallic syndrome: The cortical ribbon is thin due to significant loss of neurons (**a–d**). Severe neuronal loss of neurons is seen in the CA1 to CA4 subfields of the hippocampal formation (**e–h**). Loss of Purkinje cells and granule cells is present in the cerebellum (**i, j**)

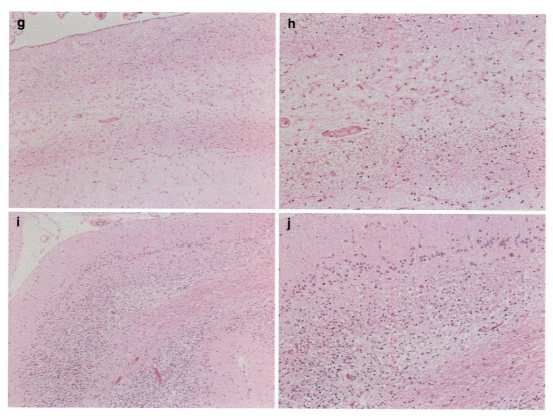

Fig. 17.8 (continued)

17.6 Molecular Neuropathology

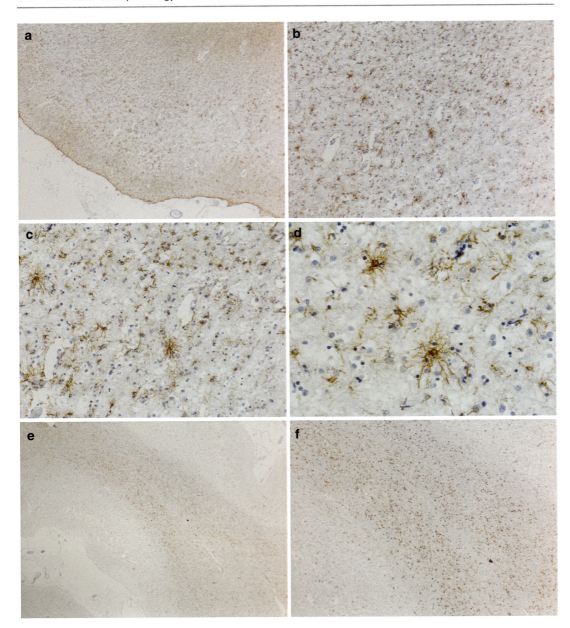

Fig. 17.9 Apallic syndrome—immunophenotype: mild to moderate reactive astrogliosis (**a–d**; GFAP) and moderate reactive microgliosis predominantly in the white matter (**e–h**; HLA-DRII)

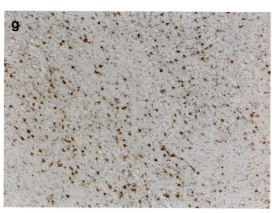
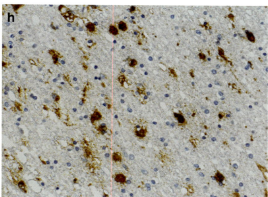

Fig. 17.9 (continued)

- Nitric oxide
- Delayed neuronal death
- Ischemic neuroprotection

17.7 Treatment and Prognosis

Treatment
- Standard intensive care
- Hemodynamic optimization
- Control dysrhythmias, hypotension, low cardiac index

Biologic Behavior–Prognosis–Prognostic Factors

Severity and extent of the pathological changes depend on:

- Severity of hypoxic event
- Duration of hypoxic event
- Body temperature
- Blood glucose concentration
  - Hyperglycemia aggravates ischemic damage.
  - Hypoglycemia protects the brain.

Selected References

Ainslie PN, Ogoh S (2010) Regulation of cerebral blood flow in mammals during chronic hypoxia: a matter of balance. Exp Physiol 95(2):251–262. https://doi.org/10.1113/expphysiol.2008.045575

Clarkson AN, Sutherland BA, Appleton I (2005) The biology and pathology of hypoxia-ischemia: an update. Arch Immunol Ther Exp 53(3):213–225

Engelhardt S, Patkar S, Ogunshola OO (2014) Cell-specific blood-brain barrier regulation in health and disease: a focus on hypoxia. Br J Pharmacol 171(5):1210–1230. https://doi.org/10.1111/bph.12489

Ferdinand P, Roffe C (2016) Hypoxia after stroke: a review of experimental and clinical evidence. Exp Transl Stroke Med 8:9. https://doi.org/10.1186/s13231-016-0023-0

Garbarino VR, Orr ME, Rodriguez KA, Buffenstein R (2015) Mechanisms of oxidative stress resistance in the brain: lessons learned from hypoxia tolerant extremophilic vertebrates. Arch Biochem Biophys 576:8–16. https://doi.org/10.1016/j.abb.2015.01.029

Ghei SK, Zan E, Nathan JE, Choudhri A, Tekes A, Huisman TA, Izbudak I (2014) MR imaging of hypoxic-ischemic injury in term neonates: pearls and pitfalls. Radiographics 34(4):1047–1061. https://doi.org/10.1148/rg.344130080

Huang BY, Castillo M (2008) Hypoxic-ischemic brain injury: imaging findings from birth to adulthood. Radiographics 28(2):417–439; quiz 617. https://doi.org/10.1148/rg.282075066

Jensen RL (2009) Brain tumor hypoxia: tumorigenesis, angiogenesis, imaging, pseudoprogression, and as a therapeutic target. J Neurooncol 92(3):317–335. https://doi.org/10.1007/s11060-009-9827-2

Johnson DR, Sherry CL, York JM, Freund GG (2008) Acute hypoxia, diabetes, and neuroimmune dysregulation: converging mechanisms in the brain. Neuroscientist 14(3):235–239. https://doi.org/10.1177/1073858407309544

LaManna JC (2007) Hypoxia in the central nervous system. Essays Biochem 43:139–151. https://doi.org/10.1042/bse0430139

Lukyanova LD, Kirova YI (2015) Mitochondria-controlled signaling mechanisms of brain protection in hypoxia. Front Neurosci 9:320. https://doi.org/10.3389/fnins.2015.00320

Selected References

Marina N, Kasymov V, Ackland GL, Kasparov S, Gourine AV (2016) Astrocytes and brain hypoxia. Adv Exp Med Biol 903:201–207. https://doi.org/10.1007/978-1-4899-7678-9_14

Millar LJ, Shi L, Hoerder-Suabedissen A, Molnar Z (2017) Neonatal hypoxia ischaemia: mechanisms, models, and therapeutic challenges. Front Cell Neurosci 11:78. https://doi.org/10.3389/fncel.2017.00078

Schmidt-Kastner R (2015) Genomic approach to selective vulnerability of the hippocampus in brain ischemia-hypoxia. Neuroscience 309:259–279. https://doi.org/10.1016/j.neuroscience.2015.08.034

Somjen GG, Aitken PG, Czeh G, Jing J, Young JN (1993) Cellular physiology of hypoxia of the mammalian central nervous system. Res Publ Assoc Res Nerv Ment Dis 71:51–65

Terraneo L, Samaja M (2017) Comparative response of brain to chronic hypoxia and hyperoxia. Int J Mol Sci 18(9):1914. https://doi.org/10.3390/ijms18091914

Thornton C, Leaw B, Mallard C, Nair S, Jinnai M, Hagberg H (2017) Cell death in the developing brain after hypoxia-ischemia. Int J Mol Sci 11:248. https://doi.org/10.3389/fncel.2017.00248

Verges S, Rupp T, Jubeau M, Wuyam B, Esteve F, Levy P, Perrey S, Millet GY (2012) Cerebral perturbations during exercise in hypoxia. Am J Physiol Regul Integr Comp Physiol 302(8):R903–R916. https://doi.org/10.1152/ajpregu.00555.2011

Yang Y, Sandhu HK, Zhi F, Hua F, Wu M, Xia Y (2015) Effects of hypoxia and ischemia on microRNAs in the brain. Curr Med Chem 22(10):1292–1301. https://doi.org/10.1016/j.abb.2015.01.029

Zhang SX, Wang Y, Gozal D (2012) Pathological consequences of intermittent hypoxia in the central nervous system. Compr Physiol 2(3):1767–1777. https://doi.org/10.1002/cphy.c100060

Vascular Disorders: Ischemia–Infarction–Stroke

18.1 Introduction

Clinical definition of stroke (WHO):

- Stroke:
  - Abrupt onset of focal neurological signs lasting more than 24 h
  - Symptoms lasting less than 24 h but with imaging evidence of an acute relevant lesion
- Transient ischemic attack (TIA)
  - Focal signs lasting less than 24 h
  - Evidence of brain infraction (imaging) in the absence of clinical signs
  - Brief episode of neurologic dysfunction caused by retinal or brain ischemia with clinical symptoms lasting less than 1 h and without evidence (by neuroimaging) of acute infraction

Stroke results from pathology of blood vessel in the CNS. The following two types of stroke are distinguished:

- Ischemic stroke (cerebral infarction):
  - Occlusion of a blood vessel with focal tissue ischemia and infarction
- Hemorrhagic stroke:
  - Rupture of a blood vessel with extravasation of blood and subsequent tissue damage

Ischemia:

- Decreased blood flow
- Hypoxia plus lack of nutrients
- Accumulation of toxic cellular metabolites

Hemorrhage

- Accumulation of blood outside the vascular channel system

18.2 Clinical Signs and Symptoms

Clinical signs and symptoms include:
- Loss of focal neurologic function
  - Motor symptoms
  - Speech/language disturbances
  - Somatosensory symptoms
  - Visual symptoms
  - Vestibular symptoms
  - Behavioral/cognitive symptoms

- Sudden onset
- Non-focal neurological symptoms
  - Generalized weakness
  - Dizziness
  - Confusion
  - Incontinence

18.3 Epidemiology

Incidence

Data generation not consistent

- Age-adjusted rate: 100–300 per 100,000 population/year

Stroke types:

- Ischemic stroke: 70–80%
- Hemorrhagic stroke: 20–30%

Stroke causes:

- Cardioembolism 15–30%
- Atherosclerotic 14–40%
- Lacunar infarcts 15–30%
- Cryptogenic 40%

Age Incidence
- Doubles per decade over age 55

Sex Incidence
- Male:Female ratio 3:1

Race ethnicity
- 2.4 fold increase for African Americans
- 2 fold increase in Hispanics
- Increasing among Asians

Localization
- By site:
  - Wedge-shaped cortical/subcortical
  - Elongated sickle-shaped strips of infarction (borderzone infarcts)
  - Small, deep lacunar infarcts
- By vascular supply
  - Anterior circulation
  - Posterior circulation

The clinical classification by the Oxfordshire Community Stroke Project (OCSP) (Bamford et al. 1991) allows anatomical and vascular location as follows:

- Total anterior circulation syndrome (20% of cases)
- Partial anterior circulation syndromes (30% of cases)
- Lacunar syndromes (25% of cases)
- Posterior circulation syndromes (25% of cases)

The territories supplied by various arteries, the ensuing clinical syndromes and involved structures in case of cessation of blood supply are depicted in Table 18.1.

18.3 Epidemiology

Table 18.1 The territories supplied by various arteries, the ensuing clinical syndromes and involved structures in case of cessation of blood supply

Territory	Artery	Clinical syndrome	Structures involved
Carotid	Ophthalmic	• Monocular blindness • Altitudinal field defect	• Retina • Optic nerve
	Anterior choroidal	• Contralateral hemiparesis • Hemisensory loss • Homonymous hemianopia with sparing of horizontal segment	• Globus pallidus (internal) • Internal capsule (posterior limb) • Choroid plexus
	Anterior cerebral	• Contralateral foot and leg weakness • Hemiparesis • Abulia • Incontinence • Grasp reflexes • Mutism • Left hand apraxia • Transcortical motor aphasia • Frontal release signs • Urinary incontinence	• Anterior medial frontal lobe • Superior medial frontal lobe
	Middle cerebral	• Contralateral central facial weakness • Hemiparesis • Global aphasia	• Frontal lobe • Parietal lobe • Superior temporal lobe
	Medial lenticulostriate	• Contralateral pure motor hemiparesis	• Internal capsule
	Lateral lenticulostriate	• Contralateral hemiparesis • Dysphasia • Visual–spatial–perceptual dysfunction • Contralateral hemisensory/motor syndrome (face/arm/leg) • Global aphasia with dominant hemisphere involvement • Visuospatial neglect (non-dominant hemisphere) • Contralateral gaze paresis • Contralateral homonymous hemianopia	• Putamen • Globus pallidus (external) • Caudate nucleus • Internal capsule • Corona radiata
Vertebral	Posterior inferior cerebellar	• Ipsilateral Horner syndrome • Ipsilateral facial sensory loss • Vertigo • Nystagmus • Ataxia • Dysphagia • Dysarthria • Gaze paresis • Pain/temperature deficits face (ipsilateral), trunk/extremities (contralateral)	• Lateral medulla • Inferior cerebellum

(continued)

Table 18.1 (continued)

Territory	Artery	Clinical syndrome	Structures involved
Basilary	Anterior inferior cerebellar	• Ipsilateral Horner syndrome • Ipsilateral facial sensory loss • Ipsilateral nuclear facial and abducens palsy • Vertigo • Vomiting • Nystagmus • Ipsilateral facial anesthesia/ • Weakness • Ipsilateral deafness • Contralateral decrease in temperature/pain sensation in limbs • Ipsilateral ataxia	• Base of pons • Rostral medulla • Rostral cerebellum • Cochlea • Vestibule
	Paramedian and circumferential basilar penetrators	• Lacunar syndromes	• Paramedian pons
	Superior cerebellar artery	• Ipsilateral Horner syndrome • Ipsilateral limb ataxia • Vertigo • Nystagmus • Contralateral fourth nerve palsy • Ipsilateral tremor/dyskinesia • Contralateral decreased sensation to pain/temperature in the trunk	• Midbrain • Superior cerebellar peduncle • Superior cerebellum
Posterior	Posterior cerebellar	• Contralateral homonymous hemianopia with macular sparing (if purely cortical) • If bilateral: Balint syndrome or cortical blindness with or without denial of blindness (Anton syndrome) • Dysnomic aphasia with alexia without agraphia (dominant hemisphere) • Memory disturbance • Color dysnomia • Agitated delirium • Hemisensory deficits with thalamic stroke	• Mammillary bodies • Thalamus • Lateral wall of third ventricle • Posterior part of the internal capsule • Posterior thalamus • Tectal plate • Pineal body • Medial geniculate body • Basilar surface of the posterior occipital lobe • Posterior temporal lobe • Medial surface of the posterior occipital lobe • Splenium corporis callosum • Cuneus • Precuneus • Occipital pole

18.4 Neuroimaging Findings

CT: Loss of gray-white matter differentiation corresponding to vessel territory
  MR: Restricted diffusion with correlating low signal in ADC map

CT non-contrast-enhanced (Figs. 18.1a–c and 18.2a)
- Without pathological findings in 50% of cases up to 6 h after onset
- Hyperdense vessel sign due to thrombus (most often seen in middle cerebral artery)
- Cytotoxic edema seen by loss of gray-white matter differentiation and obscuration of lentiform nucleus
- Focal effacement of sulci
- Over days increasing hypodense demarcation of infarct with swelling and possible hyperdense hemorrhagic transformation

CT contrast-enhanced
- Gyral enhancement day 4–7

CT-Angiography
- Demonstrates occluded vessel or stenoses.
- Status of collateralization helps to indicate mechanical recanalization.

CT-Perfusion
- Diminished CBV demonstrates irreversible damage of parenchyma.
- CBF correlates with final infarct size.
- TTP and MTT are sensitive indicators of reduced brain perfusion.

MRI-T2
- Hyperintense infarct demarcation within 12 h
- Cortical swelling

MRI-FLAIR (Fig. 18.2b)
- Hyperintense infarct demarcation 6 h after onset, helpful to evaluate onset of wake up stroke
- Hyperintense "flair sign" in occluded vessels possible

MRI-T1
- Infarction hypointense after 12 h
- Effacement of sulci

MRI-T1 contrast-enhanced (Fig. 18.2c)
- Meningeal enhancement within 12 h
- Parenchymal enhancement after days till months

MRI-T2*/SWI (Fig. 18.2e)
- Demonstrates thrombus in occluded vessel by "blooming" effect of the clot

MR-Diffusion Imaging (Fig. 18.2d)
- Restricted diffusion (high signal) with corresponding low signal on ADC maps demonstrates cytotoxic edema and correlates with infarct core although reversible DWI lesions are described.
- Most sensitive within minutes after stroke onset.

MRI-Perfusion (Fig. 18.2g, h, i, j)
- CBF correlates with final infarct size
- Diffusion/perfusion mismatch: DWI lesion demonstrates infarct core (irreversible damage), while delayed perfusion parameters (TTP/MTT) may represent "tissue at risk = penumbra" (reversible damage).

MR-Spectroscopy
- NAA reduced
- Lactate increased

MR-Angiography (Fig. 18.2f)
- Detection of vessel occlusion or stenoses

Nuclear Medicine Imaging Findings (Figs. 18.3, 18.4, and 18.5)
- CBF-SPECT demonstrates perfusion deficits by reduced tracer binding.
- FDG-PET can demonstrate reduced glucose uptake und utilization in impaired neuronal structures with a deficit in the ischemic area (and in most cases with general inhomogeneous uptake due to arteriosclerosis).
- Flumazenil PET, which shows the distribution of $GABA_A$ receptors, can demonstrate the neuronal damage caused by ischemia by presenting a deficit in tracer uptake.
- 15-O PET can demonstrate the oxygen extraction fraction.
- Presynaptic and postsynaptic SPECT and PET studies can show a reduced or lacking tracer uptake, even with a reduction in the caudate nucleus in presynaptic studies.

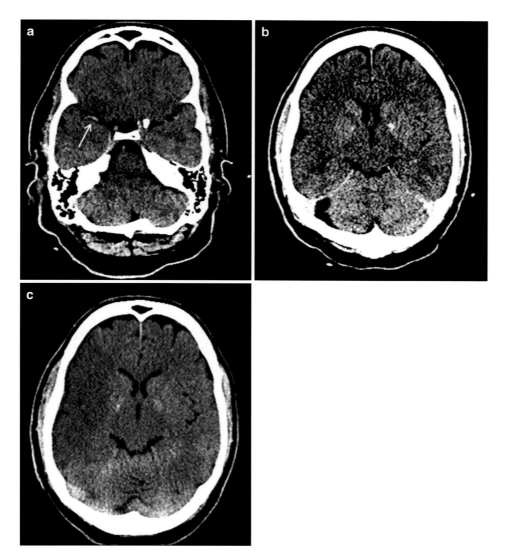

Fig. 18.1 Infarct of right middle cerebral artery with dense media sign on CT (**a**), loss of gray/white matter differentiation insular in CT (**b**) and infarct demarcation on CT after day 1 (**c**)

18.4 Neuroimaging Findings

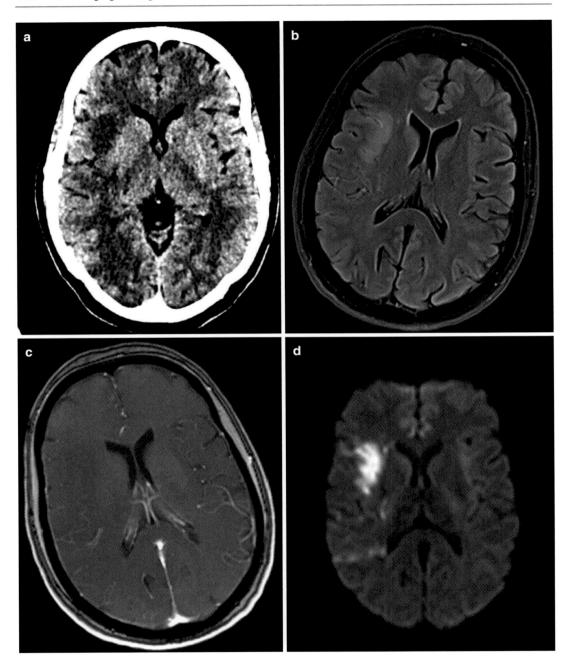

Fig. 18.2 Right middle cerebral artery infarction with CT (**a**), FLAIR (**b**), T1 contrast (**c**), DWI (**d**), SWI white arrow shows thrombus (**e**), MRA (**f**), MR-perfusion with mismatch (DWI/TTP) TTP (**g**), MTT (**h**), CBV (**i**), CBF (**j**), and DSA before and after mechanical thrombectomy of the M1 occlusion (**k, l**)

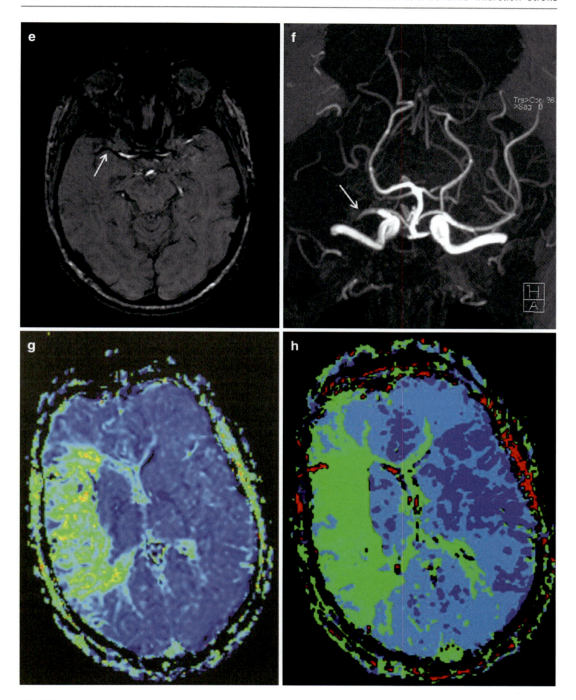

Fig. 18.2 (continued)

18.4 Neuroimaging Findings

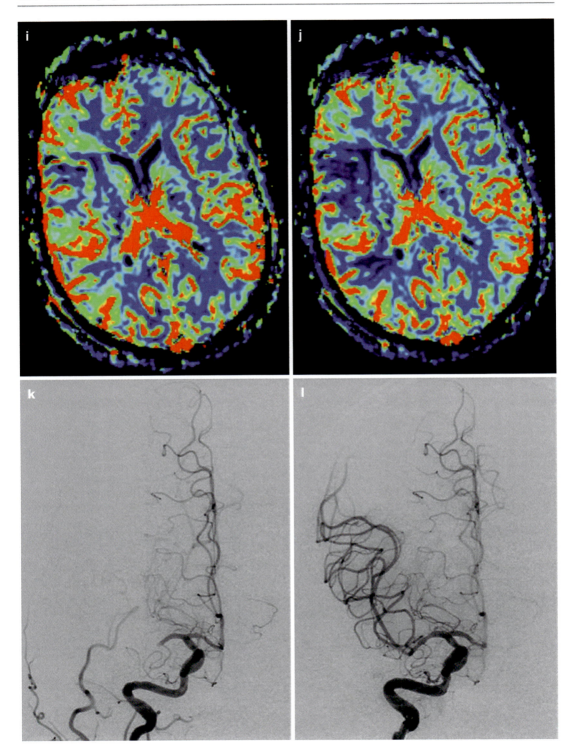

Fig. 18.2 (continued)

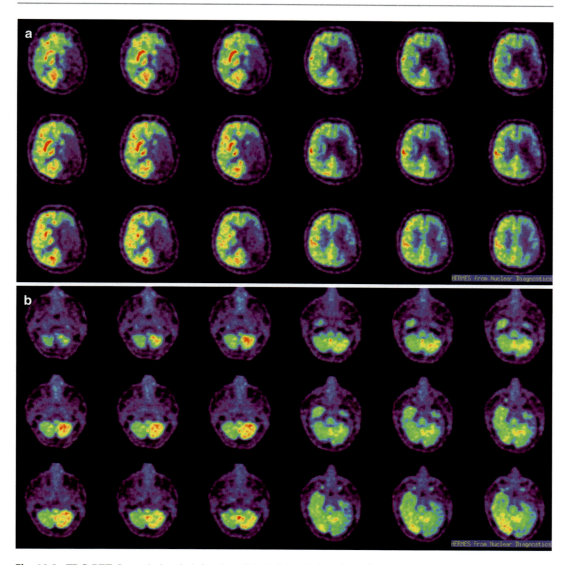

Fig. 18.3 FDG-PET: Large ischemic infarction of the left hemisphere including the cortex and the basal ganglia (**a**). The same patient with cerebellar diaschisis due to the left hemispheric ischemic infarction (**b**)

18.4 Neuroimaging Findings

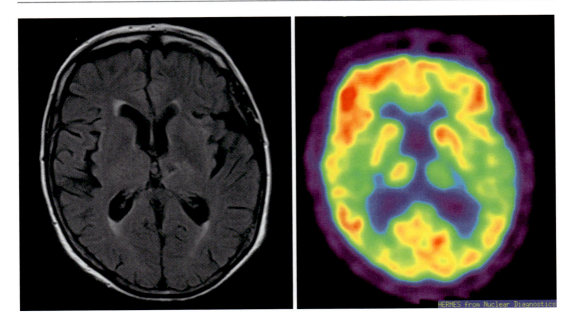

Fig. 18.4 FDG-PET: ischemic infarction affecting the left thalamus

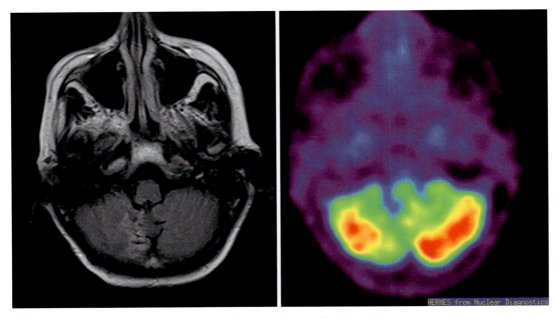

Fig. 18.5 FDG-PET: ischemic infarction located in the right cerebellum

18.5 Neuropathology Findings

Staging of infarcts is done as follows:

- Stage I: acute infarct
- Stage II: subacute infarct
- Stage III: chronic infarct

Macroscopic Features (Figs. 18.6, 18.7, and 18.8)

Stage I: acute infarct (1–4 days) (Fig. 18.7a–n)

- Mild softening of the involved brain region (palpation)
- Swelling of the involved brain region
- Discolored
- Reddish-brownish colored (when hemorrhagic)

Stage II: subacute infarct (5–30 days)

- Tissue shrinkage
- Softening of tissue
- Partial cystic change (6 weeks after incident)

Stage III: chronic infarct (weeks–months or years) (Fig. 18.8a–l)

- Cystic formation, 1 cm^3 size
- Develops 3 months after incident
- Depth of the gyrus

Microscopic Features (Figs. 18.9, 18.10, and 18.11)

Stage I: acute infarct (1–4 days) (Fig. 18.9a–f)

- Pale staining tissue.
- Pallor after 18 h.
- Zone of vacuolated neuropil separates the infarct from brain tissue 24–48 h after incident.
- Neuronal changes are irreversible and include:
  - Eosinophilic neuronal necrosis (ischemic cell change or ischemic neuronal necrosis) "red neurons"
    - Shrunken eosinophilic cell bodies
    - Pyknotic nuclei
  - Neuronal ghost
    Pale outline of the neuron
- Neuronal apoptosis
- Axonal swellings
  - At the edge of the infarct
- Immune cell infiltrates
  - Polymorphonuclear leukocytes appear between 24 and 48 h after incident.
  - Number of leukocytes is higher in hemorrhagic than anemic infarcts.
  - Correlates with reperfusion.
- Penumbra zone
  - Peri-infarct brain with reduced blood flow
  - Contains eosinophilic neuronal necrosis

Stage II: subacute infarct (5–30 days) (Fig. 18.10a–l)

- Necrotic tissue
- Numerous macrophages/microglial cells
- Reactive astrogliosis in the vicinity of the necrosis (2 weeks after incident)
  - Gemistocytic astrocytes with large pink bodies and eccentric nuclei
- Vascular endothelial proliferation
- Seldomly perivascular lymphocytic cuffing
- Dystrophic calcifications
- Neuronal ferrugination

Stage III: chronic infarct (weeks–months or years) (Fig. 18.11a–f)

- Cystic formation with nearly complete tissue loss
- Occasionally macrophages
- Gliotic adjacent brain tissue

18.5 Neuropathology Findings

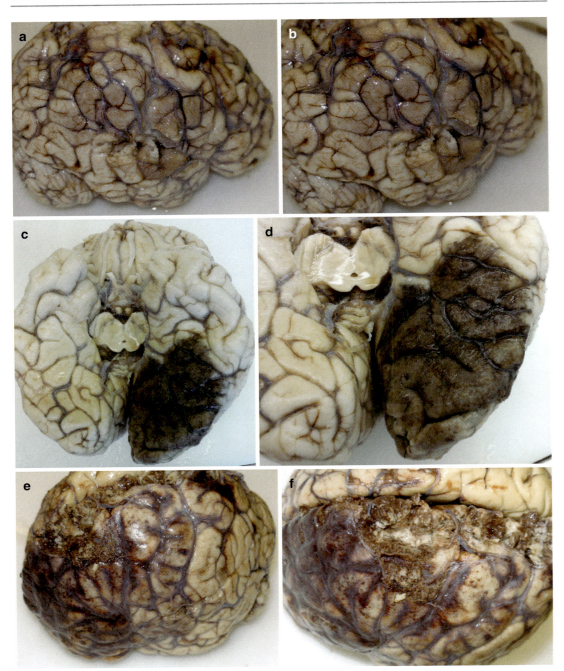

Fig. 18.6 Ischemic infarct: brownish discoloration of the outer surface in the right central region (**a**, **b**), left occipital lobe (**c**, **d**), left frontal and central region (**e**, **f**) as a sign of ischemic infarction. Infarct in the right temporoparietal region (**g**, **h**: outer surface) with corresponding tissue destruction of the coronal sections (**i**, **j**). Complete destruction of the white matter (**k**, **l**)

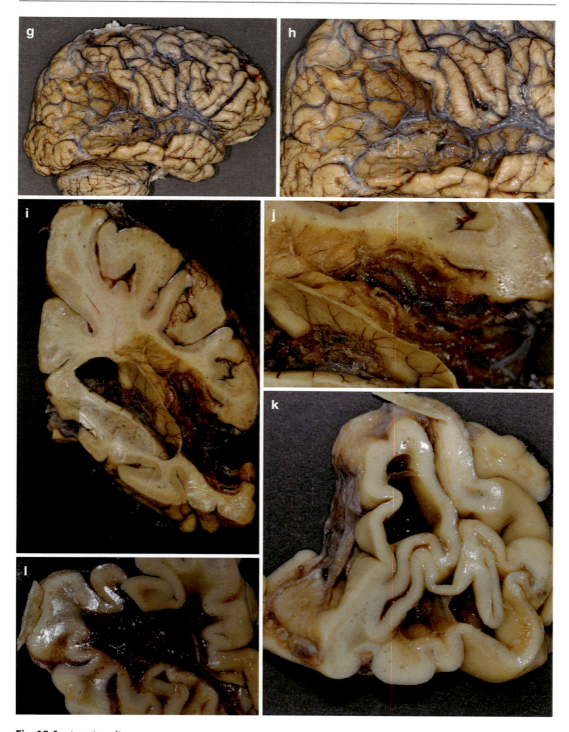

Fig. 18.6 (continued)

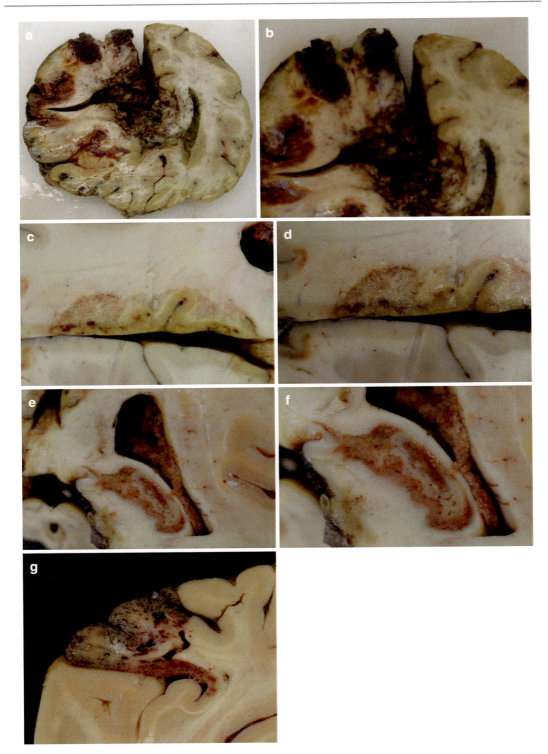

Fig. 18.7 Ischemic infarct—early stages: destruction of the left frontal lobe and parts of the corpus callosum (**a**, **b**). Cortical band necrosis (**c**, **d**); petechial hemorrhages in the posterior parts of the hippocampal formation (**e**, **f**), left parietal lobe (**g**, **h**), frontobasal cortex (**i**, **j**), left frontal lobe (**k**, **l**), and left frontal white matter (**m**, **n**)

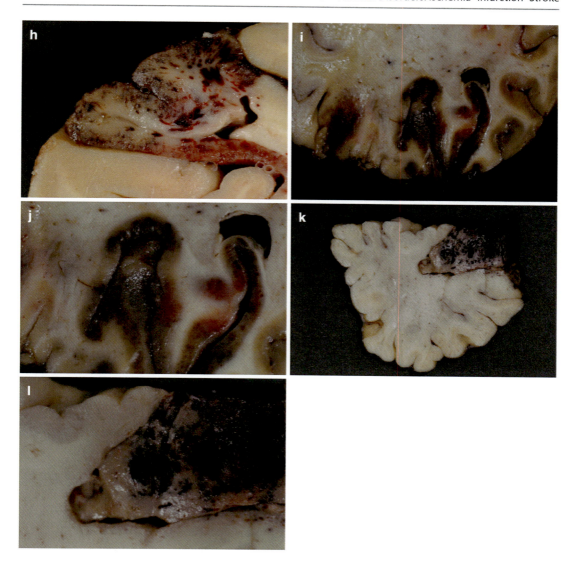

Fig. 18.7 (continued)

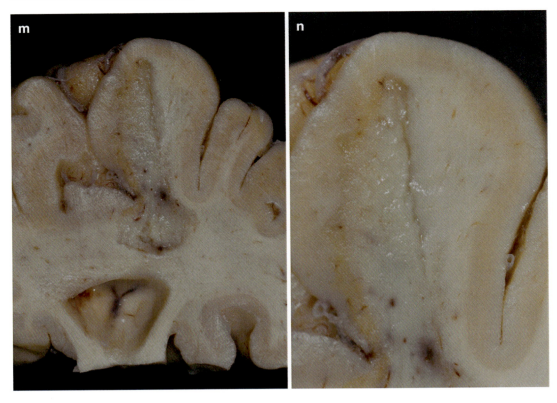

Fig. 18.7 (continued)

Hemorrhagic infarcts

- Multiple
- Of different age
- Located at border zones of arterial vascular supply

Lacunar infarct

- Small (<1–1.5 cm³) cystic infarct
- Subcortical locations (cerebral white matter, basal ganglia, thalamus, brain stem)
- Irregular shape with ragged borders

Immunohistochemical Staining Characteristics
- GFAP for astrogliosis
- CD68 and HLA-DRII for reactive microgliosis
- Lymphocytic markers

Differential Diagnosis
- Traumatic brain lesion
- Tumor necrosis
- Necrosis in infectious disease processes

18.6 Molecular Neuropathology

Pathogenesis
- Atherosclerosis
  - Large- and medium-size arteries
  - Arterial branching
  - Tortuosity
  - Confluence
- Dissection of large arteries
- Intracranial small vessel (lacunar) infarction
  - arteriolosclerosis
  - cerebral amyloid angiopathy
  - inherited or genetic small vessel disease

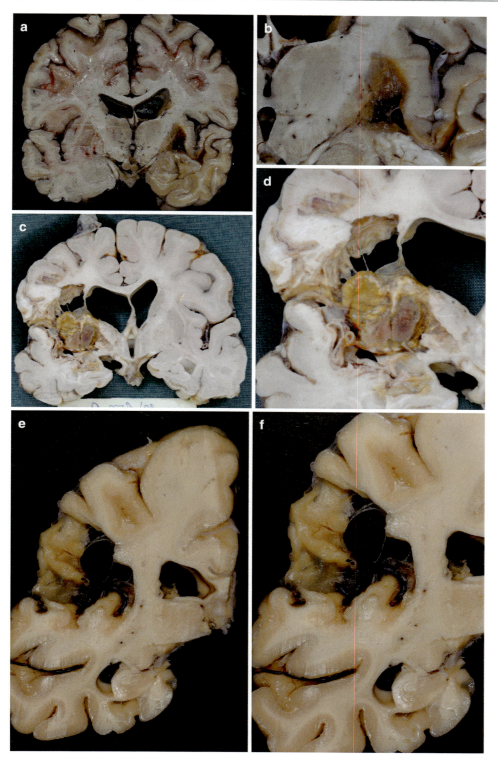

Fig. 18.8 Ischemic infarct—late stages: old ischemic infarcts manifest as brownish discolored necroses with partial to total tissue loss. Right basal ganglia (**a**, **b**); left basal ganglia (**c**, **d**), left parietal lobe (**e**, **f**), white matter of the cerebellum (**g**, **h**), coexistence of a fresh infarct in the central white matter (asterisk) and an old infarct in the left basal ganglia (**i**, **j**), and pons (**k**, **l**)

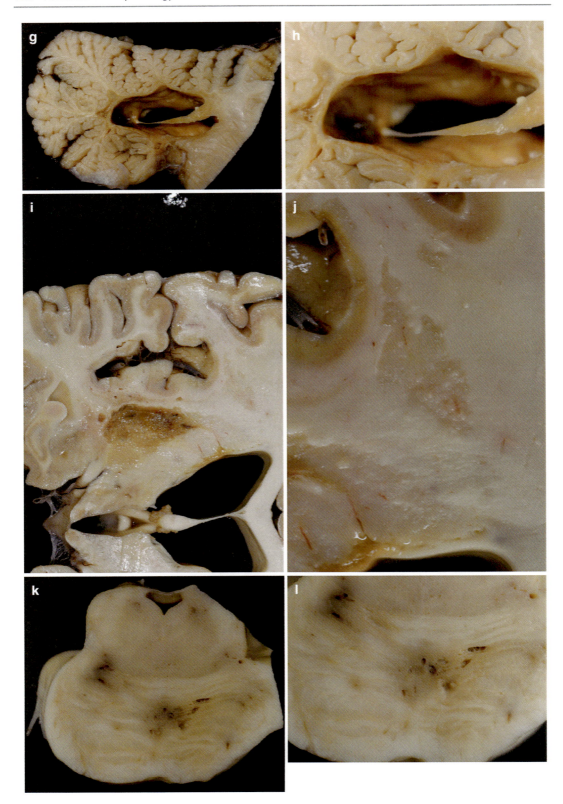

Fig. 18.8 (continued)

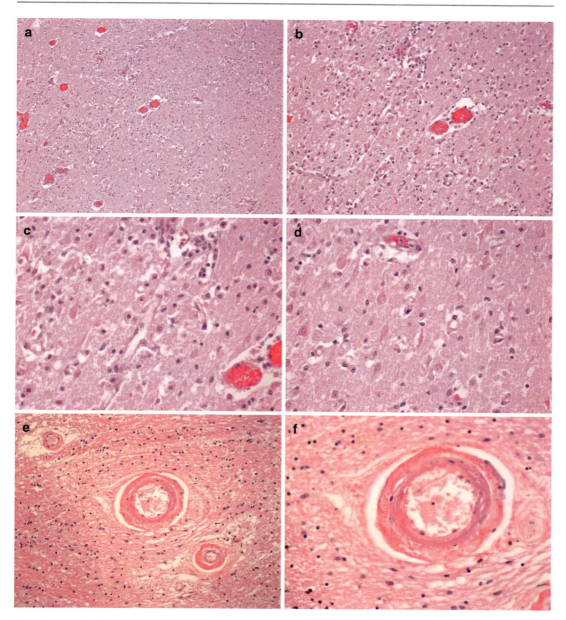

Fig. 18.9 Ischemic infarct—stage I: not-well demarcated area of beginning tissue dissolution with the presence of a few macrophages and reactive astrocytes (**a**–**d**). Note the presence of vessels with hyalinosis of the wall in close proximity of the lesion (**e**, **f**)

18.6 Molecular Neuropathology

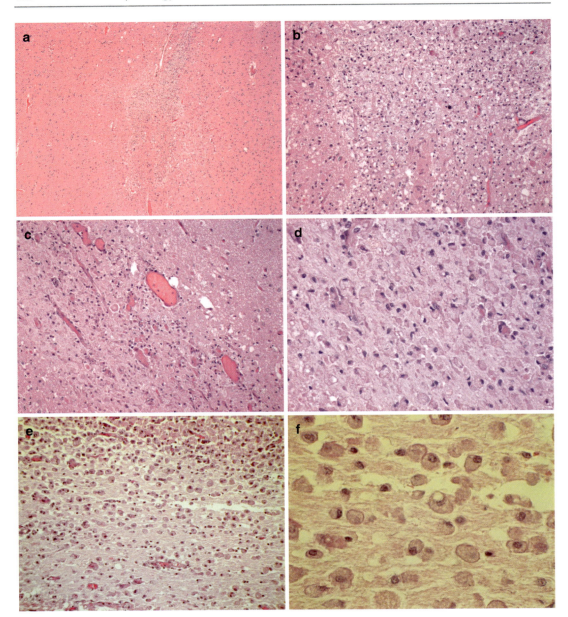

Fig. 18.10 Ischemic infarct—stage II: well-demarcated region with tissue destruction and the presence of numerous macrophages, reactive astrocytes, and endothelial proliferation (**a**–**f**). Sometimes one might not perivascular lymphocytic cuffing (**g**, **h**). Necrosis of the cerebral cortex (band necrosis) with complete destruction of layers II–VI, cellular debris, and some reactive astrocytes at the border of the lesion (**i**–**l**)

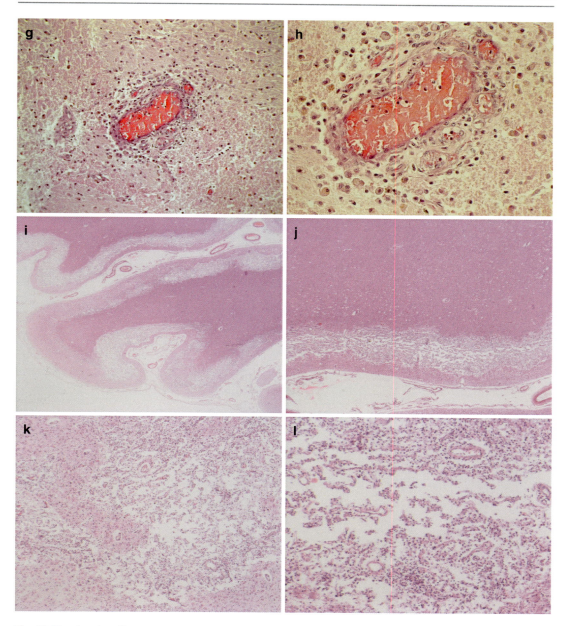

Fig. 18.10 (continued)

18.6 Molecular Neuropathology

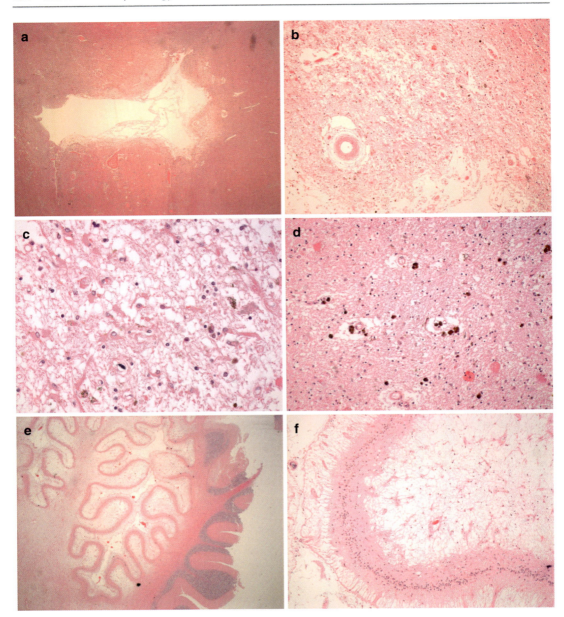

Fig. 18.11 Ischemic infarct—stage III: old necrosis with complete tissue loss (**a**); the surrounding tissue shows loosely textured tissue (**b**), reactive astrogliosis (**c**), and hemosiderinophages (**d**). Complete tissue loss in layers I and III of the cerebellar folia with preservation of layer II (**e**, **f**)

- infectious small vessel disease
- inflammatory small vessel disease
- immunologically mediated small vessel disease
- Cardiac embolism
  - Right to left shunt
  - Left atrium
  - Mitral valve
  - Left ventricle
  - Aortic valve
  - Congenital heart disease
- Other determined causes
  - Fabry disease
  - Moyamoya disease
  - Arteritis
- Cryptogenic stroke

Hemorrhagic infarcts
- Delayed breakup of the embolus allowing reperfusion into the necrotic blood vessel
- Occurs within the first 15 days of infarct onset
- Hemosiderin-laden macrophages
- Reactive astrogliosis

18.7 Treatment and Prognosis

Treatment
- Based on levels and grades of evidence
- Acute thrombolysis
- Antiplatelet therapy (aspirin/acetylsalicyclic acid)
- Anticoagulation therapy
- Recanalization
- Neuroprotection
- HemicraniectomyBiologic

Behavior–Prognosis–Prognostic Factors
- Risk factors
  - Non-modifiable factors
    - Age
    - Race ethnicity
    - Family history
  - Modifiable factors
    - Hypertension
    - Smoking
    - Physical activity
    - Diabetes
    - Depression
    - Psychosocial stress
    - Alcohol intake
- Outcome
  - 10% of all deaths in industrialized countries in persons over the age of 65 years
  - Age-adjusted stroke mortality 50–100 per 100,000 population/year
  - Fatality rates:
    - 10% at 7 days
    - 20% at 30 days
    - 30% at 1 year
    - 60% at 5 years
    - 80% at 10 years
- Prognostic factors for survival
  - Preadmission comorbidities
  - Increased age
  - Reduced level of consciousness
  - Severe/total limb weakness with aphasia or neglect
- Secondary effects
  - Cerebral edema
  - Hydrocephalus
- Wallerian degeneration

Selected References

Bamford J, Sandercock P, Dennis M, Burn J, Warlow C (1991) Classification and natural history of clinically identifiable subtypes of cerebral infarction. Lancet 337(8756):1521–1526

Bateman M, Slater LA, Leslie-Mazwi T, Simonsen CZ, Stuckey S, Chandra RV (2017) Diffusion and perfusion MR imaging in acute stroke: clinical utility and potential limitations for treatment selection. Top Magn Reson Imaging 26(2):77–82. https://doi.org/10.1097/rmr.0000000000000124

Bosetti F, Koenig JI, Ayata C, Back SA, Becker K, Broderick JP, Carmichael ST, Cho S, Cipolla MJ, Corbett D, Corriveau RA, Cramer SC, Ferguson AR, Finklestein SP, Ford BD, Furie KL, Hemmen TM, Iadecola C, Jakeman LB, Janis S, Jauch EC, Johnston KC, Kochanek PM, Kohn H, Lo EH, Lyden PD, Mallard C, McCullough LD, McGavern LM, Meschia JF, Moy CS, Perez-Pinzon MA, Ramadan I, Savitz SI, Schwamm LH, Steinberg GK, Stenzel-Poore MP, Tymianski M, Warach S, Wechsler LR, Zhang JH, Koroshetz W (2017) Translational stroke research: vision and opportunities. Stroke 48(9):2632–2637. https://doi.org/10.1161/strokeaha.117.017112

Selected References

Caldwell J, Heran MKS, McGuinness B, Barber PA (2017) Imaging in acute ischaemic stroke: pearls and pitfalls. Pract Neurol 17(5):349–358. https://doi.org/10.1136/practneurol-2016-001569

Chauhan G, Debette S (2016) Genetic risk factors for ischemic and hemorrhagic stroke. Curr Cardiol Rep 18(12):124. https://doi.org/10.1007/s11886-016-0804-z

Ferdinand P, Roffe C (2016) Hypoxia after stroke: a review of experimental and clinical evidence. Exp Transl Stroke Med 8:9. https://doi.org/10.1186/s13231-016-0023-0

Gupta A, Sattur MG, Aoun RJN, Krishna C, Bolton PB, Chong BW, Demaerschalk BM, Lyons MK, McClendon J Jr, Patel N, Sen A, Swanson K, Zimmerman RS, Bendok BR (2017) Hemicraniectomy for ischemic and hemorrhagic stroke: facts and controversies. Neurosurg Clin N Am 28(3):349–360. https://doi.org/10.1016/j.nec.2017.02.010

Harris AD, Coutts SB, Frayne R (2009) Diffusion and perfusion MR imaging of acute ischemic stroke. Magn Reson Imaging Clin N Am 17(2):291–313. https://doi.org/10.1016/j.mric.2009.02.001

Heiss WD, Zaro Weber O (2017) Validation of MRI determination of the penumbra by PET measurements in ischemic stroke. J Nucl Med 58(2):187–193. https://doi.org/10.2967/jnumed.116.185975

Kassis H, Shehadah A, Chopp M, Zhang ZG (2017) Epigenetics in stroke recovery. Genes 8(3):89. https://doi.org/10.3390/genes8030089

Khoshnam SE, Winlow W, Farzaneh M, Farbood Y, Moghaddam HF (2017) Pathogenic mechanisms following ischemic stroke. Neurol Sci 38(7):1167–1186. https://doi.org/10.1007/s10072-017-2938-1

Kim JS, Caplan LR (2016) Clinical stroke syndromes. Front Neurol Neurosci 40:72–92. https://doi.org/10.1159/000448303

Kranz PG, Eastwood JD (2009) Does diffusion-weighted imaging represent the ischemic core? An evidence-based systematic review. AJNR Am J Neuroradiol 30(6):1206–1212. https://doi.org/10.3174/ajnr.A1547

Leary MC, Kidwell CS, Villablanca JP, Starkman S, Jahan R, Duckwiler GR, Gobin YP, Sykes S, Gough KJ, Ferguson K, Llanes JN, Masamed R, Tremwel M, Ovbiagele B, Vespa PM, Vinuela F, Saver JL (2003) Validation of computed tomographic middle cerebral artery "dot" sign: an angiographic correlation study. Stroke 34(11):2636–2640. https://doi.org/10.1161/01.str.0000092123.00938.83

Mijajlovic MD, Pavlovic A, Brainin M, Heiss WD, Quinn TJ, Ihle-Hansen HB, Hermann DM, Assayag EB, Richard E, Thiel A, Kliper E, Shin YI, Kim YH, Choi S, Jung S, Lee YB, Sinanovic O, Levine DA, Schlesinger I, Mead G, Milosevic V, Leys D, Hagberg G, Ursin MH, Teuschl Y, Prokopenko S, Mozheyko E, Bezdenezhnykh A, Matz K, Aleksic V, Muresanu D, Korczyn AD, Bornstein NM (2017) Post-stroke dementia—a comprehensive review. BMC Med 15(1):11. https://doi.org/10.1186/s12916-017-0779-7

Ng GJL, Quek AML, Cheung C, Arumugam TV, Seet RCS (2017) Stroke biomarkers in clinical practice: a critical appraisal. Neurochem Int 107:11–22. https://doi.org/10.1016/j.neuint.2017.01.005

Radu RA, Terecoasa EO, Bajenaru OA, Tiu C (2017) Etiologic classification of ischemic stroke: where do we stand? Clin Neurol Neurosurg 159:93–106. https://doi.org/10.1016/j.clineuro.2017.05.019

Rangel-Castilla L, Rajah GB, Shakir HJ, Davies JM, Snyder KV, Siddiqui AH, Levy EI, Hopkins LN (2016) Acute stroke endovascular treatment: tips and tricks. J Cardiovasc Surg 57(6):758–768

Siket MS (2016) Treatment of acute ischemic stroke. Emerg Med Clin North Am 34(4):861–882. https://doi.org/10.1016/j.emc.2016.06.009

Tan R, Traylor M, Rutten-Jacobs L, Markus H (2017) New insights into mechanisms of small vessel disease stroke from genetics. Clin Sci (Lond) 131(7):515–531. https://doi.org/10.1042/cs20160825

Toyoda K, Ida M, Fukuda K (2001) Fluid-attenuated inversion recovery intraarterial signal: an early sign of hyperacute cerebral ischemia. AJNR Am J Neuroradiol 22(6):1021–1029

Trenkler J (2008) Acute ischemic stroke. Diagnostic imaging and interventional options. Radiologe 48(5):457–473. https://doi.org/10.1007/s00117-008-1663-4

Warach S, Al-Rawi Y, Furlan AJ, Fiebach JB, Wintermark M, Lindsten A, Smyej J, Bharucha DB, Pedraza S, Rowley HA (2012) Refinement of the magnetic resonance diffusion-perfusion mismatch concept for thrombolytic patient selection: insights from the desmoteplase in acute stroke trials. Stroke 43(9):2313–2318. https://doi.org/10.1161/strokeaha.111.642348

Wintermark M, Reichhart M, Cuisenaire O, Maeder P, Thiran JP, Schnyder P, Bogousslavsky J, Meuli R (2002) Comparison of admission perfusion computed tomography and qualitative diffusion- and perfusion-weighted magnetic resonance imaging in acute stroke patients. Stroke 33(8):2025–2031

Wong KS, Caplan LR, Kim JS (2016) Stroke mechanisms. Front Neurol Neurosci 40:58–71. https://doi.org/10.1159/000448302

Yoo AJ, Andersson T (2017) Thrombectomy in acute ischemic stroke: challenges to procedural success. J Stroke 19(2):121–130. https://doi.org/10.5853/jos.2017.00752

Vascular Disorders: Hemorrhage   19

19.1 General Considerations

The following types of hemorrhages are distinguished (Fig. 19.1):

- Subcutaneous hemorrhage
- Subgaleal hemorrhage
- Epidural hemorrhage
- Subdural hemorrhage
- Subarachnoid hemorrhage
- Intracerebral hemorrhage
- Intramedullary hemorrhage
- Choroid plexus hemorrhage (mainly in fetuses)
- Germinal matrix hemorrhage (in fetuses)

These types of hemorrhages are defined as accumulation of blood (Fig. 19.1):

- Subgaleal hemorrhage
  - Into the galea aponeurotica
- Epidural hemorrhage
  - Between the skull bone and the dura
- Subdural hemorrhage
  - Between the dura and the arachnoidea
- Subarachnoid hemorrhage
  - Into the leptomeninges
- Intracerebral hemorrhage
  - Into the brain parenchyme
- Intramedullary hemorrhage
  - Into the parenchyme of the brain stem

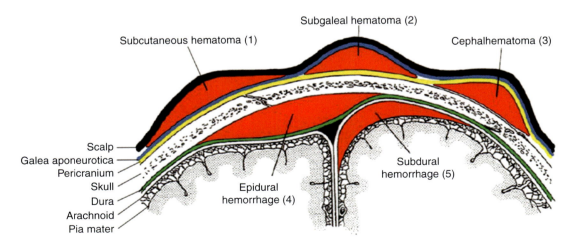

Fig. 19.1 Local-ization of blood in the different spaces of the brain coverings (reproduced from Öhmichen et al. (2006) with kind permission by Springer Nature)

- Choroid plexus hemorrhage (mainly in fetuses)
  - Into the choroid plexus
- Germinal matrix hemorrhage (in fetuses)
  - Into the germinal matrix of the developing brain

Clinical characterization of hematomas based on time elapsed after the causing event:

- Hyperacute: <6 h
- Acute: 6 h to 3 days
- Early subacute: 3–7 days
- Late subacute: 1–4 weeks
- Chronic: >4 weeks

19.2 Intracerebral Hemorrhage

19.2.1 Clinical Signs and Symptoms

Either acute onset or evolving neurological symptoms
- Headache
- Vomiting
- Neurologic deficit
- Decreased level of conscious due to raised intracranial pressure
- Damage of connecting fibers or of overlaying cortex may lead to:
  - Dysphasia
  - Visual field defects
  - Neglect

19.2.2 Epidemiology

Incidence
- 10–20 per 100,000/year
- 10–40% are the cause of stroke

Age Incidence
- Progressively increases with age

Sex Incidence
- Male:Female ratio: M > F

Localization
- Any part of the brain
- By specific region
  - Putamen or internal capsule: 30%
  - Caudate nucleus: 5%
  - Basal ganglia: 5%
  - Lobar: 30%
  - Thalamus: 15%
  - Cerebellum: 10%
  - Pons or midbrain: 5%

19.2.3 Neuroimaging Findings

General Imaging Findings
- In acute phase hyperdense mass (CT).
- MR signal varies with age, most helpful are hemosensitive sequences (T2* or SWI) with hypointense bleeding.

CT Non-Contrast-Enhanced (Figs. 19.2a–d and 19.3a, b)
- Acute: hyperdense mass, isodense rare, surrounding hypodense edema
- Subacute: over time from hyperdense to isodense, finally hypodense

CT Contrast-Enhanced
- No enhancement
- Contrast extravasation demonstrates active bleeding
- During resorption (subacute) peripheral enhancement possible

CT-Angiography
- Detects vascular malformations
- Negative in hypertensive bleeding

MRI-T2 (Figs. 19.2e and 19.3c)
- Hyperacute (<6 h): hyperintense
- Acute (6 h to 3 days): hypointense
- Early subacute (3–7 days): hypointense
- Late subacute (1–4 weeks): hyperintense
- Chronic: hypointense, with hypointense rim (hemosiderin)

MRI-FLAIR (Figs. 19.2f and 19.3d)
- Hyperacute (<6 h): hyperintense
- Acute (6 h to 3 days): hypointense
- Early subacute (3–7 days): hypointense
- Late subacute (1–4 weeks): hyperintense
- Chronic: hypointense

MRI-T1 (Figs. 19.2g and 19.3e)
- Hyperacute (<6 h): iso- to slight hypointense
- Acute (6 h to 3 days): iso- to hypointense
- Early subacute (3–7 days): hyperintense
- Late subacute (1–4 weeks): hyperintense
- Chronic: iso- to hypointense

MRI-T1 Contrast-Enhanced (Figs. 19.2h and 19.3f)
- No enhancement

MR-Diffusion Imaging (Figs. 19.2i and 19.3g)
- Hyperacute (<6 h): hypointense
- Acute (6 h to 3 days): hypointense

MRI-T2∗/SWI (Figs. 19.2j and 19.3h)
- Hyperacute (<6 h): hypointense
- Acute (6 h to 3 days): hypointense
- Early subacute (3–7 days): hypointense
- Late subacute (1–4 weeks): hypointense
- Chronic: hypointense

Nuclear Medicine Imaging Findings (Fig. 19.4a, b)
- CBF-SPECT demonstrates perfusion deficits.
- FDG-PET can demonstrate the reduced glucose uptake und utilization in impaired neuronal structures.
- Flumazenil PET which shows the $GABA_A$ receptors can demonstrate the neuronal damage caused by hemorrhage.
- 15-O PET can demonstrate oxygen extraction fraction.

19.2.4 Neuropathology Findings

Macroscopic Features (Figs. 19.5a–x)
- The macroscopic changes seen at different time points are detailed in Table 19.1.

Microscopic Features (Fig. 19.6a–n)
- The microscopic changes seen at different time points are detailed in Table 19.2.

Immunohistochemical Staining Characteristics
- β-amyloid to exclude cerebral amyloid angiopathy (CAA)

Differential Diagnosis
- Hemorrhage due to cerebral amyloid angiopathy (CAA)
- Hemorrhage into an ischemic necrosis

19.2.5 Molecular Neuropathology

- Primary
  - Arterial hypertension
  - Cerebral amyloid angiopathy
- Secondary
  - Trauma
  - Ruptured aneurysm
  - Arteriovenous malformations
  - Brain tumors
  - Medication (anticoagulant, thrombolytic, antiplatelet agents)
  - Recreational drugs (cocaine, amphetamine, ephedrine)
  - Hemorrhagic conversion of cerebral infarct
  - Vasculitis
- Less common causes include:
  - Hematological diseases (leukemia, thrombocytopenia, hemophilia)
  - Vasculitis
  - Subarachnoidal hemorrhage with intraparenchymal extension
  - Cavernous hemangioma

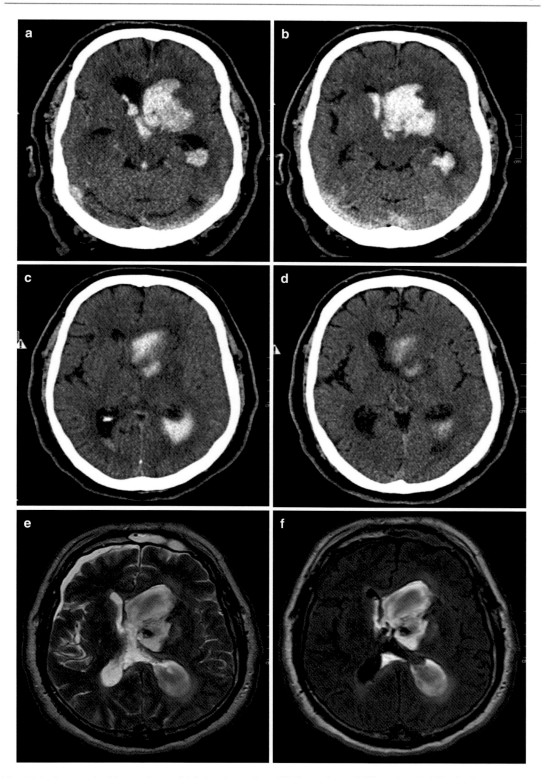

Fig. 19.2 Intracerebral hemorrhage of left basal ganglia with intraventricular blood over time CT day 1 (**a**), CT day 5 (**b**), CT day 10 (**c**), and CT day 25 (**d**). MR of day 19 (late subacute) T2 ax (**e**), FLAIR (**f**), T1 (**g**), T1 contrast (**h**), DWI (**i**), SWI (**j**)

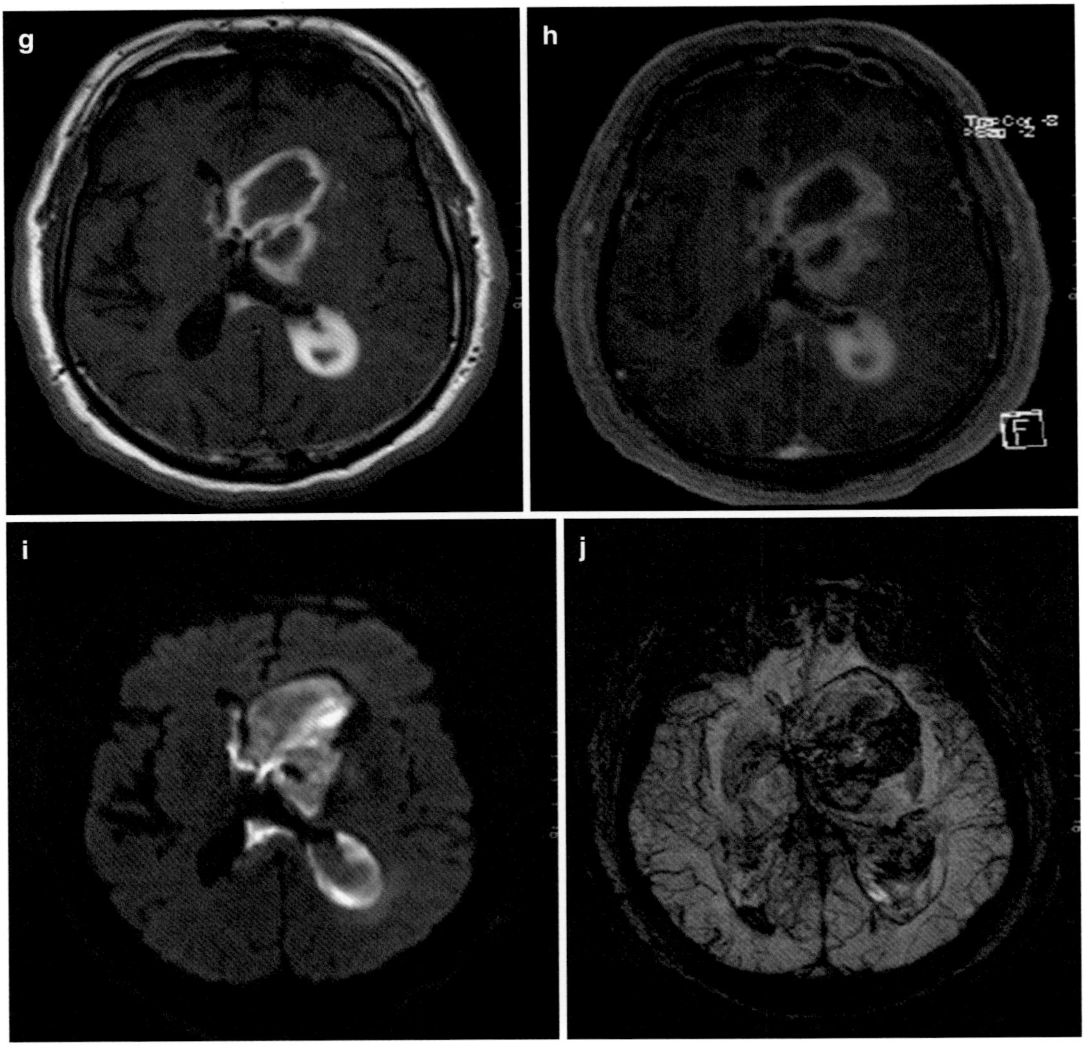

19.2 Intracerebral Hemorrhage

Fig. 19.2 (continued)

19.2.6 Treatment and Prognosis

Treatment
- Surgical evacuation of supratentorial intracerebral in selected patients
- Surgical evacuation of infratentorial intracerebellar hemorrhage
- Hemostatic drug therapy
- Blood pressure reduction

Biologic Behavior–Prognosis–Prognostic Factors
- Lethal to good outcome
- Success of rehabilitation
  - Mobility
  - Spasticity
  - Gait
- Control of risk factors
- Recurrences frequent in cerebral amyloid angiopathy

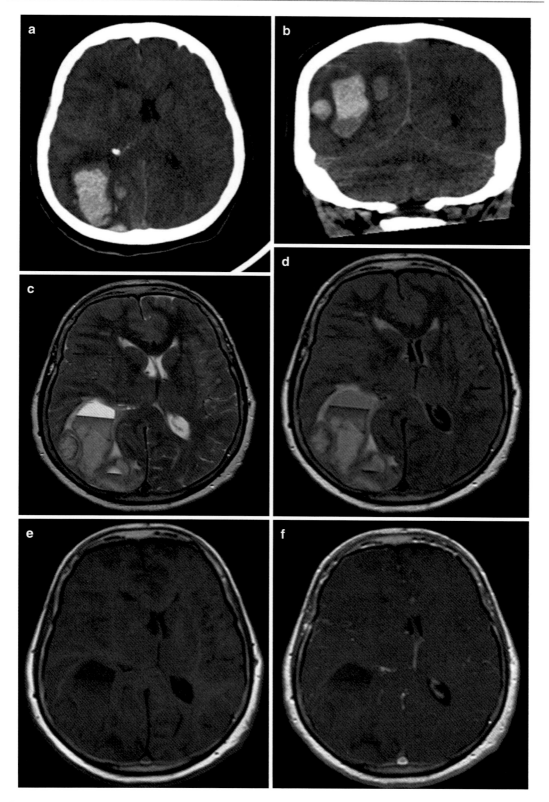

Fig. 19.3 Acute intraparenchymal hemorrhage right parieto-occipital with CT ax/cor (**a**, **b**), T2 (**c**), Flair (**d**), T1 (**e**), T1 contrast (**f**), DWI (**g**), SWI (**h**)

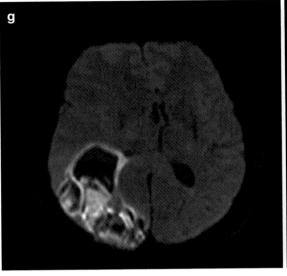
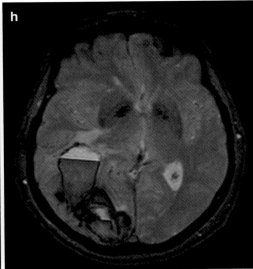

Fig. 19.3 (continued)

19.3 Subarachnoid Hemorrhage (SAH)

19.3.1 Clinical Signs and Symptoms

- Sudden onset of severe, diffuse headache
  - Peaking within minutes
  - Lasting 1–2 weeks
- Focal neurologic signs include
  - Hemiparesis
  - Paraparesis
  - Cerebellar ataxia, Wallenberg syndrome
  - IIIrd cranial nerve palsy
  - VIth cranial nerve palsy
  - IXth–XIIth cranial nerve palsy
  - Sustained downward gaze and unreactive pupils

19.3.2 Epidemiology

Incidence
- 4.1–22.7 per 100,000 person-years

Age Incidence
- Middle ages

Sex Incidence
- Male:Female ratio: 1:3

Localization
- Subarachnoidal space
- See Chap. 21 for common sites of aneurysms
  - Anterior communicating artery (ACA)
  - Middle cerebral artery (MCA)
  - Internal carotid artery (ICA)
  - Basilar artery (BA)

19.3.3 Neuroimaging Findings

General Imaging Findings
- Hyperintense CSF on CT and MRI-FLAIR
- MRA/CTA/DSA: Detection/exclusion of aneurysm mandatory

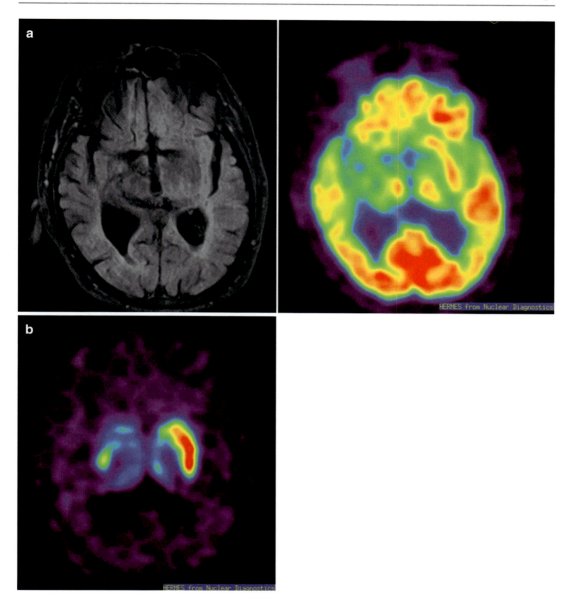

Fig. 19.4 Patient with a status post-hemorrhage into right basal ganglia—MRI, FDG-PET (**a**) and fallypride-PET (postsynaptic dopaminergic system) (**b**)

CT Non-Contrast-Enhanced (Fig. 19.7a, b)
- Hyperintense sulci and cisterns
- Helps to detect hydrocephalus

CT Contrast-Enhanced
- Reveals aneurysm

MRI-T2 (Fig. 19.7c)
- Isointense to CSF

MRI-FLAIR (Fig. 19.7d)
- Hyperintense, highly sensitive

MRI-T1 (Fig. 19.7e)
- Not sensitive for SAH, "dirty CSF"

MRI-T1 Contrast-Enhanced (Fig. 19.7f)
- No enhancement

19.3 Subarachnoid Hemorrhage (SAH)

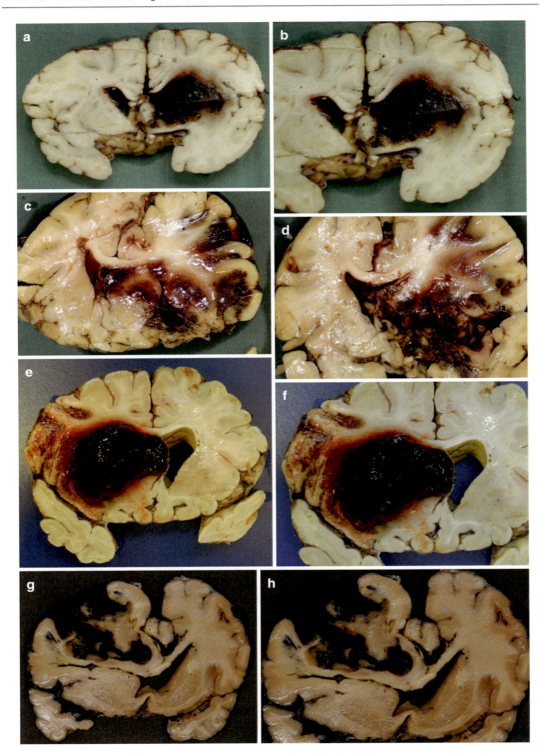

Fig. 19.5 Intracerebral hemorrhage: Brain sections show tissue destruction due to hemorrhage of the right basal ganglia (**a, b**), right frontal white matter (**c, d**), left basal ganglia with ventricular hemorrhage (**e, f**), left central region (**g, h**), left parietal lobe (**i, j**), left thalamus (**k, l**), ventricular tamponade (**m, n**), disruption of the right parietal cortical surface (**o, p**), cerebellar hemispheres (**q–t**). Secondary hemorrhages due to increased cerebral pressure in the brain stem (**u–x**)

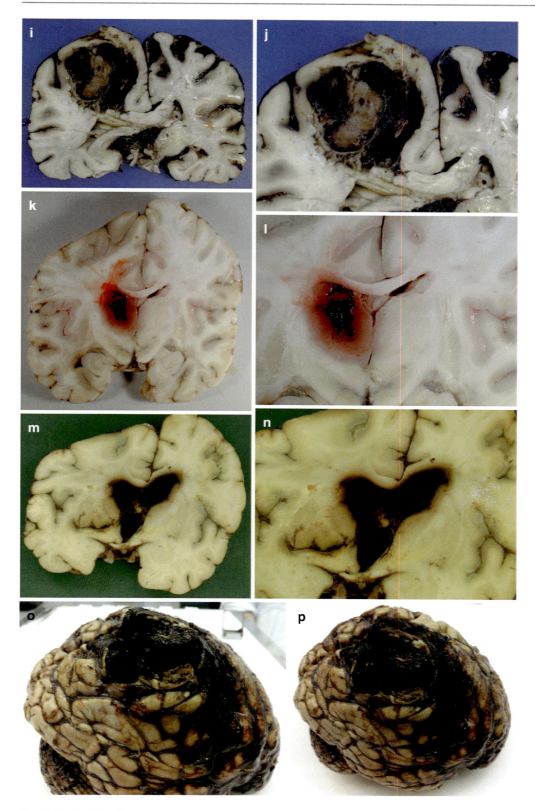

Fig. 19.5 (continued)

19.3 Subarachnoid Hemorrhage (SAH)

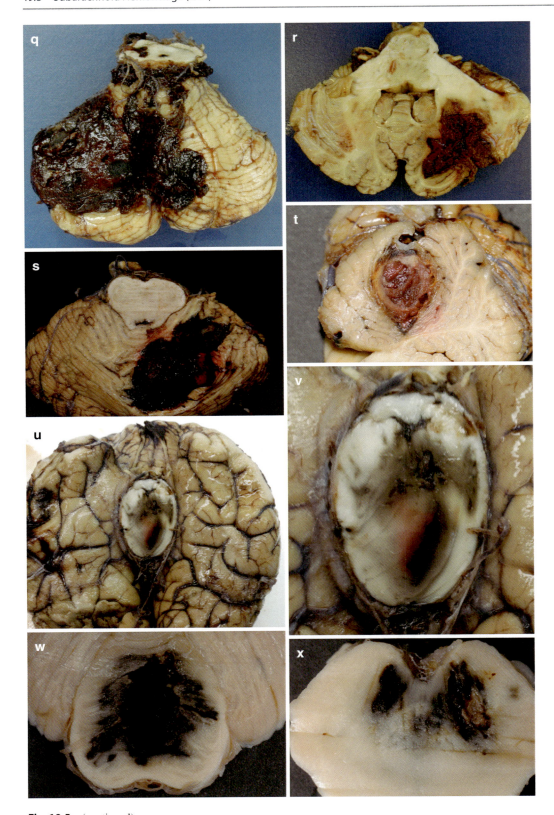

Fig. 19.5 (continued)

Table 19.1 Timing and estimation of the age of the hematoma based on macroscopic criteria

Time	Macroscopic changes
Seconds to minutes	• Hematoma formation, red colored
Minutes to hours	• Space-occupying effect • Distortion and compression of surrounding tissue
Several hours	• Peri-hematoma edema Ischemia • Increasing space-occupying effect
2–3 days to weeks	• Brown coloration of the hematoma
Weeks to months	• Friable brown clot
Months to years	• Cavity containing dark blood-stained fluid • Cavity containing clear fluid resembling CSH with brown hemosiderin-stained cavity wall

Table 19.2 Timing and estimation of the age of the hematoma based on microscopic criteria

Time	Microscopic changes
Seconds to minutes	• Rupture of blood vessel • Extravasation of blood
Minutes to hours	• Lysis of erythrocytes
Several hours	• Edema • Ischemia • Polymorph infiltrates
2–3 days to weeks	• Hemosiderin formation • Phagocytosis by macrophages • Astrocyte hypertrophy • Formation of new blood vessels
Weeks to months	• Organization of the hematoma • Phagocytosis of blood • Phagocytosis of necrotic tissue
Months to years	• Resorption of blood clot • Cavity lined by hyperplastic and hypertrophic glial cells • Hemosiderin-laden residual macrophages

MRI-T2∗/SWI
- Hypointense

Nuclear Medicine Imaging Findings
- CBF-SPECT demonstrates perfusion deficits.
- FDG-PET can demonstrate the reduced glucose uptake und utilization in impaired neuronal structures.
- Flumazenil PET which shows the $GABA_A$ receptors can demonstrate the neuronal damage caused by hemorrhage.
- 15-O PET can demonstrate oxygen extraction fraction.

19.3.4 Neuropathology Findings

Macroscopic Features (Fig. 19.8a–f)
- Hemorrhage in the leptomeningeal spaces.
- Diffusely throughout the subarachnoid space.
- Subarachnoidal hematoma.
- Hemorrhage enters and destroys the brain parenchyma.
- Can extend into the ventricles (from brain parenchyma or from subarachnoidal spaces).

Microscopic Features (Fig. 19.9a–j)
- Erythrocytes
- Fibrin
- Mononuclear cells
- Vessel walls might be thickened

Immunohistochemical Staining Characteristics
- β-amyloid to exclude cerebral amyloid angiopathy (CAA)

Differential Diagnosis
- Hemorrhage due to cerebral amyloid angiopathy (CAA)
- Hemorrhage into an ischemic necrosis

19.3 Subarachnoid Hemorrhage (SAH)

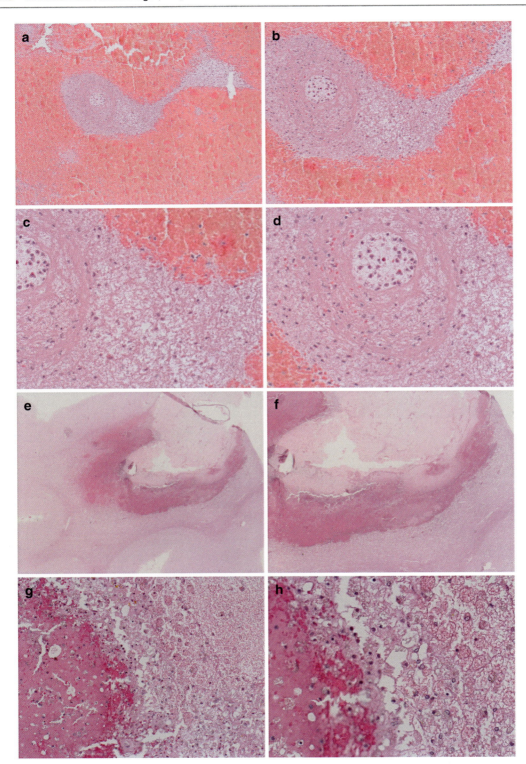

Fig. 19.6 Intracerebral hemorrhage: Between erythrocytes the presence of a vessels and fibrin is obvious (**a–d**). In the vicinity of the lesions, there is recruitment of large numbers of macrophages (**e–h**). Fibrin stains reddish while erythrocytes stain green on Elastica van Gieson stain (**i, j**). Vessels in the proximity usually show wall hyalinosis (**k, l**). Petechial reperfusion bleedings in the cerebellum (**m, n**)

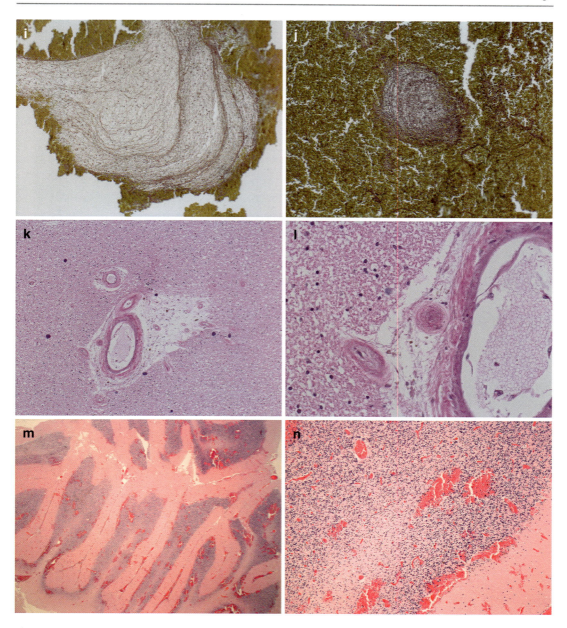

Fig. 19.6 (continued)

19.3 Subarachnoid Hemorrhage (SAH)

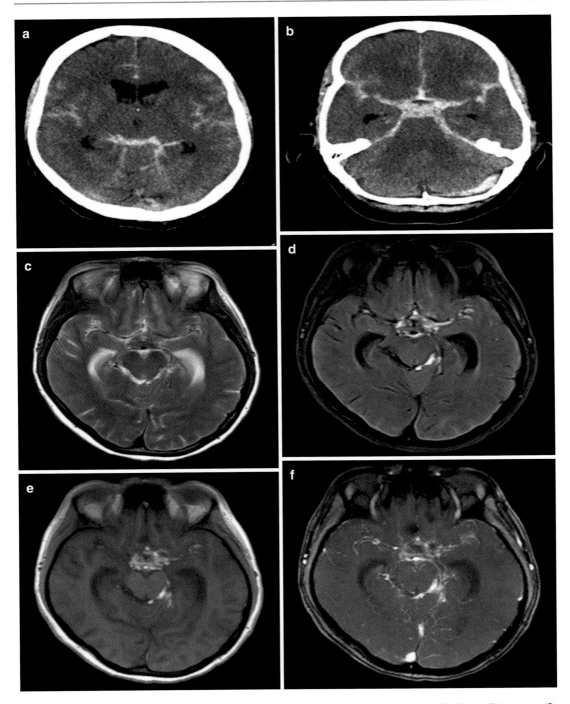

Fig. 19.7 Subarachnoidal hemorrhage with CT ax (**a**, **b**) and MR at day 7 T2 (**c**), FLAIR (**d**), T1 (**e**), T1 contrast (**f**). DSA of dissecting left vertebral aneurysm (**g**)

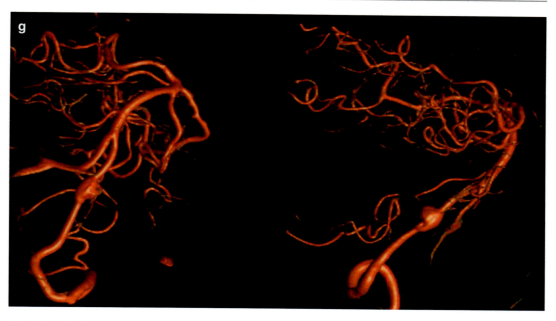

Fig. 19.7 (continued)

19.3.5 Molecular Neuropathology

- Ruptured saccular aneurysm (85%)
- Non-aneurysmal perimesencephalic hemorrhage
- Non-inflammatory lesions of intracerebral vessels
  - Arterial dissection
  - Cerebral arteriovenous malformation
- Inflammatory lesions of cerebral arteries
  - Mycotic aneurysm
  - Borreliosis
- Sickle cell disease
- Tumors
- Drugs
  - Cocaine
  - Anticoagulants
- Head trauma
- Inflammatory molecules (Table 19.3)

19.3.6 Treatment and Prognosis

Treatment
- Calcium antagonist Nimodipine
- Endovascular coiling/neurosurgical clipping of aneurysm

Biologic Behavior–Prognosis–Prognostic Factors
- Modifiable factors (Table 19.4)
  - Hypertension
  - Smoking
  - Physical activity
  - Diabetes
  - Depression
  - Psychosocial stress
  - Alcohol intake

19.3 Subarachnoid Hemorrhage (SAH)

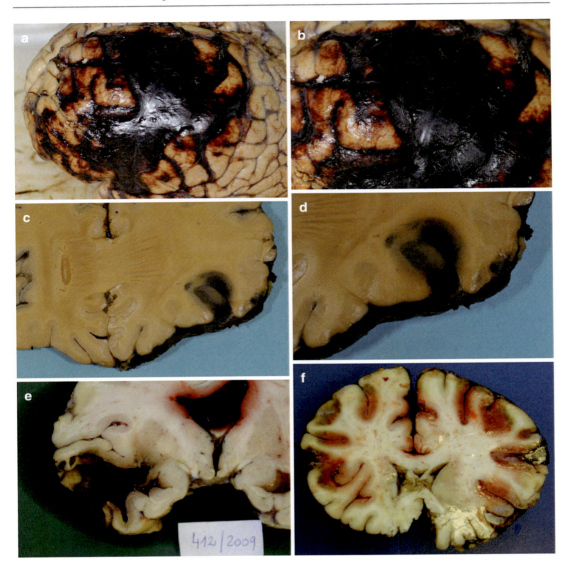

Fig. 19.8 Subarachnoidal hemorrhage: Large area of blood accumulation in the arachnoidal spaces over the left frontal lobe (**a**, **b**), extending deep into the sulci (**c**, **d**) with destruction of the right temporal cerebral tissue (**e**), and leading to intracortical petechial reperfusion bleedings (**f**)

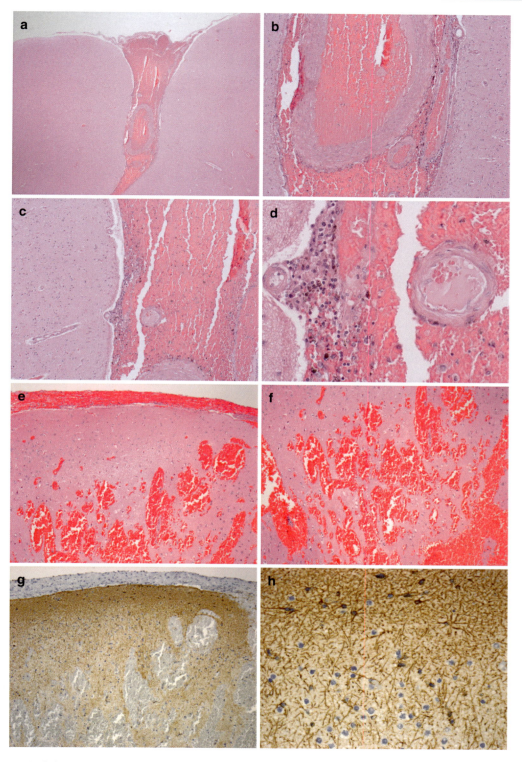

Fig. 19.9 Subarachnoidal hemorrhage: The blood fills the leptomeningeal spaces of the sulci (**a**, **b**) containing hyalinised vessels (**a**, **b**), monomorphonuclear cells (**c**, **d**). The intracortical petechial reperfusion bleedings might destroy large areas of tissue (**e**, **f**). Large areas might show strong reactive astrogliosis (**g**, **h**: GFAP) while reactive microgliosis is mild (**i**, **j**)

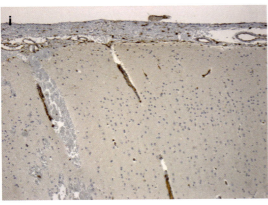
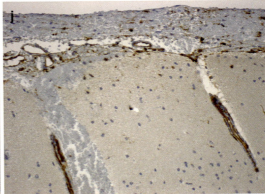

Fig. 19.9 (continued)

Table 19.3 Key inflammatory molecules implicated in the pathology of SAH (Miller et al. 2014) reproduced with kind permission from Hindawi

Molecule	Function	Roles in human studies	Roles in animal studies
Selectins	Leukocyte adhesion	• Higher levels in CSF correlate to vasospasm in some studies • Found in walls of ruptured aneurysms	• Inhibition of selectins decreases vasospasm
Integrins	Leukocyte adhesion	• Higher levels seen in patients with vasospasm	• Blocking reduces vasospasm
TNFα	Pro-inflammatory cytokine produced by leukocytes	• Found in CSF in patients after SAH • cCorrelates with vasospasm after SAH	• Induces neuronal apoptosis after SAH • Blockade reduces vasospasm
MCP-1	Macrophage chemoattractant	• Found in CSF after SAH • Associated with poor outcomes but not vasospasm	• Promotes repair of aneurysms
ICAM-1	Leukocyte adhesion	• Increased in patients with SAH	• Increased in animal SAH studies • Blockade reduces vasospasm
Interleukins	Mediate leukocyte interactions	• Peak early in SAH	• Blockade reduces vasospasm
Endothelin-1	Potent vasoconstrictor	• Produced by monocytes from SAH patients • No proved benefit in clinical trials	• Inhibition reduces vasospasm

Biomarkers associated with outcome in SAH are listed in Table 19.5.

Abbreviations used: *GOS* Glasgow Outcome Scale, *GOSE* Glasgow Outcome Scale Extended, *MMSE* Mini-Mental State Examination, *RDI* Rankin Disability Index, *mRS* Modified Rankin Score, *mTS* Modified Tardieu Scale, *BI* Barthel Index.

Table 19.4 Risk factors for subarachnoid hemorrhage, modified after Abraham and Chang (2016) with kind permission by Elsevier

Modifiable risk factors	Non-modifiable risk factors
Hypertension	Female gender
Smoking history	First-degree family member with SAH
Alcohol abuse	Autosomal-dominant PCKD
Cocaine use	Sickle cell disease
Caffeine consumption	Alpha1-antitrypsin deficiency

Table 19.5 Summary of studies reporting biomarkers associated with outcome in SAH (Hong et al. 2014)

Biomarker	Summary of findings and outcome scale used
Neuron and astrocyte-specific markers	
S100b	• Univariate analysis demonstrated increased S100b associated with poor outcome (GOS) • S100b is excellent predictor of 12-month outcome (GOS) • Increased CSF and blood S100b was associated with outcome prognosis (GOS) • S100b indicator of scale and severity as well as prognostic indicator of 1 year outcome (GOS) • Level of S100b correlated with initial SAH severity and at day 8 was an independent predictive factor for outcome at 6 months (GOS) • Elevated S100b associated with increased mortality and unfavorable outcome at 6 months (GOS) • Elevations of S100b was associated with poor outcome (GOSE) • Mean values of S100b predictor of outcome (GOS) • Elevations of S100b correlate with early neurological deficits (7 days) and worse outcome at 6 months (GOS) • iIncreased S100b associated with severity of injury, clinical course, delayed ischemic deterioration and outcome (GOS)
Neuron-specific enolase (NSE)	• Increased CSF levels of NSE associated with poor outcome at discharge from ICU (GOS) • Increased NSE levels associated with poor outcome at discharge (GOS)
Glial fibrillary acid protein (GFAP)	• Univariate analysis demonstrated increased GFAP associated with poor outcome (GOS) • GFAP-independent predictor of outcome after 1 year (GOSE) • eElevations of GFAP associated with poor outcome (GOSE)
Apolipoprotein E (ApoE)	• Decreases correlated with poor clinical outcome at 3 months (GOS) • E4 carriers trend towards detrimental long-term effect on cognitive function (10-year longitudinal study) • E4 expression prognostic for clinical VSP and higher risk of definitive neurologic deficits at least 6 months (MMSE and RDI) • E4 gene expression prognostic factor for poor outcome with a risk of unfavorable outcome 7.1 times higher noncarriers (GOS) • E4 association with unfavorable outcome at 3 months (GOS) • E4 carriers associated with poor outcome at 6 months (GOS)
Neurofilament	• Phosphorylated neurofilament subunit (pNF-H) elevations from the second week predict poorer outcome (GOSE) • Neurofilament heavy chain elevations in CSF associated with bad outcome at 3 months (GOS) • Neurofilament protein elevation in CSF correlates with neurological status in-hospital and 1-year outcome (GOSE)
Amyloid B-protein	• Decreases levels correlated with poor clinical outcome at 3 months (GOS)
Ubiquitin C-terminal hydrolase 1 (UCHL1)	• Elevation from the second week predict poorer outcome (GOSE)
Inflammatory markers	
CRP	• Early elevations of CRP prognostic for poor outcome (mRS) • Elevated CRP predict risk for poor outcome (GOS) • Elevated CRP associated with worse admission grade and poor GCS and NIHSS scores • Inverse relationship between CRP and GOS at discharge (GOS and mRS) • hsCRP in patients who had delayed cerebral ischemia and poorer outcome at 3 months (mRS) • CRP levels were inversely related to GOS and mRS scores on discharge • Increased levels of CRP were associated with delayed ischemic neurologic deficit at day 0 and day 7 after SAH

(continued)

19.3 Subarachnoid Hemorrhage (SAH)

Table 19.5 (continued)

Biomarker	Summary of findings and outcome scale used
TNFa	• Elevations of TNFa on Day 2–3 is significantly associated with poor outcome at 3 months with a similar trend at 6 months (mRS) • Increased TNFa associated with unfavorable outcome at 3 months (GOS) • Increased TNFa associated with unfavurable outcome at 12 days post SAH (GOS)
IL-1 22	• Increased IL-1Ra (IL-1 receptor antagonist) associated with unfavorable outcome at 12 days post SAH (GOS)
IL-6	• Increased IL-6 associated with unfavorable outcome at 3 months (GOS) • Increased IL-6 in CSF significantly increased in patients with poor clinical outcome (Day 11) (GOS)
IL-8	• Increased IL-8 associated with unfavorable outcome at 3 months (GOS)
High-mobility group box 1 protein (HMGB1)	• Increased HMGB1 associated with unfavorable outcome at 3 months (GOS)
Catecholamine	• Elevated CSF epinephrine-independent predictor of mortality and disability at 30 days • Elevated CSF epinephrine and norepinephrine associated with patients with focal ischemic deficits
Microalbuminuria	• High microalbumin/creatinine ration (MACR), 4200 mg/g, in first 8 days from SAH predictor of unfavorable neurological outcome at 3 months (GOS)
Molecular adhesion and extracellular matrix markers	
MMP-9	• Elevation of MMP-9 associated with poor 3-month clinical outcome (mRS)
ICAM-1, VCAM-1	• Blood increased levels of ICAM-1 and VCAM-1 were associated with delayed ischemic neurologic deficit at day 0 and day 7 after SAH • Very high CSF ICAM-1 and VCAM-1 associated with unfavorable outcome and/or symptomatic VSP (GOS at discharge) • ICAM-1 associated with patients with SAH with poor outcome at day 14 (mRS)
Selectin	• sL-selectin associated with poor outcome at 6 months (BI)
Vascular and angiogenic markers	
Endothelial microparticles	• MP higher at discharge but no significant differences after 6 months (mRS and GOS)
VEGF	• Increased levels of VEGF predict onset of delayed VSP before onset or neurological deterioration
Caspase-3	• Regression analysis demonstrated early C3a strong independent predictor of functional outcome
Coagulation factor markers	
vWF	• Early levels of vWF associated with delayed cerebral ischemia and poor outcome at 12–14 weeks (mTS)
Fibrinogen	• Elevated fibrinogen correlated with worse Barthel scores at 14 days and trended to worse Barthel index at 3 months (BI) • Elevated levels strongly correlated with mortality
Thrombin-antithrombin complex (TAT)	• Elevated levels strongly correlated with mortality
Cardiac markers	
Cardiac troponin I (cTnI)	• Neurologic outcome during hospital stay was adversely related to increased cTnI and wall motion abnormalities, predicting poor GCS on admission and increased hospital stay (GOS) • Patients with elevated cTnI more severe aSAH symptoms and levels 0.3 ng/mL independent predictor of poor functional outcome at 2 months (GOS and mRS) • In-hospital mortality significantly increased with increased • Elevated cTnI predictor of in-hospital mortality • Strong association between TnI and in-patient mortality • cTnI elevations independent prognostic indicator of poor outcome at 3 months (mRS)

(continued)

Table 19.5 (continued)

Biomarker	Summary of findings and outcome scale used
Other markers	
Malondialdehyde (MDA)	• At 2 weeks, elevations of MDA predictor of poor neurological outcome at 6 months (GOS)
Kallikrein-related peptidase-6 (KLK6)	• Kallikrein-related peptidase 6 (KLK6) was significantly lower in patients with severe disability or death
Creatine kinase-BB (CK-BB)	• Increased levels of CK-BB4 greater than 40 U/L were associated with unfavorable outcome at 1 week and 2 months (GOS)
Microdialysis (MD)	
Lactate	• Significantly higher in patients with acute focal neurological deficits and correlated with neurological worsening at 6 and 12 months (GOS) • Elevations significantly correlated with poor outcome at 3 months (GOS)
Pyruvate	• Decreased levels in patients with acute focal neurological deficits and correlated with neurological worsening at 6 and 12 months (GOS)
Excitatory amino acids (EAA)	• Significantly higher in patients with acute focal neurological deficits and correlated with neurological worsening at 6 and 12 months (GOS) • Elevations significantly correlated with poor outcome at 3 months (GOS)
Nitrate	• Elevations significantly correlated with poor outcome at 3 months (GOS)

19.4 Subdural Hemorrhage

- acute
- chronic

19.4.1 Clinical Signs and Symptoms

- gradually increasing headache and confusion
- loss of consciousness
- dizziness
- disorientation
- nausea and vomiting

19.4.2 Epidemiology

Incidence
- 7.35 per 100.000 population

Age Incidence
- newborn
- fifth to seventh decade

Sex Incidence
- Male:Female ratio: 3:1

Localization
- Inner layer of dura mater and arachnoid mater
  - Cerebral hemispheric convexities

19.4.3 Neuroimaging Findings

General Imaging Findings
- Crescent-shaped extra-axial bleeding, can cross sutures but not duplications of dura (falx and tentorium).

CT Non-Contrast-Enhanced (Fig. 19.10a, b)
- Hyperacute: hypodense
- Acute: hyperdense, or mixed hyper-hypodense
- Chronic: isodense (2–3 week), hypodense with age

CT Contrast-Enhanced
- Membranes enhance

MRI-T2 (Fig. 19.11a)
- Hyperacute: Iso- to hyperintense
- Acute: Hypointense
- Chronic: Iso- to hyperintense

MRI-FLAIR (Fig. 19.11b)
- Hyperintense

19.4 Subdural Hemorrhage

MRI-T1 (Fig. 19.11c)
- Hyperacute: Isointense
- Acute: Iso- to hypointense
- Chronic: Iso- to hyperintense

MRI-T1 Contrast-Enhanced (Fig. 19.11d)
- Enhancement of dura in chronic stage

MRI-T2∗/SWI (Fig. 19.11f)
- Hypointense

MR-Diffusion Imaging (Fig. 19.11e)
- Heterogeneous, nonspecific

Nuclear Medicine Imaging Findings
- CBF-SPECT demonstrates perfusion deficits.
- FDG-PET can demonstrate the reduced glucose uptake und utilization in impaired neuronal structures.
- Flumazenil PET which shows the $GABA_A$ receptors can demonstrate the neuronal damage caused by hemorrhage.
- 15-O PET can demonstrate oxygen extraction fraction.

19.4.4 Neuropathology Findings

Macroscopic Features (Fig. 19.12a–l)
- Accumulation of blood beneath the dura mater
- Can reach large extension
- Might be firm in consistency (chronic hemorrhagic pachymeningeosis)

Microscopic Features (Fig. 19.13a–n) (Table 19.6)
- Acute SDH
  - Fresh coagulated blood between the arachnoid and dura mater.
  - Most cases of SDH are accompanied by laceration and/or contusion injuries of the cerebral cortex.
  - A concomitant old SDH is often found.
  - Spontaneous or mechanically induced rebleeding into an old SDH is not uncommon.
  - The bleeding has its source in the sinusoidal vessels of the granulation tissue organizing the pre-existing hematoma.
  - The presence of hemosiderin-containing macrophages or of macrophages of different ages in different layers of the bleeding indicates that multiple bleeds have occurred at different times.
- Subacute SDH
  - Coagulation of the blood has usually occurred.
  - Signs of leukocyte emigration.
  - Ingestion of erythrocytes and/or digestion as demonstrated by Fe-containing macrophages.
  - Formation of granulation tissue comprised of
    o fibroblasts
    o collagenous fibers
    o macrophages
    o endothelial cells
  - A dense network of precipitated fibrin holds the hematoma together.
- Chronic SDH
  - By a clearly delineated collection of a clot between the dura mater and arachnoid.
  - The SDH is typically encapsulated by a neomembrane.
  - Neomembrane
    o Formed by the dura mater as a nonspecific reaction to blood or its degradation products
    o Outer membrane contains giant neovessels.
    o The inner membrane is only poorly vascularized.
  - The neomembrane that forms on the inner aspect creates a small space or a cavity into which recurrent bleeding may occur.

Immunohistochemical Staining Characteristics
- β-amyloid to exclude cerebral amyloid angiopathy (CAA)

Differential Diagnosis
- Hemorrhage due to cerebral amyloid angiopathy (CAA)
- Hemorrhage into an ischemic necrosis

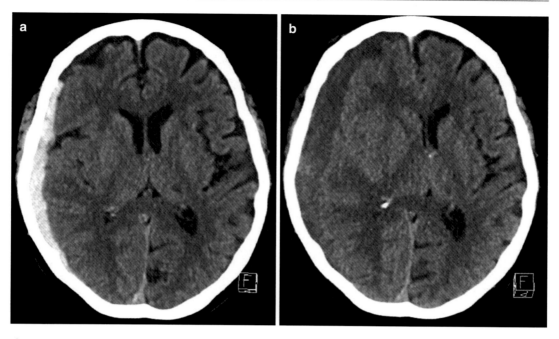

Fig. 19.10 Right hemispheric subdural hemorrhage with CT day 3 (**a**) and day 10 (**b**)

19.4.5 Molecular Neuropathology

- Spontaneous SDH
- Traumatic brain injuries
    - Contusion-induced
    - Cortical lacerations associated with fissures, linear fractures, or depressed fractures of the skull
    - Acceleration/rotational mechanisms
    - High speed acceleration or deceleration injuries
    - Motor vehicle collisions, falls, assaults, accidents
- Arterial origin
    - Rupture of small pial artery
    - Saccular aneurysm of major intracerebral artery
    - Arteriovenous malformation
    - Aneurysm of the middle meningeal artery
- Rupture of a bridging vein (chronic)
    - Anticoagulant or thrombolytic treatment
    - Coagulation defects
    - Rupture of arachnoidal cyst
    - Dural metastases
- Coagulopathy or medical anticoagulation
    - Warfarin, heparin, hemophilia, liver disease, thrombocytopenia
- Nontraumatic hemorrhage
    - Cerebral aneurysm
    - Arteriovenous malformation
    - Tumor (especially meningioma or dural metastasis)
- Postsurgical
    - Craniotomy
    - CSF shunting
- Intracranial hypotension
    - Lumbar puncture, lumbar CSF leak, lumboperitoneal shunt, spinal epidural anesthesia
- Inflicted injury
    - Usually pediatric age group; also can be seen in the elderly
- Spontaneous or unknown
- Rare

The clinical progression of CSDH can be generally categorized into three periods:

- the initial period of traumatic event
- the latency period of hematoma expansion
- the clinical period of CSDH manifestation

19.4 Subdural Hemorrhage

The initial period may present as

- either 1 or multiple clinical or subclinical traumatic events
- causing the initial formation of the hematoma
- which is referred as the "seed" for CSDH development

Immediately after the initial phase is the latent phase

- The hematoma matures slowly.
- Increases in volume.
- The neomembrane formation on the dural side as well as on the arachnoid side facilitated the encapsulation of the hematoma.
- Microhemorrhages owing to fragility of vessels formed by extensive neovascularization.
- The hyperactivation of the fibrinolytic system has also been proposed to play a role in the extension of hematoma.

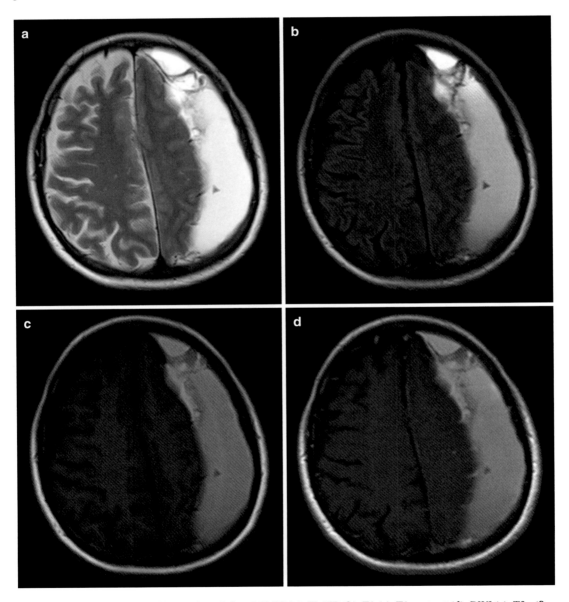

Fig. 19.11 Subacute, subdural hemorrhage left on MR T2 (**a**), FLAIR (**b**), T1 (**c**), T1 contrast (**d**), DWI (**e**), T2∗ (**f**)

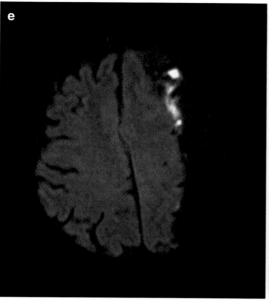 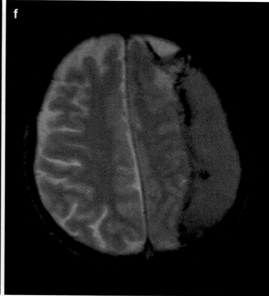

Fig. 19.11 (continued)

- During this period, patients may be asymptomatic.
- This may last for weeks to years.

After the latency period,

- Progressive decompensation of intracranial capacity occurs as a result of continuous growing of the hematoma capsule.
- A constellation of symptoms may appear from increased intracranial pressure.
- At clinical presentation, patients have:
  - seizures (10–20%)
  - coma (2–15%)
  - herniation (2%)
- Less than 1% of all reported cases were discovered incidentally.

19.4.6 Treatment and Prognosis

Treatment
- Surgical removal of hemorrhage.
- Without any treatment, few CSDHs have been reported to regress spontaneously.

- Forty percent of all patients may eventually recover on medical management without surgical intervention.
- However, 20% of patients undergoing conservative management experience clinical deterioration and require surgical intervention.

Biologic Behavior–Prognosis–Prognostic Factors
- Age of patient.
- Acute subdural hematoma
  - high mortality rate if not rapidly treated with surgical decompression.
- Chronic subdural hematoma.
- A rapidly developing SDH becomes life threatening in adults once its volume has attained 50 mL.
  - If the SDH develops slowly, a considerably larger volume can be tolerated.

19.4 Subdural Hemorrhage

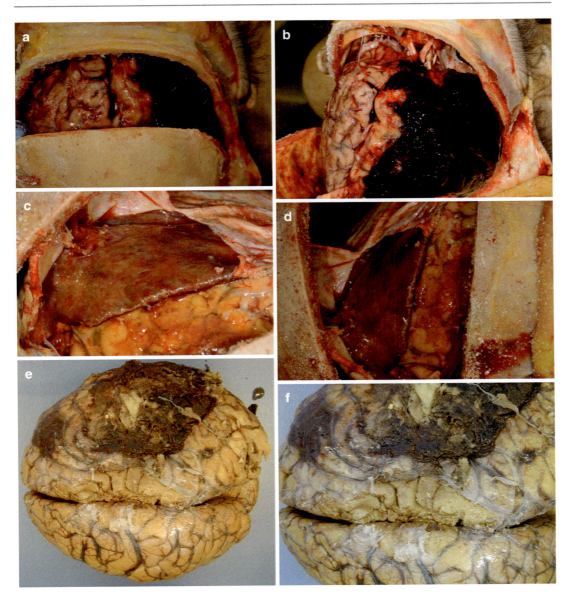

Fig. 19.12 Subdural hemorrhage: A large amount of fresh blood (**a**, **b**) and old blood (**c**, **d**) accumulates between the brain and dura mater upon opening the skull. The subdural hematoma can extend over nearly the total surface of the telencephalon (**e–f**) with indwelling of the cortical surface (**g–j**). Subdural hematoma affecting the spinal cord (**k**, **l**)

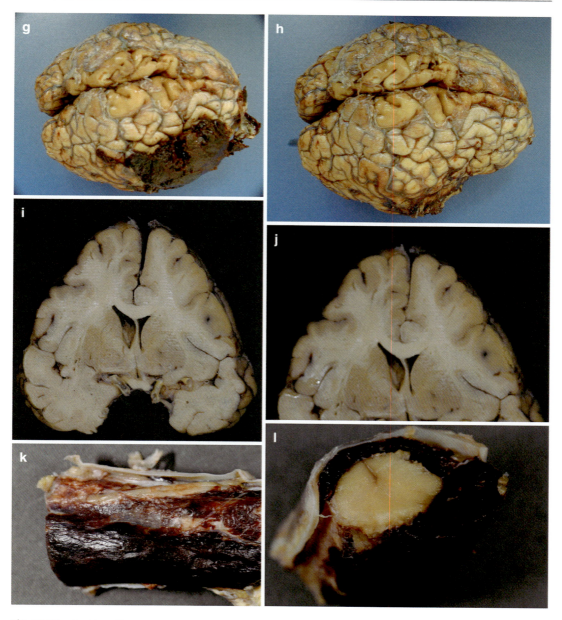

Fig. 19.12 (continued)

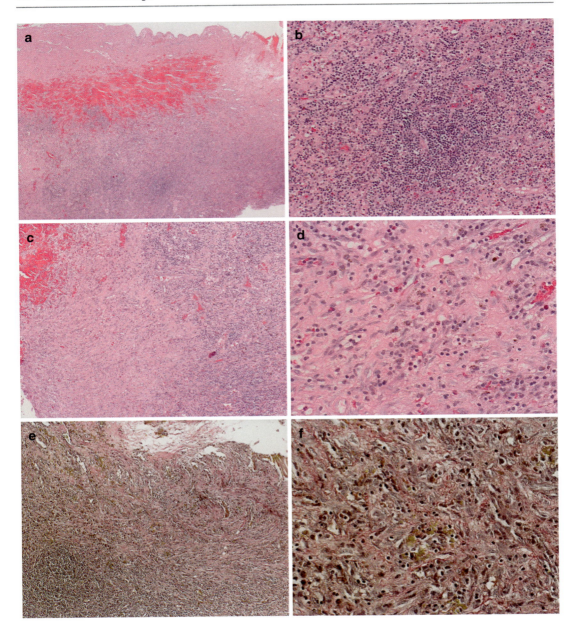

Fig. 19.13 Subdural hemorrhage: The chronic subdural hematoma consists microscopically of monomorphonuclear cells, and erythrocytes (**a–d**), connective tissue (**a–f**; **e, f**: EvG stain), extensive reticular network (**g, h**: Reticulin stain); old hemorrhages (**i, j**: blue color in Prussian blue stain). Monomorphonuclear cells are immunohistochemically identified as CD3-positive T-lymphocytes (**k, l**), while connective tissue is vimentin-positive (**m, n**)

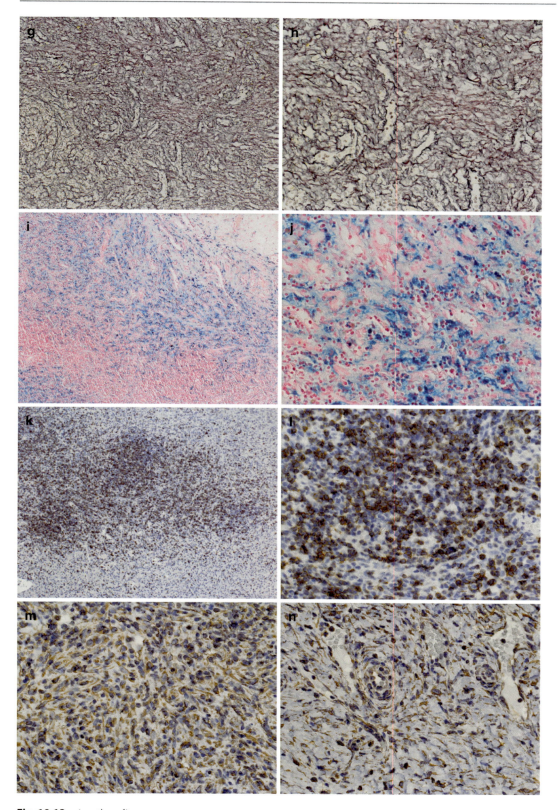

Fig. 19.13 (continued)

Table 19.6 Histologic features of subdural hematoma

Time after injury	Hematoma	Dural side	Arachnoidal side
To 24 h	Fresh erythrocytes	Fibrin	Fibrin
24–48 h	Fresh erythrocytes polymorphonuclear cells and fibrin	Fibrin	Fibrin
2–5 days	Macrophages replace polymorphonuclear cells	Fibroblasts seen at dural junction	Fibrin
4–5 days	Mixture of intact and lysed erythrocytes and pigment (iron)-laden macrophages are found	Fibroblastic layer is 2–5 cell layers thick	Fibrin
1 week	Erythrocytes lysed; early angiofibroblastic proliferation seen	Fibroblastic layer is up to 12 cell layers thick	A single layer of fibroblastic cells appears
2 weeks	Hematoma liquifies; sinusoids ("giant capillaries") appear	Fibroblastic layer is about one-half thickness of dura	Fibroblastic layer is a few cells thick and has a rare capillary
3 weeks	Vascular sinusoids are well developed		
4 weeks	Hematoma liquifies	Fibroblastic layer is as thick as the dura. Pigment-laden macrophages are apparent	Fibrous membrane and a few capillaries seen
1–3 months	The fibroblastic layers are hyalinized and form membranes of both the dural and arachnoidal sides. Large (giant) capillaries appear early and secondary hemorrhages often develop.		
3–12 month	The neomembranes usually fuse and contain mature fibrous tissue and scattered pigment-laden macrophages. After 3 months, it is no longer possible to accurately date (age) the hematoma.		
>1 year	The neomembrane forms a distinct fibrous connective tissue layer that closely resembles the adjacent dura mater. Occasionally, calcification and/or ossification appears.		

19.5 Epidural Hemorrhage (EDH)

19.5.1 Clinical Signs and Symptoms

- Variable.
- Concomitant injury of the brain parenchyma:
  - Clouding of consciousness with neurological deficits will develop either immediately (in approximately 25–30% of cases) or after an interval of minutes or hours (usually within 4–8 h).
  - With focal ipsilateral mydriasis and hemiplegia.
  - Skull fractures may be associated with EDH, the incidence of EDH being 20 times higher in cases with skull fracture than in cases without fracture.

19.5.2 Localization

- Temporal: 70–90%
- Frontal: 5–25%
- Parietal: 1–3%
- Occipital: 3–14%
- Posterior fossa: 3–12%

19.5.3 Neuroimaging Findings

General Imaging Findings
- Biconvex extra-axial bleeding, does not cross sutures

CT Non-Contrast-Enhanced (Figs. 19.14a, b and 19.15a, b)
- Hyperdense, recent bleeding hypodense
- Fracture?

CT Contrast-Enhanced
- Contrast extravasation in acute bleeding possible

MRI-T2 (Fig. 19.15c)
- Acute: Hyper- to hypointense
- Late subacute: Hyperintense

MRI-FLAIR (Fig. 19.15d)
- Hyperintense

MRI-T1 (Fig. 19.15e)
- Acute: Isointense
- Late subacute: Hyperintense

MRI-T1 Contrast-Enhanced (Fig. 19.15f)
- Contrast extravasation rare

MRI-T2∗/SWI (Fig. 19.15h)
  – Hypointense

19.5.4 Neuropathology Findings

Macroscopic Features
- Accumulation of blood between the inner table of the skull and dura mater.
- Tightly attached to the skull and dura mater at the borders of the sutures.
- Hematoma has thick lenticular, convex appearance.
  – Blood fills the space and causes further stripping of the dura from the skull.
- The volume of blood varies greatly, but amounts to at least 100 mL in most fatal cases.
- Usually located beneath the fracture in the cranial vault, i.e., on the side of the impact, in most cases in the region of the temporal bone.
- EDH rarely develops contralateral to the impact site.
- A space-occupying EDH will displace the brain resulting in compression of the brain stem (herniation syndrome).

Microscopic Features
  – The histological features resemble those of SDH and vary according to the survival time.

19.5.5 Molecular Neuropathology

Pathogenesis
- Trauma
  – Traffic accident.
  – Focal impact almost always associated with a nearby skull fracture and stripping of the dura from the inner table of the skull.
  – EDH arises from injury of the middle meningeal artery and its branches near the impact site.

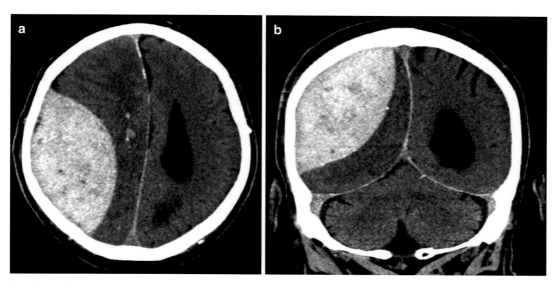

Fig. 19.14 Massive right hemispheric epidural hemorrhage with CT ax (**a**) and cor (**b**)

19.5 Epidural Hemorrhage (EDH)

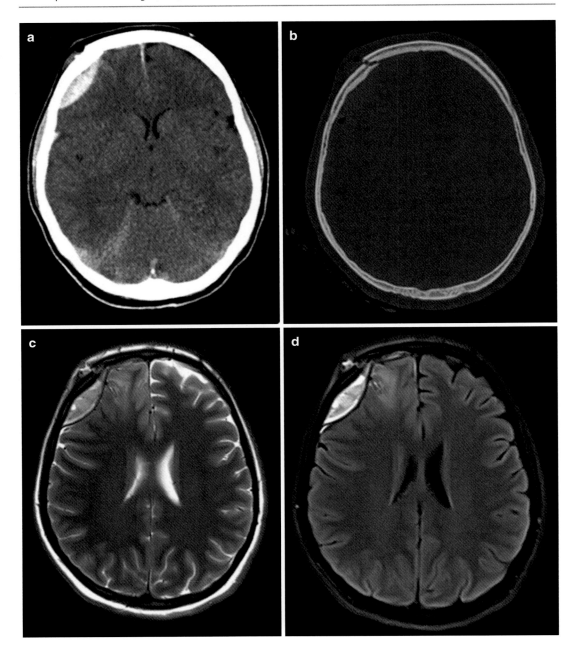

Fig. 19.15 Right frontal epidural hemorrhage with CT (**a**) and CT bone demonstrating the adjacent fracture (**b**) and MR day 10 T2 (**c**), FLAIR (**d**), T1 (**e**), T1 contrast (**f**), DWI (**g**), SWI (**h**)

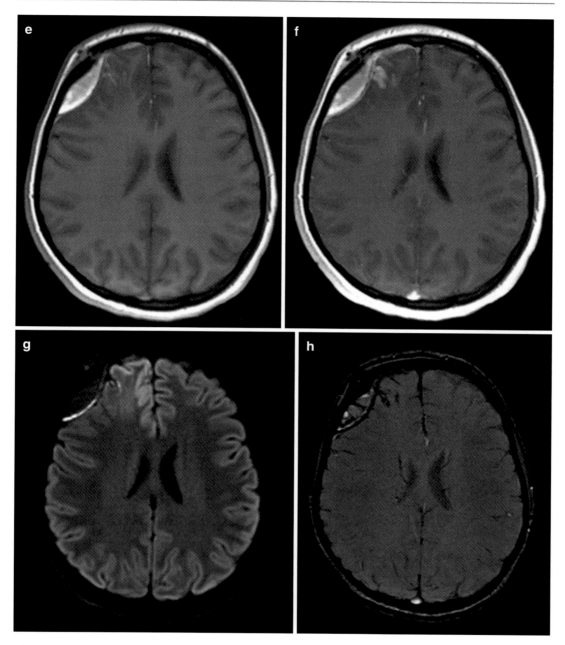

Fig. 19.15 (continued)

- About 24% of all instances of skull fracture are associated with EDH; only about 1% of EDH are not associated with a fracture.
- Edges of fractured bone can cause laceration of underlying dural arteries and, less frequently, veins.
- In rare cases, EDH is caused by lacerations of one or more branches of the venous sinuses or emissary veins.
- EDH rarely occurs spontaneously.
- EDH is less likely to produce cerebral contusion injuries than SDH.

Table 19.7 Comparison of acute subdural and epidural hematoma

	Subdural hematoma	Epidural hematoma
Pathology	• Trauma in ~75% of cases • Blood dyscrasias • Hemodialysis • Ruptured aneurysms, etc.	• Trauma in 95% of cases • Blood dyscrasias • Other: rare
Associated clinical condition	• Alcoholism • Pneumoencephalography • Ventricular decompression for hydrocephalus • Battered child syndrome • Boxing	• Ventricular decompression for hydrocephalus • Battered child syndrome
Sex	• Males predominate	• Males predominate
Bleeding source	• Bridging cortical veins	• Middle meningeal artery, vein, or venous sinuses
Location	• Frontoparietal most common • Bilateral: 20% adults, 80% children • Posterior fossa neonate: rare • Spinal canal: rare	• Temporal: 80%; do not respect suture line • Unilateral: 97% • Spinal canal: uncommon
Size	• Significant: >50 mL blood • Lethal: >100 mL blood • Maximum: ~300 mL blood	• Significant: 25–50 mL blood • Lethal: 75–100 mL blood • Maximum: ~300 mL blood
Associated neuropathologic conditions	• Skull fracture: 67% adults • Edema: Ggeneralized, common • Ipsilateral cerebrum, common • Contusions: common • Hematoma: intracerebral and subarachnoid common; extradural, infrequent • Herniation: brain stem in 33% • Infarcts: posterior cerebral artery, distribution, occasional	• Skull fracture: 90% adults • Edema: Ggeneralized, common • Ipsilateral cerebrum, common • Contusions: uncommon • Hematoma: subdural, subarachnoid and/or intracerebral in 33%; epicranial, uncommon • Herniation: brain stem, near 100% • Infarcts: posterior cerebral artery, distribution, common
Mortality	• Untreated: dependent on size and rapidity of onset • Treated: subacute, 24% • Treated: chronic, 6%	• Untreated: dependent on size and rapidity of onset • Treated: average about 30%

19.5.6 Treatment and Prognosis

Treatment
• surgery craniotomy

Biologic Behavior–Prognosis–Prognostic Factors
• Timely diagnosis and treatment are essential to a favorable prognosis.
• Clinical deterioration can be rapid.
• Mortality decreases in recent decades.
• Interval between onset of the space-occupying EDH-induced cerebral compression and the start of surgical decompression.
• Mortality of EDH ranges between 0 and 43%.

A comparison between subdural and epidural hematoma with regard to pathology, location, mortality is given in Table 19.7.

Selected References

Abraham MK, Chang WW (2016) Subarachnoid hemorrhage. Emerg Med Clin North Am 34(4):901–916. https://doi.org/10.1016/j.emc.2016.06.011

Al-Mufti F, Amuluru K, Smith B, Damodara N, El-Ghanem M, Singh IP, Dangayach N, Gandhi CD (2017) Early emerging markers of delayed cerebral ischemia following aneurysmal subarachnoid hemorrhage: a literature review. World Neurosurg 107:148–159. https://doi.org/10.1016/j.wneu.2017.07.114

Al-Mufti F, Mayer SA (2017) Neurocritical care of acute subdural hemorrhage. Neurosurg Clin N

Am 28(2):267–278. https://doi.org/10.1016/j.nec.2016.11.009

An SJ, Kim TJ, Yoon BW (2017) Epidemiology, risk factors, and clinical features of intracerebral hemorrhage: an update. J Stroke 19(1):3–10. https://doi.org/10.5853/jos.2016.00864

Ariesen MJ, Claus SP, Rinkel GJ, Algra A (2003) Risk factors for intracerebral hemorrhage in the general population: a systematic review. Stroke 34(8):2060–2065. https://doi.org/10.1161/01.str.0000080678.09344.8d

Bauer AM, Rasmussen PA (2014) Treatment of intracranial vasospasm following subarachnoid hemorrhage. Front Neurol 5:72. https://doi.org/10.3389/fneur.2014.00072

Catana D, Koziarz A, Cenic A, Nath S, Singh S, Almenawer SA, Kachur E (2016) Subdural hematoma mimickers: a systematic review. World Neurosurg 93:73–80. https://doi.org/10.1016/j.wneu.2016.05.084

Chau M, Chen JC, Levy ML (2000) Causes, epidemiology, and risk factors of chronic subdural hematoma. Neurosurg Clin N Am 11(3):399–406

Chen S, Wu H, Tang J, Zhang J, Zhang JH (2015a) Neurovascular events after subarachnoid hemorrhage: focusing on subcellular organelles. Acta Neurochir Suppl 120:39–46. https://doi.org/10.1007/978-3-319-04981-6_7

Chen Y, Li Q, Tang J, Feng H, Zhang JH (2015b) The evolving roles of pericyte in early brain injury after subarachnoid hemorrhage. Brain Res 1623:110–122. https://doi.org/10.1016/j.brainres.2015.05.004

Ciurea AV, Palade C, Voinescu D, Nica DA (2013) Subarachnoid hemorrhage and cerebral vasospasm - literature review. J Med Life 6(2):120–125

Dabdoub CB, Adorno JO, Urbano J, Silveira EN, Orlandi BM (2016) Review of the management of infected subdural hematoma. World Neurosurg 87:663.e661–663.e668. https://doi.org/10.1016/j.wneu.2015.11.015

de Lima Oliveira M, Kairalla AC, Fonoff ET, Martinez RC, Teixeira MJ, Bor-Seng-Shu E (2014) Cerebral microdialysis in traumatic brain injury and subarachnoid hemorrhage: state of the art. Neurocrit Care 21(1):152–162. https://doi.org/10.1007/s12028-013-9884-4

Domenicucci M, Signorini P, Strzelecki J, Delfini R (1995) Delayed post-traumatic epidural hematoma. A review. Neurosurg Rev 18(2):109–122

Dority JS, Oldham JS (2016) Subarachnoid hemorrhage: an update. Anesthesiol Clin 34(3):577–600. https://doi.org/10.1016/j.anclin.2016.04.009

Dubosh NM, Bellolio MF, Rabinstein AA, Edlow JA (2016) Sensitivity of early brain computed tomography to exclude aneurysmal subarachnoid hemorrhage: a systematic review and meta-analysis. Stroke 47(3):750–755. https://doi.org/10.1161/strokeaha.115.011386

Durrant JC, Hinson HE (2015) Rescue therapy for refractory vasospasm after subarachnoid hemorrhage. Curr Neurol Neurosci Rep 15(2):521. https://doi.org/10.1007/s11910-014-0521-1

Edjlali M, Rodriguez-Regent C, Hodel J, Aboukais R, Trystram D, Pruvo JP, Meder JF, Oppenheim C, Lejeune JP, Leclerc X, Naggara O (2015) Subarachnoid hemorrhage in ten questions. Diagn Interv Imaging 96(7-8):657–666. https://doi.org/10.1016/j.diii.2015.06.003

Edlow JA, Figaji A, Samuels O (2015) Emergency neurological life support: subarachnoid hemorrhage. Neurocrit Care 23(suppl 2):S103–S109. https://doi.org/10.1007/s12028-015-0183-0

Egashira Y, Hua Y, Keep RF, Xi G (2015) Intercellular cross-talk in intracerebral hemorrhage. Brain Res 1623:97–109. https://doi.org/10.1016/j.brainres.2015.04.003

Figueroa J, DeVine JG (2017) Spontaneous spinal epidural hematoma: literature review. J Spine Surg 3(1):58–63. https://doi.org/10.21037/jss.2017.02.04

Flaherty ML, Beck J (2013) Surgery for intracerebral hemorrhage: moving forward or making circles? Stroke 44(10):2953–2954. https://doi.org/10.1161/strokeaha.113.002533

Francoeur CL, Mayer SA (2016) Management of delayed cerebral ischemia after subarachnoid hemorrhage. Crit Care 20(1):277. https://doi.org/10.1186/s13054-016-1447-6

Gulati D, Dua D, Torbey MT (2017) Hemostasis in intracranial hemorrhage. Front Neurol 8:80. https://doi.org/10.3389/fneur.2017.00080

Hayakawa M (2015) Reperfusion-related Intracerebral hemorrhage. Front Neurol Neurosci 37:62–77. https://doi.org/10.1159/000437114

Hayman EG, Patel AP, James RF, Simard JM (2017) Heparin and heparin-derivatives in post-subarachnoid hemorrhage brain injury: a multimodal therapy for a multimodal disease. Molecules 22(5). https://doi.org/10.3390/molecules22050724

Heit JJ, Iv M, Wintermark M (2017) Imaging of intracranial hemorrhage. J Stroke 19(1):11–27. https://doi.org/10.5853/jos.2016.00563

Heyman R, Heckly A, Magagi J, Pladys P, Hamlat A (2005) Intracranial epidural hematoma in newborn infants: clinical study of 15 cases. Neurosurgery 57(5):924–929;discussion 924-929

Hong CM, Tosun C, Kurland DB, Gerzanich V, Schreibman D, Simard JM (2014) Biomarkers as outcome predictors in subarachnoid hemorrhage–a systematic review. Biomarkers 19(2):95–108. https://doi.org/10.3109/1354750x.2014.881418

Inagawa T (2016) Risk factors for cerebral vasospasm following aneurysmal subarachnoid hemorrhage: a review of the literature. World Neurosurg 85:56–76. https://doi.org/10.1016/j.wneu.2015.08.052

James RF, Kramer DR, Aljuboori ZS, Parikh G, Adams SW, Eaton JC, Abou Al-Shaar H, Badjatia N, Mack WJ, Simard JM (2016) Novel treatments in neuroprotection for aneurysmal subarachnoid hemorrhage. Curr Treat Options Neurol 18(8):38. https://doi.org/10.1007/s11940-016-0421-6

Karibe H, Hayashi T, Hirano T, Kameyama M, Nakagawa A, Tominaga T (2014) Surgical management of traumatic acute subdural hematoma in adults: a review. Neurol Med Chir 54(11):887–894

Killeffer JA, Killeffer FA, Schochet SS (2000) The outer neomembrane of chronic subdural hematoma. Neurosurg Clin N Am 11(3):407–412

Koch S, Gonzalez N (2013) Preconditioning the human brain: proving the principle in subarachnoid hemorrhage. Stroke 44(6):1748–1753. https://doi.org/10.1161/strokeaha.111.000773

Lawton MT, Vates GE (2017) Subarachnoid hemorrhage. N Engl J Med 377(3):257–266. https://doi.org/10.1056/NEJMcp1605827

Lindbohm JV, Kaprio J, Korja M (2016) Cholesterol as a risk factor for subarachnoid hemorrhage: a systematic review. PLoS One 11(4):e0152568. https://doi.org/10.1371/journal.pone.0152568

Liu B, Zhang L, Yang Q (2012) Genetics of intracerebral hemorrhage: insights from candidate gene approaches. Neurol India 60(1):3–8. https://doi.org/10.4103/0028-3886.93581

Liu W, Bakker NA, Groen RJ (2014) Chronic subdural hematoma: a systematic review and meta-analysis of surgical procedures. J Neurosurg 121(3):665–673. https://doi.org/10.3171/2014.5.jns132715

Macellari F, Paciaroni M, Agnelli G, Caso V (2014) Neuroimaging in intracerebral hemorrhage. Stroke 45(3):903–908. https://doi.org/10.1161/strokeaha.113.003701

Mangla R, Drumsta D, Alamst J, Mangla M, Potchen M (2015) Cerebral convexity subarachnoid hemorrhage: various causes and role of diagnostic imaging. Biomed Res Int 22(2):181–195. https://doi.org/10.1007/s10140-014-1251-z

Marder CP, Narla V, Fink JR, Tozer Fink KR (2014) Subarachnoid hemorrhage: beyond aneurysms. AJR Am J Roentgenol 202(1):25–37. https://doi.org/10.2214/ajr.12.9749

Milinis K, Thapar A, O'Neill K, Davies AH (2017) History of aneurysmal spontaneous subarachnoid hemorrhage. Stroke 48(10):e280–e283. https://doi.org/10.1161/strokeaha.117.017282

Miller BA, Turan N, Chau M, Pradilla G (2014) Inflammation, vasospasm, and brain injury after subarachnoid hemorrhage. Biomed Res Int 2014:384342. https://doi.org/10.1155/2014/384342

Mittal MK, LacKamp A (2016) Intracerebral hemorrhage: perihemorrhagic edema and secondary hematoma expansion: from bench work to ongoing controversies. Front Neurol 7:210. https://doi.org/10.3389/fneur.2016.00210

Morotti A, Goldstein JN (2016) Diagnosis and management of acute intracerebral hemorrhage. Emerg Med Clin North Am 34(4):883–899. https://doi.org/10.1016/j.emc.2016.06.010

Naidech AM (2015) Diagnosis and management of spontaneous intracerebral hemorrhage. Continuum (Minneap, Minn) 21(5 Neurocritical Care):1288–1298. https://doi.org/10.1212/con.0000000000000222

Öhmichen M, Auer R, König H (2006) Forensic neuropathology and associated neurology. Springer, Berlin

Parizel PM, Makkat S, Van Miert E, Van Goethem JW, van den Hauwe L, De Schepper AM (2001) Intracranial hemorrhage: principles of CT and MRI interpretation. Eur Radiol 11(9):1770–1783

Prabhakaran S, Naidech AM (2012) Ischemic brain injury after intracerebral hemorrhage: a critical review. Stroke 43(8):2258–2263. https://doi.org/10.1161/strokeaha.112.655910

Pradilla G, Righy C, Bozza MT, Oliveira MF, Bozza FA (2016) Molecular, cellular and clinical aspects of intracerebral hemorrhage: are the enemies within? Curr Neuropharmacol 14(4):392–402

Sahyouni R, Mahboubi H, Tran P, Roufail JS, Chen JW (2017) Membranectomy in chronic subdural hematoma: meta-analysis. World Neurosurg 104:418–429. https://doi.org/10.1016/j.wneu.2017.05.030

Schlunk F, Greenberg SM (2015) The pathophysiology of intracerebral hemorrhage formation and expansion. Transl Stroke Res 6(4):257–263. https://doi.org/10.1007/s12975-015-0410-1

Sieswerda-Hoogendoorn T, Postema FAM, Verbaan D, Majoie CB, van Rijn RR (2014) Age determination of subdural hematomas with CT and MRI: a systematic review. Eur J Radiol 83(7):1257–1268. https://doi.org/10.1016/j.ejrad.2014.03.015

Squier W, Mack J, Green A, Aziz T (2012) The pathophysiology of brain swelling associated with subdural hemorrhage: the role of the trigeminovascular system. Childs Nerv Syst 28(12):2005–2015. https://doi.org/10.1007/s00381-012-1870-1

Stippler M, Ramirez P, Berti A, Macindoe C, Villalobos N, Murray-Krezan C (2013) Chronic subdural hematoma patients aged 90 years and older. Neurol Res 35(3):243–246. https://doi.org/10.1179/1743132813y.0000000163

Stoodley M, Weir B (2000) Contents of chronic subdural hematoma. Neurosurg Clin N Am 11(3):425–434

Suarez JI (2015) Diagnosis and management of subarachnoid hemorrhage. Continuum (Minneap, Minn) 21(5 Neurocritical Care):1263–1287. https://doi.org/10.1212/con.0000000000000217

Tanaka Y, Ohno K (2013) Chronic subdural hematoma—an up-to-date concept. J Med Dent Sci 60(2):55–61

Thabet AM, Kottapally M, Hemphill JC 3rd (2017) Management of intracerebral hemorrhage. Handb Clin Neurol 140:177–194. https://doi.org/10.1016/b978-0-444-63600-3.00011-8

van Lieshout JH, Dibue-Adjei M, Cornelius JF, Slotty PJ, Schneider T, Restin T, Boogaarts HD, Steiger HJ, Petridis AK, Kamp MA (2018) An introduction to the pathophysiology of aneurysmal subarachnoid hemorrhage. Neurosurg Rev 41(4):917–930. https://doi.org/10.1007/s10143-017-0827-y

Vega RA, Valadka AB (2017) Natural history of acute subdural hematoma. Neurosurg Clin N Am 28(2):247–255. https://doi.org/10.1016/j.nec.2016.11.007

Wilberger JE (2000) Pathophysiology of evolution and recurrence of chronic subdural hematoma. Neurosurg Clin N Am 11(3):435–438

Williams VL, Hogg JP (2000) Magnetic resonance imaging of chronic subdural hematoma. Neurosurg Clin N Am 11(3):491–498

Wilson CD, Shankar JJ (2014) Diagnosing vasospasm after subarachnoid hemorrhage: CTA and CTP. Can J Neurol Sci 41(3):314–319

Yadav YR, Parihar V, Namdev H, Bajaj J (2016) Chronic subdural hematoma. Asian J Neurosurg 11(4):330–342. https://doi.org/10.4103/1793-5482.145102

Yang W, Huang J (2017) Chronic subdural hematoma: epidemiology and natural history. Neurosurg Clin N Am 28(2):205–210. https://doi.org/10.1016/j.nec.2016.11.002

Zheng VZ, Wong GKC (2017) Neuroinflammation responses after subarachnoid hemorrhage: a review. J Clin Neurosci 42:7–11. https://doi.org/10.1016/j.jocn.2017.02.001

Vascular Disorders: Arteriosclerosis

20.1 Introduction

Arteriosclerosis is

- a hardening or "sclerosis" of the arteries
- characterized by
    - thickening of the arterial wall
    - loss of elasticity

Arteriosclerosis occurs in the following forms:

- Arteriolosclerosis
    - Affects small arteries and arterioles
    - Causes downstream ischemic injury
    - Two forms:
        - hyaline
        - hyperplastic
- Atherosclerosis
    - affects large- and medium-sized arteries
    - is cause of coronary, cerebral, and peripheral vascular disease
    - is cause of high morbidity and mortality
- Mönckeberg medial calcification (sclerosis)
    - Medial calcification ("pipestem rigidity") of muscular arteries
    - In elderly men
    - Non-stenotic condition usually without clinical significance

20.2 Epidemiology

Incidence
- 2.27 per 1,000 per year

Age Incidence
- Middle to higher age

Sex Incidence
- Male:Female ratio: 1.5:1

Localization
- Elastic to medium-sized muscular arteries
- Most severely at ostia where laminar flow is disrupted
- Descending order of prominence:
    - Abdominal aorta
    - Coronary arteries
    - Popliteal arteries
    - Internal carotid arteries
    - Circle of Willis
- Cerebral vessels:
    - Carotid arteries (external and internal)
    - Vertebral arteries
    - Basilary artery
    - Medial cerebral artery

20.3 Neuroimaging Findings

General Imaging Findings:
- Cerebral imaging demonstrates secondary signs of arteriosclerosis.
- Plaque morphology: thickening of intima, fatty core, subintimal hemorrhage, and rupture of fibrous cap.
- Evaluation of degree of stenosis.
- Sonography is method of choice.

CT non-contrast-enhanced
- Calcification of plaques along vessel wall

CTA/MRA/DSA (Fig. 20.1a–h)
- Demonstrates degree of stenosis and ulcerations
- DSA: Gold standard
- DSA: Differentiation of occlusion versus pseudoocclusion

Nuclear Medicine Imaging Findings (Figs. 20.2 and 20.3)
- CBF-SPECT demonstrates perfusion deficits. Patients present with inhomogeneous tracer uptake not only in the cortex but also in basal ganglia without larger defect zones.
- FDG-PET can demonstrate the reduced glucose uptake und utilization in impaired neuronal structure, typically resulting in inhomogeneous uptake especially also in the basal ganglia.
- Flumazenil PET which shows the $GABA_A$ receptors can demonstrate the neuronal damage and correlating to CBF-SPECT and FDG-PET shows inhomogeneous tracer uptake.
- 15-O PET can demonstrate oxygen extraction fraction.
- Presynaptic and postsynaptic SPECT and PET studies can show an inhomogeneous tracer uptake, even with a reduction in caudate nucleus in presynaptic studies or a symmetric reduction in tracer binding in the dorsal putamen

20.4 Neuropathology Findings

Macroscopic Features (Fig. 20.4a–n)
- Fatty streak
  - Minute flat yellow spots
- Atherosclerotic plaque (fibrous or atheromatous plaque or atheroma)
  - Protrude into the vessel lumen
  - White-yellow
  - Variable size
- Fibroatheroma
  - Atheroma with development of a fibrous cap

Microscopic Features (Fig. 20.5a–l)
- Fatty streaks
  - Focal accumulations of subendothelial smooth muscle cells
  - Foamy macrophages containing lipid
- Atherosclerotic plaques
  - Thickening of the intima
  - Intimal accumulation of foam cells and extracellular lipid (cholesterol and cholesterol esters)
  - Components of atherosclerotic plaque:
    ○ Smooth muscle cells, macrophages, T-cells
    ○ Extracellular matrix (collagen, elastic fibers, proteoglycans)
    ○ Intracellular and extracellular lipid
  - Atheromatous core contains:
    ○ extracellular lipid
    ○ macrophages with intracellular lipid
    ○ necrotic tissue
    ○ calcium
  - Shoulder of plaque composed of:
    ○ Macrophages
    ○ Leukocytes
    ○ Blood vessels
- The components of a fibroatheroma are as follows:
  - Fibrous cap composed of:
    ○ smooth muscle cells
    ○ macrophages

20.4 Neuropathology Findings

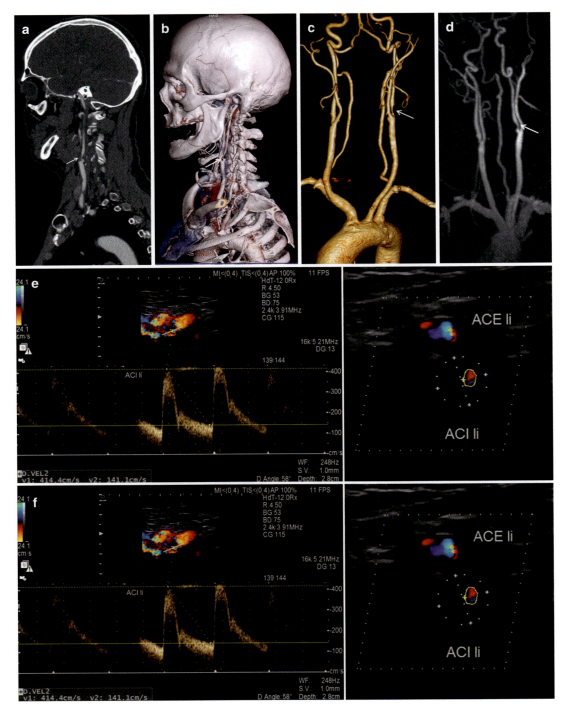

Fig. 20.1 Arteriosclerotic high-grade stenosis of left internal carotid artery on sag CTA (**a**), volume rendering of CTA (**b, c**), MRA (**d**), ultrasound (**e, f**), DSA before and after stenting (**g, h**)

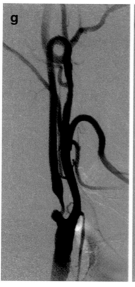
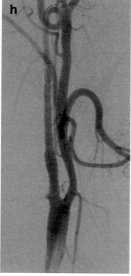

Fig. 20.1 (continued)

- foam cells
- lymphocytes
- extracellular matrix proteins (e.g., collagen, elastin, proteoglycans)
• Hyaline arteriosclerosis
  – Homogeneous hyaline thickening of the arteriolar wall
  – Deposition of protein (leakage of plasma proteins across injured endothelial cells)
  – Markedly narrowed lumen
• Hyperplastic arteriosclerosis
  – Concentric, laminated (onion-skin) thickening of vascular wall
  – Reduplicated basement membrane
  – Luminal obliteration

Immunohistochemical Staining Characteristics
• Smooth muscle actin (SMA)
• Collagen type I
• CD68

Ultrastructural Features
• Affected cells: smooth muscle cells, endothelial cells, stromal cells.
• Lesional smooth muscle cells and endothelial cells generate membranous microvesicles within specific compartments of the cell, called multivesicular bodies.
• Mucodegeneration: homogeneous granular mucopolysaccharides surround arterial smooth muscle cells.
• Calcification: calcium deposits on elastic fibers are dense, granular, and irregular.
• Deposition of fibrous material.
• Increase of mesenchymal matrix material.
• Collagen deposition by myocytes.
• Accumulation of collagen and elastin.
• Fibrous plaque:
  – modified smooth muscle cells surrounded by increased amounts of extracellular matrix
  – thickened basement membrane
  – reduplication of and breaks in the internal elastic membrane
  – hyperplastic smooth muscle cells

Differential Diagnosis
• Vasculitis
• Arteritis
• Vascular malformation

20.5 Molecular Neuropathology

The evolution of arterial wall changes leading to the formation of the atheromatous plaques following the injury hypothesis is as follows:
• Chronic endothelial injury caused by:
  – Hyperlipidemia
  – Hypertension
  – Smoking
  – Elevated levels of homocysteine

20.4 Neuropathology Findings

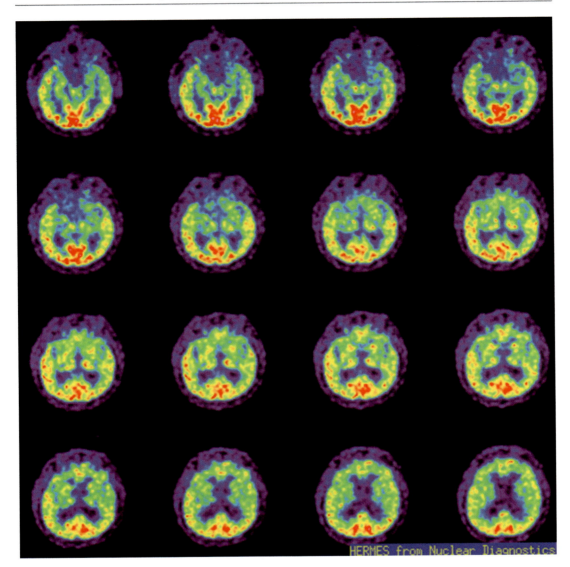

Fig. 20.2 FDG-PET of a patient with subcortical arteriosclerotic encephalopathy (SAE)—inhomogeneous FDG uptake in the cortex and basal ganglia

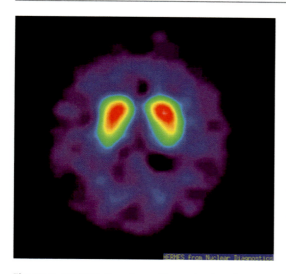

Fig. 20.3 FP-CIT of a patient with arteriosclerosis—symmetrical reduction of tracer uptake in the dorsal putamen

- Hemodynamic factors/forces
- Toxins
- Immune reactions
- Viruses
- Chronic endothelial injury leads to endothelial cell dysfunction.
- Endothelial dysfunction promotes:
  - Thrombosis
  - Increased permeability
  - Adherence of monocytes and lymphocytes to vessel surface
  - Migration of monocytes and lymphocytes into the intima
- Macrophages produce enzymes to oxidize low density lipoproteins in the intima.
- Engulfment of lipids by macrophages and smooth muscle cells.
- Migration of smooth muscle cells into the intima:
  - Converts to a secretory role producing extracellular matrix (e.g., collagen).
- Leads to the development of plaques.
- Smooth muscle cells are able to engulf oxidized LDL.
- Various changes:
  - Proliferation of smooth muscles
  - Deposition of collagen and other extracellular matrix proteins
  - Debris of extracellular lipid

20.6 Treatment and Prognosis

Treatment
- Pharmacologic
  - Statins
- Diet
- Surgical (carotid artery)

Biologic Behavior–Prognosis–Prognostic Factors
- Major and modifiable risk factors include:
  - Smoking, diabetes mellitus, hypertension, hyperlipidemia, inflammation
- Major and non-modifiable risk factors include:
  - Male gender, advanced age, family history, genetic abnormalities
- Other risk factors include:
  - Chlamydia pneumonia infection, elevated levels of homocysteine, elevated levels of lipoprotein-a
- Complications include:
  - Occlusion of vessel
    - Ischemic stroke
  - Disruption of plaque
    - Hemorrhage
  - Emboli and thrombosis
  - Aneurysm formation
  - Peripheral vascular disease

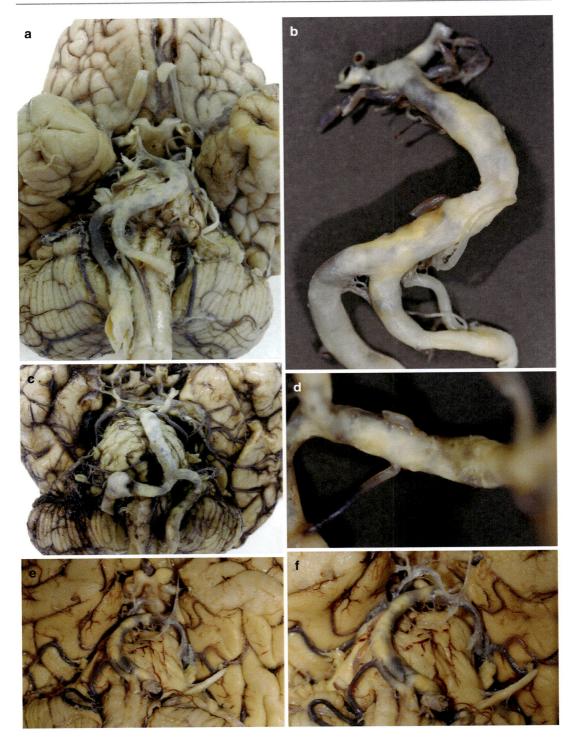

Fig. 20.4 Arteriosclerosis: arteriosclerotic plaques in the basilar artery (**a–h**), internal carotid artery (**i, j**), and pericallosal artery (**k, l**). Parts of a plaque removed upon surgery (**m, n**)

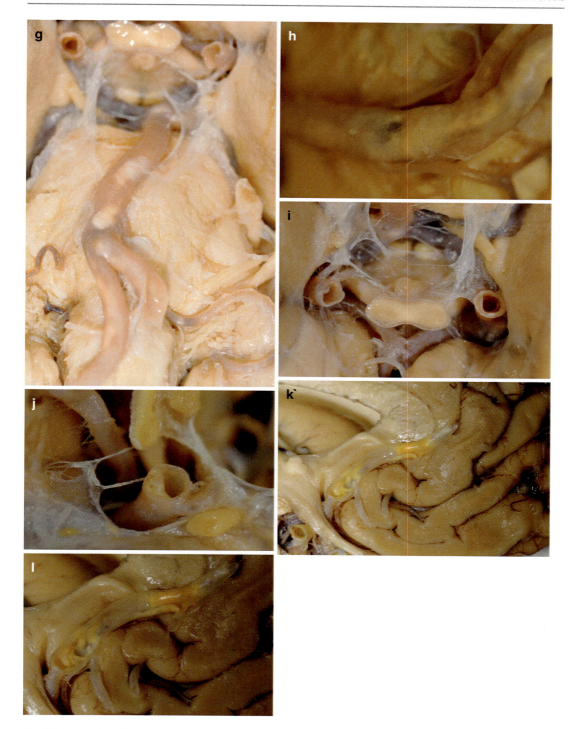

Fig. 20.4 (continued)

20.6 Treatment and Prognosis

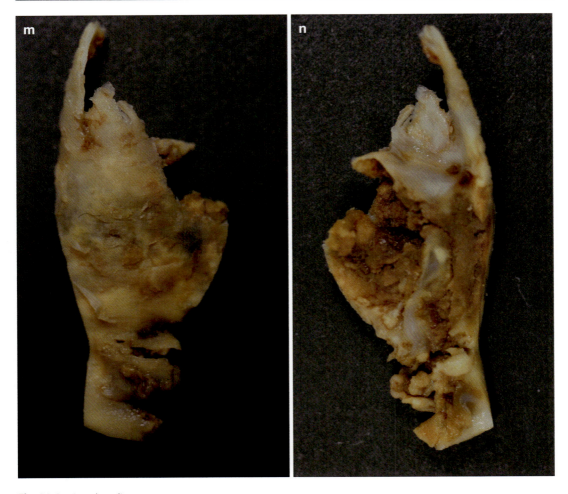

Fig. 20.4 (continued)

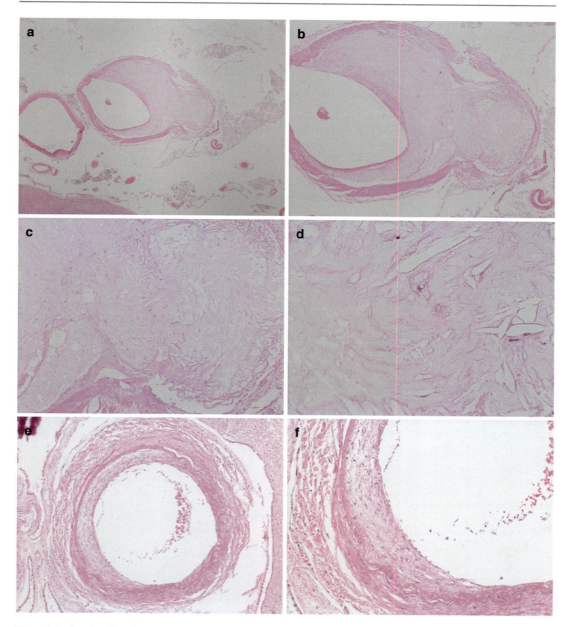

Fig. 20.5 Arteriosclerosis: artery with thickened wall and aneurysmatic sack; the lumen is narrowed by deposits of cholesterin crystal and cholesterin clefts (**a–d**). Initial stage of plaque formation (**e, f**); advanced stage of plaque formation with 50% narrowing of the lumen (**g–j**); end stage of plaque formation with nearly complete closure of the lumen (**k, l**)

20.6 Treatment and Prognosis

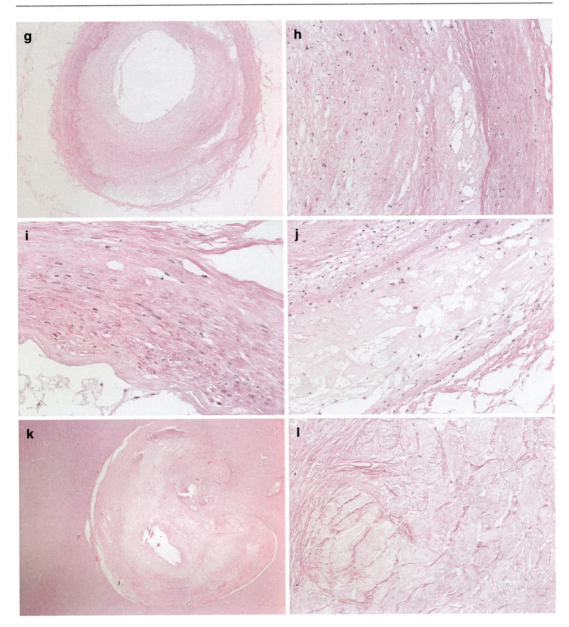

Fig. 20.5 (continued)

Selected References

Ali A, Tawakol A (2016) FDG PET/CT imaging of carotid atherosclerosis. Neuroimaging Clin N Am 26(1):45–54. https://doi.org/10.1016/j.nic.2015.09.004

Arning C, Widder B, von Reutern GM, Stiegler H, Gortler M (2010) Revision of DEGUM ultrasound criteria for grading internal carotid artery stenoses and transfer to NASCET measurement. Ultraschall Med 31(3):251–257. https://doi.org/10.1055/s-0029-1245336

Bories GFP, Leitinger N (2017) Macrophage metabolism in atherosclerosis. FEBS Lett 591(19):3042–3060. https://doi.org/10.1002/1873-3468.12786

Chistiakov DA, Melnichenko AA, Myasoedova VA, Grechko AV, Orekhov AN (2017) Mechanisms of foam cell formation in atherosclerosis. J Mol Med (Ber) 95(11):1153–1165. https://doi.org/10.1007/s00109-017-1575-8

Choromanska B, Mysliwiec P, Choromanska K, Dadan J, Chabowski A (2017) The role of CD36 receptor in the pathogenesis of atherosclerosis. Adv Clin Exp Med 26(4):717–722. https://doi.org/10.17219/acem/62325

Conti P, Shaik-Dasthagirisaeb Y (2015) Atherosclerosis: a chronic inflammatory disease mediated by mast cells. Cent Eur J Immunol 40(3):380–386. https://doi.org/10.5114/ceji.2015.54603

Dahal U, Sharma D, Dahal K (2017) An unsettled debate about the potential role of infection in pathogenesis of atherosclerosis. J Clin Med Res 9(7):547–554. https://doi.org/10.14740/jocmr3032w

Das T, Dron JS, Hegele RA (2017) Genetics of triglycerides and the risk of atherosclerosis. Curr Atheroscler Rep 19(7):31. https://doi.org/10.1007/s11883-017-0667-9

Fishbein GA, Fishbein MC (2009) Arteriosclerosis: rethinking the current classification. Arch Pathol Lab Med 133(8):1309–1316. https://doi.org/10.1043/1543-2165-133.8.1309

Fishbein MC, Fishbein GA (2015) Arteriosclerosis: facts and fancy. Cardiovasc Pathol 24(6):335–342. https://doi.org/10.1016/j.carpath.2015.07.007

Forstermann U, Xia N, Li H (2017) Roles of vascular oxidative stress and nitric oxide in the pathogenesis of atherosclerosis. Circ Res 120(4):713–735. https://doi.org/10.1161/circresaha.116.309326

Gillard JH, Gistera A, Hansson GK (2017) The immunology of atherosclerosis. Nat Rev Nephrol 13(6):368–380. https://doi.org/10.1038/nrneph.2017.51

Goncharov NV, Avdonin PV, Nadeev AD, Zharkikh IL, Jenkins RO (2015) Reactive oxygen species in pathogenesis of atherosclerosis. Curr Pharm Des 21(9):1134–1146

Graves MJ, Hai Z, Zuo W (2016) Aberrant DNA methylation in the pathogenesis of atherosclerosis. Clin Chim Acta 456:69–74. https://doi.org/10.1016/j.cca.2016.02.026

Jia SJ, Gao KQ, Zhao M (2017) Epigenetic regulation in monocyte/macrophage: a key player during atherosclerosis. Cardiovasc Ther 35(3). https://doi.org/10.1111/1755-5922.12262

Jonsson AL, Backhed F (2017) Role of gut microbiota in atherosclerosis. Nat Rev Cardiol 14(2):79–87. https://doi.org/10.1038/nrcardio.2016.183

Kattoor AJ, Pothineni NVK, Palagiri D, Mehta JL (2017) Oxidative stress in atherosclerosis. Curr Atheroscler Rep 19(11):42. https://doi.org/10.1007/s11883-017-0678-6

Khyzha N, Alizada A, Wilson MD, Fish JE (2017) Epigenetics of atherosclerosis: emerging mechanisms and methods. Trends Mol Med 23(4):332–347. https://doi.org/10.1016/j.molmed.2017.02.004

Kraml P (2017) The role of iron in the pathogenesis of atherosclerosis. Physiol Res 66(Suppl 1):S55–s67

Laffont B, Rayner KJ (2017) MicroRNAs in the pathobiology and therapy of atherosclerosis. Can J Cardiol 33(3):313–324. https://doi.org/10.1016/j.cjca.2017.01.001

Li F, Guo X, Chen SY (2017) Function and therapeutic potential of mesenchymal stem cells in atherosclerosis. Mediat Inflamm 4:32. https://doi.org/10.3389/fcvm.2017.00032

Linton MF, Babaev VR, Huang J, Linton EF, Tao H, Yancey PG (2016) Macrophage apoptosis and efferocytosis in the pathogenesis of atherosclerosis. Int J Inflamm 80(11):2259–2268. https://doi.org/10.1253/circj.CJ-16-0924

Meschia JF, Klaas JP, Brown RD Jr, Brott TG (2017) Evaluation and management of atherosclerotic carotid stenosis. Mayo Clin Proc 92(7):1144–1157. https://doi.org/10.1016/j.mayocp.2017.02.020

Osborn EA, Kessinger CW, Tawakol A, Jaffer FA (2017) Metabolic and molecular imaging of atherosclerosis and venous thromboembolism. J Nucl Med 58(6):871–877. https://doi.org/10.2967/jnumed.116.182873

Pace NP, Patterson AJ, Roshan MH, Tambo A (2016) The role of TLR2, TLR4, and TLR9 in the pathogenesis of atherosclerosis. Int J Inflam 2016:1532832

Saba L, Yuan C (2018) Carotid artery wall imaging: perspective and guidelines from the ASNR Vessel Wall Imaging Study Group and expert consensus recommendations of the American Society of Neuroradiology. AJNR Am J Neuroradiol 39(2):E9–e31. https://doi.org/10.3174/ajnr.A5488

Shimizu Y, Kuge Y (2016) Recent advances in the development of PET/SPECT probes for atherosclerosis imaging. AJNR Am J Neuroradiol 50(4):284–291. https://doi.org/10.3174/ajnr.A5026

Spence JD (2016) Recent advances in pathogenesis, assessment, and treatment of atherosclerosis. F1000Res. 5. https://doi.org/10.12688/f1000research.8459.1

Tolle M, Reshetnik A, Schuchardt M, Hohne M, van der Giet M (2015) Arteriosclerosis and vascular calcification: causes, clinical assessment and therapy. Eur J Clin Investig 45(9):976–985. https://doi.org/10.1111/eci.12493

Wang D, Wang Z (2017) Roles of cells from the arterial vessel wall in atherosclerosis. Mediat Inflamm 2017:8135934. https://doi.org/10.1155/2017/8135934

Selected References

Wang Y, Xie W, Li L, Zheng XL, Yin WD, Tang CK (2017) The role of Kruppel-like factor 14 in the pathogenesis of atherosclerosis. Atherosclerosis 263:352–360. https://doi.org/10.1016/j.atherosclerosis.2017.06.011

Yang X, Li Y, Li Y, Ren X, Zhang X, Hu D, Gao Y, Xing Y, Shang H (2017) Oxidative stress-mediated atherosclerosis: mechanisms and therapies. Front Physiol 8:600. https://doi.org/10.3389/fphys.2017.00600

Yoneyama K, Venkatesh BA, Bluemke DA, McClelland RL, Lima JAC (2017) Cardiovascular magnetic resonance in an adult human population: serial observations from the multi-ethnic study of atherosclerosis. J Cardiovasc Magn Reson 19(1):52. https://doi.org/10.1186/s12968-017-0367-1

Yuan J, Usman A (2017) Imaging carotid atherosclerosis plaque ulceration: comparison of advanced imaging modalities and recent developments. AJNR Am J Neuroradiol 38(4):664–671. https://doi.org/10.3174/ajnr.A5026

Zhang L, Zhou B, Margariti A, Zeng L, Xu Q (2011) Role of histone deacetylases in vascular cell homeostasis and arteriosclerosis. Cardiovasc Res 90(3):413–420. https://doi.org/10.1093/cvr/cvr003

Zhang J, Zhou HJ, Ji W, Min W (2015) AIP1-mediated stress signaling in atherosclerosis and arteriosclerosis. Curr Atheroscler Rep 17(5):503. https://doi.org/10.1007/s11883-015-0503-z

Vascular Disorders: Aneurysms

21.1 Definition

An aneurysm is a localized pathological dilatation of a blood vessel (or of the cardiac wall) involving all layers.

The following types of aneurysm are distinguished:

- Saccular (berry) aneurysms
- Fusiform aneurysms
- Inflammatory/infective "mycotic" (septic) aneurysms
- Dissecting aneurysms (arterial dissections)
- Dolichoectasia
- False aneurysm "pseudoaneurysm"

21.2 Epidemiology

Incidence
- Prevalence of unruptured aneurysms: 3%

Age Incidence
- 40–70 years of age

Sex Incidence
- Male:Female ratio: 1:3

Localization
- Anterior communicating artery (ACA)
- Middle cerebral artery (MCA)
- Internal carotid artery (ICA)
- Basilar artery (BA)

21.3 Neuroimaging Findings

General Imaging Findings
Focal abnormal enlargement of a blood vessel
  Imaging of choice: DSA gold standard > CTA > MRA

CT Non-Contrast-Enhanced (Fig. 21.2a, b)
- Well defined, slightly hyperdense, subarachnoidal mass
- Small aneurysm invisible
- Calcifications of aneurysm wall possible
- If partial thrombosis: hyperdense inclusions

CT Contrast-Enhanced
- Intraluminal enhancement of aneurysm
- Thrombosed aneurysm: enhancement of wall possible

CTA (Fig. 21.1a)
- high sensitivity for aneurysm >2 mm

MRI-T2/FLAIR (Figs. 21.1b–d and 21.2c, d)
- Hypointense flow void

MRI-T1 (Figs. 21.1e and 21.2e)
- Flow void
- Variable signal

MRI-T1 contrast-enhanced (Figs. 21.1f, g and 21.2f)
- Intraluminal enhancement

MRA (Fig. 21.1j, k)
- high sensitivity for aneurysm >2 mm

DSA (Figs. 21.1l–n and 21.2h, i)
- Gold standard, including rotational 3D DSA
- For evaluation of treatment options

Nuclear Medicine Imaging Findings
- No indication for examination

21.4 Neuropathology Findings

Macroscopic Features (Figs. 21.3, 21.4, 21.5, and 21.6)
- Saccular (berry) aneurysms
  - Saccular outpouching from one side of the affected vessel
- Fusiform aneurysms (arterial dolichoectasia)
  - Generalized dilatation of the entire circumference of the affected vessel along its length
- Inflammatory/infective "mycotic" (septic) aneurysms
  - Result of an infection from septic emboli or an aneurysm that has subsequently become infected
- Dissecting aneurysms (arterial dissections)
  - In extracranial and/or intracranial branches of the carotid or vertebro-basilar system.
  - Between the internal elastic lamina and the media.
  - Intravascular thrombosis might occur.
  - Transmural dissection is possible in the posterior circulation.
- Buried in blood clot
- Ruptured wall
- Coils in the aneurysmal sac
- Clip around neck of aneurysm

Microscopic Features (Fig. 21.7a–d)
- Aneurysmal sac is formed.
  - Thin fibrous tissue
  - Attenuation of the elastic laminae
  - Thinning of the media
- Mycotic aneurysm (Fig. 21.8).
  - accumulation of inflammatory cells
  - fibrin matrix
  - extensive capillary network
  - hemosiderinophages
  - perivascular lymphocytic infiltrates

Immunophenotype
- Smooth muscle actin
- CD68

Ultrastructural Features
- basement membranes with
  - thickening
  - lamination
  - redundancy
  - separation
- abundant cellular debris
- paucity or absence of elastic
- extracellular lipid and lipophages

Differential Diagnosis
- Subdural hematoma
- Subarachnoidal hemorrhage
- Intracerebral hemorrhage

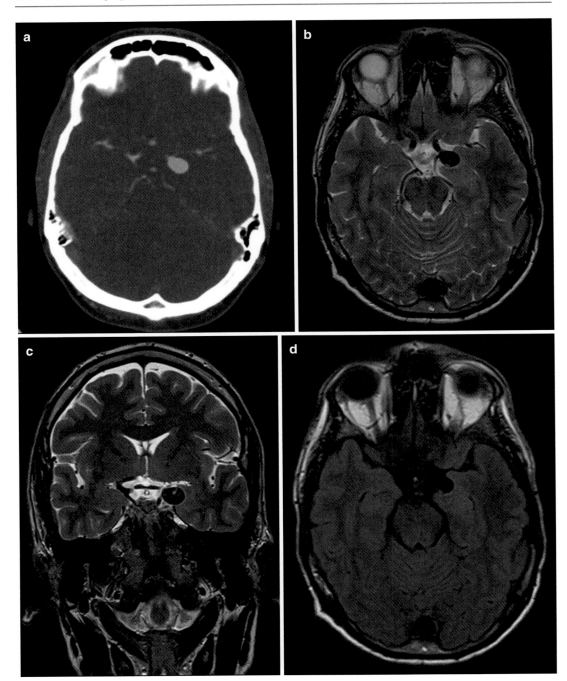

Fig. 21.1 Incidental aneurysm of the left communicating posterior artery in CTA (**a**), T2 ax/cor (**b**, **c**), FLAIR (**d**), T1 (**e**), T1 contrast ax/cor (**f**, **g**), DWI (**h**), SWI (**i**), MRA TOF (**j**, **k**), VR-DSA (**l**), DSA before and after coiling (**m**, **n**)

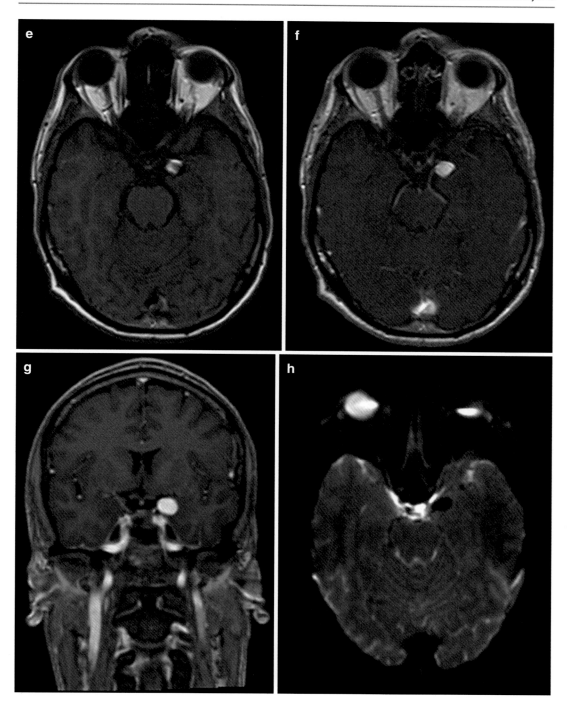

Fig. 21.1 (continued)

21.2 General Imaging Findings

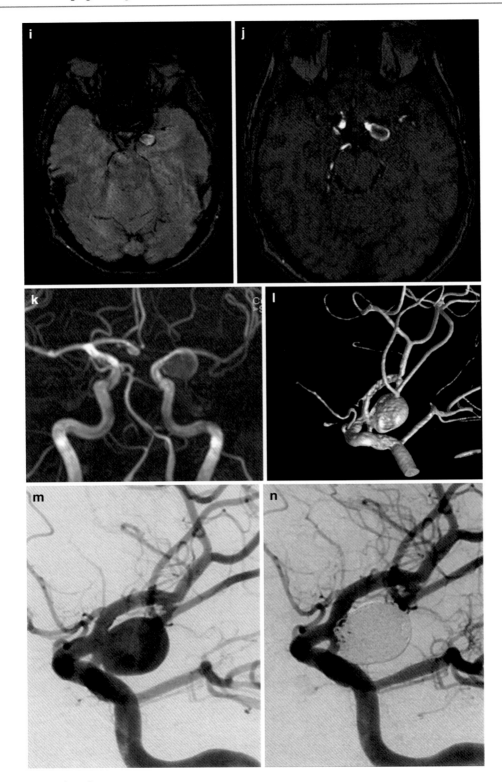

Fig. 21.1 (continued)

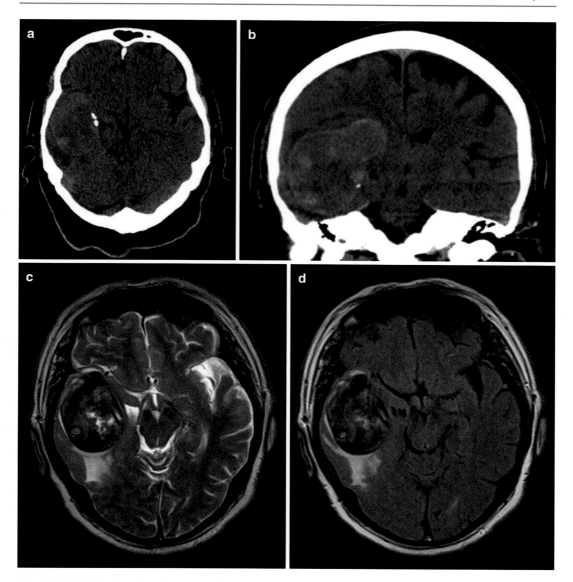

Fig. 21.2 Partially thrombosed aneurysm of the bifurcation of left middle cerebral artery in CT ax/cor (**a**, **b**), T2 (**c**) FLAIR (**d**), T1 (**e**), T1 contrast (**f**), SWI (**g**), DSA ap (**h**), VR-DSA (**i**)

21.2 General Imaging Findings

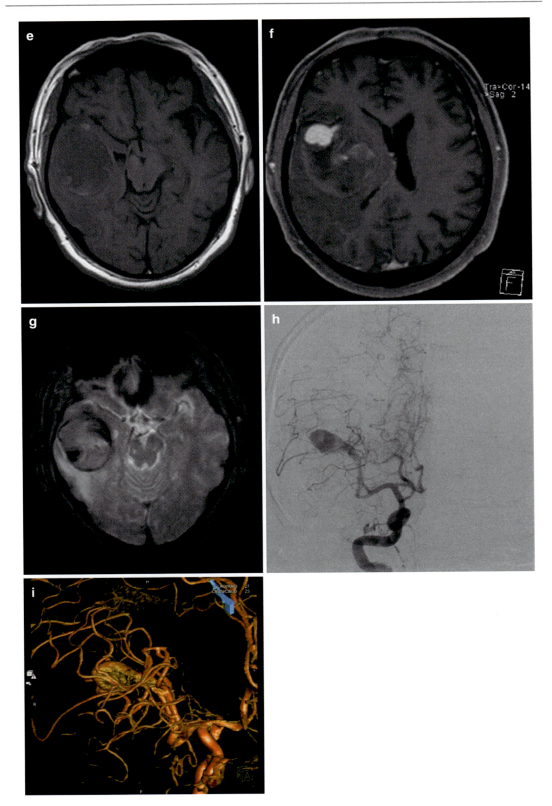

Fig. 21.2 (continued)

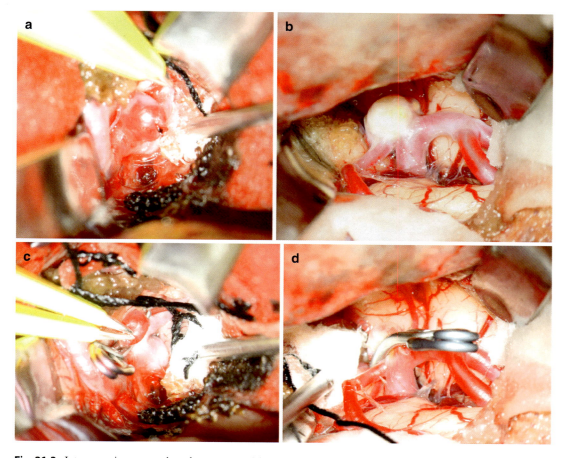

Fig. 21.3 Intraoperative approach to the aneurysm (**a**), exposure of the aneurysm (**b**), the clip is positioned (**c, d**)

21.5 Molecular Neuropathology

Pathogenesis
- Weakness of the media due to primary intimal changes of atherosclerosis
- Cystic medial degeneration
- Congenital weakness
- Tertiary syphilis leading to luetic aortic aneurysm

Cerebral aneurysm (CA) formation and rupture.

- Increased mechanical stress in aneurysm-prone regions is believed to trigger events that culminate in vascular dysfunction, leaving the endothelium nude from antithrombotic protection.
- Aneurysm formation is initiated by hemodynamically triggered endothelial dysfunction.
- An inflammatory response implicating several cytokines and inflammatory mediators as well as macrophages, T-cells, and mast cells ensues.
- The inflammatory cascade then begins (Table 21.1).
  - Expression of chemoattractants and pro-inflammatory cytokines.
  - Burgeoning of cell adhesion molecules at the surface of endothelial cells.
  - Attraction of peripheral blood mononuclear cells, including monocytes and T-cells.
  - The complement is also activated through the classic pathway.
  - Monocytes are able to adhere and transmigrate into the endothelium, which they would not do under normal conditions.

21.2 General Imaging Findings

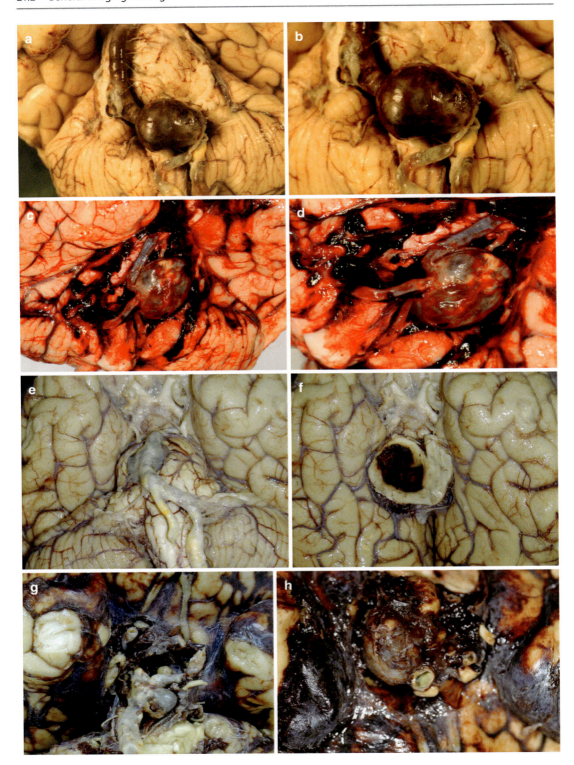

Fig. 21.4 Gross-anatomical appearances of aneurysms (**a–r**). (**a, b**) Basilar artery, caudal part, fixed brain, (**c, d**) basilar artery, caudal part, unfixed brain, (**e, f**) basilar artery with grooving of the aneurysm into the mesencephalon, (**g**) basilar artery, cranial part, (**h**) internal carotid artery, (**i, j**) internal carotid artery with impression on the optic nerves, (**k, l**) middle cerebral artery, (**m, n**) posterior inferior cerebellar artery, (**o**) anterior communicating artery, (**p**) middle cerebral artery, (**q, r**) coronal section through a medial cerebral artery aneurysm

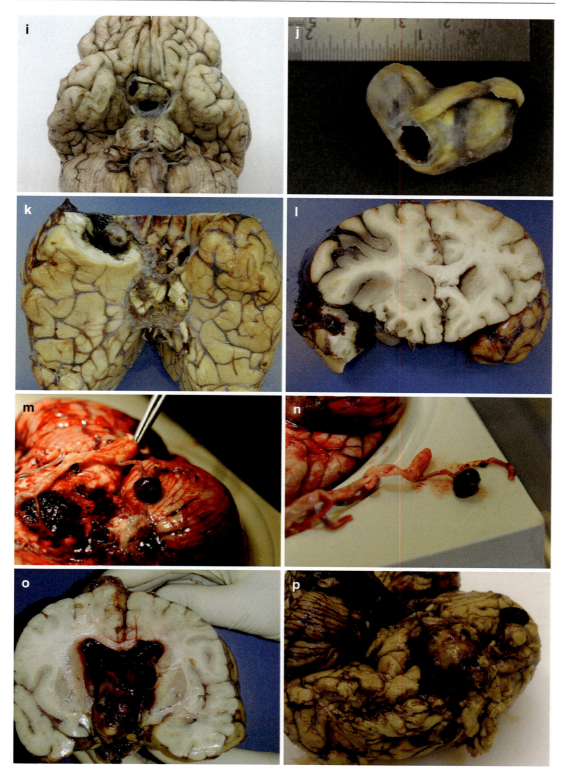

Fig. 21.4 (continued)

21.2 General Imaging Findings

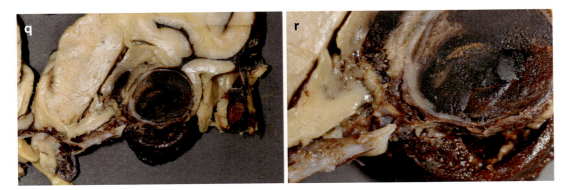

Fig. 21.4 (continued)

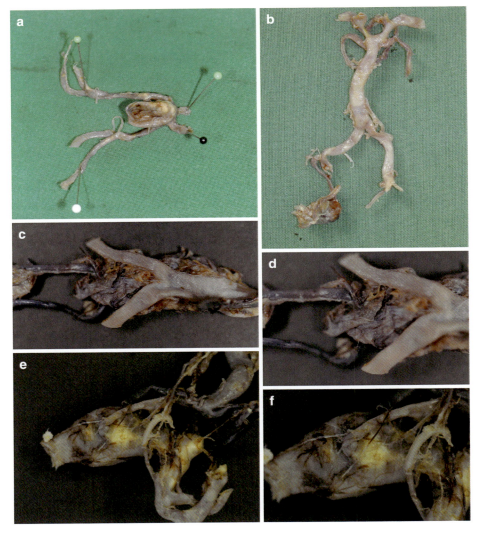

Fig. 21.5 Macroscopic appearances of aneurysms after preparation: (**a**) anterior communicating artery, (**b**) posterior inferior cerebellar artery, (**c, d**) posterior communicating artery, (**e, f**) basilar artery, (**g, h**) giant aneurysms of the basilar artery, (**i, j**) giant aneurysm (7 cm in diameter) of the basilar artery with flow diverter, (**k, l**) stent in an artery

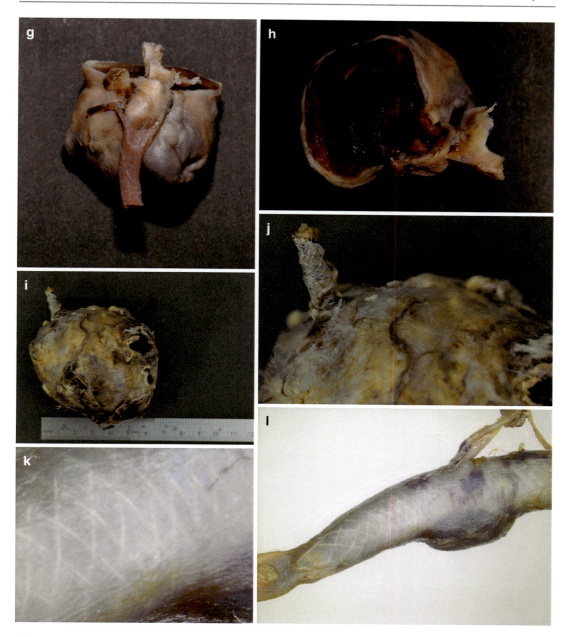

Fig. 21.5 (continued)

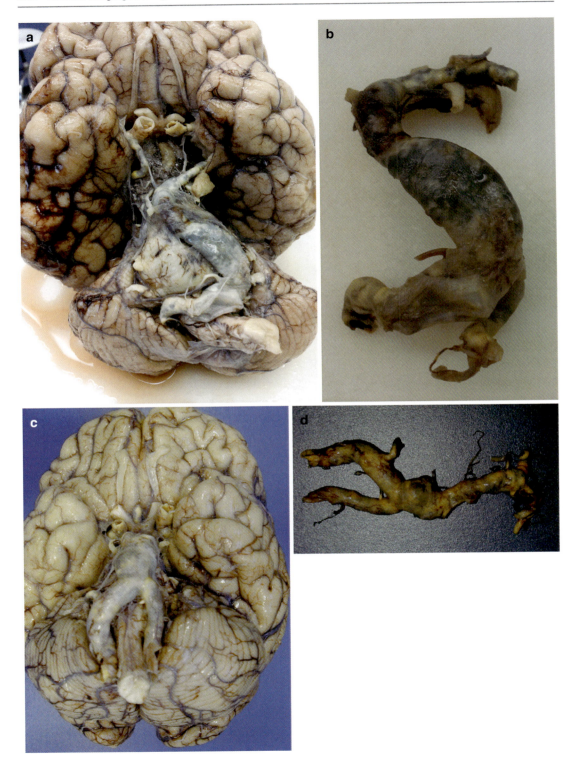

Fig. 21.6 Megadolichocephalic basilar artery (**a–d**)

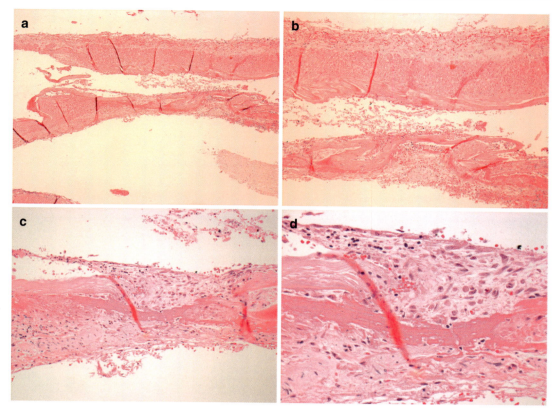

Fig. 21.7 Microscopic appearance of an aneurysmal wall (**a–d**) with wall thinning (**a**, **b**) and accumulation of monomorphonuclear cells in the wall (**c**, **d**)

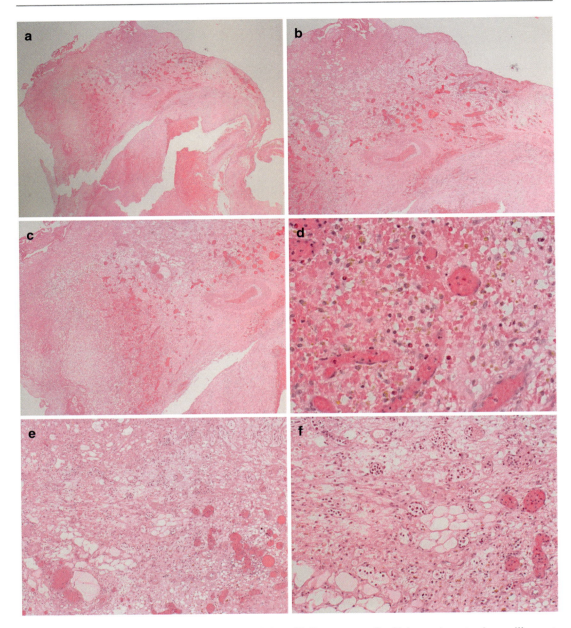

Fig. 21.8 Mycotic aneurysm consists of an accumulation of inflammatory cells, fibrin matrix, extensive capillary network, hemosiderinophages, perivascular lymphocytic infiltrates (**a–l**; **k**, **l**: EvG stain)

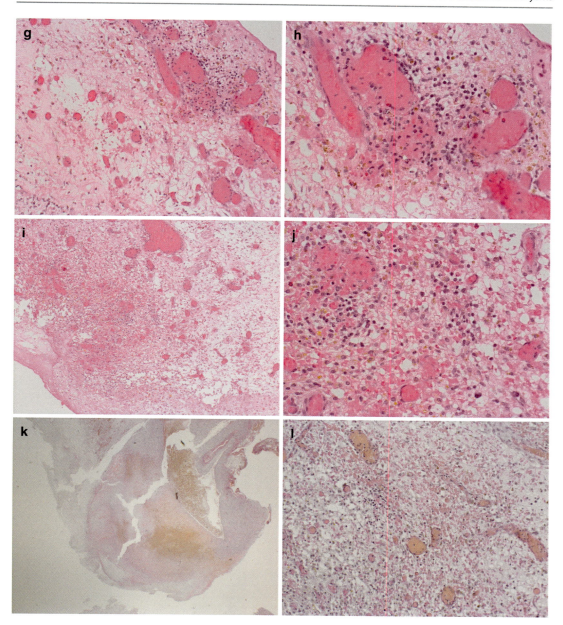

Fig. 21.8 (continued)

21.2 General Imaging Findings

- Monocytes subsequently differentiate into macrophages, as observed in morphological studies of intracranial aneurysm wall.
- The level of proteases in aneurysmal wall is increased.
- Macrophages are responsible for the imbalance of proteases.
- Concurrently, smooth muscle cells (SMCs) undergo phenotypic modulation to a pro-inflammatory phenotype.
- The inflammatory response in vessel wall leads to
  - disruption of internal elastic lamina
  - extracellular matrix digestion
  - aneurysm formation
- Loss of mural cells and further inflammation and vessel wall degeneration ultimately lead to CA rupture.

Molecular pathways include:

- Inflammation (Table 21.1)
- Oxidative stress
- Genes
- Gene polymorphisms (Tables 21.2 and 21.3)

Major pathways of **oxidative stress** in cerebral aneurysm pathogenesis include (Starke et al. 2013):

- Atherosclerosis
  - Oxidized LDL
  - NADPH
  - Myeloperoxidase
  - COX
  - LIPOX
  - NOS
  - IL1β
  - TNFα
  - IL-6
  - MCP-1
  - Selectins and adhesion molecules
- Endothelial dysfunction, hemodynamic stress, and hypertension
  - NADPH
  - NF-κB
  - COX
  - NOS
  - VCAM
  - IL-8
  - mPGEs-1
  - angiotensin II
- VSMC pro-inflammatory, pro-matrix remodeling phenotypic modulation. Apoptotic cell death
  - NADPH
  - NOS
  - NF-κB
  - KLF4
  - TNFα
  - VCAM
  - MMP
  - MCP
- Chronic inflammatory reaction, vessel wall remodeling and damage, apoptotic cell death
  - NADPH
  - NOS
  - MCP-1
  - MMP
  - VCAM
  - IL-1β, IL-8, IL-12
  - NF-κB

Table 21.1 Inflammatory pathways and mediators implicated in aneurysm formation and rupture (Chalouhi et al. 2013) reproduced with kind permission by Lippincott

Pathway	Mediators
Endothelial dysfunction	• IL-1β (interleukin 1β) • NF-κB (nuclear factor-κB) • Ets-1 • MCP-1 (monocyte chemoattractant protein) • Reactive oxygen species • Nitric oxide (NO), endothelial NO synthase, inducible NO synthase • Angiotensin II • Phosphodiesterase-4 • Prostaglandin E2 • E selectin, P selectin, vascular cell adhesion protein 1 (VCAM1), intercellular adhesion molecule 1 (ICAM1)
Phenotypic modulation and loss of SMCs	• TNFα tumor necrosis factor-α • Kruppel-like transcription factor 4 (KLF-4) • Interleukin 1β (IL-1β) • P47phox • MCP-1 monocyte chemoattractant protein • MMPs matrix metalloproteinase • Adhesion molecules
Macrophages, M1/M2 imbalance, leukocyte infiltration	• MCP-1 monocyte chemoattractant protein • NF-κB nuclear factor-κB • Ets-1 • MMPs matrix metalloproteinase • IL-1β interleukin 1β • TNF-α tumor necrosis factor-α • Normal T-cell expressed and secreted • Monokine induced by γ-interferon • Interferon-γ-induced protein-10 • Eotaxin • IL-8 • IL-17
Vascular remodeling, cell death	• MMP matrix metalloproteinase and cathepsins • TNFα tumor necrosis factor-α • IL-1β interleukin 1β • IL-6 • Toll-like receptor 4 • Fas • NO • Complement • IgG, IgM • Basic fibroblast growth factor • Transforming growth factor α and β • Vascular endothelial growth factor • Reactive oxygen species

Genes associated with **aneurysm formation** have been identified (Theodotou et al. 2017) and include:

- IQSEC1—Cell adhesion activator protein ARF-GEP100
- ARHGEF11—Rho-dependent signaling
- TMEM195—Fatty acid hydroxylase
- COL3A1—Type III collagen
- SAP130—Sin3A-associated protein 130
- CDKN2BAS—Associated with atherosclerotic disease
- BTBD16—BTB domain containing 16
- C12orf75—Chromosome 12 open reading frame 75, protein coding
- SOX17—Transcription factor
- Chromosome 7 SNP—Near HDAC9; associated with ischemic stroke; TWIST1, FERD3L
- COL1A2—Type 1 collagen
- eNOS—Endothelial nitric oxide synthase
- JDP2—Transcription repressor
- IL-12A/B—Interleukin 12
- miR-34b/c—MicroRNA
- Endoglin—Co-receptor of the TGF-β family
- IL-6-572—IL-6
- LIMK1—Kinase for actin cytoskeleton
- MMP2—Matrix metalloproteinase; ECM remodeling in blood vessels
- TNF-α - TNF-α; pro-inflammatory cytokine
- EDNRA—Endothelin-1 Receptor
- CDKN2BAS—Associated with atherosclerotic disease
- ALDH2—Mitochondrial aldehyde dehydrogenase
- CSPG2—Versican (ECM structure)
- HSPG2—Perlecan (ECM structure)
- TGFBR1—TGF-β receptor
- KLK—Kallikrein (serine protease; basement membrane components, remodeling)
- RBBP8—Retinoblastoma-binding protein 8
- STARD13/KL—StAR-related lipid transfer; suppresses cell proliferation
- CNNM2—Cyclin M2
- SOX17—Transcription factor
- CDKN2A/B—Associated with CAD

21.2 General Imaging Findings

Table 21.2 Most significant associations in candidate gene studies (Tromp et al. 2014) (reproduce with kind permission by Taylor & Francis, open access)

Gene symbol	Polymorphism	Region	Context	Genetic model	Potential biological
ACE	rs4646994	17q23.3	Intron	Recessive	Vascular endothelium
COL1A2	rs42524	7q21	Missense (p.549P-A)	Dominant	Extracellular matrix
COL3A1	rs1800255	2q32	Missense (p.698A-T)	Dominant	Extracellular matrix
ELN	rs8326	7q11.2	3'-UTR	Allelic	Vascular endothelium
HSPG2	rs3767137	1p36.1	Intron	Additive	Extracellular matrix
IL6	rs1800796	7p15	Intergenic	Recessive	Inflammatory mediator
JDP2	rs175646	14q24	Intron	Allelic	Apoptosis
KLK8	rs1722561	19q13.3	Intron	Additive	Extracellular matrix
LIMK1	rs6460071	7q11.2	Intergenic	Dominant	Actin depolymerization
SERPINA3	rs4934	14q32	Missense (p.9A-T)	Dominant	Extracellular matrix
TCN2	rs1801198	22q12	Missense (p.259R-P)	Genotypic	Methionine metabolism
TNFRSF13B	rs4985754	17p11.2	Promoter	Haplotype	Immunity
	rs2274892	17p11.2	Intron		
	rs34562254	17p11.2	Missense (p.251P-L)		
	rs11078355	17p11.2	Synonymous		
VCAN	rs173686	5q14	Intron	Additive	Extracellular matrix
VCAN	rs251124	5q14	Intron	Additive	Extracellular matrix

Table 21.3 Most significant associations from genome-wide association studies (Tromp et al. 2014) (reproduce with kind permission by Taylor & Francis, open access)

Gene symbol	Polymorphism	Region	Context	OR
CDKN2B-AS1 (ANRIL)	rs1333040	9p21	Intron	1.24
CDKN2B-AS1 (ANRIL)	rs10757278	9p21	Intergenic	1.29
CDKN2B-AS1 (ANRIL)	rs6475606	9p21	Intron	1.35
CNNM2	rs12413409	10q24.3	Intron	1.29
EDNRA	rs6841581	4q31.23	Intergenic	1.22
FGD6	rs6538595	12q22	Intron	1.16
RRBP1	rs1132274	20p12.1	Missense (p.891R > L)	1.19
SOX17	rs10958409	8q11.23	Intergenic (5')	1.20
SOX17	rs9298506	8q11.23	Intergenic (3')	1.21
STARD13	rs9315204	13q13	Intron	1.20

- EDNRA—Endothelin-1 receptor Rs6841581 1.22 1.14-1.31 < 0.001
- NDUFA12INR2C1/FGD61VEZT—Ubiquinone 1 alpha-12, nuclear receptor
- RRBP1—Ribosome-binding protein

Genes associated with **aneurysm rupture** have been identified (Theodotou et al. 2017) and include:

- GpIIIa—Platelet-mediated thrombosis receptor
- AGTR1/A116C—Angiotensin II type 1 receptor
- ADAMTS13—Thrombus inhibition (cleaves vWF)
- 9p21—Associated with atherosclerotic disease
- MMP2—Matrix metalloproteinase
- MMP9—Matrix metalloproteinase
- IL-6—Inflammatory cytokine
- Factor V—Leiden Increased thrombosis
- Prothrombin—Coagulation
- MTHFR—Methylenetetrahydrofolate reductase
- Factor XIII subunit A—Coagulation factor
- Factor XIII subunit B—Coagulation factor
- ACE—ACE
- eNOS3—Endothelial nitric oxide synthase
- COL6A3—Collagen

- ITM2C—Integral membrane protein 2C, protein coding
- MAPKAP1—Mitogen-activated protein kinase-associated protein 1, protein coding
- NVL—Nuclear VCP-like, protein coding
- WNT3—Wnt family member 3, protein coding
- TBL3—Transducin beta like 3, protein coding

21.6 Treatment and Prognosis

Treatment
- Clipping (neurosurgery) (Fig. 21.9)
- Coiling (interventional neuroradiology) (Fig. 21.10)
- Coiling: Clipping ratio: 70:30

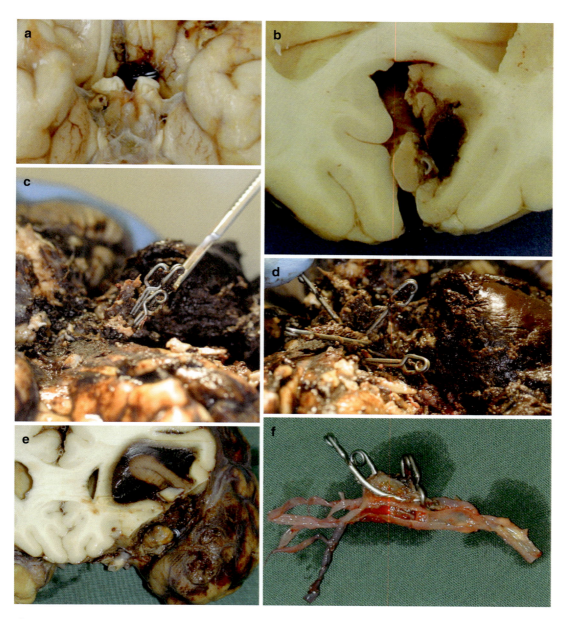

Fig. 21.9 Examples of clipped aneurysms: anterior communicating artery (**a, b**), middle cerebral artery (**c–l**), multiple aneurysms (**m–p**). (The specimens were trimmed by Anja Grimmer, MD and Christian Auer, MD, consultants in neurosurgery, Neuromed Campus, Kepler University Hospital during their rotation in neuropathology)

21.2 General Imaging Findings

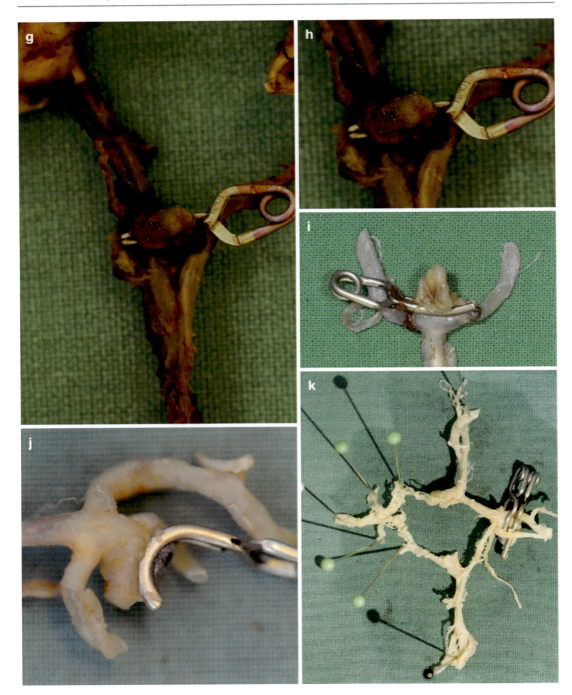

Fig. 21.9 (continued)

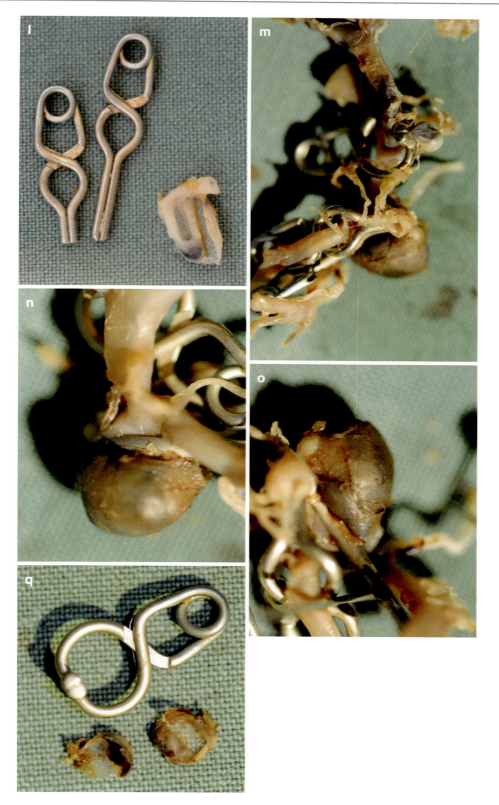

Fig. 21.9 (continued)

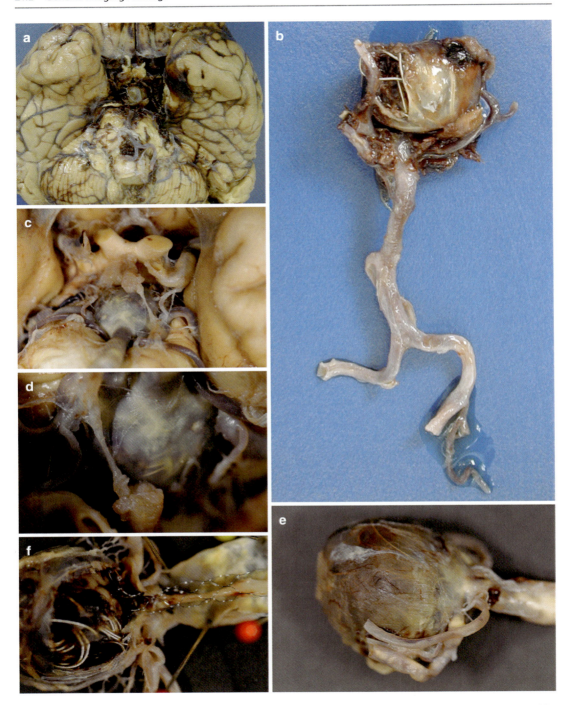

Fig. 21.10 Examples of coiled aneurysms. Basilar artery (**a–f**), anterior communicating artery (**g, h**), basilar artery (**i, j**), posterior cerebellar artery (**k, l**), anterior communicating artery (**m**), anterior cerebral artery (**n**), anterior cerebral artery (**o, p**). (The specimens were trimmed by Anja Grimmer, MD and Christian Auer, MD, consultants in neurosurgery, Neuromed Campus, Kepler University Hospital during their rotation in neuropathology)

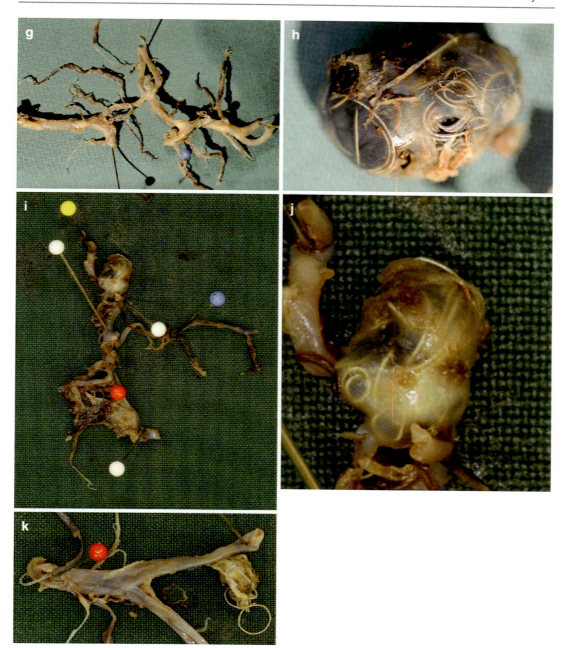

Fig. 21.10 (continued)

21.2 General Imaging Findings

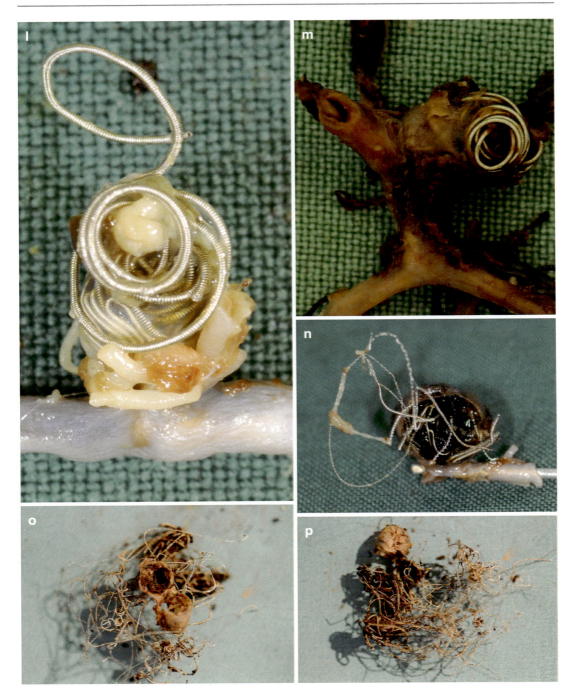

Fig. 21.10 (continued)

Biologic Behavior–Prognosis–Prognostic Factors

- Complications include:
  - Emboli
  - Thrombosis
  - Rupture with resultant subarachnoidal and/or intracerebral hemorrhage
  - Obstruction of branch vessels
  - Impingement on neighboring structures (e.g., cranial nerves, optic nerve)

Selected References

Bourcier R, Redon R, Desal H (2015) Genetic investigations on intracranial aneurysm: update and perspectives. Mediat Inflamm 42(2):67–71. https://doi.org/10.1016/j.neurad.2015.01.002

Castro MA (2013) Understanding the role of hemodynamics in the initiation, progression, rupture, and treatment outcome of cerebral aneurysm from medical image-based computational studies. ISRN Radiol 2013:602707. https://doi.org/10.5402/2013/602707

Chalouhi N, Hoh BL, Hasan D (2013) Review of cerebral aneurysm formation, growth, and rupture. Stroke 44(12):3613–3622. https://doi.org/10.1161/strokeaha.113.002390

Dorsch N (2011) A clinical review of cerebral vasospasm and delayed ischaemia following aneurysm rupture. Acta Neurochir Suppl 110(Pt 1):5–6. https://doi.org/10.1007/978-3-7091-0353-1_1

Frosen J, Tulamo R, Paetau A, Laaksamo E, Korja M, Laakso A, Niemela M, Hernesniemi J (2012) Saccular intracranial aneurysm: pathology and mechanisms. Acta Neuropathol 123(6):773–786. https://doi.org/10.1007/s00401-011-0939-3

Henkes H, Weber W (2015) The past, present and future of endovascular aneurysm treatment. Clin Neuroradiol 25(Suppl 2):317–324. https://doi.org/10.1007/s00062-015-0403-1

Lai LT, O'Neill AH (2017) History, evolution, and continuing innovations of intracranial aneurysm surgery. World Neurosurg 102:673–681. https://doi.org/10.1016/j.wneu.2017.02.006

Li MH, Li YD, Gu BX, Cheng YS, Wang W, Tan HQ, Chen YC (2014) Accurate diagnosis of small cerebral aneurysms </=5 mm in diameter with 3.0-T MR angiography. Radiology 271(2):553–560. https://doi.org/10.1148/radiol.14122770

McFadden JT (2012) Magnetic resonance imaging and aneurysm clips. J Neurosurg 117(1):1–11. https://doi.org/10.3171/2012.1.jns111786

Menke J, Larsen J, Kallenberg K (2011) Diagnosing cerebral aneurysms by computed tomographic angiography: meta-analysis. Ann Neurol 69(4):646–654. https://doi.org/10.1002/ana.22270

Numminen J, Tarkiainen A, Niemela M, Porras M, Hernesniemi J, Kangasniemi M (2011) Detection of unruptured cerebral artery aneurysms by MRA at 3.0 tesla: comparison with multislice helical computed tomographic angiography. Acta Radiol 52(6):670–674. https://doi.org/10.1258/ar.2011.100421

Pritz MB (2011) Cerebral aneurysm classification based on angioarchitecture. J Stroke Cerebrovasc Dis 20(2):162–167. https://doi.org/10.1016/j.jstrokecerebrovasdis.2009.11.018

Raabe A, Seidel K (2016) Prevention of ischemic complications during aneurysm surgery. J Neurosurg Sci 60(1):95–103

Sadasivan C, Fiorella DJ, Woo HH, Lieber BB (2013) Physical factors effecting cerebral aneurysm pathophysiology. Ann Biomed Eng 41(7):1347–1365. https://doi.org/10.1007/s10439-013-0800-z

Sailer AM, Wagemans BA, Nelemans PJ, de Graaf R, van Zwam WH (2014) Diagnosing intracranial aneurysms with MR angiography: systematic review and meta-analysis. Stroke 45(1):119–126. https://doi.org/10.1161/strokeaha.113.003133

Sawyer DM, Amenta PS, Medel R (2015) Inflammatory mediators in vascular disease: identifying promising targets for intracranial aneurysm research. Mediators Inflamm 2015:896283. https://doi.org/10.1155/2015/896283

Sorenson T, Lanzino G (2016) Trials and tribulations: an evidence-based approach to aneurysm treatment. J Neurosurg Sci 60(1):22–26

Starke RM, Chalouhi N, Ali MS, Jabbour PM, Tjoumakaris SI, Gonzalez LF, Rosenwasser RH, Koch WJ, Dumont AS (2013) The role of oxidative stress in cerebral aneurysm formation and rupture. Curr Neurovasc Res 10(3):247–255

Starke RM, Chalouhi N, Ding D, Raper DM, McKisic MS, Owens GK, Hasan DM, Medel R, Dumont AS (2014a) Vascular smooth muscle cells in cerebral aneurysm pathogenesis. Transl Stroke Res 5(3):338–346. https://doi.org/10.1007/s12975-013-0290-1

Starke RM, Raper DM, Ding D, Chalouhi N, Owens GK, Hasan DM, Medel R, Dumont AS (2014b) Tumor necrosis factor-alpha modulates cerebral aneurysm formation and rupture. Transl Stroke Res 5(2):269–277. https://doi.org/10.1007/s12975-013-0287-9

Theodotou CB, Snelling BM, Sur S, Haussen DC, Peterson EC, Elhammady MS (2017) Genetic associations of intracranial aneurysm formation and sub-arachnoid hemorrhage. Asian J Neurosurg 12(3):374–381. https://doi.org/10.4103/1793-5482.180972

Tromp G, Weinsheimer S, Ronkainen A, Kuivaniemi H (2014) Molecular basis and genetic predisposition to intracranial aneurysm. Ann Med 46(8):597–606. https://doi.org/10.3109/07853890.2014.949299

Tsyben A, Paldor I, Laidlaw J (2016) Cerebral vasospasm and delayed ischaemic deficit following elective aneurysm clipping. J Clin Neurosci 34:33–38. https://doi.org/10.1016/j.jocn.2016.06.006

Tulamo R, Frosen J, Hernesniemi J, Niemela M (2010) Inflammatory changes in the aneurysm wall: a review. J Neurointerv Surg 2(2):120–130. https://doi.org/10.1136/jnis.2009.002055

Turjman AS, Turjman F, Edelman ER (2014) Role of fluid dynamics and inflammation in intracranial aneurysm formation. Circulation 129(3):373–382. https://doi.org/10.1161/circulationaha.113.001444

Vascular Disorders: Malformations

22.1 Introduction

Malformations of intracranial vessels include:
- Arteriovenous malformation
- Cavernous hemangioma
- Capillary telangiectasis
- Capillary hemangioma
- Venous angioma
- Varix of the vein of Galen

22.2 Arteriovenous Malformation (AVM)

22.2.1 Epidemiology

Incidence
- 0.001% in adults

Age Incidence
- Median age at diagnosis: 34 years

Sex Incidence
- Male:Female ratio: 1:1

Localization
- Brain
- Spinal cord

22.2.2 Neuroimaging Findings

General Imaging Findings
- Conglomerate of vessels (arterial feeders, nidus, and dilated veins) without mass effect

CT Non-Contrast-Enhanced (Fig. 22.1a)
- Iso- to hyperdense vessels.
- Calcifications are possible.

CT Contrast-Enhanced
- Enhancement of enlarged arterial feeders, nidus, and draining veins

MRI-T2 (Fig. 22.1b, c)
- Conglomerate of hypointense flow voids due to dilated vessels

MRI-FLAIR (Fig. 22.1d)
- Flow voids

MRI-T1 (Fig. 22.1e)
- Variable signal of vessels

MRI-T1 contrast-enhanced (Fig. 22.1f)
- Strong enhancement of the AVM vessels

MR-Diffusion Imaging (Fig. 22.1h)
- Normal

MRI-T2∗/SWI (Fig. 22.1g)
- Hypointense signal in case of bleeding

Angiography (Fig. 22.1i–k)
- Gold standard for the detection and strategy of therapy

Nuclear Medicine Imaging Findings
- No indication for examination

22.2.3 Neuropathology Findings

Macroscopic Features (Fig. 22.2a–d)
- Areas of hemorrhages
- Broad base near surface
- Aggregates of blood vessels of varying sizes

Microscopic Features (Fig. 22.3a–n)
- Mass of vascular channels of variable mural thickness and diameter.
- Embedded within abnormal, gliotic, and occasionally malformed brain parenchyma.
- More veins than arteries.
- Internal elastic lamina can be duplicated in arteries.
- Old hemorrhage in brain parenchyma.
- Thrombosed and recanalized vascular channels.
- Hyalinized sometimes calcified arterial walls.

Ultrastructural Features
- Vessel wall architecture of arteries and veins

Immunohistochemical Staining Characteristics (Fig. 22.3i–l)
- CD31
- CD34
- Smooth muscle actin

Differential Diagnosis
- Cavernous hemangioma
- Normal but compacted vessels usually in the leptomeninges

Distinct differential diagnostic features of cerebral vascular malformations include (Frischer et al. 2008):

- **Cerebral cavernous malformations**
  - Mulberry-like assembly of thin-walled vascular sinusoids
  - Low flow dynamics
  - Single layer of endothelium, collagenous adventitia
  - No smooth muscle, no elastic fibers
  - No intervening brain parenchyma
  - Peripheral rim of hemosiderin deposits
  - Gliomatous reaction in surrounding parenchyma
  - Hyalinization, thrombosis, calcification, cholesterol crystals possible within lesion
- **Arteriovenous malformations**
  - Tangled, serpiginous mass of abnormally dilated vessels corresponding to arteries and veins
  - High flow dynamics
  - Arteries with muscular and elastic laminae
  - Veins "arterialized," thickened collagenous walls with increased cellularity due to proliferation of fibroblasts
  - Intervening gliomatous brain parenchyma within the interstices of the nidus
  - Hemosiderin pigmentation often present
  - Gliomatous reaction
  - Foci of calcification possible
- **Venous malformations**
  - Single dilated or conglomerates of varicose veins drained by a single large vein
  - Venous walls mostly normal or thickened by muscular hyperplasia and hyalinization
  - Normal intervening brain parenchyma
  - No hemosiderin pigmentation
  - No gliomatous reaction
  - Thrombosis possible
- **Capillary telangiectases**
  - Dilated capillaries of differing caliber
  - Occasionally petechial hemorrhage appearance

22.2 Arteriovenous Malformation (AVM)

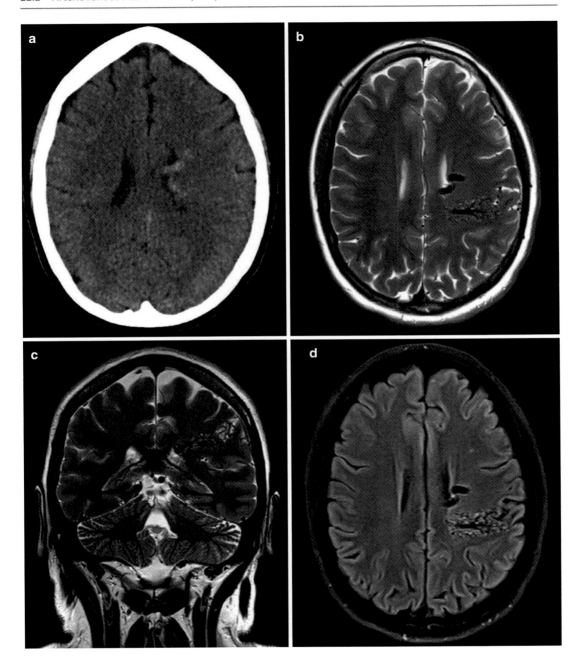

Fig. 22.1 Left hemispheric AVM: CT (**a**), T2 ax/cor (**b**, **c**), FLAIR (**d**), T1 (**e**), T1 contrast (**f**), SWI (**g**), DWI (**h**), MRA (**i**), DSA ap/sag (**j**, **k**)

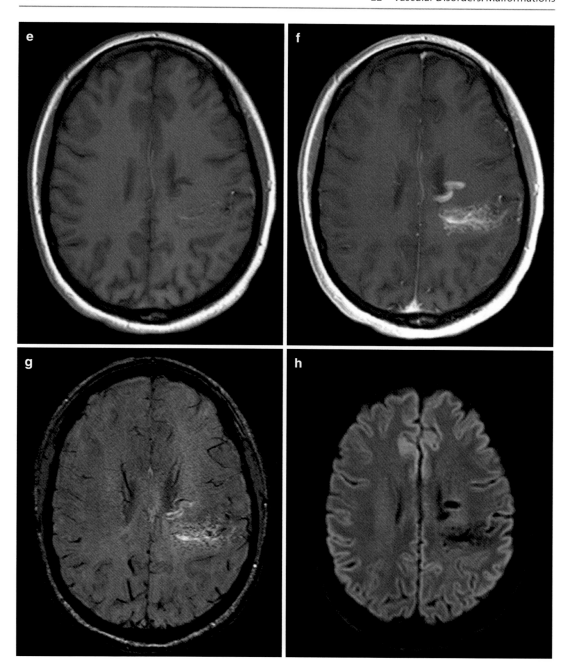

Fig. 22.1 (continued)

22.2 Arteriovenous Malformation (AVM)

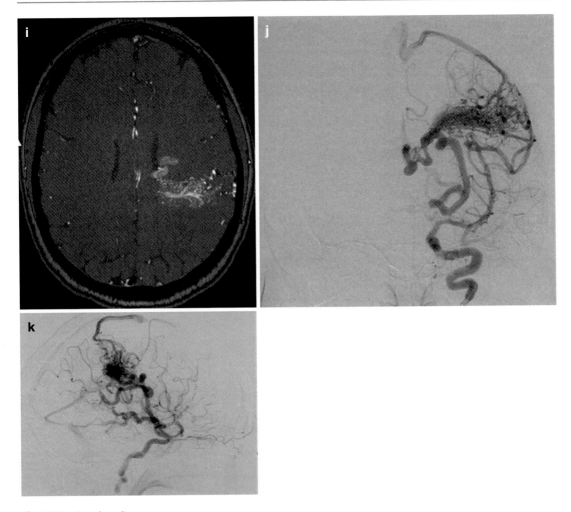

Fig. 22.1 (continued)

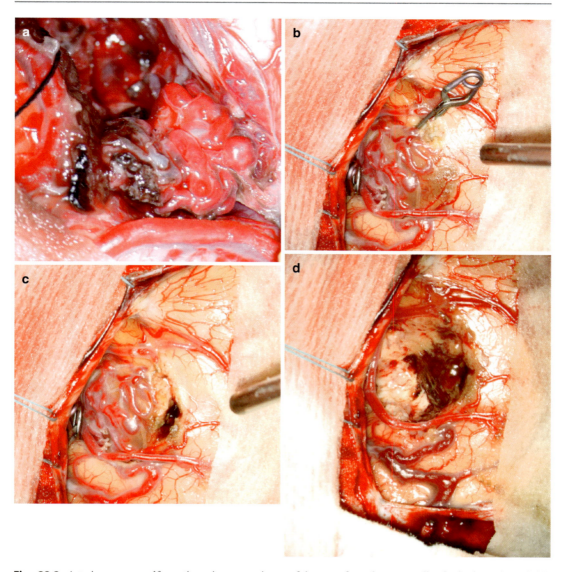

Fig. 22.2 Arteriovenous malformation: intraoperative appearance of AVM as a mass of tortuous vascular channels (**a**, **b**); clipping of major branches (**b**); mobilization of the mass from the surrounding brain tissue (arrow) (**c**); resection cavity (**d**)

22.2 Arteriovenous Malformation (AVM)

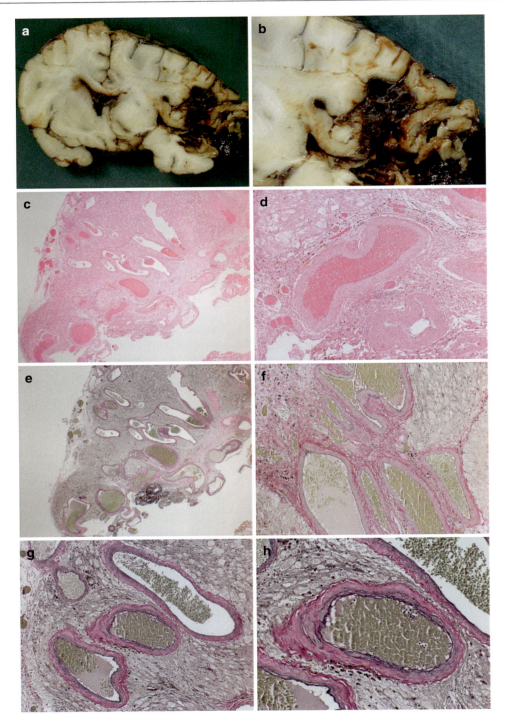

Fig. 22.3 Arteriovenous malformation: autopsy specimen showing in the centro-parietal region aggregates of blood vessels of varying sizes and tissue destruction due to hemorrhage (**a, b**). The AVM consists histologically of a mass of vascular channels of variable mural thickness and diameter embedded within abnormal, gliotic brain parenchyma (**c–h**; **e–h**: EvG stain). The walls of vessels stain positive for actin (**i, j**); endothelial cells are positive for CD4 (**k, l**). Vascular walls can be hyalinized (**m, n**). Thrombosed vascular channels and old hemorrhage in brain parenchyma are evident (**m, n**)

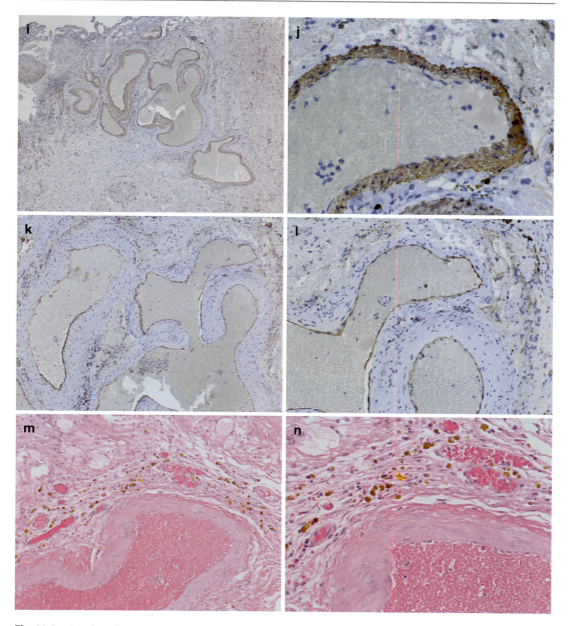

Fig. 22.3 (continued)

- Walls consist of basement membrane and endothelium
- No smooth muscle, no elastic fibers
- Normal intervening brain parenchyma
- No hemosiderin pigmentation
- Rarely gliomatous reaction

22.2.4 Molecular Neuropathology

Pathogenesis
- Congenital origin
- Reduced expression of integrin αvß8
  - Rarely associated with hereditary hemorrhagic telangiectasia (Rendu-Osler-Weber syndrome)

22.2.5 Treatment and Prognosis

Treatment (Table 22.1)
- Embolization
- Resection
- Radiosurgery

Biologic Behavior–Prognosis–Prognostic Factors
- Risk of hemorrhage: 2–4% per year
- Hemorrhage might lead to death in 5–10%

22.3 Cavernous Hemangioma (Cavernoma)

22.3.1 Epidemiology

Incidence
- Rare
- prevalence: 0.1–0.5%

Age Incidence
- birth
- elderly

Sex Incidence
- Male:Female ratio: 1:1

Localization
- Any brain location (Frischer et al. 2008)
  - Frontal 24.1%
  - Parietal 13.8%
  - Temporal 23.0%
  - Occipital 10.3%
  - Basal ganglia/Thalamus 1.1%
  - Corpus callosum 1.1%
  - Brain stem 17.2%
  - Cerebellum 9.2%
- Pons
- Subcortical white matter

22.3.2 Neuroimaging Findings

General Imaging Findings
Popcorn-like mass, developmental venous anomaly (DVA) can be associated.

CT Non-Contrast-Enhanced (Figs. 22.4j and 22.5a, b)
- Normal in most of the cases.
- Or hyperdense mass.
- Calcifications are possible.

CT Contrast-Enhanced
- No or slight enhancement
- May reveal DVA

MRI-T2 (Figs. 22.4a–c and 22.5c, k–m)
- Mixed signal
- Typically hypointense rim of hemosiderin

MRI-FLAIR (Figs. 22.4d and 22.5d)
- Mixed signal

Table 22.1 Treatment approaches for cerebral arteriovenous malformations (Asif et al. 2013) reproduced with kind permission by Thieme Verlag

	Approach	Benefits	Limitations
Endovascular embolization	Catheter delivery of • Liquid embolics (n-butylcyanoacrylate glue, onyx) • Coils	• Minimally invasive • Real-time angiography	• Obliteration rate can be lower depending on characteristics • Risk of ischemic complications during treatment
Surgical resection	• Microsurgical excision	• High rates of complete obliteration	• Invasive due to craniotomy
Radiotherapy	• Focal radiation is administered to the lesion	• Noninvasive	• 1–3 year latency for obliteration • Parenchymal radiation injury • Limited to smaller lesions

MRI-T1 (Figs. 22.4e and 22.5e)
- Mixed signal depending on blood products

MRI-T1 contrast-enhanced (Figs. 22.4f, g and 22.5f)
- No enhancement

MRI-T2∗/SWI (Figs. 22.4h and 22.5g, h)
- Method of choice in detection of cavernomas
- Hypointense "blooming" lesions due to susceptibility effect of hemosiderin

MR-Diffusion Imaging
- No restricted diffusion

DSA
- Angiographically occult

The differentiation of four types of cavernomas based on MRI features is shown in Table 22.2.

Nuclear Medicine Imaging Findings
- No indication for examination

22.3.3 Neuropathology Findings

Macroscopic Features (Figs. 22.6a–h and 22.7a)
- Tightly compacted dilated vessels
- Reddish-brownish discoloration due to acute and subacute blood products, hemosiderin

Microscopic Features (Fig. 22.7b–j)
- Closely packed and juxtaposed (dos-à-dos position) blood vessels
- Varying wall thickness
- Little or no intervening CNS parenchyma between blood vessels
- Deposits of hemosiderin
- Variable hyalinization of vessel walls
- Calcification
- Gliosis

Immunophenotype (Fig. 22.7k–n)
- CD31
- CD34

Differential Diagnosis
- AVM
- Capillary telangiectasia
- See Table in Sect. 22.1

22.3.4 Molecular Neuropathology

Neuropathogenesis
- Familial forms with autosomal-dominant inheritance
- Three known genes
    - CCT1 (*KRIT1*)
    - CCT2 (malcavernin, *MG4707*)
    - CCT3 (programmed cell death 10, *PCD10*)
- 2-hit hypothesis (familial forms)
    - Germline mutation in first gene
    - Somatic mutation in second gene within endothelial cells

22.3.5 Treatment and Prognosis

Treatment
- Surgical removal
- Beware of the developmental venous anomaly (DVA)

Biologic Behavior–Prognosis–Prognostic Factors
- May cause hemorrhages
- May present with seizures

22.3 Cavernous Hemangioma (Cavernoma)

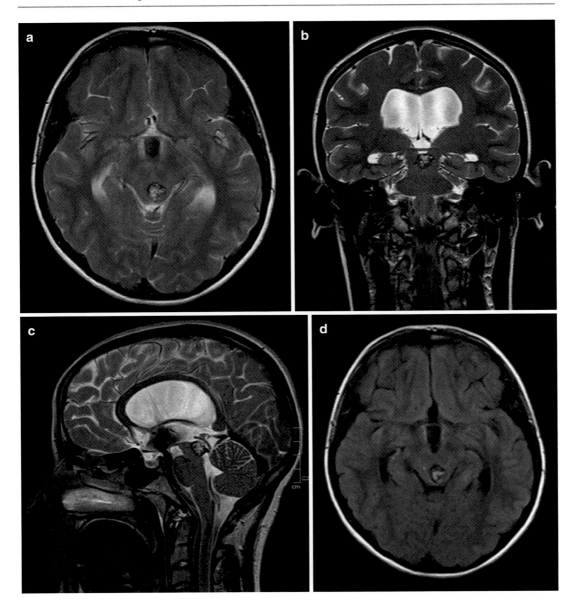

Fig. 22.4 Exophytic brain stem cavernoma T2 ax/cor/sag (**a–c**), FLAIR (**d**), T1 (**e**), T1 contrast (**f**), T1 contrast cor with associated developmental venous anomaly (**g**), SWI (**h**), DWI (**i**). Acute ventral bleeding of the cavernoma in CT sag (**j**), T2 ax and sag (**k–m**)

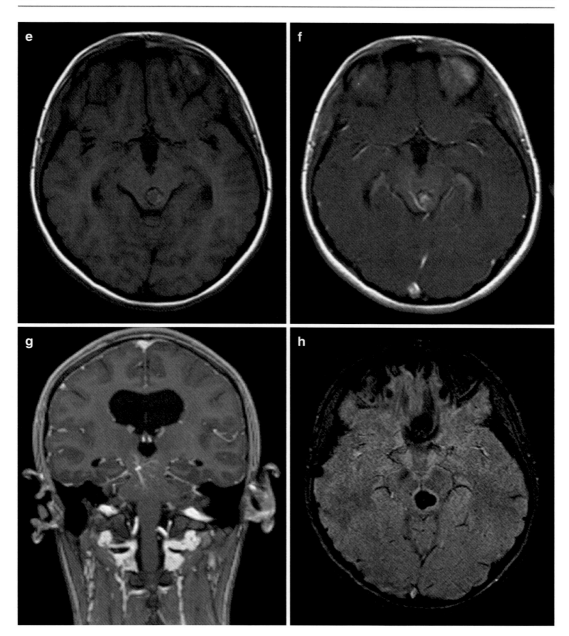

Fig. 22.4 (continued)

22.3 Cavernous Hemangioma (Cavernoma)

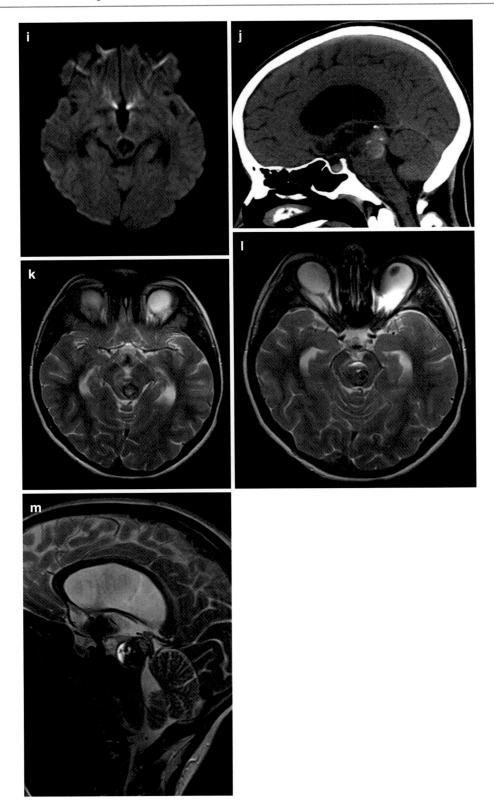

Fig. 22.4 (continued)

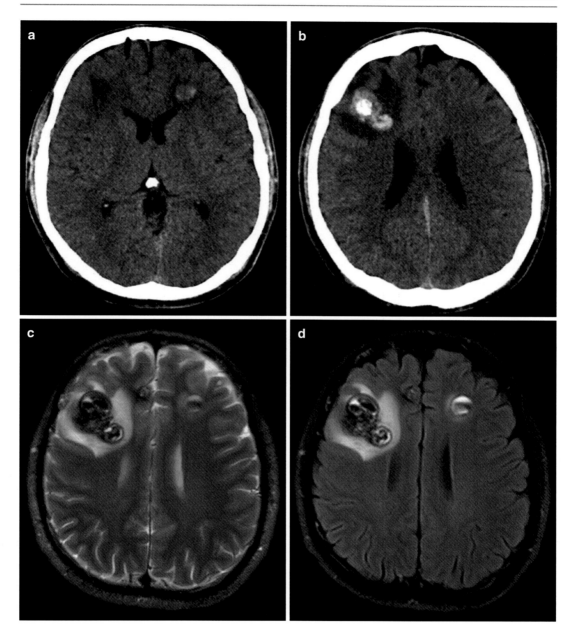

Fig. 22.5 Multiple cavernoma hemorrhages on CT ax (**a**, **b**), T2 (**c**), FLAIR (**d**), T1 (**e**), T1 contrast (**f**), T2∗ (**g**), SWI (**h**)

22.3 Cavernous Hemangioma (Cavernoma)

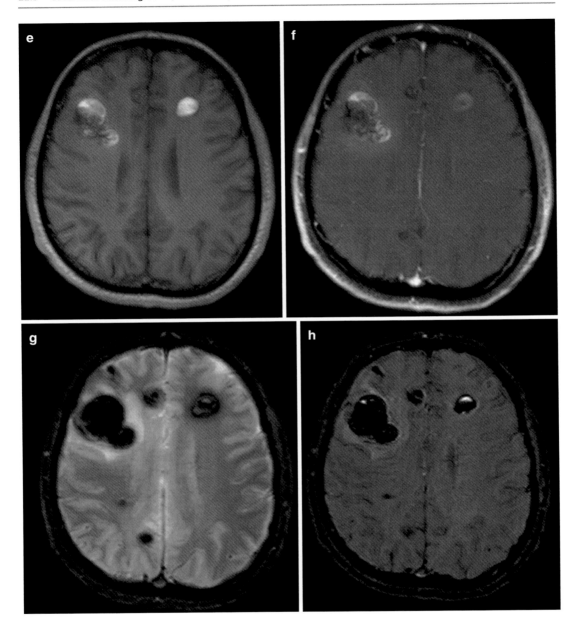

Fig. 22.5 (continued)

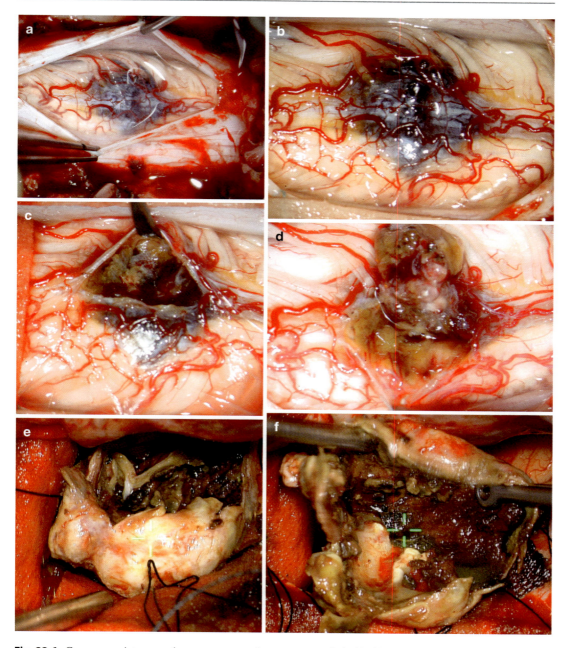

Fig. 22.6 Cavernoma: intraoperative appearances of cavernoma as dark, blackish masses (**a–g**). Resection site after removal of cavernoma (**h**)

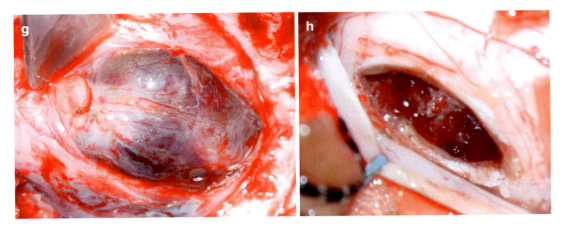

Fig. 22.6 (continued)

Table 22.2 Four types of cavernomas can be differentiated based on MRI features

Type	MRI signal characteristics
IA	• T1: hyperintense focus of hemorrhage • T2: hyper- or hypointense focus of hemorrhage extending through at least one wall of the hypointense rim that surrounds the lesion. Focal edema present
IB	• T1: hyperintense focus of hemorrhage • T2: hyper- or hypointense focus of hemorrhage surrounded by a hyperintense rim
II	• T1: reticulated mixed signal • T2: reticulated mixed signal core surrounded by a hyperintense rim
III	• T1: iso- or hypointense • T2: hypointense with a hypointense rim that magnifies size of the lesion
IV	• T1: poorly seen or not visualized at all • T2: poorly visualized at all • Gradient-echo sequences: punctate hypointense lesions

22.4 Capillary Telangiectasia

22.4.1 Epidemiology

Incidence
- Usually accidental finding (mainly at autopsy)
- 15–20% of all vascular malformations

Age Incidence
- any age

Sex Incidence
- Male:Female ratio: 1:1

Localization
- Pons
- Spinal cord
- Cerebral white matter
- Brain stem

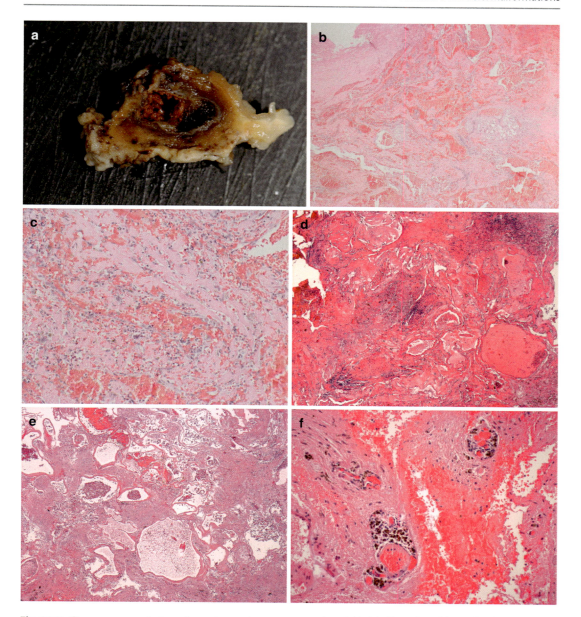

Fig. 22.7 Cavernoma: surgical specimen shows a brownish lesion (**a**). Histologically, cavernoma consists of closely packed and juxtaposed (dos-à-dos position) blood vessels of varying wall thickness and variable hyalinization of vessel walls (**b–i**; **g–i**: EvG stain). Little or no intervening CNS parenchyma between blood vessels is seen (asterisk) (**e**). Deposits of hemosiderin are evident (**f**). Cavernoma of the orbita might have large amounts of connective tissue between the vascular channels (**j**). The endothelial lining of the vascular channels are immunopositive for CD 34 (**k, l**) and CD31 (**m, n**)

22.3 Cavernous Hemangioma (Cavernoma)

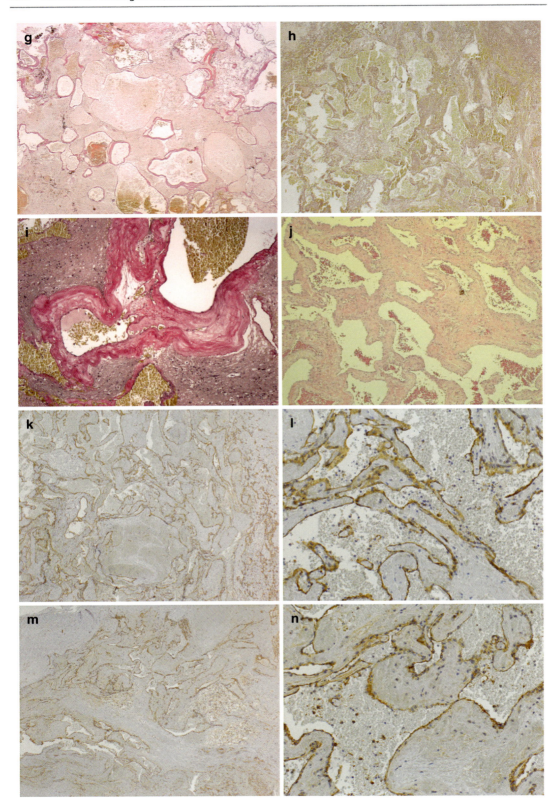

Fig. 22.7 (continued)

22.4.2 Neuroimaging Findings

General Imaging Findings
- Small hypointense lesion in hemosensitive sequences with slight enhancement
- In most of the cases located at the brain stem

CT Non-Contrast-Enhanced
- Normal

CT Contrast-Enhanced
- Normal

MRI-T2 (Fig. 22.8a)
- Normal or moderate hyperintense

MRI-FLAIR (Fig. 22.8b)
- Normal

MRI-T1 (Fig. 22.8c)
- Normal or hypointense

MRI-T1 contrast-enhanced (Fig. 22.8d)
- Low enhancement

MRI-T2*/SWI (Fig. 22.8e)
- Slightly hypointense

MR-Diffusion Imaging (Fig. 22.8f)
- Hypointense or normal

DSA
- Angiographically occult

Nuclear Medicine Imaging Findings
- No indication for examination

22.4.3 Neuropathology Findings

Macroscopic Features (Fig. 22.9a, b)
- small hyperemic lesion
- prominent, accumulation of congested vessels
- usually no surrounding acute hemorrhage
- seldom, small, fairly well-defined hemorrhagic lesions indicative of localized bleeding

Microscopic Features (Fig. 22.9c–f)
- Multiple, thin-walled, dilated capillaries without alterations of the surrounding brain substance
- No vessel wall hyalinization
- No vessel wall calcification
- No thrombosis

Immunophenotype (Fig. 22.9g, h)
- CD31
- CD34

Ultrastructural Features
- Thin-walled capillaries

Differential Diagnosis
- AVM
- Cavernoma
- Venous angioma
- Focal petechial hemorrhage
- See Table in Sect. 22.1

22.4.4 Molecular Neuropathology

Pathogenesis
- Sporadic anomaly
- No genetic association
- Rarely found in hereditary hemorrhagic telangiectasia (Rendu-Osler-Weber syndrome)

22.4.5 Treatment and Prognosis

Treatment
- accidental finding at autopsy

Biologic Behavior–Prognosis–Prognostic Factors
- No risk of hemorrhage

22.4 Capillary Telangiectasia

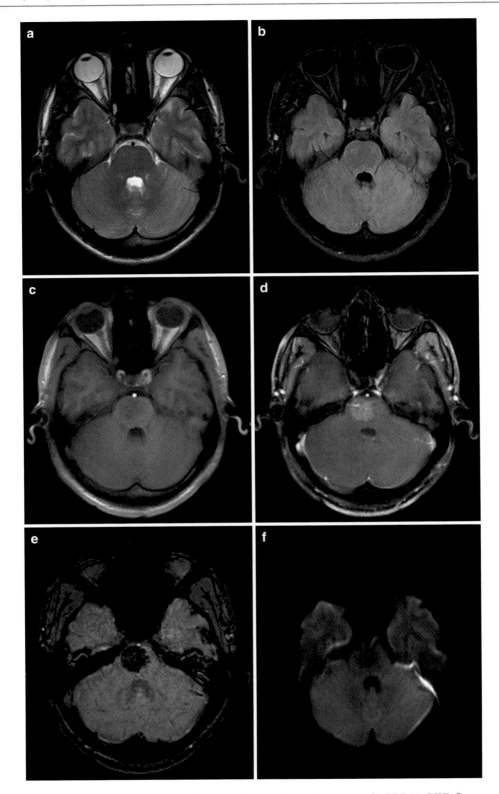

Fig. 22.8 Pontine capillary teleangiectasia: T2 (**a**), FLAIR (**b**), T1 (**c**), T1 contrast (**d**), SWI (**e**), DWI (**f**)

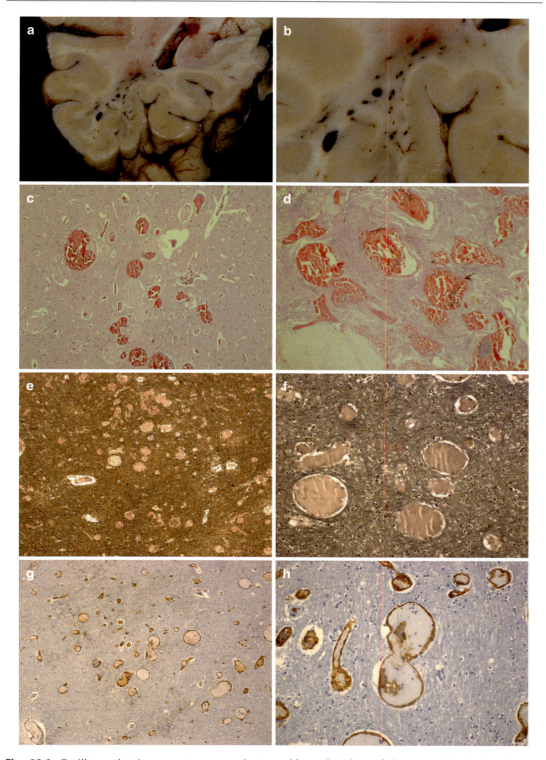

Fig. 22.9 Capillary telangiectasy: autopsy specimen shows prominent, accumulation of congested, ecstatic vessels in the white matter of the temporal lobe (**a**, **b**). Histology reveals multiple, thin-walled, dilated capillaries without alterations of the surrounding brain substance (**c–f**; **e**, **f**: EvG stain). The endothelial lining is CD34-positive (**g**, **h**)

22.5 Dural AV-Fistula

22.5.1 Neuroimaging Findings

General Imaging Findings
- Multiple tiny arteriovenous shunts in wall of sinus

CT Non-Contrast-Enhanced (Fig. 22.10a, b)
- Usually normal in case of no bleeding

CT Contrast-Enhanced
- May detect dural feeders, thrombosed sinus, and dilated cortical or superior ophthalmic veins

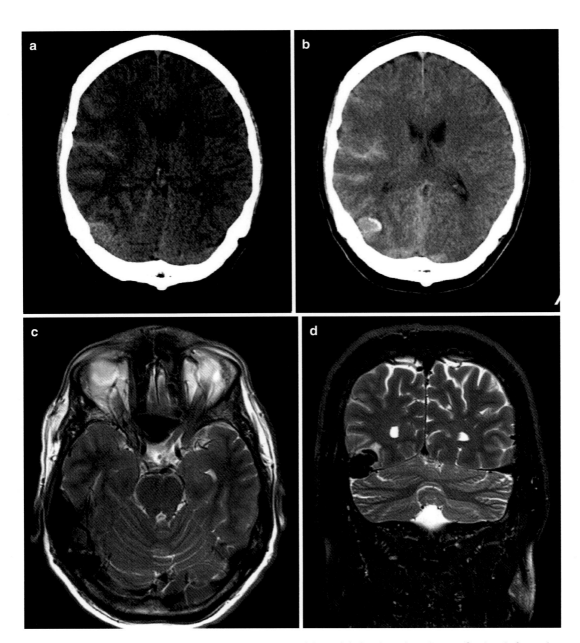

Fig. 22.10 Right occipital d-AV Fistula: CT (**a**, **b**), T2 ax/cor (**c**, **d**), FLAIR (**e**), T1 (**f**), T1 contrast (**g**), SWI (**h**), DWI (**i**), MRA (**j**, **k**), DSA ap/sag showing feeders from right occipital and meningeal artery (**l**, **m**) and after embolization with onyx (**n**, **o**)

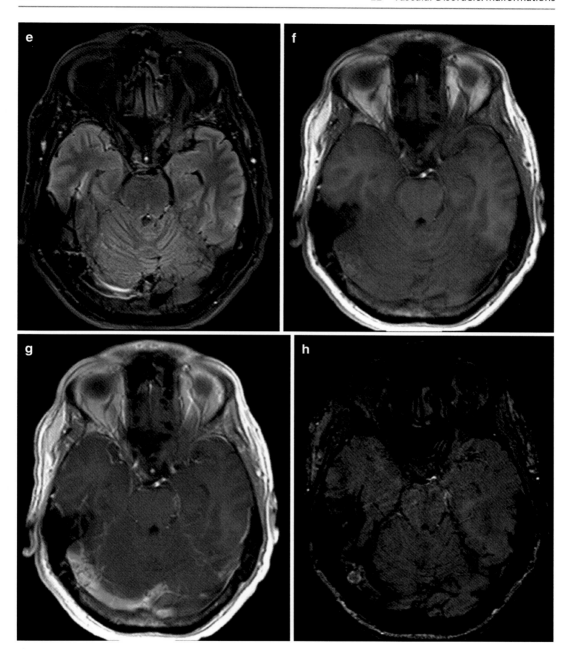

Fig. 22.10 (continued)

22.4 Capillary Telangiectasia

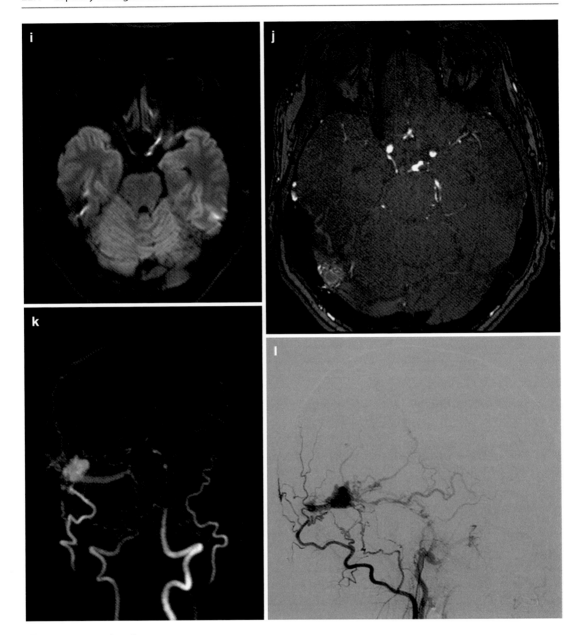

Fig. 22.10 (continued)

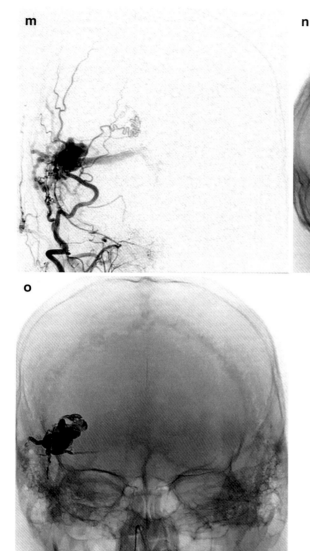

Fig. 22.10 (continued)

MRI-T2/FLAIR (Fig. 22.10c–e)

- Normal
- Or hyperintense parenchymal edema due to venous congestion

MRI-T1 (Fig. 22.10f)

- Normal

MRI-T1 contrast-enhanced (Fig. 22.10g)

- No enhancement

MR-T2*/SWI (Fig. 22.10h)

- Normal
- Or hypointense bleeding in case of venous infarction

MR-Diffusion Imaging (Fig. 22.10i)

- Usually normal

Angiography (Fig. 22.10j–p)

- Gold standard for detection of feeders and cortical drainage

Selected References

Asif K, Leschke J, Lazzaro MA (2013) Cerebral arteriovenous malformation diagnosis and management. Semin Neurol 33(5):468–475. https://doi.org/10.1055/s-0033-1364212

Chen W, Choi EJ, McDougall CM, Su H (2014) Brain arteriovenous malformation modeling, pathogenesis, and novel therapeutic targets. Transl Stroke Res 5(3):316–329. https://doi.org/10.1007/s12975-014-0343-0

Cossu M, Raneri F, Casaceli G, Gozzo F, Pelliccia V, Lo Russo G (2015) Surgical treatment of cavernoma-related epilepsy. J Neurosurg Sci 59(3):237–253

Dammann P, Schaller C, Sure U (2017) Should we resect peri-lesional hemosiderin deposits when performing lesionectomy in patients with cavernoma-related epilepsy (CRE)? Neurosurg Rev 40(1):39–43. https://doi.org/10.1007/s10143-016-0797-5

Dao I, Akhaddar A, El-Mostarchid B, Boucetta M (2012) Giant cerebral cavernoma. Case report with literature review. Neurosciences (Riyadh) 17(1):69–73

Essig M (2007) [Multimodal magnetic resonance diagnostics of arteriovenous malformations]. Radiologe 47 (10):884–892. https://doi.org/10.1007/s00117-007-1568-7

Frischer JM, Pipp I, Stavrou I, Trattnig S, Hainfellner JA, Knosp E (2008) Cerebral cavernous malformations: congruency of histopathological features with the current clinical definition. J Neurol Neurosurg Psychiatry 79(7):783–788. https://doi.org/10.1136/jnnp.2007.132316

Gross BA, Puri AS, Popp AJ, Du R (2013) Cerebral capillary telangiectasias: a meta-analysis and review of the literature. Neurosurg Rev 36(2):187–193. ; discussion 194. https://doi.org/10.1007/s10143-012-0435-9

Lee RR, Becher MW, Benson ML, Rigamonti D (1997) Brain capillary telangiectasia: MR imaging appearance and clinicohistopathologic findings. Radiology 205(3):797–805. https://doi.org/10.1148/radiology.205.3.9393538

Maruyama K, Koga T, Niranjan A, Kondziolka D, Flickinger JC, Lunsford LD (2013) Radiosurgery for brainstem arteriovenous malformation. Prog Neurol Surg 27:67–72. https://doi.org/10.1159/000341639

Mohr JP, Yaghi S (2015) Management of unbled brain arteriovenous malformation study. Neurol Clin 33(2):347–359. https://doi.org/10.1016/j.ncl.2014.12.006

Sackey FNA, Pinsker NR, Baako BN (2017) Highlights on cerebral arteriovenous malformation treatment using combined embolization and stereotactic radiosurgery: why outcomes are controversial? Cureus 9(5):e1266. https://doi.org/10.7759/cureus.1266

Serulle Y, Miller TR, Gandhi D (2016) Dural arteriovenous fistulae: imaging and management. Neuroimaging Clin N Am 26(2):247–258. https://doi.org/10.1016/j.nic.2015.12.003

Stevens J, Leach JL, Abruzzo T, Jones BV (2009) De novo cerebral arteriovenous malformation: case report and literature review. AJNR Am J Neuroradiol 30(1):111–112. https://doi.org/10.3174/ajnr.A1255

Strozyk D, Nogueira RG, Lavine SD (2009) Endovascular treatment of intracranial arteriovenous malformation. Neurosurg Clin N Am 20(4):399–418. https://doi.org/10.1016/j.nec.2009.07.004

Tranvinh E, Heit JJ, Hacein-Bey L, Provenzale J, Wintermark M (2017) Contemporary imaging of cerebral arteriovenous malformations. AJR Am J Roentgenol 208(6):1320–1330. https://doi.org/10.2214/ajr.16.17306

Vilanova JC, Barcelo J, Smirniotopoulos JG, Perez-Andres R, Villalon M, Miro J, Martin F, Capellades J, Ros PR (2004) Hemangioma from head to toe: MR imaging with pathologic correlation. Radiographics 24(2):367–385. https://doi.org/10.1148/rg.242035079

Wilms G, Bleus E, Demaerel P, Marchal G, Plets C, Goffin J, Baert AL (1994) Simultaneous occurrence of developmental venous anomalies and cavernous angiomas. AJNR Am J Neuroradiol 15(7):1247–1254; discussion 1255–1247

Xu M, Xu H, Qin Z (2015) Animal models in studying cerebral arteriovenous malformation. Biomed Res Int 2015:178407. https://doi.org/10.1155/2015/178407

Vascular Disorders: Angiopathies

23.1 Introduction

Other angiopathies include:

- Sporadic.
  - Hypertensive angiopathy.
  - Amyloid (congophilic) angiopathy.
  - Fibromuscular dysplasia.
  - Moyamoya angiopathy.
  - Binswanger disease.
  - Fahr disease.
  - Marfan syndrome.
  - Sneddon syndrome.
  - Kohlmeier Degos syndrome.
  - Cerebroretinal vasculopathy.
- Familial.
  - Familial CAA.
  - CADASIL Cerebral autosomal dominant arteriopathy with subcortical infarcts and leukoencephalopathy.
  - CARASIL Cerebral recessive dominant arteriopathy with subcortical infarcts and leukoencephalopathy.
  - CARASAL Cathepsin A-related arteriopathy with strokes and leukoencephalopathy.
  - Hereditary vascular retinopathy.
  - HERNS Hereditary endotheliopathy with retinopathy, nephropathy, and stroke.
  - COL4A1 mutations (combined small vessel and large arterial disease).

23.2 Cerebral Amyloid Angiopathy

Cerebral amyloid angiopathy (CAA) is a heterogeneous disease clinically characterized by ischemic or hemorrhagic changes. Amyloid deposits in the wall of leptomeningeal and cortical vessels is the histopathological hallmark.

23.2.1 Clinical Signs and Symptoms

The following three clinical groups of sporadic CAA may be identified:
- Recurrent, multiple hemorrhages affecting the telencephalic lobes with acute focal neurological signs or sudden coma or death
- Transient focal neurologic signs leading to the diagnosis of transient ischemic attack or focal epilepsy

Dementia with acute beginning or progression

Criteria for diagnosis of CAA-related hemorrhage

- Definite CAA
  - Full postmortem examination demonstrating:
    - Lobar, cortical, or cortico-subcortical hemorrhage
    - Severe CAA with vasculopathy
    - Absence of other diagnostic lesions

- Probable CAA with supporting pathology
  - Clinical data and pathologic tissue (evacuated hematoma or cortical biopsy) demonstrating:
    ○ Lobar, cortical, or cortico-subcortical hemorrhage
    ○ Some degree of CAA in the specimen
    ○ Absence of other diagnostic lesions
- Probable CAA
  - Clinical data and MRI or CT demonstrating:
    ○ Multiple hemorrhages restricted to lobar, cortical, or cortico-subcortical regions (cerebellar hemorrhage allowed)
    ○ [or Single lobar, cortical, or cortical-subcortical hemorrhage, and focal or
    ○ Disseminated II superficial siderosis]
    ○ Age ≥55 years
    ○ Absence of other causes of hemorrhage [or superficial siderosis]
- Possible CAA
  - Clinical data and MRI or CT demonstrating:
    ○ Single lobar, cortical, or cortico-subcortical hemorrhage [or focal or disseminated superficial siderosis]
    ○ Age ≥55 years
    ○ Absence of other causes of hemorrhage [or superficial siderosis]

23.2.2 Epidemiology

Incidence
- Common in the elderly

Age Incidence
- Elderly patients
- 65–74 year olds: 2.3%
- 75–84 year olds: 8.0%
- Over 85 years: 12.1%

Sex Incidence
- Male:Female ratio 1:1

Localization
- Leptomeningeal, cerebellar, and neocortical arteries.
- Veins and/or capillaries.
- Cerebral lobes (lobar hemorrhages).
- White matter and deep gray matter are usually spared.

23.2.3 Neuroimaging Findings

General Imaging Findings (Table 23.1)
- Micro- and macrobleedings, cortical siderosis, leukoencephalopathy

CT Non-Contrast-Enhanced (Fig. 23.1a)
- Lobar hematomas (irregular borders are described) with subarachnoidal extension or focal subarachnoidal hemorrhages
- Hypodense leukoencephalopathy

CT Contrast-Enhanced
- No enhancement

MRI-T2/FLAIR (Fig. 23.1b, c)
- Hemorrhages, signal depends on age
- Hyperintense leukoencephalopathy

MRI-T1 (Fig. 23.1d)
- Hemorrhage

MRI-T1 Contrast-Enhanced
- No enhancement

MRI-T2*/SWI (Fig. 23.1f)
- Hemorrhage
- Most sensitive for microbleeds, seen as multiple black dots
- Superficial siderosis with curvilinear cortical hemosiderin depositions

Nuclear Medicine Imaging Findings (Fig. 23.2a, b)
- Today the impact of amyloid PET in CAA is being discussed.

- FDG-PET and CBF studies can be used to assess the extent of the damage caused by bleedings.

23.2.4 Neuropathology Findings

Macroscopic Features (Fig. 23.3a–d)
- Associated with intracerebral hemorrhage

Microscopic Features (Fig. 23.4a–l)
- Amyloid deposition in the media and/or adventitia of leptomeningeal and cortical small arteries, arterioles, and venules
- Acellular amorphous eosinophilic substance in the vessel wall
- Double-barrel appearance
- Amyloid stains:
  - Congo red: apple-green birefringence under polarized light
  - Thioflavin T: bright-green fluorescence under ultraviolet light
- Thal classification of CAA (Thal et al. 2002):
  - Thal Type 1: dysphoric angiopathy: amyloid leaks from the capillary wall into the brain parenchyma
  - Thal Type 2: amyloid deposition in the media and/or adventitia of leptomeningeal and cortical small arteries, arterioles, and venules
- Stages of CAA (Thal et al. 2003)
  - Stage 1: leptomeningeal and neocortical vessels
  - Stage 2: allocortical regions (hippocampus, entorhinal and cingulate cortex, amygdala), the hypothalamus, the cerebellum, and midbrain vessels
  - Stage 3: the basal ganglia, thalamus, lower brain stem, and white matter (Thal et al. 2003).
- Miscellaneous changes of vessels include:
  - Fibrosis
  - Microaneurysm formation
  - Chronic granulomatous inflammation
  - Fibrinoid necrosis
  - Thrombosis
  - Calcification
  - Splitting of the internal elastic lamina elastica interna
  - Hyaline non-amyloidogenic arteriolar degeneration

Immunophenotype (Fig. 23.5a–h)
- β-amyloid

Ultrastructural Features
- vascular amyloid is composed of
  - Fibrils identical to those in systemic amyloid disease.
  - Mixed with a large amount of vesicular debris.
  - Amyloid appears to be derived from circulating protein and is deposited in areas of vascular basement membrane degeneration.
- initiating degenerative change
  - thickening of basement membrane with accumulation of debris

Differential Diagnosis
- Hypertensive hemorrhage
- Other amyloid angiopathies

Neuropathological, clinical, and neuroimaging characteristics between CAA and "hypertensive arteriopathy" are given in Table 23.1.

23.2.5 Molecular Neuropathology

- deposition of Aβ-protein which is 42 amino acids long and cleaved from the amyloid precursor protein (see Table 23.2)
- damage of the medial smooth muscle cell
  - disrupting the vascular architecture
  - weakening the arterial wall

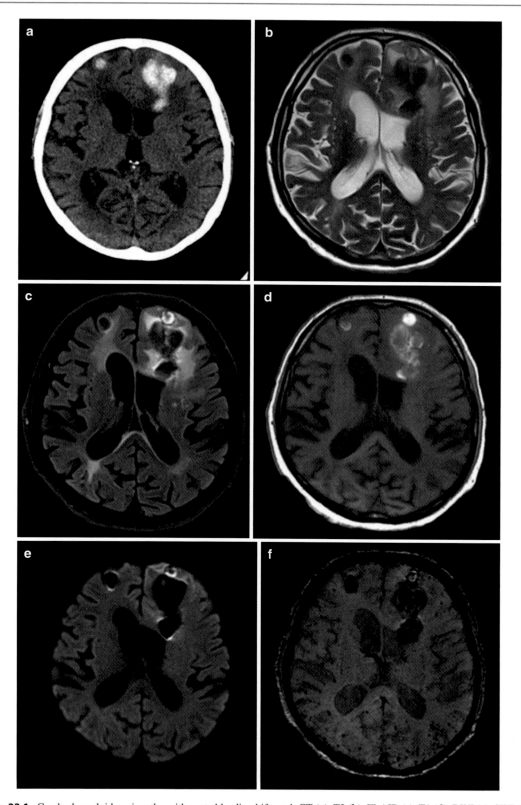

Fig. 23.1 Cerebral amyloid angiopathy with acute bleeding bifrontal: CT (**a**), T2 (**b**), FLAIR (**c**), T1 (**d**), DWI (**e**), SWI (**f**)

- dose-dependent association between APOE ε4 and sporadic CAA
- no significant association between APOE ε2 and CAA
- various types of deposited amyloid (Table 23.2)
- non-APOE polymorphism
  - TGFβ1 (transforming growth factor β1): positive association between T allele and CAA
  - TOMM40 (translocase of outer mitochondrial membrane 40): SNPs associated with vascular amyloid burden
  - CR1 (complement component receptor 1): associated with severity of CAA pathology
- no significant associations of non-APOE polymorphism

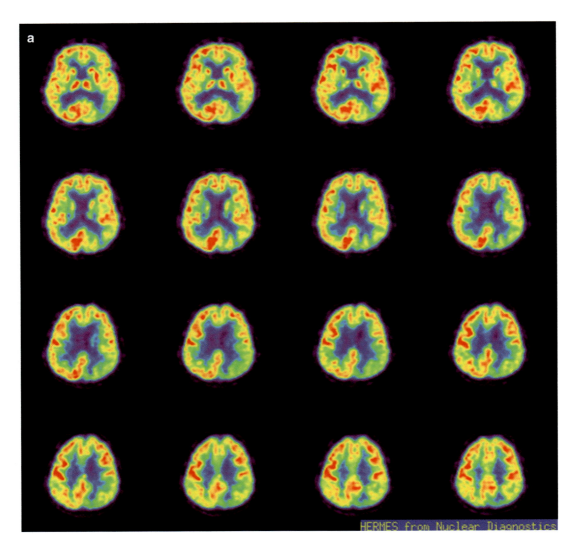

Fig. 23.2 FDG-PET shows hypometabolism in the left occipital lobe where the hemorrhage occurred (**a**). Increased amyloid load in the right occipital lobe (**b**) as visualized with the f-18 flutemetamol tracer

Fig. 23.2 (continued)

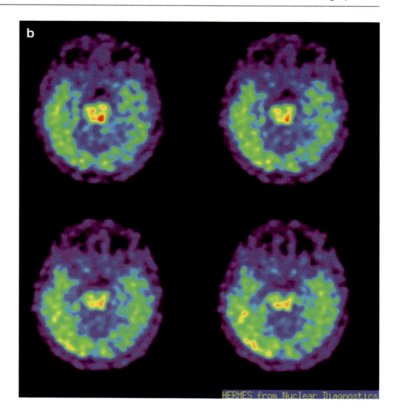

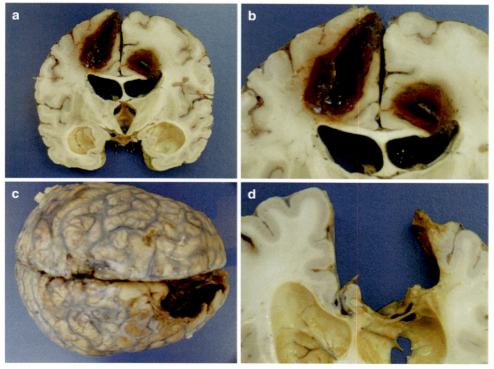

Fig. 23.3 Cerebral amyloid angiopathy (CAA): autopsy specimens showing lobar hemorrhage affecting the left frontal lobe and right cingulated gyrus (**a**, **b**). The blot clot affecting the right frontal lobe was operatively removed (**c**, **d**)

23.1 Cerebral Amyloid Angiopathy

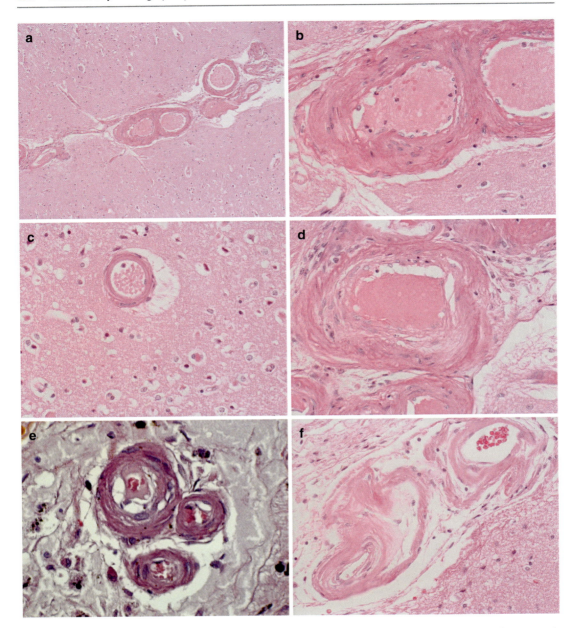

Fig. 23.4 Cerebral amyloid angiopathy (CAA): Microscopy reveals leptomeningeal vessels with thickened walls (**a–d**), deposition of acellular amorphous eosinophilic substance in the vessel wall (**e**: PAS stain). Some vessels have double-barrel appearance (**f**). Amyloid deposited in the vessel wall is visualized under polarized light (**g–l**)

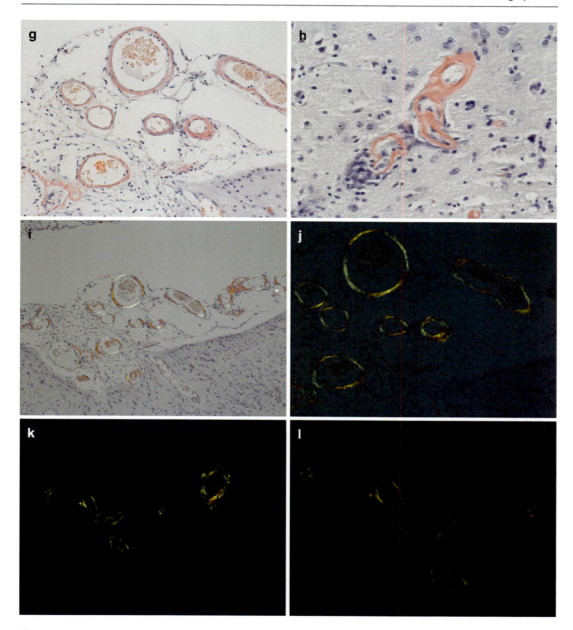

Fig. 23.4 (continued)

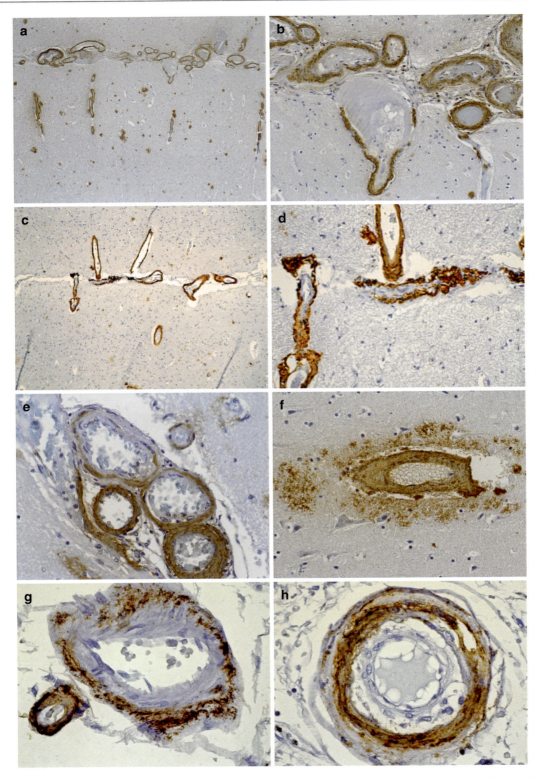

Fig. 23.5 Cerebral amyloid angiopathy (CAA): Immunohistochemical demonstration of amyloid deposition in the media and/or adventitia of leptomeningeal and cortical small arteries, arterioles, and venules (**a–h**)

Table 23.1 Key neuropathological, clinical, and neuroimaging characteristics of the two major sporadic cerebral small vessel diseases: CAA and "hypertensive arteriopathy" (Charidimou et al. 2017) reproduced with kind permission by Oxford University Press

Characteristics	CAA	Sporadic non-amyloid microangiopathy ("hypertensive arteriopathy")
Small vessel pathology	Amyloid-b deposition and associated vasculopathy in cortical and leptomeningeal vessels	A range of different features, e.g., arteriolosclerosis, fibrinoid necrosis, mural damage.
Risk factors	Age, APOE e4 and e2	Age, hypertension, diabetes, smoking
Associated clinical syndromes		
ICH	Lobar (cortical-subcortical), cerebellar?	Typically deep: basal ganglia, thalamus, pons cerebellum; sometimes lobar
Associated with high risk of recurrence (7–12% per year)		
Ischemic stroke	Not typically associated with lacunes	Lacunar syndromes
Uncertain role other than affecting treatment decisions, e.g., antithrombotic drugs, thrombolysis.		
Other clinical syndromes	Transient focal neurological episodes ("amyloid spells"), cognitive impairment and dementia, inflammatory CAA	Vascular cognitive impairment and dementia
MRI markers of small vessel disease		
Cerebral microbleed CMBs	Strictly lobar	Predominantly deep, with or without lobar
Cortical superficial siderosis (cSS)	Very common: 40% in symptomatic CAA	Rare: 55% of deep ICH
MRI-visible perivascular spaces	Centrum semiovale (i.e., cerebral white matter)	Basal ganglia
White matter hyperintensities	Posterior predominance, white matter spots	No predilection for brain region, peribasal ganglia
Lacunes	Not typically present, more superficial in the cerebral white matter	Common, usually in the basal ganglia or deep white matter
Diagnosis	Boston criteria, based on the presence of multiple strictly lobar cerebral microbleeds (CMBs) or macrobleeds and cortical superficial siderosis (cSS)	No established criteria available; diagnosed in patients not fulfilling Boston criteria for CAA, in the appropriate clinical context and based on MRI markers of small vessel damage
Therapeutic implications	Acute treatment according to the clinical syndrome at presentation. Main long-term goal is prevention of new lobar ICH (recurrent or incident), by blood pressure management and avoiding antithrombotics unless a completing indication exists. Cognitive rehabilitation in mild cognitive impairment/dementia.	Acute treatment according to the clinical syndrome at presentation. Control of vascular risk factors. Cognitive rehabilitation in vascular cognitive impairment/ dementia. Safety of antithrombotic use is of lesser concern compared to CAA patients.

Table 23.2 Amyloid angiopathies

Disease	Type of amyloid	Gene involved
Sporadic Aβ-CAA (associated with Alzheimer disease)	Aß	Amyloid precursor protein (APP)
Hereditary Aβ-CAA (Dutch and Flemish types, familial AD)	Aß	Amyloid precursor protein (APP) (codon 693 Dutch type, codons 692 and 694 Flemish type)
Hereditary cerebral hemorrhage with amyloid angiopathy—Icelandic type	ACys	Cystatin C/gamma trace
Familial amyloidosis-Finnish type	AGel	Gelsolin
Familial British dementia	ABri	BRI2/ABri
Familial Danish dementia	ADan	BRI2/ADan
Familial amyloidotic polyneuropathy/meningovascular amyloidosis	ATTR	Transthyretin
Prion protein CAA	APrP	Prion protein (PRNP)

- LRP1 (low density lipoprotein receptor 1)
- ACT (α1 antichymotrypsin)
- CYP46
- ACE (angiotensin 1 converting enzyme)
- others

23.2.6 Treatment and Prognosis

Treatment

- surgical removal of hemorrhage (tissue procurement for diagnosis)

Biologic Behavior–Prognosis–Prognostic Factors

- poor as recurrent hemorrhages are frequent

23.3 Binswanger Disease

Binswanger disease is a rare neurodegenerative disorder.

23.3.1 Clincal Signs and Symptoms

- Dementia must be established by clinical examination and confirmed by neuropsychological tests.
- One finding from two of the following three groups must be present:
  - the presence of a vascular risk factor or evidence of systemic vascular disease (e.g., hypertension, diabetes, a history of myocardial infarction, cardiac arrhythmia, or congestive heart failure)
  - evidence of focal cerebrovascular disease (e.g., a history of stroke, or demonstration of a focal pyramidal or sensory sign)
  - evidence of "subcortical" cerebral dysfunction (e.g., a Parkinsonian, magnetic, or "senile" gait, Parkinsonian or rigidity, or a history of incontinence secondary to a spastic bladder)
- The radiological criteria requires bilateral leuko-araiosis on computed tomography (CT), or bilateral and, multiple or diffuse, subcortical high signal T2-weighted lesions greater than 2×2 mm on magnetic resonance (MR) scan.
- The proposed criteria lose their validity in the presence of:
  - 1 multiple or bilateral cortical lesions on CT or MR; or
  - 2 severe dementia (e.g., MMS < 10)

23.3.2 Epidemiology

Incidence
- Unknown
- Rare
- Elderly

Age Incidence
- 50–70 years

Sex Incidence
- Male:Female ratio 1:1

Localization
- White matter

23.3.3 Neuroimaging Findings

General Imaging Findings
- Leukoencephalopathy, lacunar infarcts, and microbleeds

CT Non-Contrast-Enhanced (Fig. 23.6a)
- Hypodense leukoencephalopathy predominantly in deep white matter and centrum semiovale
- Hypodense lacunar lesions

CT Contrast-Enhanced
- No enhancement

MRI-T2/FLAIR (Fig. 23.6b, c)
- Confluent or focal subcortical and periventricular hyperintensities
- Hyperintense lacunar lesions in basal ganglia and thalamus

MRI-T1 (Fig. 23.6d)
- Hypointnese signal of leukoencephalopathic and lacunar lesions

MRI-T1 Contrast-Enhanced (Fig. 23.6e)
- Subacute ischemic lesions enhance

MRI-T2*/SWI (Fig. 23.6g)
- Multifocal microbleeds

MR-Diffusion Imaging (Fig. 23.6f)
- Restricted diffusion in acute infarcts

Nuclear Medicine Imaging Findings
- FDG-PET (and CBF-SPECT) demonstrates an inhomogeneous metabolizing (perfusion) pattern not only in all cortical regions but also in the basal ganglia.
- Rare reports state a statistical particular frontal reduced uptake.

23.3.4 Neuropathology Findings

Macroscopical Findings (Fig. 23.7a–f)
- Usually normal brain weight
- Significant changes of the white matter include
  - Reduced volume
  - Discoloration
  - Hardening
  - Foci with infarcts
- Enlargement of the lateral ventricular system as well as the third ventricle
- Presence of lacunar changes in the gray matter and pons

Microscopical Findings (Fig. 23.7g–n)
- Myelin pallor
  - bilateral not always symmetrical
  - degeneration of myelin sheats
- Region of necrotic tissue damage
- Axonal damage
  - Numerical reduction of axons and oligodendrocytes
- Variable degree of reactive astrogliosis
- Rare lipid-laden macrophages

23.2 Binswanger Disease

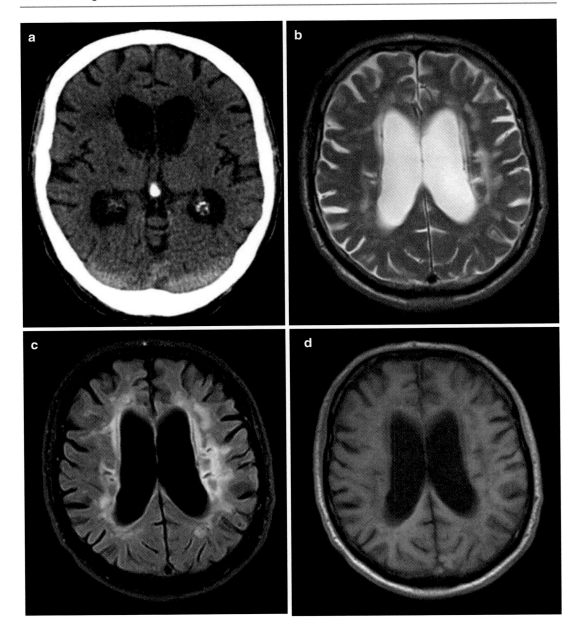

Fig. 23.6 Morbus Binswanger: CT (**a**), T2 (**b**), FLAIR (**b**), T1 (**d**), T1 contrast (**e**), DWI (**f**), SWI (**g**)

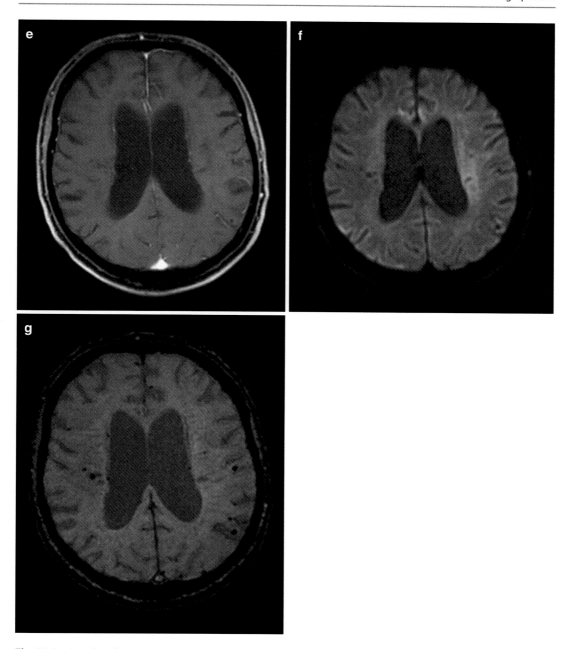

Fig. 23.6 (continued)

23.2 Binswanger Disease

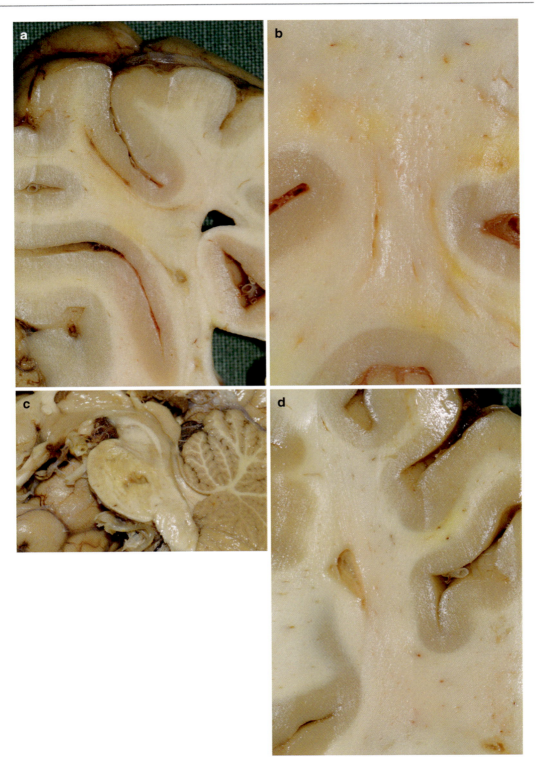

Fig. 23.7 Binswanger disease: autopsy specimen showing significant changes of the white matter consisting of ischemic lacunar changes (**a, b**) and necrotic foci (**c–e**), and petechial hemorrhages (**f**). Microscopically, myelin pallor is evident (**g–l**; **h, l**: LFB stain) whereby the white matter vessels show wall thickening (**j, l**). Area of necrotic tissue damage (**m, n**)

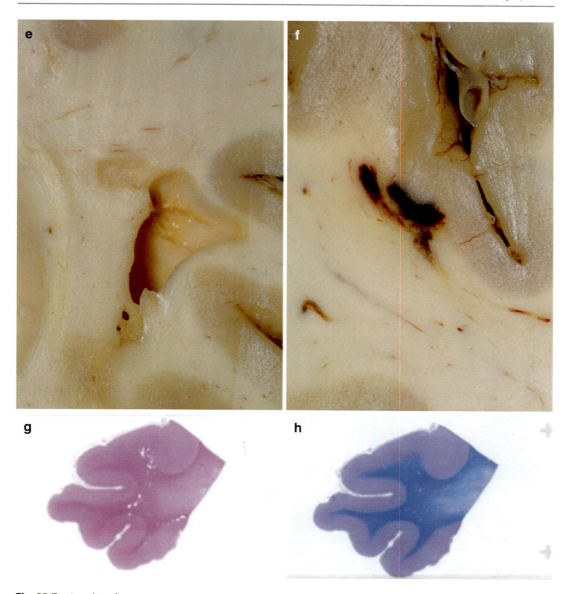

Fig. 23.7 (continued)

23.2 Binswanger Disease

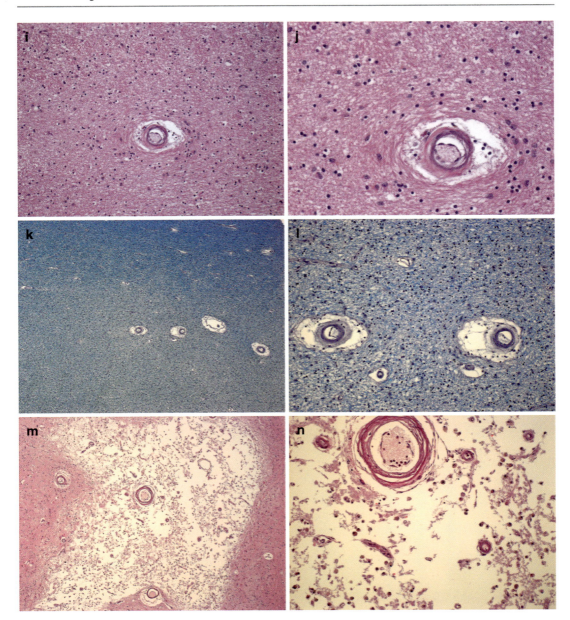

Fig. 23.7 (continued)

- Arterioles of the white matter show:
  - Hyalinotic thickening of the vessel wall
  - Widening of the perivascular spaces

23.3.5 Molecular Neuropathology

Pathogenesis
- Reduced, non-adequate blood supply due to vessel wall damage

23.3.6 Treatment and Prognosis

Treatment
- management of hypertension and diabetes
- avoidance of processes associated with vascular damage (e.g., cigarette smoking)
- salutary effects
  - calcium channel blocker nimodipine
  - cerebral vasodilators

Biologic Behavior–Prognosis–Prognostic Factors
- variable

23.4 Fahr Disease

Familial idiopathic basal ganglia calcification (Fahr disease) is a rare neurodegenerative disorder characterized by symmetrical and bilateral calcification of the basal ganglia.

23.4.1 Clinical Signs and Symptoms

- Neuropsychiatric features
- Movement disorders
- Psychiatric features include:
  - cognitive impairment, depression, hallucinations, delusions, manic symptoms, anxiety, schizophrenia-like psychosis, and personality change
- Other clinical features include:
  - Parkinsonism, ataxia, headache, seizures, vertigo, stroke-like events, orthostatic hypotension, tremor, dysarthria, and paresis

23.4.2 Localisation

Localization
- Basal ganglia
- Cerebellar dentate nucleus
- Thalamus
- Cerebral cortex

23.4.3 Neuroimaging Findings

General Imaging Findings
- Symmetric calcifications of basal ganglia

CT Non-Contrast-Enhanced (Fig. 23.8a, b)
- No enhancement

CT Contrast-Enhanced
- Method of choice to detect hyperdense calcifications of basal ganglia and dentate nuclei

MRI-T2/FLAIR (Fig. 23.8c, d)
- Hypo- or hyperintense calcifications

MRI-T1 (Fig. 23.8e)
- No enhancement

MRI-T2∗/SWI (Fig. 23.8h)
- Calcifications usually hyperintense

MRI-T1 Contrast-Enhanced (Fig. 23.8f)
- No enhancement

Nuclear Medicine Imaging Findings
- CBF-SPECT can demonstrate hypoperfusion correlated with clinical findings.
- FDG-PET can demonstrate hypometabolism in basal ganglia.

23.4.4 Neuropathology Findings

Macroscopic Changes (Fig. 23.9a, b)
- Usually none are noted.
- Rarely rough appearance on touch (like an unshaved beard) (Fig. 23.9a, b).

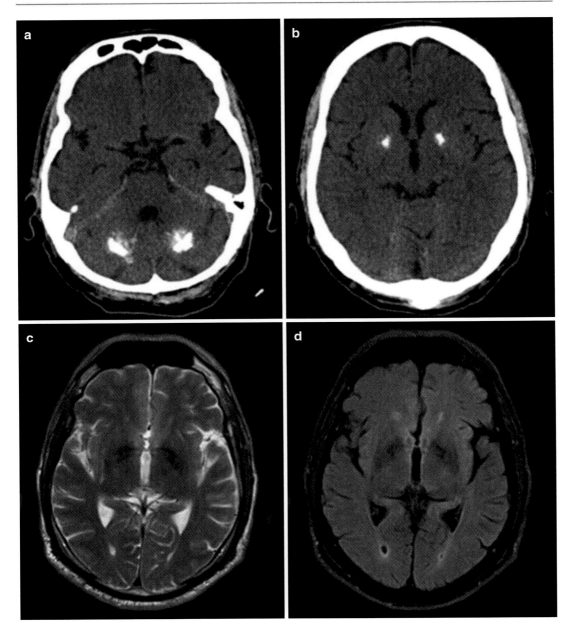

Fig. 23.8 Morbus Fahr: CT (**a**, **b**), T2 (**c**), FLAIR (**d**), T1 (**e**), T1 contrast (**f**), DWI (**g**), SWI (**h**)

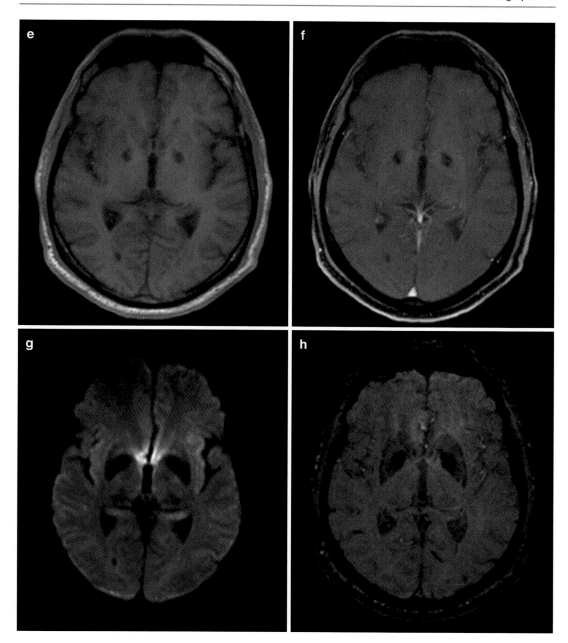

Fig. 23.8 (continued)

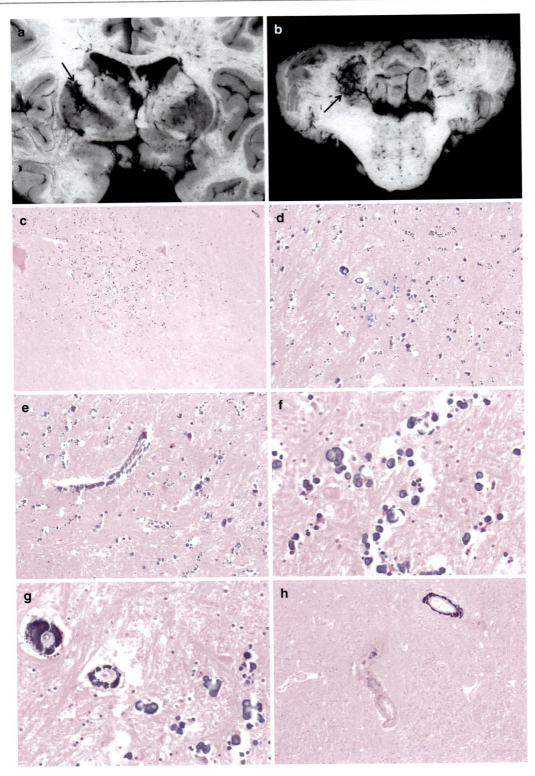

Fig. 23.9 Idiopathic basal ganglia calcification (IBGC) or Fahr disease: Gross-anatomical appearance of calcium deposits in the basal ganglia and in the dentate nucleus of the cerebellum (**a**). Calcium deposits in the basal ganglia (**b–h**), dentate nucleus (**g**), and vascular wall (**d, f, h**)

Microscopic Changes (Fig. 23.9c–h)
- within the vessel wall (capillaries and small arteries)
- as small extra-parenchymal droplet-like, globular to mulberry-like basophilic structures

23.4.5 Molecular Neuropathology

Pathogenesis
- encountered in patients presenting with hypo- or hyperparathyroid disorders

Genetics
- Predominantly with autosomal dominant fashion
- Genetic heterogeneity
- Phosphate imbalance disorder
- Associated genes
  - SLC20A2
  - PDGFRß (encodes a member of the platelet-derived growth factor receptor family type β)
  - PDGF (the specific ligand of PDGFRβ)
  - ISG15
  - XPR1
- Loss-of-function mutations in these genes have been associated
  - with disturbance in phosphate homeostasis in brain regions
  - the dysfunction of blood–brain barrier
  - enhanced IFN-α/β immunity
  - have an effect through haploinsufficiency (Wang et al. 2012)
- The mutations might
  - suppress PDGFRβ autophosphorylation
  - result in partial loss of autophosphorylation
  - involve reduced protein levels
  - no kinase activity and failed to activate any of the pathways normally stimulated by PDGF
  - activated Akt and MAP kinases, but did not induce the phosphorylation of signal transducer and activator of transcription 3 (STAT3)

23.4.6 Treatment and Prognosis

Biologic Behavior–Prognosis–Prognostic Factors
- variable

23.5 Cerebral Autosomal Dominant Arteriopathy (CADASIL)

CADASIL: Cerebral autosomal dominant arteriopathy with subcortical infarcts and leukoencephalopathy (CADASIL).
  Synonyms used:

- subcortical dementia with arteriopathic leukoencephalopathy
- chronic familial vascular encephalopathy
- hereditary multi-infarct dementia
- subcortical ischemic strokes with dementia and leukoencephalopathy

23.5.1 Clinical Signs and Symptoms

- highly variable
- migraine
- infarcts/stroke
  - motoric
  - sensible
  - senso-motoric
  - atactic-hemiparetic
  - brain stem
- dementia

Typical and atypical clinical manifestations of CADASIL (Di Donato et al. 2017)

- Typical manifestations
  - Migraine, usually with aura, as the first symptom in the third decade of life (40% of cases)
  - Recurrent subcortical ischemic events (transient ischemic attack/stroke) in adulthood
  - Mood disturbances, apathy, and depression among other psychiatric symptoms

- Progressive cognitive decline, especially of executive functioning
- Seizures, in a smaller but well-defined portion of patients
• Atypical manifestations
  - Pathological gambling
  - Recurrent status epilepticus
  - Schizophreniform organic psychosis
  - Neuropathy
  - Myopathy
  - "CADASIL coma"
  - Early-onset
  - Late-onset
  - Bipolar disorder
  - Inflammatory-like presentation
  - Acute vestibular syndrome
  - Spinal cord involvement
  - Acute confusional migraine
  - Sporadic hemiplegic migraine with normal imaging
  - Postpartum psychiatric disturbances
  - Parkinsonism
  - Recurrent transient global amnesia

23.5.2 Epidemiology

Incidence
• at least 4.6 per 100,000 adults

Age Incidence
• 30–50 years

Sex Incidence
• Male:Female ratio 1:1

Localization
• Leptomeningeal vessels

23.5.3 Neuroimaging Findings

General Imaging Findings
• Leukoencephalopathy and lacunar infarcts including temporopolar white matter and internal/external capsule

CT Non-Contrast-Enhanced (Fig. 23.10a)
• Hypodense white matter lesions

CT Contrast-Enhanced
• No enhancement

MRI-T2 (Fig. 23.10b)
• Confluent periventricular and subcortical white matter hyperintensities
• Hyperintense lacunar lesions in basal ganglia, thalamus, and pons

MRI-FLAIR (Fig. 23.10c)
• Confluent and lacunar white matter hyperintensities

MRI-T1 (Fig. 23.10d)
• Isointense confluent white matter lesions
• Hypointense lacunar lesions

MRI-T1 Contrast-Enhanced (Fig. 23.10e)
• Lesions do not enhance.

MRI-T2∗/SWI
• Microbleeds are possible.

MR-Diffusion Imaging (Fig. 23.10f, g)
• Recent lesions show restricted diffusion.

MR-Diffusion Tensor Imaging
• May be reduced due to white matter damage

Nuclear Medicine Imaging Findings
• FDG-PET can demonstrate severe changes in glucose metabolism in CADASIL patients.
• Overall glucose metabolism is reduced in these patients and statistically the caudate nucleus and the frontal cortex show the lowest uptake rates compared to healthy people. The findings correlate with the cognitive and psychiatric symptoms.
• Crossed cerebellar diaschisis can be observed.

23.5.4 Neuropathology Findings

Macroscopic Features
- diffuse leukoencephalopathy with rarefication of the white matter
- multiple small- to medium-sized infarcts affecting
  - basal ganglia
  - thalamus

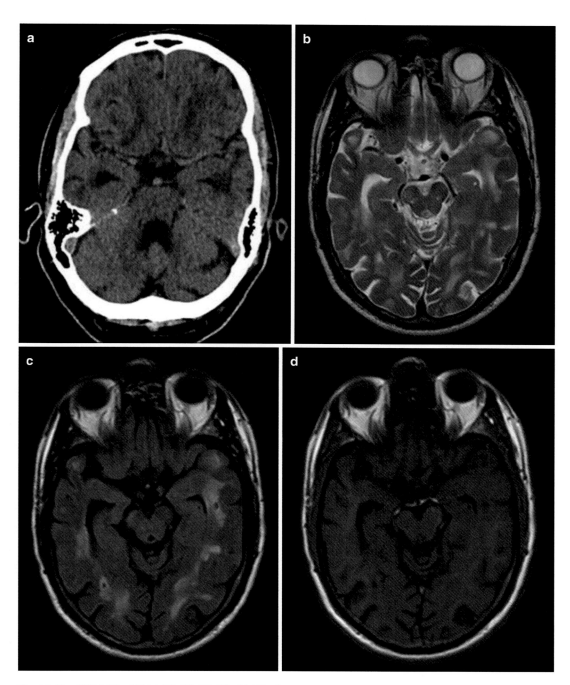

Fig. 23.10 CADASIL: CT (**a**), T2 (**b**), FLAIR (**b**), T1 (**d**), T1 contrast (**e**), DWI (**f**), SWI (**g**)

23.4 Cerebral Autosomal Dominant Arteriopathy (CADASIL)

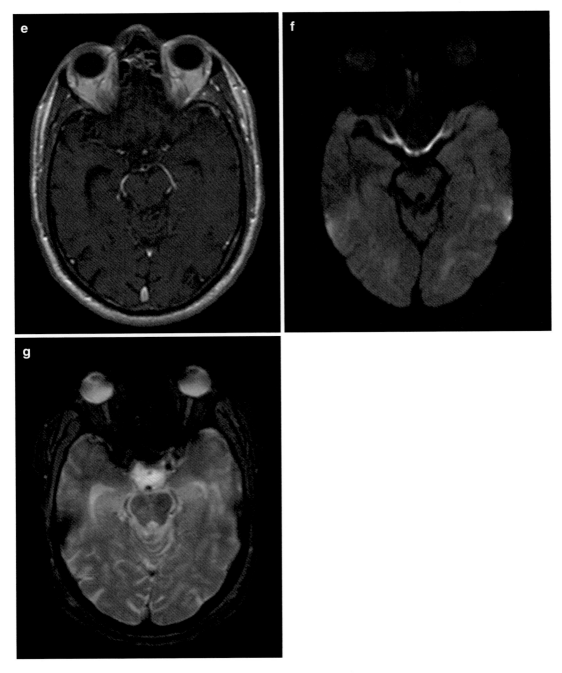

Fig. 23.10 (continued)

- cerebral cortex and subcortical U-fibers not affected

Microscopic Features (Fig. 23.11a–l)
- Luminal narrowing of small vessels
- Progressive wall thickening due to
  - degenerated smooth muscle cells
  - thickening of the media
  - fragmentation and reduplication of the internal elastic lamina

- deposition of granular, eosinophilic PAS-positive material
- Multiple small infarcts
- Lesions not present include:
  - Arteriosclerotic changes
  - Diffuse amyloid deposits
  - Amyloid plaques
  - Neurofibrillary tangles

Ultrastructural Features
- Excision biopsy of skin from the upper arm is usually used.

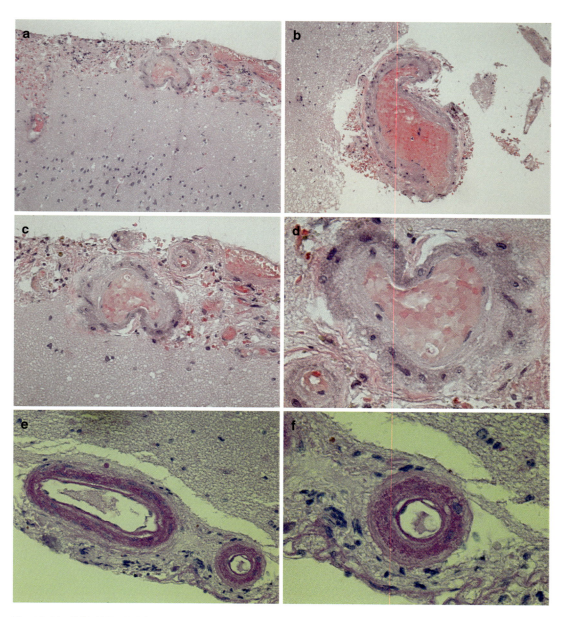

Fig. 23.11 CADASIL: Thickening of the walls of leptomeningeal vessels (**a–d**) with deposits of PAS-positive (**e, f**) pathognomonic granular osmiophilic material (GOM) in the media (including dermal vessels) around smooth muscle cells. Ultrastructurally GOM are commonly found in small-sized arterioles and contain extracellular electron-dense granular material located in small indentations of the cytoplasmic membrane of pericytes and vascular smooth muscle cells (**g–l**). They are oval shape with a tail extending into the intercellular matrix (**h, j, l**)

23.4 Cerebral Autosomal Dominant Arteriopathy (CADASIL)

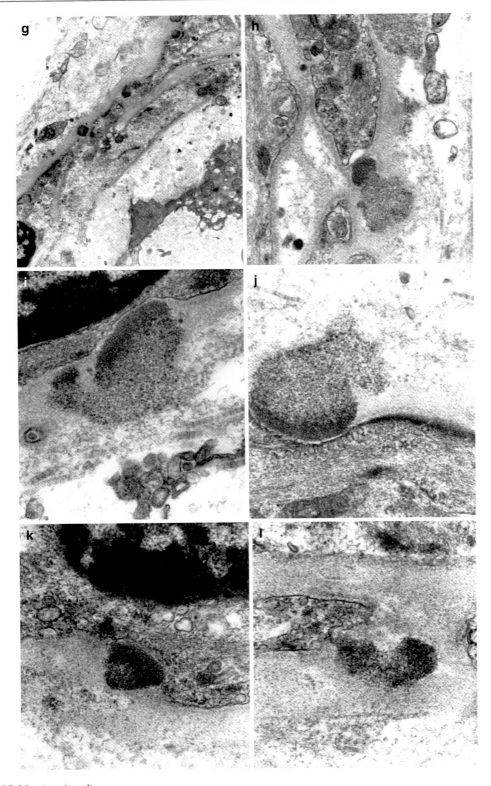

Fig. 23.11 (continued)

- GOM: granular osmiophilic material
  - commonly found in small-sized arterioles (seldomly small capillaries or veins)
  - contain the Notch3 receptor extracellular domain
  - extracellular electron-dense granular material located in small indentations of the cytoplasmic membrane of pericytes and vascular smooth muscle cells
  - oval shape with a tail extending into the intercellular matrix

Immunophenotype
- Notch3: accumulation of the extracellular domain cleaved in response to ligand binding

Differential Diagnosis
- Arteriosclerosis
- Arteriolosclerosis

23.5.5 Molecular Neuropathology

- Notch3
  - located on chromosome 19 q12
  - encodes a transmembrane receptor with a 97 kDa intracellular domain and a 210 kDa extracellular domain containing 34 epidermal growth factor-like repeats
  - plays a key role in cell differentiation during embryogenesis
- Mutations of the gene encoding the transmembrane receptor Notch3
  - lead to the loss or gain of a cysteine residue in 1 of the 34 EGFR domains of the NOTCH3 protein. The majority are missense mutations, but small deletions, insertions, and splice-site mutations have been reported, which typically also lead to a numerical cysteine alteration (Rutten et al. 2014).
  - more than 180 mutations described.
  - clustered in exons 3–6, 8, and 11.
- Cerebral autosomal dominant arteriopathy with subcortical infarcts and leukoencephalopathy (CADASIL) is caused by gain-of-function mutations in NOTCH3, leading to toxic NOTCH3 accumulation in the vessel wall (Rutten et al. 2014).

- Only NOTCH3 mutations that alter the number of cysteines in 1 of the 34 EGFr domains of the NOTCH3 protein have been proven to cause CADASIL:
  - The great majority are missense mutations.
  - Mutations are found only in EGFr-encoding exons (2–24).
  - Most mutations are located in exon 4.
- Some CADASIL patients with homozygous and compound heterozygous mutations have been described. The symptoms of these patients seem to be within the normal CADASIL spectrum.
- Small NOTCH3 in-frame deletions, insertions, or splice-site mutations can also cause CADASIL. These typically also alter the number of cysteines in 1 of the 34 EGFr of NOTCH3.
- Mutations in NOTCH3 leading to loss of NOTCH3 function do not cause CADASIL. These rare mutations include mutations leading to a frameshift and stop mutations.
- Missense mutations in NOTCH3 not altering a cysteine residue are unlikely to be pathogenic, and should be considered coincidental findings, until proven otherwise. If such a mutation is detected, the following should be considered:
  - A coinciding cysteine-altering mutation may have been missed due to technical reasons or incomplete sequencing analysis.
- The clinical diagnosis of CADASIL may be incorrect and should be confirmed by electron microscopy and NOTCH3 immunohistochemistry on a skin biopsy.

23.5.6 Treatment and Prognosis

Treatment
- Symptomatic
- Migraine
  - Acetazolamide
    - As prophylaxis, reduces the frequency of migraine attacks

- Sodium valproate
- Anecdotal cases
- Cognitive decline
  - Acetylcholinesterase inhibitor
    - Not efficacious on the primary endpoint (Vascular Dementia Assessment Scale after 18 weeks), but some improvement in relation to frontal subcortical dysfunction
- Primary and secondary stroke prevention
  - Antiplatelet drugs
    - Unproven and debated benefits

Biologic Behavior–Prognosis–Prognostic Factors
- variable

Selected References

Andre C (2010) CADASIL: pathogenesis, clinical and radiological findings and treatment. Arq Neuropsiquiatr 68(2):287–299

Attems J, Jellinger K, Thal DR, Van Nostrand W (2011) Review: sporadic cerebral amyloid angiopathy. Neuropathol Appl Neurobiol 37(1):75–93. https://doi.org/10.1111/j.1365-2990.2010.01137.x

Auer DP, Putz B, Gossl C, Elbel G, Gasser T, Dichgans M (2001) Differential lesion patterns in CADASIL and sporadic subcortical arteriosclerotic encephalopathy: MR imaging study with statistical parametric group comparison. Radiology 218(2):443–451. https://doi.org/10.1148/radiology.218.2.r01fe24443

Auriel E, Greenberg SM (2012) The pathophysiology and clinical presentation of cerebral amyloid angiopathy. Curr Atheroscler Rep 14(4):343–350. https://doi.org/10.1007/s11883-012-0254-z

Bottcher J, Sauner D, Jentsch A, Mentzel HJ, Becker H, Reichenbach JR, Kaiser WA (2004) [Visualization of symmetric striopallidodentate calcinosis by using high-resolution susceptibility-weighted MR imaging. An account of the impact of different diagnostic methods of M. Fahr]. Nervenarzt 75(4):355–361. https://doi.org/10.1007/s00115-003-1667-2

Carare RO, Hawkes CA, Jeffrey M, Kalaria RN, Weller RO (2013) Review: cerebral amyloid angiopathy, prion angiopathy, CADASIL and the spectrum of protein elimination failure angiopathies (PEFA) in neurodegenerative disease with a focus on therapy. Neuropathol Appl Neurobiol 39(6):593–611. https://doi.org/10.1111/nan.12042

Chabriat H, Joutel A, Dichgans M, Tournier-Lasserve E, Bousser MG (2009) Cadasil. Lancet Neurol 8(7):643–653. https://doi.org/10.1016/s1474-4422(09)70127-9

Chao CP, Kotsenas AL, Broderick DF (2006) Cerebral amyloid angiopathy: CT and MR imaging findings. Radiographics 26(5):1517–1531. https://doi.org/10.1148/rg.265055090

Charidimou A, Boulouis G, Gurol ME, Ayata C, Bacskai BJ, Frosch MP, Viswanathan A, Greenberg SM (2017) Emerging concepts in sporadic cerebral amyloid angiopathy. Brain J Neurol 140(7):1829–1850. https://doi.org/10.1093/brain/awx047

Choi EJ, Choi CG, Kim JS (2005) Large cerebral artery involvement in CADASIL. Neurology 65(8):1322–1324. https://doi.org/10.1212/01.wnl.0000180965.79209.50

Di Donato I, Bianchi S, De Stefano N, Dichgans M, Dotti MT, Duering M, Jouvent E, Korczyn AD, Lesnik-Oberstein SA, Malandrini A, Markus HS, Pantoni L, Penco S, Rufa A, Sinanovic O, Stojanov D, Federico A (2017) Cerebral autosomal dominant arteriopathy with subcortical infarcts and leukoencephalopathy (CADASIL) as a model of small vessel disease: update on clinical, diagnostic, and management aspects. BMC Med 15(1):41. https://doi.org/10.1186/s12916-017-0778-8

Federico A, Bianchi S, Dotti MT (2005) The spectrum of mutations for CADASIL diagnosis. Neurol Sci 26(2):117–124. https://doi.org/10.1007/s10072-005-0444-3

Grinberg LT, Korczyn AD, Heinsen H (2012) Cerebral amyloid angiopathy impact on endothelium. Exp Gerontol 47(11):838–842. https://doi.org/10.1016/j.exger.2012.08.005

Jang SH, Seo YS (2015) Injuries of neural tracts in a patient with CADASIL: a diffusion tensor imaging study. BMC Neurol 15:176. https://doi.org/10.1186/s12883-015-0434-x

Kalaria RN, Viitanen M, Kalimo H, Dichgans M, Tabira T (2004) The pathogenesis of CADASIL: an update. J Neurol Sci 226(1-2):35–39. https://doi.org/10.1016/j.jns.2004.09.008

Kirshner HS, Bradshaw M (2015) The inflammatory form of cerebral amyloid Angiopathy or "Cerebral Amyloid Angiopathy-Related Inflammation" (CAARI). Curr Neurol Neurosci Rep 15(8):54. https://doi.org/10.1007/s11910-015-0572-y

Linn J, Halpin A, Demaerel P, Ruhland J, Giese AD, Dichgans M, van Buchem MA, Bruckmann H, Greenberg SM (2010) Prevalence of superficial siderosis in patients with cerebral amyloid angiopathy. Neurology 74(17):1346–1350. https://doi.org/10.1212/WNL.0b013e3181dad605

Lotz PR, Ballinger WE Jr, Quisling RG (1986) Subcortical arteriosclerotic encephalopathy: CT spectrum and pathologic correlation. AJR Am J Roentgenol 147(6):1209–1214. https://doi.org/10.2214/ajr.147.6.1209

Love S, Miners S, Palmer J, Chalmers K, Kehoe P (2009) Insights into the pathogenesis and pathogenicity of cerebral amyloid angiopathy. Front Biosci (Landmark edition) 14:4778–4792

Miller-Thomas MM, Sipe AL, Benzinger TL, McConathy J, Connolly S, Schwetye KE (2016) Multimodality review of amyloid-related diseases of the central nervous system. Radiographics 36(4):1147–1163. https://doi.org/10.1148/rg.2016150172

Miller JH, Wardlaw JM, Lammie GA (1999) Intracerebral haemorrhage and cerebral amyloid angiopathy: CT features with pathological correlation. Clin Radiol 54(7):422–429

Oide T, Takahashi H, Yutani C, Ishihara T, Ikeda S (2003) Relationship between lobar intracerebral hemorrhage and leukoencephalopathy associated with cerebral amyloid angiopathy: clinicopathological study of 64 Japanese patients. Amyloid 10(3):136–143

Rannikmae K, Samarasekera N, Martinez-Gonzalez NA, Al-Shahi Salman R, Sudlow CL (2013) Genetics of cerebral amyloid angiopathy: systematic review and meta-analysis. J Neurol Neurosurg Psychiatry 84(8):901–908. https://doi.org/10.1136/jnnp-2012-303898

Rutten JW, Haan J, Terwindt GM, van Duinen SG, Boon EM, Lesnik Oberstein SA (2014) Interpretation of NOTCH3 mutations in the diagnosis of CADASIL. Expert Rev Mol Diagn 14(5):593–603. https://doi.org/10.1586/14737159.2014.922880

Safriel Y, Sze G, Westmark K, Baehring J (2004) MR spectroscopy in the diagnosis of cerebral amyloid angiopathy presenting as a brain tumor. AJNR Am J Neuroradiol 25(10):1705–1708

Samarasekera N, Rodrigues MA (2017) Imaging features of intracerebral hemorrhage with cerebral amyloid angiopathy: systematic review and meta-analysis. PLoS One 12(7):e0180923. https://doi.org/10.1371/journal.pone.0180923

Schrag M, Kirshner H (2016) Neuropsychological effects of cerebral amyloid angiopathy. Curr Neurol Neurosci Rep 16(8):76. https://doi.org/10.1007/s11910-016-0674-1

Tang SC, Jeng JS, Lee MJ, Yip PK (2009) Notch signaling and CADASIL. Acta Neurol Taiwanica 18(2):81–90

Thal DR, Ghebremedhin E, Orantes M, Wiestler OD (2003) Vascular pathology in Alzheimer disease: correlation of cerebral amyloid angiopathy and arteriosclerosis/lipohyalinosis with cognitive decline. J Neuropathol Exp Neurol 62(12):1287–1301

Thal DR, Ghebremedhin E, Rub U, Yamaguchi H, Del Tredici K, Braak H (2002) Two types of sporadic cerebral amyloid angiopathy. J Neuropathol Exp Neurol 61(3):282–293

Tikka S, Baumann M, Siitonen M, Pasanen P, Poyhonen M, Myllykangas L, Viitanen M, Fukutake T, Cognat E, Joutel A, Kalimo H (2014) CADASIL and CARASIL. Brain Pathol (Zurich, Switzerland) 24(5):525–544. https://doi.org/10.1111/bpa.12181

Wang C, Li Y, Shi L, Ren J, Patti M, Wang T, de Oliveira JR, Sobrido MJ, Quintans B, Baquero M, Cui X, Zhang XY, Wang L, Xu H, Wang J, Yao J, Dai X, Liu J, Zhang L, Ma H, Gao Y, Ma X, Feng S, Liu M, Wang QK, Forster IC, Zhang X, Liu JY (2012) Mutations in SLC20A2 link familial idiopathic basal ganglia calcification with phosphate homeostasis. Nat Genet 44(3):254–256. https://doi.org/10.1038/ng.1077

Yamada M (2004) Cerebral amyloid angiopathy and gene polymorphisms. J Neurol Sci 226(1-2):41–44. https://doi.org/10.1016/j.jns.2004.09.009

Yamada M (2013) Brain hemorrhages in cerebral amyloid angiopathy. Semin Thromb Hemost 39(8):955–962. https://doi.org/10.1055/s-0033-1357489

Yamada M (2015) Cerebral amyloid angiopathy: emerging concepts. J Stroke 17(1):17–30. https://doi.org/10.5853/jos.2015.17.1.17

Yamada M, Naiki H (2012) Cerebral amyloid angiopathy. Prog Mol Biol Transl Sci 107:41–78. https://doi.org/10.1016/b978-0-12-385883-2.00006-0

Zhu S, Nahas SJ (2016) CADASIL: imaging characteristics and clinical correlation. Curr Pain Headache Rep 20(10):57. https://doi.org/10.1007/s11916-016-0584-6

Vascular Disorders: Vasculitis

24.1 Definition

Vasculitis is an inflammation of blood vessel walls.

The following types of vasculitis can be distinguished (Table 24.1):

- Infectious vasculitis
  - caused by direct invasion and proliferation of pathogens in vessel walls with resultant inflammation
  - rickettsial vasculitis, syphilitic aortitis, and *Aspergillus* arteritis
- Non-infectious vasculitis
  - not known to be caused by direct vessel wall invasion by pathogens
  - categorizes non-infectious vasculitis by integrating knowledge about etiology, pathogenesis, pathology, demographics, and clinical manifestations

Inflammation of blood vessel walls at least at some time during the course of the disease is a shared defining feature of all categories of vasculitis. Some categories of vasculitis also have characteristic tissue injury unrelated to the vasculitis.

The categorization level is based on (Table 24.2)

- the predominant type of vessels involved (Fig. 24.1)
  - large vessel vasculitis
  - medium vessel vasculitis
  - small vessel vasculitis
- vessel type
  - capillaries in different organs (e.g., in brain, kidney, and lung)
  - different segments of the aorta (e.g., arch, thoracic, abdominal)

The definitions for vasculitides as given by the 2012 International Chapel Hill Consensus Conference on the Nomenclature of Vasculitides (CHCC2012) are shown in Table 24.3 (Jennette et al. 2013).

Different types of vasculitides affecting the central nervous system include:

- Non-infectious
  - Primary vasculitis involving the CNS
  - Vasculitis due to systemic disease
  - Vasculitis associated with malignancy
  - Drug-induced vasculitis
- Infectious
  - Bacterial vasculitis
  - Viral vasculitis
  - Fungal vasculitis
  - Other infectious agents

Table 24.1 Classification of vasculitis

Non-infectious	Primary vasculitis involving the CNS	• Giant cell or temporal arteritis (GCA) • Primary angiitis of CNS (PACNS) • Takayasu arteritis • Kawasaki arteritis • Aß-related angiitis
	Vasculitis due to systemic disease	• Systemic lupus erythematosus (SLE) • Polyarteritis nodosa (PAN) • Wegener's granulomatosis • Churg–Strauss syndrome • Sjögren's syndrome • Behçet's syndrome • Rheumatoid arteritis
	Vasculitis associated with malignancy	• Hodgkin disease • Non-Hodgkin lymphoma
	Drug-induced vasculitis	• Cocaine • Amphetamines • Phenylpropanolamine
Infectious	Bacterial vasculitis	• Streptococcus • Mycobacteria • Spirochetes
	Viral vasculitis	• Herpes zoster • HIV • Hepatitis B and C • EBV • ZVZ
	Fungal vasculitis	• Aspergillus • Candida • Coccidioides • Mucor sp.
	Other infectious agents	• Protozoa • Mycoplasma • Rickettsia sp.

24.2 Clinical Signs and Symptoms

Variable symptoms include (Table 24.4):

- Ischemia
- Intracerebral or subarachnoidal hemorrhage
- Persistent headache
- Focal epilepsy
- Progressive focal neurologic signs
- Dementia
- Cranial nerve palsies

Table 24.2 Names for vasculitides adopted by the 2012 International Chapel Hill Consensus Conference on the Nomenclature of Vasculitides modified after Jennette et al. (2013) reproduced with kind permission by Wiley Publishing Company

Type of vessel	Name of disease
Large vessel vasculitis (LVV)	• Takayasu arteritis (TAK) • Giant cell arteritis (GCA)
Medium vessel vasculitis (MVV)	• Polyarteritis nodosa (PAN) • Kawasaki disease (KD)
Small vessel vasculitis (SVV)	• Antineutrophil cytoplasmic antibody (ANCA)-associated vasculitis (AAV) • Microscopic polyangiitis (MPA) • Granulomatosis with polyangiitis (Wegener's) (GPA) • Eosinophilic granulomatosis with polyangiitis (Churg–Strauss) (EGPA) • Immune complex SVV • Anti-glomerular basement membrane (anti-GBM) disease • Cryoglobulinemic vasculitis (CV) • IgA vasculitis (Henoch-Schönlein) (IgAV) • Hypocomplementemic urticarial vasculitis (HUV) (anti-C1q vasculitis)
Variable vessel vasculitis (VVV)	• Behçet's disease (BD) • Cogan's syndrome (CS)
Single-organ vasculitis (SOV)	• Cutaneous leukocytoclastic angiitis • Cutaneous arteritis • Primary central nervous system vasculitis • Isolated aortitis • Others
Vasculitis associated with systemic disease	• Lupus vasculitis • Rheumatoid vasculitis • Sarcoid vasculitis • Others
Vasculitis associated with probable etiology	• Hepatitis C virus-associated cryoglobulinemic vasculitis • Hepatitis B virus-associated vasculitis • Syphilis-associated aortitis • Drug-associated immune complex vasculitis • Drug-associated ANCA-associated vasculitis • Cancer-associated vasculitis • Others

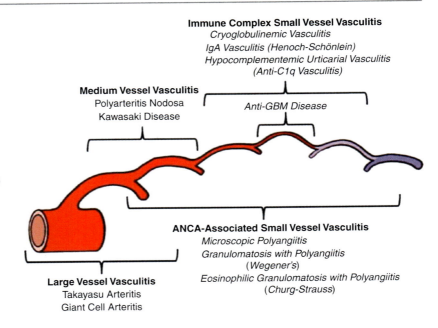

Fig. 24.1 Distribution of vessel involvement by large vessel vasculitis, medium vessel vasculitis, and small vessel vasculitis. *Anti-GBM* antiglomerular basement membrane; *ANCA* antineutrophil cytoplasmic antibody after Jennette et al. (2013) (with permission)

- Meningism
- Myelopathy
- Cauda equina syndrome

Criteria for primary CNS vasculitis (PCNSV) are given by Calabrese and Mallek (1988) and include:

- Clinical criteria
  - The patient has a history or clinical findings of an acquired neurological deficit, which remains unexplained after a thorough initial basic evaluation.
- Imaging/histopathologic criteria
  - The patient demonstrates either classic angiographic findings or histopathologic features of angiitis within CNS.
- Criteria of exclusion
  - There is no evidence of systemic vasculitis or of any other condition to which the angiographic or pathologic features could be secondary.

24.3 Epidemiology

Incidence
- 2.4 cases per 1,000,000

Age Incidence
 – fourth to fifth decade

Sex Incidence
- M > F

Localization
- Leptomeninges
- Subcortical areas

24.4 Neuroimaging Findings

General Imaging Findings
- Intra- or extracranial irregularities of vessels atypical for atherosclerosis with secondary signs of ischemia

Table 24.3 Definitions for vasculitides adopted by the 2012 International Chapel Hill Consensus Conference on the Nomenclature of Vasculitides (CHCC2012) modified after Jennette et al. (2013) reproduced with kind permission by Wiley Publishing Company

CHCC 2012 name	CHCC 2012 definition
Large vessel vasculitis (LVV)	• Vasculitis affecting large arteries more often than other vasculitides. • Large arteries are the aorta and its major branches. • Any size artery may be affected.
Takayasu arteritis (TAK)	• Arteritis, often granulomatous, predominantly affecting the aorta and/or its major branches. • Onset usually in patients younger than 50 years.
Giant cell arteritis (GCA)	• Arteritis, often granulomatous, usually affecting the aorta and/or its major branches, with a predilection for the branches of the carotid and vertebral arteries. • Often involves the temporal artery. • Onset usually in patients older than 50 years and often associated with polymyalgia rheumatic.
Medium vessel vasculitis (MVV)	• Vasculitis predominantly affecting medium arteries defined as the main visceral arteries and their branches. • Any size artery may be affected. Inflammatory aneurysms and stenosis are common.
Polyarteritis nodosa (PAN)	• Necrotizing arteritis of medium or small arteries without glomerulonephritis or vasculitis in arterioles, capillaries, or venules. • Not associated with antineutrophil cytoplasmic antibodies (ANCAs).
Kawasaki disease (KD)	• Arteritis associated with the mucocutaneous lymph node syndrome and predominantly affecting medium and small arteries. • Coronary arteries are often involved. Aorta and large arteries may be involved. • Usually occurs in infants and young children.
Small vessel vasculitis (SVV)	• Vasculitis predominantly affecting small vessels, defined as small intraparenchymal arteries, arterioles, capillaries, and venules. • Medium arteries and veins may be affected.
ANCA-associated vasculitis (AAV)	• Necrotizing vasculitis, with few or no immune deposits, predominantly affecting small vessels (i.e., capillaries, venules, arterioles, and small arteries). • Associated with myeloperoxidase (MPO) ANCA or proteinase 3 (PR3) ANCA. • Not all patients have ANCA. Add a prefix indicating ANCA reactivity, e.g., MPO-ANCA, PR3-ANCA, ANCA negative.
Microscopic polyangiitis (MPA)	• Necrotizing vasculitis, with few or no immune deposits, predominantly affecting small vessels (i.e., capillaries, venules, or arterioles). • Necrotizing arteritis involving small and medium arteries may be present. • Necrotizing glomerulonephritis is very common. • Pulmonary capillaritis often occurs. • Granulomatous inflammation is absent.
Granulomatosis with polyangiitis (Wegener's) (GPA)	• Necrotizing granulomatous inflammation usually involving the upper and lower respiratory tract. • Necrotizing vasculitis affecting predominantly small to medium vessels (e.g., capillaries, venules, arterioles, arteries, and veins). • Necrotizing glomerulonephritis is common.
Eosinophilic granulomatosis with polyangiitis (Churg–Strauss) (EGPA)	• Eosinophil-rich and necrotizing granulomatous inflammation often involving the respiratory tract. • Necrotizing vasculitis predominantly affecting small to medium vessels. • Associated with asthma and eosinophilia. • ANCA is more frequent when glomerulonephritis is present.
Immune complex vasculitis	• Vasculitis with moderate to marked vessel wall deposits of immunoglobulin and/or complement components. • Predominantly affecting small vessels (i.e., capillaries, venules, arterioles, and small arteries). • Glomerulonephritis is frequent.
Anti-glomerular basement membrane (anti-GBM) disease	• Vasculitis affecting glomerular capillaries, pulmonary capillaries, or both. • With GBM deposition of anti-GBM autoantibodies. • Lung involvement causes pulmonary hemorrhage. • Renal involvement causes glomerulonephritis with necrosis and crescents.

24.4 Neuroimaging Findings

Table 24.3 (continued)

CHCC 2012 name	CHCC 2012 definition
Cryoglobulinemic vasculitis (CV)	• Vasculitis with cryoglobulin immune deposits affecting small vessels (predominantly capillaries, venules, or arterioles). • Associated with serum cryoglobulins. • Skin, glomeruli, and peripheral nerves are often involved.
IgA vasculitis (Henoch-Schönlein) (IgAV)	• Vasculitis, with IgA1-dominant immune deposits. • Affects small vessels (predominantly capillaries, venules, or arterioles). • Often involves skin and gastrointestinal tract, and frequently causes arthritis. • Glomerulonephritis indistinguishable from IgA nephropathy may occur.
Hypocomplementemic urticarial vasculitis (HUV) (anti-C1q vasculitis)	• Vasculitis accompanied by urticaria and hypocomplementemia affecting small vessels (i.e., capillaries, venules, or arterioles). • Associated with anti-C1q antibodies. • Glomerulonephritis, arthritis, obstructive pulmonary disease are common. • Ocular inflammation common.
Variable vessel vasculitis (VVV)	• Vasculitis with no predominant type of vessel involved that can affect vessels of any size (small, medium, and large) and type (arteries, veins, and capillaries).
Behçet's disease (BD)	• Vasculitis occurring in patients with Behçet's disease that can affect arteries or veins. • Behçet's disease is characterized by recurrent oral and/or genital aphthous ulcers accompanied by cutaneous, ocular, articular, gastrointestinal, and/or central nervous system inflammatory lesions. • Small vessel vasculitis, thromboangiitis, thrombosis, arteritis, and arterial aneurysms may occur.
Cogan's syndrome (CS)	• Vasculitis occurring in patients with Cogan's syndrome. • Cogan's syndrome characterized by ocular inflammatory lesions, including interstitial keratitis, uveitis, and episcleritis, and inner ear disease, including sensorineural hearing loss and vestibular dysfunction. • Vasculitic manifestations may include arteritis (affecting small, medium, or large arteries), aortitis, aortic aneurysms, and aortic and mitral valvulitis.
Single-organ vasculitis (SOV)	• Vasculitis in arteries or veins of any size in a single organ that has no features that indicate that it is a limited expression of a systemic vasculitis. • The involved organ and vessel type should be included in the name (e.g., cutaneous small vessel vasculitis, testicular arteritis, central nervous system vasculitis). • Vasculitis distribution may be unifocal or multifocal (diffuse) within an organ. • Some patients originally diagnosed as having SOV will develop additional disease manifestations that warrant redefining the case as one of the systemic vasculitides (e.g., cutaneous arteritis later becoming systemic polyarteritis nodosa).
Vasculitis associated with systemic disease	• Vasculitis that is associated with and may be secondary to (caused by) a systemic disease. • The name (diagnosis) should have a prefix term specifying the systemic disease (e.g., rheumatoid vasculitis, lupus vasculitis).
Vasculitis associated with probable etiology	• Vasculitis that is associated with a probable specific etiology. • The name (diagnosis) should have a prefix term specifying the association (e.g., hydralazine-associated microscopic polyangiitis, hepatitis B virus-associated vasculitis, hepatitis C virus-associated cryoglobulemic vasculitis).

CT Non-Contrast-Enhanced (Fig. 24.2a)
- Less sensitive
- Multifocal hypodense lesions/infarcts

CT Contrast-Enhanced
- Subacute ischemic lesions enhance
- Meningeal enhancement possible

MRI-T2/FLAIR (Fig. 24.2b, c)
- Hyperintense, multifocal lesions, predominantly in basal ganglia and subcortical

MRI-T1 (Fig. 24.2d)
- Multifocal hypointensities

Table 24.4 Ocular and neurologic signs based on disease type

Disease type	Ocular	Neurologic
Takayasu disease	• Amaurosis fugax • Progressive ischemic oculopathy	• Cerebral infarction • Transient ischemic attack • Seizures • Vascular dementia
Giant cell arteritis	• Amaurosis fugax • Monocular or binocular blindness	• Cerebral infarction • Transient ischemic attack
Polyarteritis nodosa	• Anterior ischemic optic neuropathy • Posterior ischemic optic neuropathy • Central retinal artery occlusion • Branch retinal artery occlusion • Choroidal ischemia • Diplopia • Ptosis • Tonic pupil • Internuclear ophthalmoplegia • Nystagmus	• Mononeuropathy multiplex • Headache • Seizures • Encephalopathy • Intracranial hemorrhage • Spinal cord infarction
Cogan's syndrome	• Uveitis • Interstitial keratitis • Lacrimation • Eye pain • Visual loss	• Meningoencephalitis • Personality changes • Encephalopathy
Wegener disease	• Uveitis • Corneal ulcers • Orbital mass • Retinal infarction or hemorrhage	• Isolated cranial neuropathy • Mononeuropathy multiplex • Peripheral neuropathy • Meningoencephalitis • Cerebral hemorrhage • Cerebral infarction
Churg–Strauss angiitis	• Anterior ischemic optic neuropathy • Retinal ischemia	• Mononeuropathy multiplex • Polyneuropathy • Cranial nerve palsies • Cerebral hemorrhage • Cerebral infarction
Microscopic polyangiitis		• Mononeuropathy • Cerebral infarction • Cerebral hemorrhage

MRI-T1 Contrast-Enhanced (Fig. 24.2e)
- Subacute ischemic lesions enhance
- Meningeal enhancement described

MR-Diffusion Imaging (Fig. 24.2f)
- Restricted diffusion in acute infarcts

MRI-T2∗/SWI (Fig. 24.2g)
- Detects hemorrhages

MRI-Perfusion
- Delayed perfusion due to hemodynamic stenosis

DSA/MRA and CT-Angiography (Fig. 24.2h, i)
- Vessel irregularities with stenosis, occlusion, and poststenotic dilatation

MR-Black Blood Imaging
- Enhancement of thickened vessel wall

Nuclear Medicine Imaging Findings (Fig. 24.3a, b)

- FDG-PET is of high value detecting inflammation in the large vessels.

- Due to the limited spatial resolution, visualization of the small carotid branches like temporal arteries is not frequently possible but FDG-PET of the brain demonstrates hypometabolism in several brain areas in patients with vasculitis and neurological symptoms.
- FDG-PET showed comparable results with MRI in the diagnosis of aortitis but FDG identified more vascular regions involved in the inflammatory process than did MRI.
- Normalization of FDG uptake correlates with clinical improvement and normalization of laboratory findings. Regions of interest (ROI) analysis with aorta to liver maximal standardized value (SUV) ratio with a cutoff ratio of 1.0 is described in the literature for semi-quantification.
• 15O-PET can demonstrate altered cerebral blood flow at multiple sites in patients with vasculitis and neurological symptoms.

24.5 Neuropathology Findings

Macroscopic Features

- No obvious changes
- Segmental dilation
- Thickening of arterial wall

Microscopic Features (Fig. 24.4a–p)
- Small-medium sized arteries and veins, especially those located in leptomeninges and subcortical areas.
- Inflammatory infiltration of vessel walls by T-lymphocytes.
- Inflammatory cells infiltrate the adventitia.
- Fragmentation of the internal elastic lamina.
- Intimal proliferation.
- Intimal fibrosis.
- Vascular occlusion.
- Activated macrophages which undergo granulomatous differentiation with giant cell formation.
- Multinucleated giant might be found (not necessary for final diagnosis).
- Granulomatous changes possible.
- B-lymphocytes and plasma cells can also be observed.
- Vascular ß amyloid deposits may be found.

Immunophenotype (Fig. 24.5a–d)
- CD45
- CD3
- CD4

Differential Diagnosis
- Perivascular lymphocytic infiltrates
- Lymphoma
- Leptomeningitis
- Sarcoidosis
- Carcinomatous meningitis
- Acute disseminated encephalomyelitis

24.6 Molecular Neuropathology

- Infectious
  - Viruses (varicella-zoster virus)
- Autoimmune
- Immunologic reaction directed at elastin
- Release of cytokines
  - Interleukin-1, interleukin-6
- Association between human leukocyte antigen (HLA)-B∗51 and Behçet's disease
  - model of five amino acids of the HLA-B molecule involved in the binding of the antigen
  - the interactions with receptors on CD8 T-cells and natural killer cells
  - the signal peptide of HLA-B

- Vasculitis predisposition, most of them representing
  - Important players in the immune and inflammatory response. These associations include ERAP1, CCR1-CCR3, STAT4, KLRC4, GIMAP4, and TNFAIP3 in Behçet's disease; BLK and CD40 in Kawasaki disease.
  - SERPINA1 and SEMA6A in antineutrophil cytoplasmic antibody-associated vasculitides.
  - IL12B and FCGR2A/ FCGR2A in Takayasu arteritis.
  - CECR1 in a newly defined vascular inflammatory syndrome associated with adenosine deaminase (ADA2) deficiency.

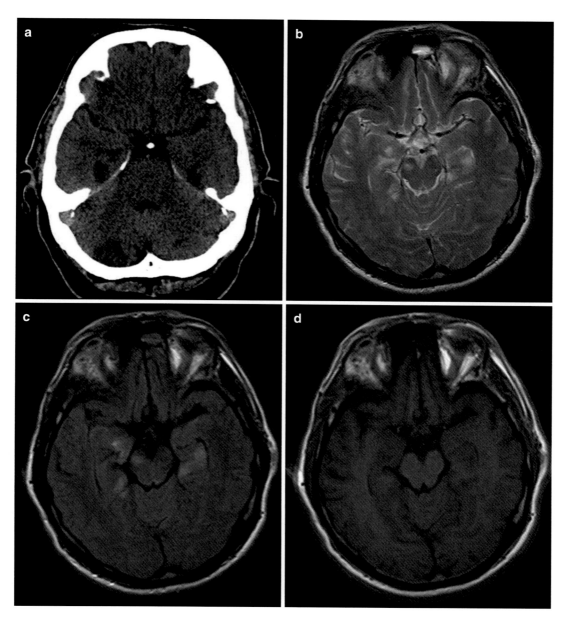

Fig. 24.2 Vasculitis with multiple infarcts in CT ax (**a**), T2 (**b**) FLAIR (**c**), T1 (**d**), T1 contrast (**e**), DWI (**f**), SWI (**g**), MRA TOF (**h**), and DSA lateral with narrowing of distal branches of the pericallosal artery (**i**)

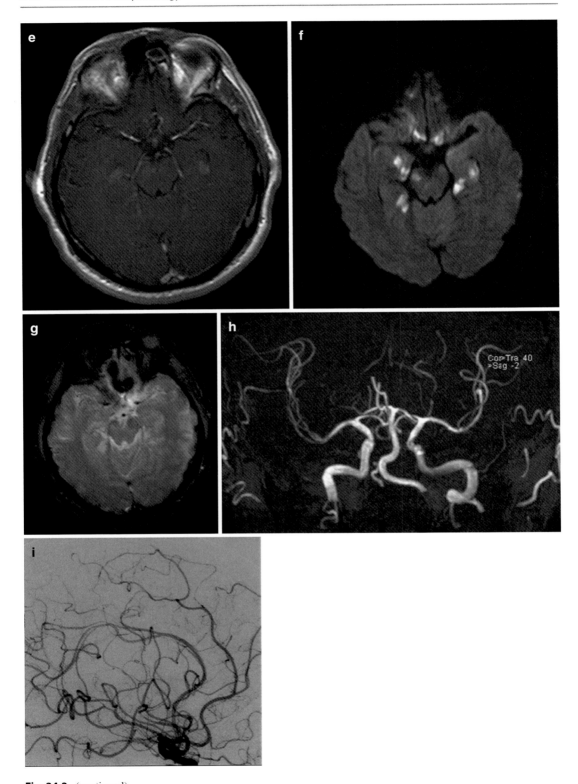

Fig. 24.2 (continued)

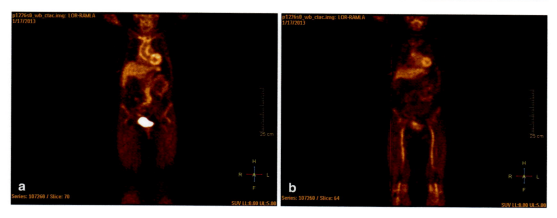

Fig. 24.3 Patient with vasculitis of the large vessels (**a**: aorta, **b**: femoral arteries)

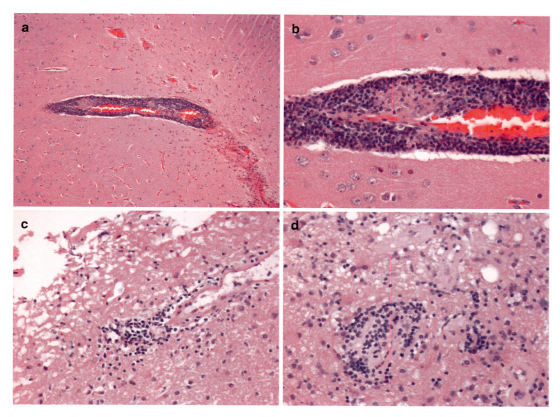

Fig. 24.4 Vasculitis: accumulation of lymphocytes within the vessel wall (**a**, **b**), in perivascular spaces (**c–e**), vessels are thrombosed (**f–l**) with perivascular petechial hemorrhages (**h–j**). Lymphocytes are also located in the adventitia (**k–m**). The vasa vasorum have thickened walls and show mild lymphocytic cuffing (**n**). Infiltration of the adventitia by lymphocytes is shown in EvG stain (**o**, **p**)

24.6 Molecular Neuropathology

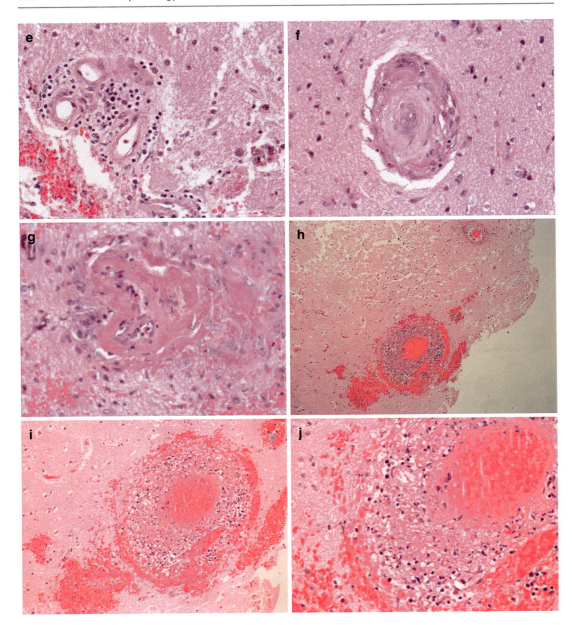

Fig. 24.4 (continued)

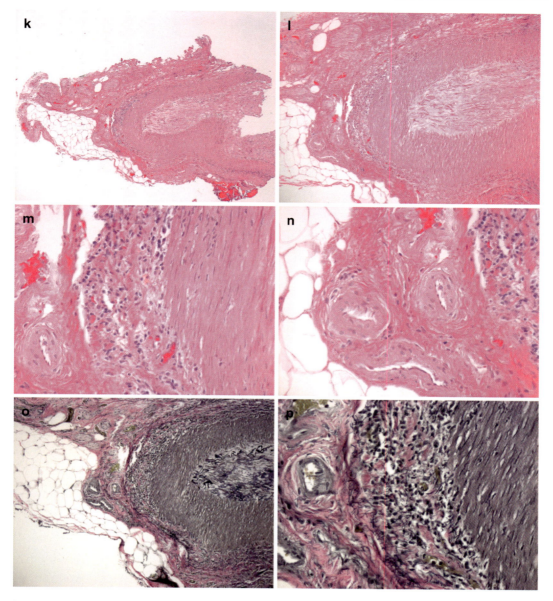

Fig. 24.4 (continued)

- Genetic factors
  - Germline mutations
    - Adenosine deaminase 2 deficiency
  - Monogenic immune dysregulation
    - Familiar hemophagozytic histiocytosis/perforin mutation
    - Hyper-IgE syndrome/DOCK8 deficiency
- Polymorphism in the I-κ B-like protein
- Histone modifications (Table 24.5)
- DNA methylation (Table 24.6)
- MicroRNA dysregulation (Table 24.7)

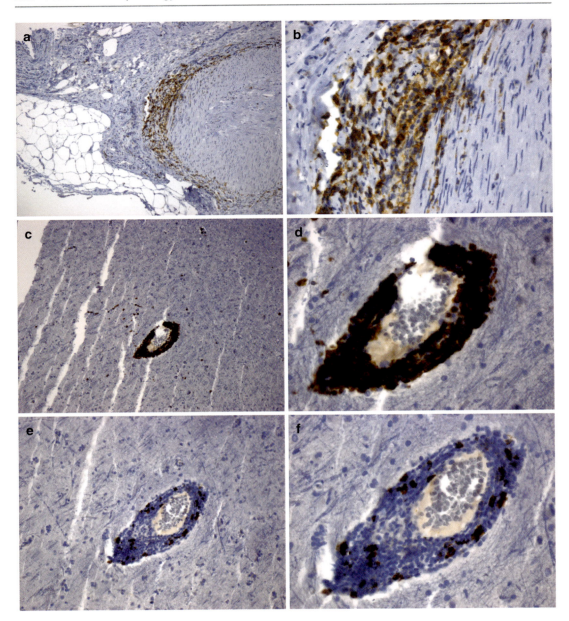

Fig. 24.5 Vasculitis—immunophenotype: presence of CD3-positive T-lymphocytes in the vascular wall (**a–d**); a few CD20-positive B-lymphocytes are contained in the infiltrate (**e, f**)

Table 24.5 Aberrant **histone modifications** in vasculitis, modified after Renauer et al. (2016) reproduced with kind permission by Springer Nature

Disease	Affected genes	Modification	Modification difference	Function	Disease contribution
ANCA-associated vasculitis	MPO (promoter and intron 7)	H3K27me3	↓	Neutrophil granule protein	Increased production of MPO-ANCA auto-antigen
	PR3 (promoter and exon 3)	H3K27me3	↓	Neutrophil granule protein	Increased production of PR3-ANCA auto-antigen
IgA vasculitis	Global	H3 acetylation	↑	Chromatin structure	Global increase in transcriptional accessibility correlating with increased CRP and ESR
	Global	H3K4 methylation	↑	Chromatin structure	Global increase in transcriptional accessibility correlating with increased serum IL-4 and disease severity
	IL4 (promoter, DNase I hypersensitivity site, and intronic enhancer)	H3K27me3 and H3 acetylation	↑	Th2 differentiation	Th2-mediated inflammatory response

Table 24.6 Aberrant **DNA methylation** in vasculitis, modified after Renauer et al. (2016) reproduced with kind permission by Springer Nature

Disease	Affected genes	Methylation difference	Disease contribution
ANCA-associated vasculitis	MPO (CpG island spanning exons 2 and 3)	↓	Increased production of MPO auto-antigen
	RUNX3 (promoter)	↑	Ineffective silencing of MPO and PR3 auto-antigen
Kawasaki disease	FCGR2A	↓	Pro-inflammatory response
Behçet's disease	Microtubule-associated proteins (TBCD, KIF1B, DNAH3, TUBB8, and RSG14)	Differential methylation	Regulation of cytoskeletal dynamics and cell migration
	Myosin genes (MYH15, MYO1C, MYO1D, and MPRIP)	Differential methylation	Regulation of cytoskeletal dynamics and cell migration
	Actin processing genes (FSCN2, BAIAP2L1, ANK1, FILIP1L, and SSH)	Differential methylation	Regulation of cytoskeletal dynamics and cell migration
Giant cell arteritis	CaN/NFAT signaling (PPP3CC, NFATC2, NFATC1)	↓	Enhanced T-cell activation and differentiation
	Pro-inflammatory genes (TNF, IL1B, IL2, IL18, LTA, LTB, NLRP1, CD40LG, CD6, IL6, IL21, IL21R, IL23R, IL17RA, RUNX3, IFNG)	↓	Pro-inflammatory disease environment. Prominent role for T-cell activation (Th1 and Th17) in GCA

Table 24.7 Aberrant **miRNA regulation** in vasculitis, modified after Renauer et al. (2016) reproduced with kind permission by Springer Nature

Disease	miRNA	miRNA expression	miRNA target functions	Disease contribution
Kawasaki disease	miR-21	↓	Promotes FOXP3 expression	Decreased Treg differentiation and function
	miR-155	↓	Inhibits SOCS-1/STAT-5 signaling pathway	Decreased Treg differentiation and function
	miR-31	↑	Inhibits FOXP3 expression	Decreased Treg differentiation and function
	miR-145	↑	TGF-β pathway	Regulates TGF-β signaling
	miR-200c	↑	TGF-β pathway	Regulates TGF-β and oxidative stress pathways
	miR-371-p	↑	TGF-β pathway	Regulates the TGF-β pathway and epithelial–mesenchymal transition
Behçet's disease	miR-155	↓	Inflammatory response	Regulates Th17 function and pro-inflammatory pathways
	miR-146a	↑	Type I interferon pathway	Regulates pro-inflammatory cytokine production
	miR-196a	↓	Inflammatory response	Regulates pro-inflammatory cytokine production

24.7 Treatment and Prognosis

Treatment
- Infectious
  - Antiviral agents
  - Antibacterial agents
- Autoimmune
  - Corticosteroids
  - Immune suppressants (cyclophosphamide, methotrexate, azathioprine)
- Antithrombotic

Biologic Behavior–Prognosis–Prognostic Factors
- involvement of other organs
  - skin, kidney, lung, sinuses, cardiovascular system, joints
- pre-existing illnesses
  - malignancy, acquired immune deficiency syndrome, transplant
- 5 year survival: 70–90%

Selected References

Adams HP Jr (2014) Cerebral vasculitis. Handb Clin Neurol 119:475–494. https://doi.org/10.1016/b978-0-7020-4086-3.00031-x

Brogan P, Eleftheriou D (2018) Vasculitis update: pathogenesis and biomarkers. Pediatr Nephrol (Berlin, Germany) 33(2):187–198. https://doi.org/10.1007/s00467-017-3597-4

Bucerius J (2016) Monitoring vasculitis with 18F-FDG PET. Q J Nucl Med Mol Imaging 60(3):219–235

Calabrese LH, Mallek JA (1988) Primary angiitis of the central nervous system. Report of 8 new cases, review of the literature, and proposal for diagnostic criteria. Medicine 67(1):20–39

Carmona FD, Martin J, Gonzalez-Gay MA (2015) Genetics of vasculitis. Curr Opin Rheumatol 27(1):10–17. https://doi.org/10.1097/bor.0000000000000124

Dutra LA, de Souza AW, Grinberg-Dias G, Barsottini OG, Appenzeller S (2017) Central nervous system vasculitis in adults: an update. Autoimmun Rev 16(2):123–131. https://doi.org/10.1016/j.autrev.2016.12.001

Elefante E, Monti S, Bond M, Lepri G, Quartuccio L, Talarico R, Baldini C (2017) One year in review 2017: systemic vasculitis. Clin Exp Rheumatol 35 Suppl 103(1):5–26

Giannini C, Salvarani C, Hunder G, Brown RD (2012) Primary central nervous system vasculitis: pathology and mechanisms. Acta Neuropathol 123(6):759–772. https://doi.org/10.1007/s00401-012-0973-9

Gutierrez-Gonzalez LA (2016) Biological therapy-induced systemic vasculitis. Curr Rheumatol Rep 18(7):39. https://doi.org/10.1007/s11926-016-0588-6

Hajj-Ali RA, Calabrese LH (2014) Diagnosis and classification of central nervous system vasculitis. J Autoimmun 48–49:149–152. https://doi.org/10.1016/j.jaut.2014.01.007

Jennette JC, Falk RJ, Bacon PA, Basu N, Cid MC, Ferrario F, Flores-Suarez LF, Gross WL, Guillevin L, Hagen EC, Hoffman GS, Jayne DR, Kallenberg CG, Lamprecht P, Langford CA, Luqmani RA, Mahr AD, Matteson EL, Merkel PA, Ozen S, Pusey CD, Rasmussen N, Rees AJ, Scott DG, Specks U, Stone JH, Takahashi K, Watts RA (2013) 2012 revised international chapel hill consensus conference nomenclature of vasculitides. Arthritis Rheum 65(1):1–11. https://doi.org/10.1002/art.37715

John S, Hajj-Ali RA (2014) CNS vasculitis. Semin Neurol 34(4):405–412. https://doi.org/10.1055/s-0034-1390389

Koster MJ, Warrington KJ (2016) Recent advances in understanding and treating vasculitis. F1000Res 5. https://doi.org/10.12688/f1000research.8403.1

Legendre P, Regent A, Thiebault M, Mouthon L (2017) Anti-endothelial cell antibodies in vasculitis: a systematic review. Autoimmun Rev 16(2):146–153. https://doi.org/10.1016/j.autrev.2016.12.012

Loricera J, Blanco R, Hernandez JL, Martinez-Rodriguez I, Carril JM, Lavado C, Jimenez M, Gonzalez-Vela C, Gonzalez-Gay MA (2015) Use of positron emission tomography (PET) for the diagnosis of large-vessel vasculitis. Rev Esp Med Nucl Imagen Mol 34(6):372–377. https://doi.org/10.1016/j.remn.2015.07.002

Misra DP, Agarwal V (2016) Innate immune cells in the pathogenesis of primary systemic vasculitis. Rheumatol Int 36(2):169–182. https://doi.org/10.1007/s00296-015-3367-1

Mossa-Basha M, Alexander M, Gaddikeri S (2016) Vessel wall imaging for intracranial vascular disease evaluation. J Neurointerv Surg 8(11):1154–1159. https://doi.org/10.1136/neurintsurg-2015-012127

Muratore F, Pipitone N, Salvarani C, Schmidt WA (2016) Imaging of vasculitis: state of the art. Best Pract Res Clin Rheumatol 30(4):688–706. https://doi.org/10.1016/j.berh.2016.09.010

Nocton JJ (2017) Usual and unusual manifestations of systemic and central nervous system vasculitis. Pediatr Clin N Am 64(1):185–204. https://doi.org/10.1016/j.pcl.2016.08.013

Peleg H, Ben-Chetrit E (2017) Vasculitis in the autoinflammatory diseases. Curr Opin Rheumatol 29(1):4–11. https://doi.org/10.1097/bor.0000000000000347

Prieto-Gonzalez S, Arguis P, Cid MC (2015) Imaging in systemic vasculitis. Curr Opin Rheumatol 27(1):53–62. https://doi.org/10.1097/bor.0000000000000130

Prieto-Gonzalez S, Espigol-Frigole G, Garcia-Martinez A, Alba MA, Tavera-Bahillo I, Hernandez-Rodriguez J, Renu A, Gilabert R, Lomena F, Cid MC (2016) The expanding role of imaging in systemic vasculitis. Rheum Dis Clin N Am 42(4):733–751. https://doi.org/10.1016/j.rdc.2016.07.009

Renauer P, Coit P, Sawalha AH (2016) Epigenetics and vasculitis: a comprehensive review. Clin Rev Allergy Immunol 50(3):357–366. https://doi.org/10.1007/s12016-015-8495-6

Salvarani C, Brown RD Jr, Hunder GG (2017) Adult primary central nervous system vasculitis. Israel Med Assoc J 19(7):448–453

Shirai T, Hilhorst M, Harrison DG, Goronzy JJ, Weyand CM (2015) Macrophages in vascular inflammation—from atherosclerosis to vasculitis. Autoimmunity 48(3):139–151. https://doi.org/10.3109/08916934.2015.1027815

Silva de Souza AW (2015) Autoantibodies in systemic vasculitis. Front Immunol 6:184. https://doi.org/10.3389/fimmu.2015.00184

Teng GG, Chatham WW (2015) Vasculitis related to viral and other microbial agents. Best Pract Res Clin Rheumatol 29(2):226–243. https://doi.org/10.1016/j.berh.2015.05.007

Thomas K, Vassilopoulos D (2017) Infections and vasculitis. Curr Opin Rheumatol 29(1):17–23. https://doi.org/10.1097/bor.0000000000000348

Twilt M, Benseler SM (2016) Central nervous system vasculitis in adults and children. Handb Clin Neurol 133:283–300. https://doi.org/10.1016/b978-0-444-63432-0.00016-5

Watanabe R, Zhang H, Berry G, Goronzy JJ, Weyand CM (2017) Immune checkpoint dysfunction in large and medium vessel vasculitis. Am J Phys Heart Circ Phys 312(5):H1052–h1059. https://doi.org/10.1152/ajpheart.00024.2017

Yates M, Watts R (2017) ANCA-associated vasculitis. Clin Med (Lond) 17(1):60–64. https://doi.org/10.7861/clinmedicine.17-1-60

Part V

The Brain Diseases: Infections

Infections: Bacteria

25.1 Clinical Signs and Symptoms

The signs and symptoms in bacterial infections of the nervous system can be grouped into (Table 25.1):

- Meningitis
- Encephalitis
- Brain abscess
- Subdural empyema

Acute Bacterial Meningitis
- Fever
- Nuchal rigidity
- Altered mental status
- Headache

Brain Abscess
- Fever
- Headache
- Focal neurologic deficit
- Signs and symptoms of space-occupying lesion
- Papilledema

Clinical signs and symptoms, laboratory and CSF findings (Table 25.2) as well predisposing conditions (Table 25.3) in patients with brain abscess are manyfold.

25.2 Classification of Bacteria

Classification criteria of bacteria are as follows:

- Morphologic groups
  - Cocci
  - Rods
  - Curved
  - Spiral
- Microscopic appearance
  - Size
  - Shape
  - Configuration
- Reaction of Gram staining
  - Gram-positive
  - Gram-negative
- Growth characteristics
  - Colonies
    - Color
    - Size
    - Shape
    - Smell
- Functional characteristics
  - Resistance to antibiotics
  - Fermentation of specific sugars
  - Lysis of erythrocytes
  - Hydrolization of lipids

Table 25.1 Neurologic signs and syndromes related to affected regions

Localization	Syndrome	Neurologic signs
Meninges	• Meningitis • Sub- or epidural empyema	• Headache • Vomiting • Photophobia • Focal neurologic deficits • Alterations in consciousness
Brain parenchyma diffuse	• Encephalitis	• Alterations in consciousness • Seizures • Multifocal neurologic deficits
Brain parenchyma focal	• Encephalitis • Cerebritis • Abscess	• Focal neurologic deficits • Seizures
Brain stem and posterior cranial fossa	• Brain stem encephalitis • Cerebellitis	• Opto- and pupillomotor disturbances • Nuclear cranial nerve lesions • Dysarthria • Bilateral pyramidal tract signs • Alterations in consciousness • Breathing insufficiency • Vegetative signs
Spinal cord	• Myelitis • Paraspinal empyema/abscess	• Paraplegia • Brown Séquard syndrome
Arteries	• Arteriitis	• Sudden focal neurologic deficit
Veins	• Septic veinous sinus thrombosis	• Headache • Seizures • Raised brain pressure • Focal neurologic deficits

Table 25.2 Clinical characteristics and laboratory and CSF examinations in patients with brain abscess (Brouwer et al. 2014a) reproduced with kind permission by Wolters Kluwer Health

Symptoms and signs	Frequency (in percent)
Headache	69
Nausea/vomiting	47
Fever	53
Altered consciousness	43
Neurologic deficits	48
Seizures	25
Nuchal rigidity	32
Papilloedema	35
Mean duration of symptoms	8.3 days
Triad of fever, headache, focal neurologic deficits	20
Leukocytosis	60
Elevated CRP	60
Elevated ESR	72
Positive blood culture	28
CSF investigation	35
LP	99
Normal CSF	16
Pleocytosis	71
Elevated CSF protein	58
Culture positive	24
Clinical deterioration attributed to LP	7

Table 25.3 Predisposing conditions in patients with brain abscess (Brouwer et al. 2014a) reproduced with kind permission by Wolters Kluwer Health

Predisposing conditions	Frequency (in percent)
Otitis/mastoiditis	32
Sinusitis	10
Heart disease	13
Posttraumatic	14
Hematogenous	13
Pulmonary disease	8
Postoperative	9
Odontogenic	5
Immunocompromise	9
Meningitis	6
Unknown	19
Other	5

A selection of bacterial pathogens (Table 25.4) and a short characterization of bacteria (Table 25.5) are provided.

25.3 General Aspects

Based on morphologic criteria, pyogenic infections of the brain can be grouped as (Table 25.6):

- Epidural abscess
- Subdural abscess or empyema
- Purulent leptomeningitis
- Brain abscess
- Septic embolism
- Suppurative intracranial phlebitis

Identification of bacterial pathogens in adults as compared to children is given in Table 25.7.

The neurological findings, location of brain abscess and its primary source in children are shown in Table 25.8.

25.4 Epidemiology

Incidence
- 1.2 million cases per year worldwide
- 135.00 deaths
- 1.5 cases per 100,000
- Infants: 0.25 per 1000 births

Table 25.4 Selected bacterial pathogens

Bacterial types	Organism
Aerobic and facultatively Gram-positive cocci	• Enterococcus faecalis • Staphylococcus aureus • Streptococcus pneumoniae
Aerobic and facultatively Gram-positive rods	• Bacillus anthracis • Listeria monocytogenes
Aerobic Gram-negative cocci	• Neisseria meningitides • Neisseria gonorrhea
Aerobic and facultatively anaerobic Gram-negative rods	• Campylobacter jejuni • Escherichia coli • Helicobacter pylori • Pseudomonas aeruginosa • Vibrio cholerae
Acid-fast bacteria	• Mycobacterium tuberculosis • Mycobacterium leprae • Mycobacterium avium • Nocardia
Anaerobes	• Actinomyces • Clostridium botulinum
Spirochetes	• Borrelia burgdorferi • Leptospira interrogans • Treponema pallidum
Chlamydiae	• Chlamydia trachomatis

Table 25.5 A short characterization of bacteria

Organism	Gram stain	Shape	Disease
Staphylococcus	pos	Cocci	Scalded skin syndrome, food poisoning, toxic shock, impetigo, folliculitis, furuncles, carbuncles, bacteremia and endocarditis, pneumonia and empyema, osteomyelitis, septic arthritis, wound infections, urinary tract infections, catheter and shunt infections, prosthetic device infection
Streptococcus	pos	Cocci	Pharyngitis, scarlet fever, pyoderma, erysipelas, cellulitis, necrotizing fasciitis, toxic shock syndrome, rheumatic fever, acute glomerulonephritis, pneumonia, bacteremia
Enterococcus	pos	Cocci	Urinary tract infection, peritonitis, bacteremia, endocarditis
Bacillus	Pos and neg	Cocci and rods	Anthrax (cutaneous, gastrointestinal, inhalation), gastroenteritis, ocular infections, sever pulmonary disease
Listeria	pos	Rods	Neonatal disease, influenza-like, gastroenteritis
Corynebacterium	pos	Rods	Diphtheria (respiratory, cutaneous)
Nocardia	pos	Rods	Bronchopulmonary disease, mycetoma, lymphocutaneous disease, cellulitis and subcutaneous abscesses, brain abscess
Mycobacterium	Pos, Acid-fast	Rods	Tuberculosis, leprosy
Neisseria	neg	Diplococci	Sexually transmitted gonorrhea, disseminated infections, ophthalmia neonatorum, meningitis, meningococcemia, pneumonia
Enterobacteriaceae	neg	Rods	Gastroenteritis, urinary tract infections, neonatal meningitis, enteric fever,
Vibrio	neg	Rods	Cholera, gastroenteritis, wound infection
Campylobacter, Helicobacter	neg	Rods	Guillain-Barré syndrome, enteritis, gastritis
Pseudomonas	neg	Rods	Pulmonary infections, skin and soft tissue infections, urinary tract infections, ear and eye infections, endocarditis
Haemophilus	neg	Rods	Meningitis, epiglottitis, pneumonia, conjunctivitis, chancroid, endocarditis
Bordetella	neg	Coccobacilli	Pertussis
Francisella and Brucella	neg	Coccobacilli	Brucellosis, tularemia
Legionella	neg	Rods	Legionnaires' disease, Pontiac fever
Clostridium	pos	Rods	Cellulitis, suppurative myositis, myonecrosis, food poisoning, necrotizing enteritis, tetanus, botulism, pseudomembranous colitis
Treponema, Borrelia, and Leptospira		Coiled spirochete	Syphilis, Lyme disease, relapsing fever, leptospirosis
Mycoplasma			Pneumonia, tracheobronchitis, pharyngitis
Rickettsia and Orientia	poor	Rods	Rocky Mountain spotted fever, typhus
Ehrlichia			Human monocytic ehrlichiosis, human anaplasmosis
Chlamydia	neg	Rods	Trachoma, adult inclusion conjunctivitis, pneumonia, urogenital infections, lymphogranuloma venereum, atherosclerosis

25.4 Epidemiology

Table 25.6 Bacteria associated with central nervous system infections

Clinical entity	Pathogens
Meningitis	• Group B streptococcus • Streptococcus pneumoniae • Neisseria meningitidis • Listeria monocytogenes • Haemophilus influenza • Escherichia coli • Staphylococcus aureus • Nocardia species • Mycobacterium tuberculosis • Borrelia burgdorferi • Leptospira species • Treponema pallidum • Brucella species
Encephalitis	• Listeria monocytogenes • Treponema pallidum • Leptospira species • Actinomyces species • Nocardia species • Borrelia species • Rickettsia rickettsii • Mycoplasma pneumonia • Mycobacterium tuberculosis
Brain abscess	• Staphylococcus aureus • Fusobacterium species • Peptostreptococcus species • Enterobacteriaceae • Actinomyces species • Clostridium perfringens • Listeria monocytogenes • Nocardia species • Mycobacterium tuberculosis
Subdural empyema	• Staphylococcus aureus • Streptococcus pneumoniae • Group B streptococcus • Neisseria meningitidis • Mixed anaerobes and aerobes

Table 25.7 Culture results (in %) and major groups of causative microorganisms (in %) (Brouwer et al. 2014a) reproduced with kind permission by Wolters Kluwer Health

Characteristic	All patients	Children
Positive culture	68	63
Monomicrobial	77	73
Polymicrobial	23	27
Cultured microorganisms		
Streptococcus spp.	34	36
Viridans streptococci	13	6
S. pneumoniae	2	4
Enterococcus	0.8	0.3
Other/not specified	18	24
Staphylococcus spp.	18	18
S. aureus	13	11
S. epidermidis	3	4
Not specified	2	2
Gram-negative enteric	15	16
Proteus spp.	7	8
Klebsiella pneumoniae	2	2
Escherichia coli	2	2
Enterobacteria	2	1
Pseudomonas spp.	2	2
Actinomycetales	3	2
Nocardia	1	0
Corynebacterium	0.8	1
Actinomyces	0.8	1
Mycobacterium tuberculosis	0.7	0.2
Haemophilus spp.	2	6
Peptostreptococcus spp.	3	6
Bacteroides spp.	6	5
Fusobacterium spp.	2	2
Parasites	0.1	0
Fungi	1	1
Other	13	7

Age. Incidence
- Any age

Sex Incidence
- Males 70%

Localization (Table 25.9)
- Epidural
- Subdural
- Meninges
- Brain

25.5 Imaging Features

25.5.1 Meningitis

General Imaging Findings
- Imaging findings often normal or unspecific
- Leptomeningeal enhancement and exudate in subarachnoidal space

Table 25.8 Primary source, usual location of lesion, and associated neurological findings in children with brain abscess, modified after Saez-Llorens and Nieto-Guevara (2013) with permission by Elsevier

Primary source	Location of abscess	Associated neurological findings
Upper respiratory site Sinusitis	Frontal lobe	• Headache • Behavioral changes • Motor speech disorders • Depressed consciousness • Forced grasping and sucking • Hemiparesis
Chronic otitis/mastoiditis	Temporal lobe	• Dyspraxia and aphasia (dominant hemisphere) • Ipsilateral third cranial nerve palsy • Ipsilateral headache • Upper homonymous hemianopsia • Motor dysfunction of face and arm
	Cerebellum	• Dizziness • Vomiting, ipsilateral ataxia, and tremor • Sixth cranial nerve palsy • Nystagmus (towards lesion)
Dental infection	Frontal lobe	• Headache • Behavioral changes • Motor speech disorders • Depressed consciousness • Forced grasping and sucking • Hemiparesis
Head trauma	Related to injured site	• Variable by region involved
Postoperative	At operative site	• Variable by region involved
Metastatic spread	Multiple lesions	• Variable by region involved
	If parietal lobe involved	• Visual field defects in inferior quadrant • Homonymous hemianopsia, dysphasia (dominant hemisphere) • Dyspraxia and contralateral spatial neglect (no dominant hemisphere)

Table 25.9 Brain abscess location (Brouwer et al. 2014a) reproduced with kind permission by Wolters Kluwer Health

Abscess location	Frequency (in percent)
Frontal	31
Temporal	27
Parietal	20
Occipital	6
Basal ganglia	3
Cerebellum and brain stem	13
Extra-axial	7
Single abscess	82
Multiple abscesses	18

CT Non-Contrast-Enhanced (Fig. 25.1a)
- Commonly normal
- Eventually narrowed outer CSF spaces and basal cisterns
- Hydrocephalus possible

CT Contrast-Enhanced (Fig. 25.1b)
- Leptomeningeal enhancement

25.5 Imaging Features

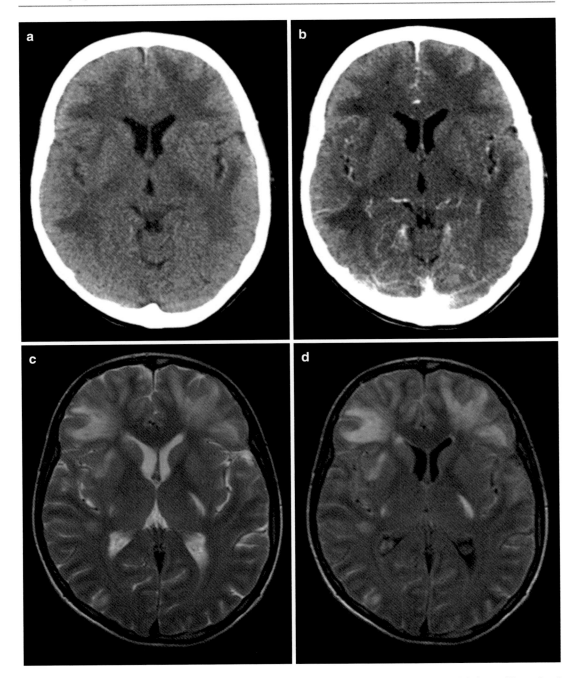

Fig. 25.1 Bacterial meningoencephalitis—leptomeningeal enhancement and bifrontal parenchymal lesions with restricted diffusion; CT non-contrast (**a**), CT contrast (**b**), T2 (**c**), FLAIR (**d**), T1 (**e**), T1 contrast (**f**), DWI (**g**), ADC (**h**)

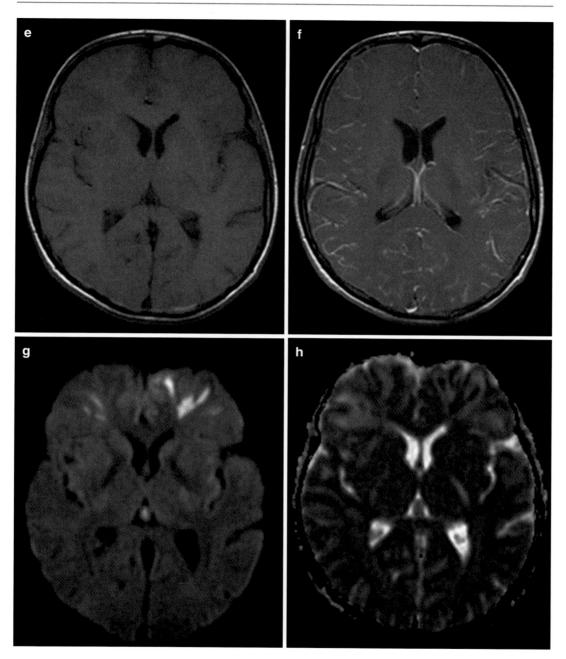

Fig. 25.1 (continued)

MRI-T2/FLAIR (Fig. 25.1c, d)
- Exudate in CSF hyperintense
- Flair most sensitive

MRI-T1 (Fig. 25.1e)
- Exudate isointense

MRI-T1 Contrast-Enhanced (Fig. 25.1f)
- Enhancement of leptomeninges and exudate in sulci

MR-Diffusion Imaging (Fig. 25.1g, h)
- Restricted diffusion possible

25.5.2 Encephalitis

General Imaging Features
- Unspecific T2-hyperintense white matter lesions, may show enhancement (see imaging features of viral infections in Chap. 26)

25.5.3 Brain Abscess

General Imaging Findings
- Ring-enhancing lesion with peripheral edema
- Brain abscess results from cerebritis, typically there are four stages:
  - early cerebritis
  - late cerebritis
  - early capsule
  - late capsule

CT Non-Contrast-Enhanced (Fig. 25.2a)
- Ring-shaped lesion with low attenuation in center surrounded by hypodensity (edema)

CT Contrast-Enhanced (Fig. 25.2b)
- Ring enhancement

MRI-T2 (Fig. 25.2c)
- Hyperintense center with hypointense rim
- Surrounding hyperintensity (edema)

MRI-FLAIR (Fig. 25.2d)
- Hyperintense center
- Peripheral edema hyperintense

MRI-T1 (Fig. 25.2e)
- Center hypo- or hyperintense depending on stage
- Capsule: iso- to hyperintense
- Peripheral edema hypointense

MRI-T1 Contrast-Enhanced (Fig. 25.2f)
- Ring enhancement of capsule

MR-Diffusion Imaging (Fig. 25.2g, h)
- Restricted diffusion in center (DWI ↑, ADC↓)

MRI-Perfusion (Fig. 25.2i)
- Low rCBV on rim

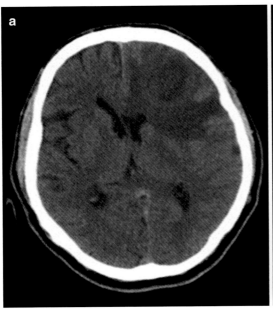 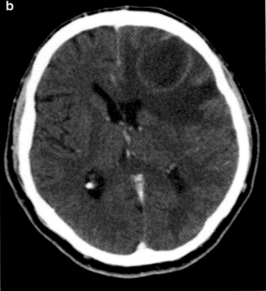

Fig. 25.2 Brain abscess in right frontal lobe with ring enhancement and perifocal edema, restricted diffusion and lactate peak in center; CT non-contrast (**a**), CT contrast (**b**), T2 (**c**), FLAIR (**d**), T1 (**e**), T1 contrast (**f**), DWI (**g**), ADC (**h**), rCBV (**i**), spectroscopy (**j**)

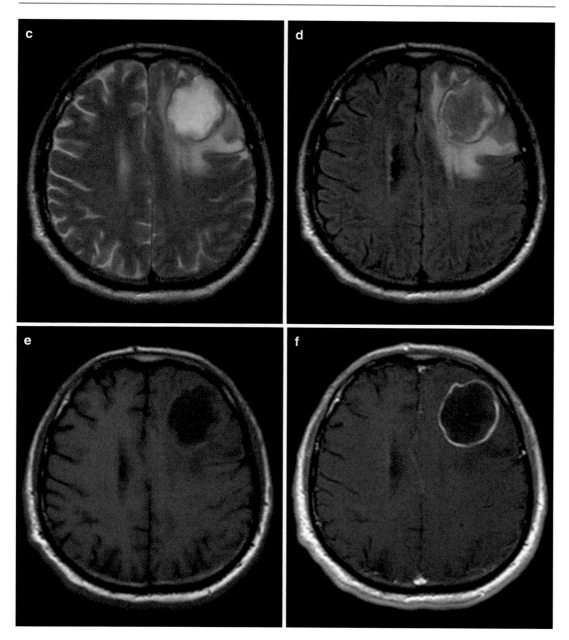

Fig. 25.2 (continued)

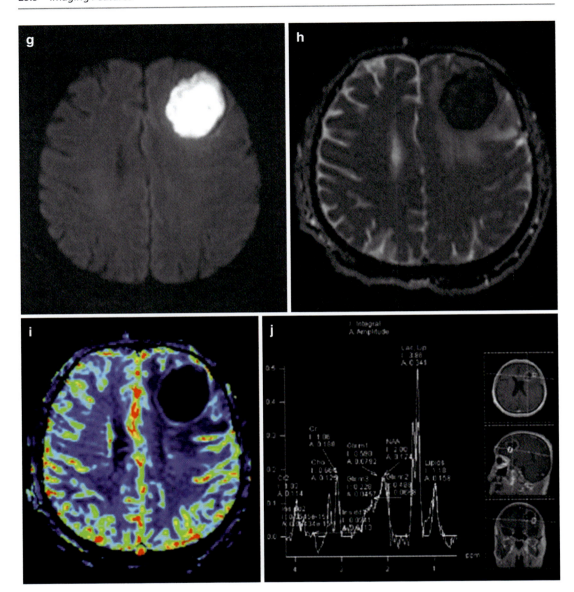

Fig. 25.2 (continued)

MR-Spectroscopy (Fig. 25.2j)
- High values of lactate and amino acids in necrotic center

25.5.4 Subdural Empyema

General Imaging Findings
- Subdural collection with enhancement of surrounding membrane

CT Non-Contrast-Enhanced (Fig. 25.3a)
- Iso- or hypodense extra-axial crescent-shaped collection

CT Contrast-Enhanced
- Rim enhancement

MRI-T2 (Fig. 25.3b)
- Iso- or hyperintense to CSF

MRI-FLAIR (Fig. 25.3c)
- Hyperintense to CSF

MRI-T1 (Fig. 25.3d)
- Hyperintense to CSF

MRI-T1 Contrast-Enhanced (Fig. 25.3e)
- Enhancement of surrounding membrane

MR-Diffusion Imaging (Fig. 25.3f, g)
- Diffusion restriction

Typical MRI imaging findings as found in tuberculosis, neuroborreliosis, and listeriosis are shown in Table 25.10.

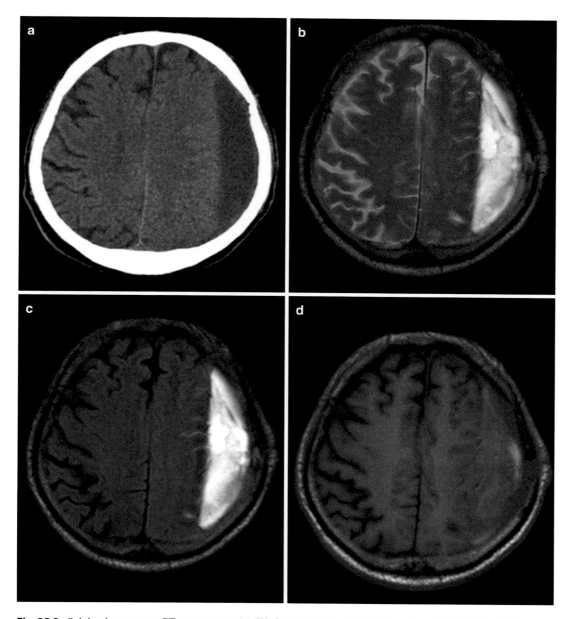

Fig. 25.3 Subdural empyema; CT non-contrast (**a**), T2 (**b**), FLAIR (**c**), T1 (**d**), T1 contrast (**e**), DWI (**f**), ADC (**g**)

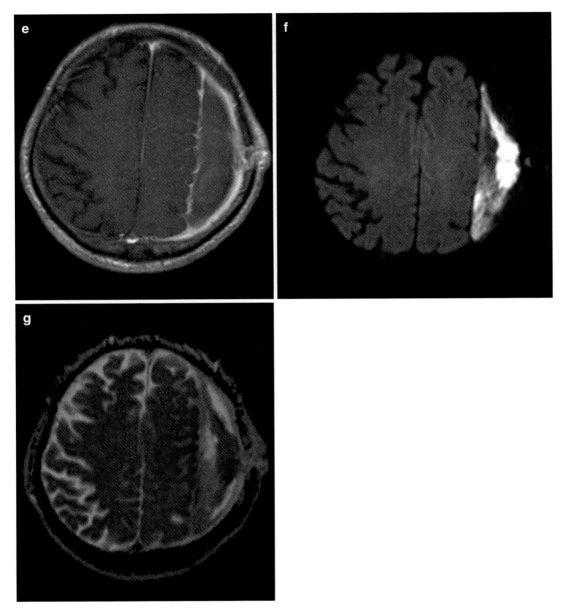

Fig. 25.3 (continued)

Nuclear Medicine Imaging Findings (Fig. 25.4)
- Abscesses caused by bacteria can be seen with FDG-PET.
- MET-PET is also reported to be (false) positive in abscesses.
- FET-PET seems to be less positive in non-neoplastic ring-enhancing intracerebral lesions caused by abscess than MET.
- FET is less accumulated in activated microglia and macrophages in experimental brain abscesses (in contrast to MET and HDG (an analog to FDG)), but taken up by reactive astrocytosis in these patients.
- Case reports state a reduction of CBF and glucose metabolism in patients with neurolues with potentially reversible findings after therapy.
- Historically it is reported that ^{111}indium-granulocyte scintigraphy can be used to address brain abscesses.
- Studies with various imaging agents are performed to assess different pathologic steps in neuroinflammation.

Table 25.10 Typical imaging features of specific bacterial infections

Tuberculosis	Tuberculous meningitis: • Basal pronounced leptomeningeal enhancement • Obstructive hydrocephalus • Infarctions (predominantly in basal ganglia and internal capsule) Tuberculomas: • Non-caseating granuloma: T2-hyperintense and T1-hypointense with solid enhancement • Caseating granuloma: T1- and T2-hypointense with rim enhancement • MR-Spectroscopy shows lactate and lipid peaks, no amino acid peaks (in contrast to pyogenic abscess)
Neuroborreliosis	• Focal or confluent white matter lesions (supratentorial and brain stem) • Leptomeninges and cranial nerves may enhance
Listeriosis	• Focal T2-hyperintensities in brain stem, cerebellum, or medulla oblongata (rhombencephalitis) • Cranial nerves may enhance • Small-seized abscesses with nodular or ring enhancement

25.6 Neuropathology Findings

Macroscopic Features (Figs. 25.5, 25.6, 25.7, 25.8, 25.9, 25.10, and 25.11)
Meningitis/Encephalitis and Abscess
- Epidural abscess (Fig. 25.9a–d)
  – Rare
  – Circumscribed abscess
  – Located in the epidural space of the vertebral canal
- Subdural abscess or empyema
  – Originates from purulent leptomeningitis
  – Extends from adjacent sinusitis, otitis, osteomyelitis
  – Spread over the convexities
- Purulent leptomeningitis (Figs. 25.5a–t, 25.6a–f, and 25.7a–d)
  – Purulent exudate in the leptomeninges
  – Yellowish, reddish, whitish discoloration
- Brain abscess (Figs. 25.8a–l and 25.10a–f)
  – Space-occupying lesion
  – Stages of formation
    ○ Focal cerebritis (day 1–3)
      • Ill-defined region of hyperemia surrounded by edema
    ○ Late cerebritis (day 4–9)
      • Necrotic purulent center
    ○ Early abscess capsule (day 10–13)
      • Poorly defined capsule
    ○ Firm capsule (day 14–later)
      • Firm capsule can be stripped from surrounding edematous tissue
- Ventriculitis (Fig. 25.7a–d)
- Septic embolism
- Cerebral infarction

Microscopic Features (Figs. 25.12, 25.13, 25.14, and 25.15)
- Epidural abscess
- Subdural abscess or empyema
- Purulent leptomeningitis (Fig. 25.12a–n)
  – Bacteria seen either free or in polymorphs
  – Early:
    ○ Polymorphic inflammatory cell infiltrates

25.6 Neuropathology Findings

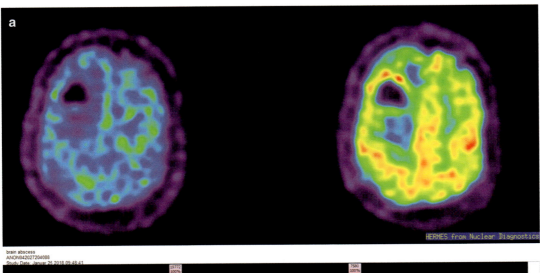

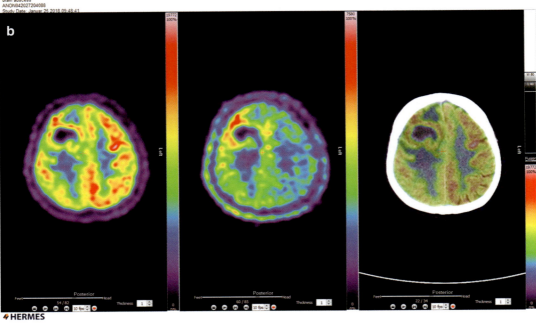

Fig. 25.4 Abscess formation in the right frontal lobe (**a**-left) FET-PET shows a defect without significant surrounding uptake, (**a**-right) FDG-PET shows a central defect with surrounding uptake. (**c**) FDG (left), FET (middle), and fused FDG/CT (right) in a right frontal lobe abscess. (**d**) Slices of FDG-PET and (**e**) slices of FET-PET of an abscess formation

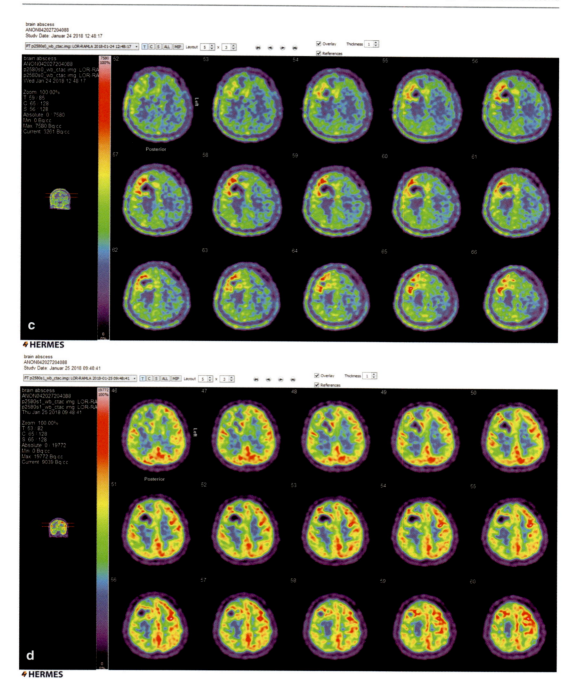

Fig. 25.4 (continued)

25.6 Neuropathology Findings

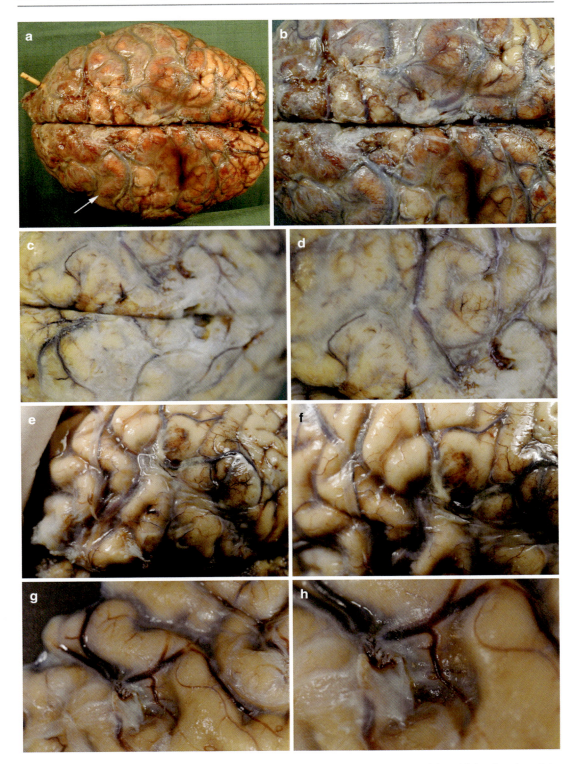

Fig. 25.5 Gross-anatomical appearance of leptomeningitis (**a–t**). Note the whitish-grayish-reddish coloration of the leptomeninges (arrow) reaching deep into the sulcus

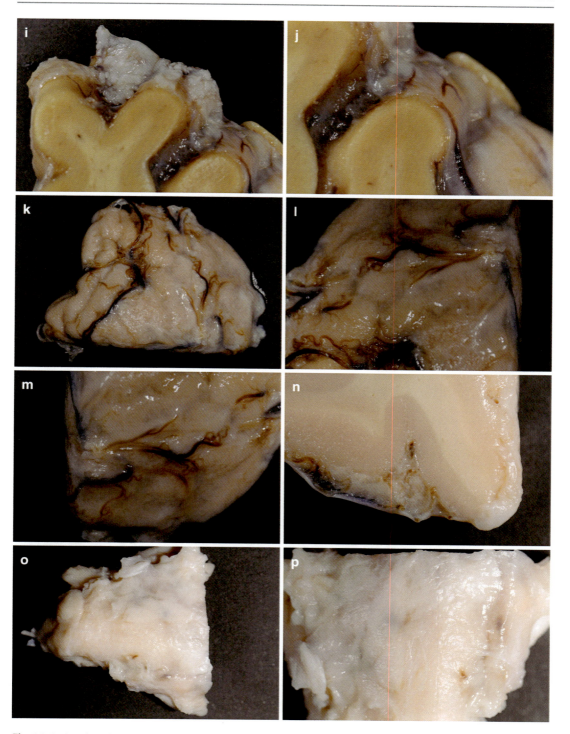

Fig. 25.5 (continued)

25.6 Neuropathology Findings

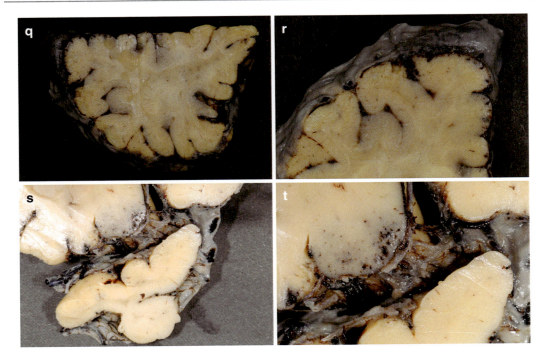

Fig. 25.5 (continued)

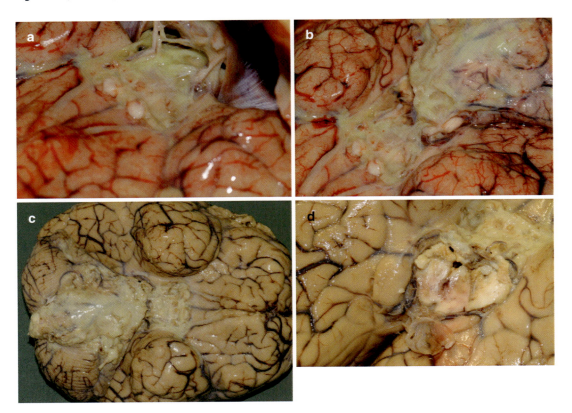

Fig. 25.6 Gross-anatomical appearance of basal leptomeningitis (**a–f**). Fresh unfixed brain with yellowish pus covering the optic chiasm, basal cisterns, and cerebellum (**a**, **b**). Fixed brain (**c–f**) with damage of the mesencephalon (**d**)

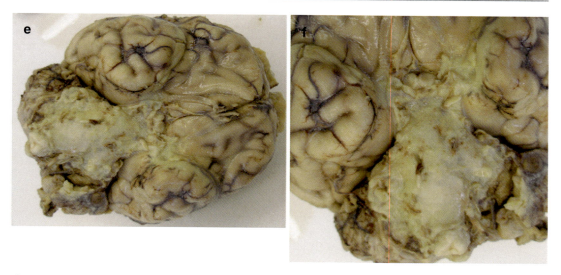

Fig. 25.6 (continued)

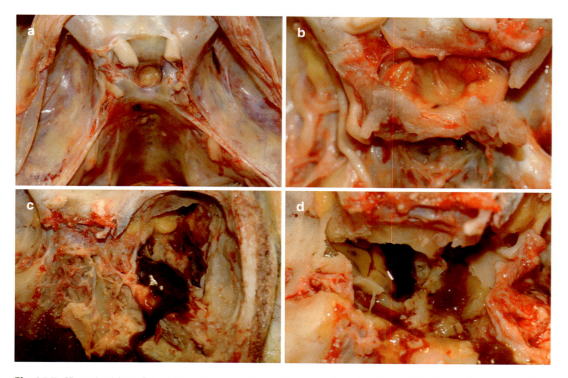

Fig. 25.7 Hypophysitis (**a**, **b**) resulting from spreading and bone eroding sinusitis (**c**, **d**) leading to leptomeningitis

25.6 Neuropathology Findings

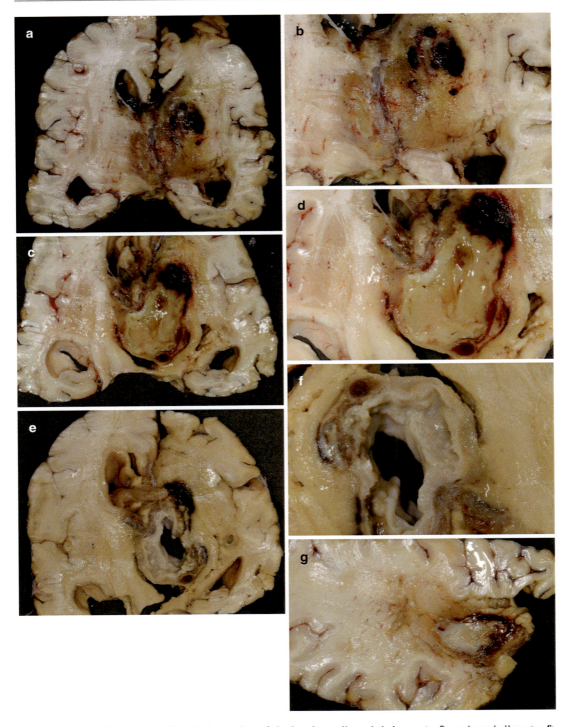

Fig. 25.8 Large abscesses (**a–h**) with destruction of the basal ganglia and thalamus (**a–f**), and cerebellum (**g, f**). Smaller abscesses located in the white matter (**i–l**)

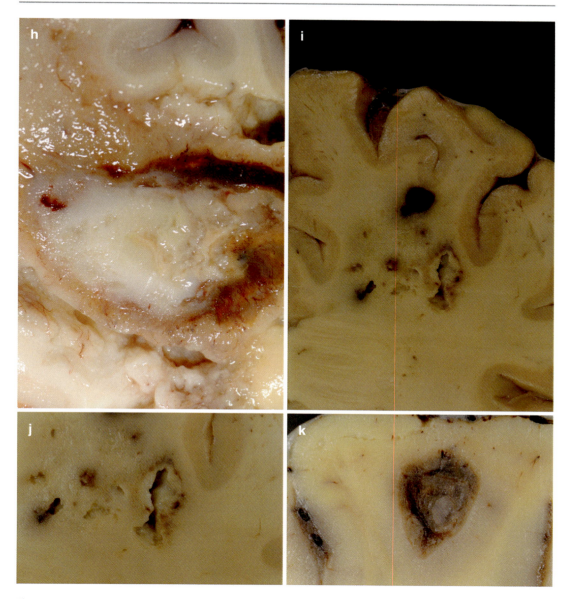

Fig. 25.8 (continued)

25.6 Neuropathology Findings

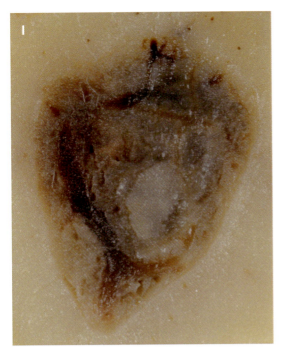

- Later:
  - Fibrinous exudate with lymphocytes, plasma cells, histiocytes, macrophages
- After weeks:
  - Organization into fibrous connective tissue
- Spread of infectious process:
  - Walls of leptomeningeal blood vessels
  - Cranial nerves, spinal roots (Fig. 25.15a–r)
  - Ventricular walls (ventriculitis)
  - Subpial, brain tissue along the Virchow-Robin spaces (leptomeningoencephalitis)
- Brain abscess (Fig. 25.13a–t)
  - Stages of formation
    - Focal cerebritis (day 1–3)
      - Early parenchymal necrosis
      - Vascular congestion
      - Petechial hemorrhages
      - Microthromboses
      - Perivascular fibrinous exudate
      - Infiltration of polymorphs

Fig. 25.8 (continued)

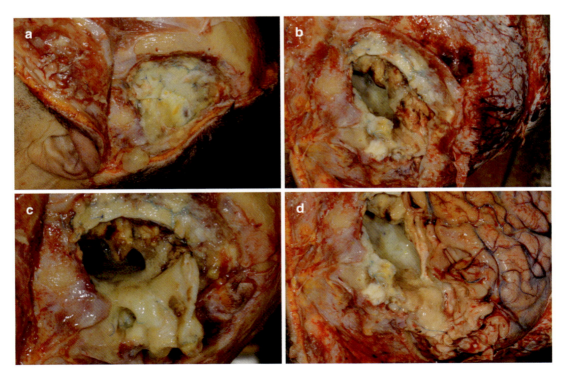

Fig. 25.9 Epidural abscess (**a, b**) resulting from intracerebral abscess (**c, d**) after surgery of meningioma

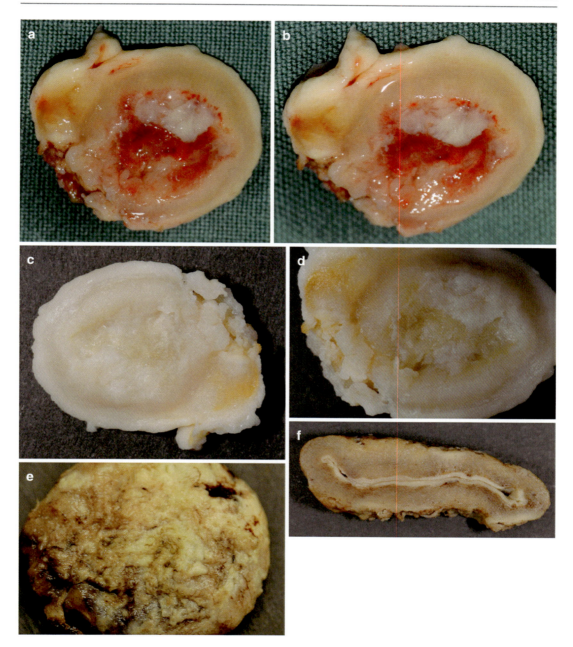

Fig. 25.10 Gross appearance of a resected abscess (**a–f**), fresh unfixed specimen (**a, b**), fixed specimen (**c–f**)

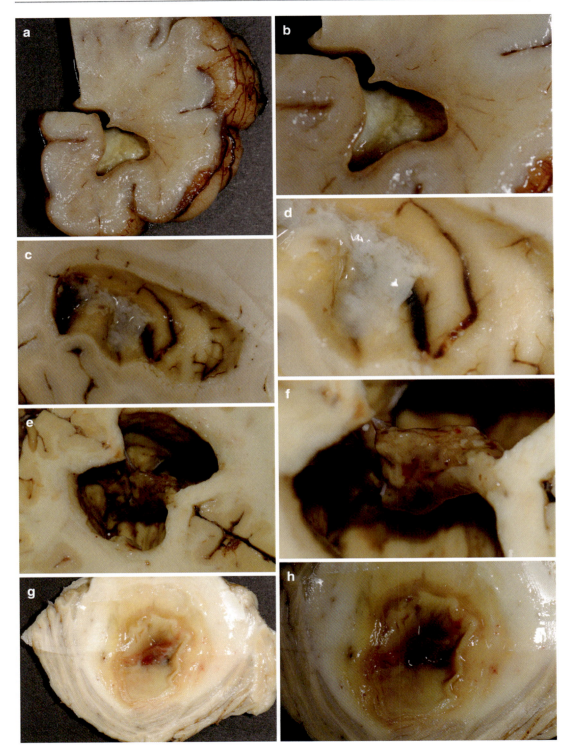

Fig. 25.11 Ventriculitis (**a–j**) in an infant brain (**a, b**), in the posterior-lateral ventricle (**c, d**), third ventricle (**e, f**), cerebral aqueduct and fourth ventricle (**g–j**)

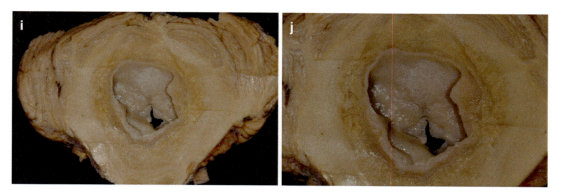

Fig. 25.11 (continued)

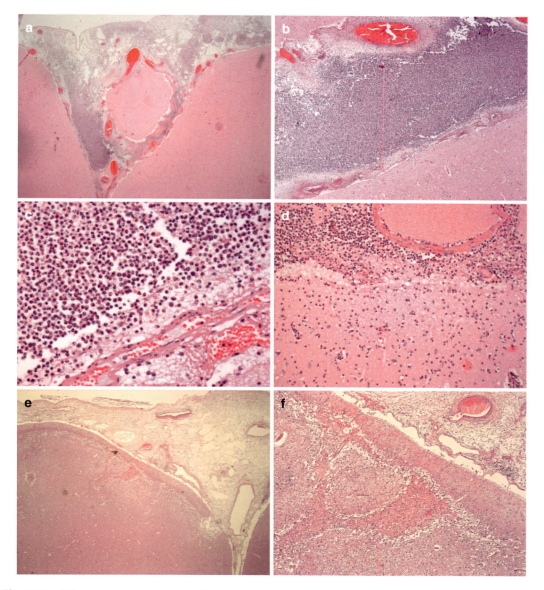

Fig. 25.12 Microscopical appearance of leptomeningitis (**a–n**). Accumulation of lymphocytes, monocytes, and granulocytes in the leptomeningeal space (**a–h**)

25.6 Neuropathology Findings

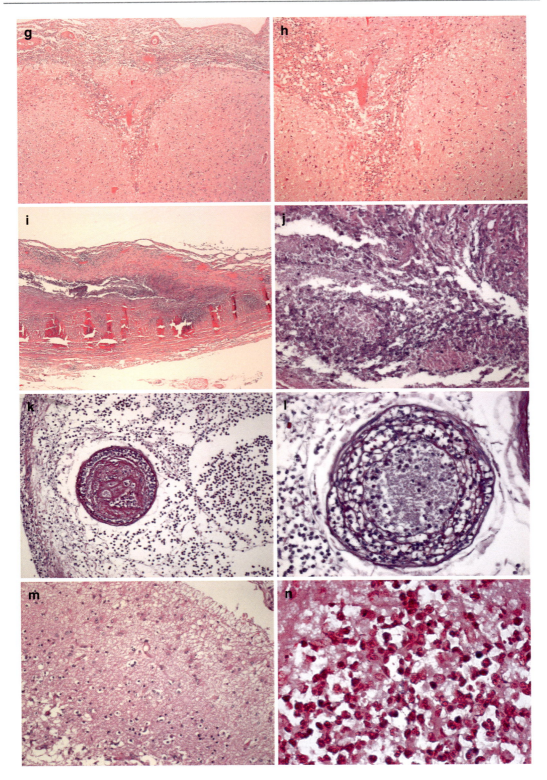

Fig. 25.12 (continued)

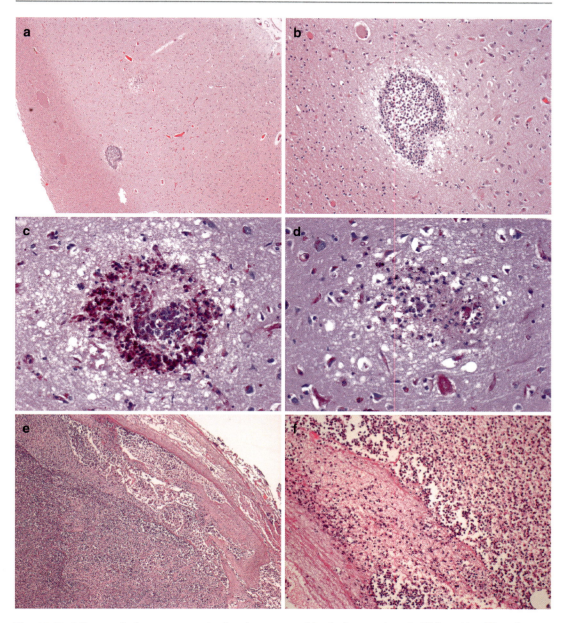

Fig. 25.13 Microscopical appearance of microabscess (**a–d**; **c**, **d**: PAS) and abscesses (**g–l**) with the presence of multinucleated giant cells (**k**, **l**). Immunoprofile: CD45-positive leukocytes (**m**, **n**), CD3-positive T-lymphocytes (**o**, **p**), macrophages (**q**, **r**), and GFAP-positive reactive astrocytes (**s**, **t**)

25.6 Neuropathology Findings

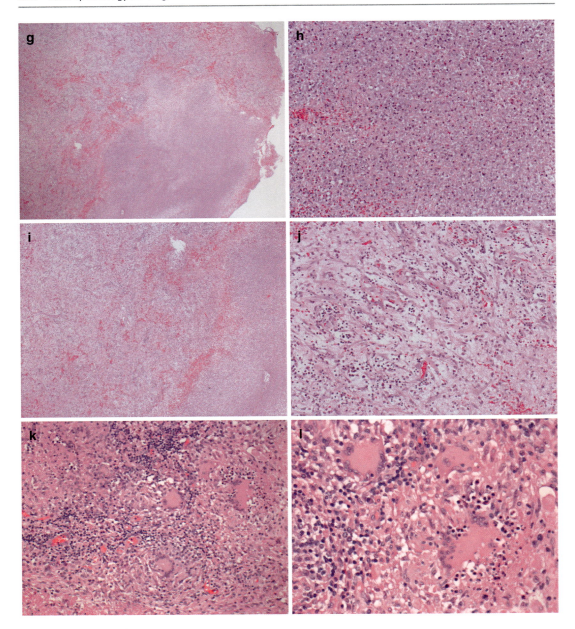

Fig. 25.13 (continued)

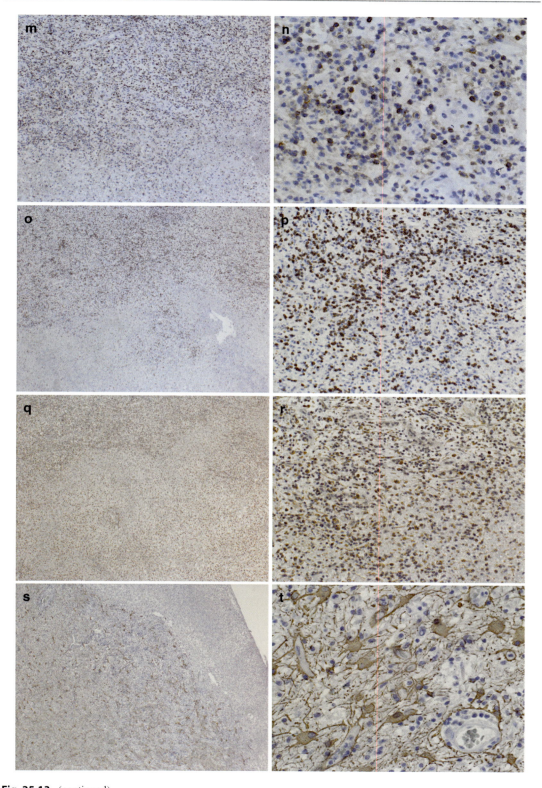

Fig. 25.13 (continued)

25.6 Neuropathology Findings

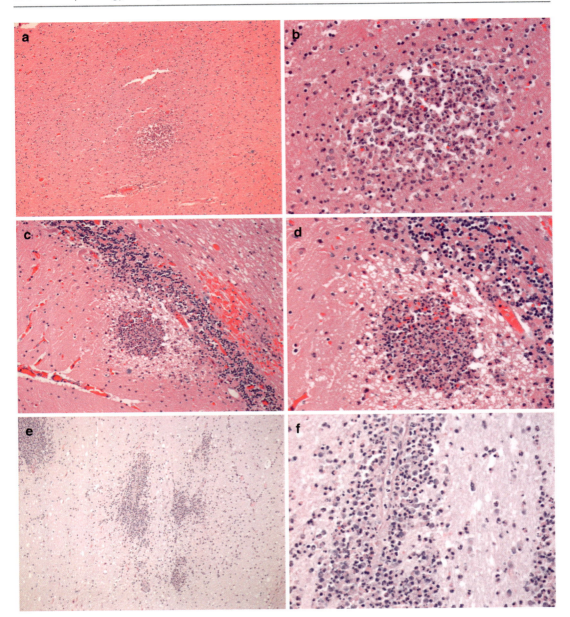

Fig. 25.14 Septic embolic encephalitis. Histological appearances of septic embolic encephalitic foci (**a–f**), in the form of gliomesenchymal nodules in the white matter (**g, h**) and in the substantia nigra (**i**), and as thromboembolus (**j**)

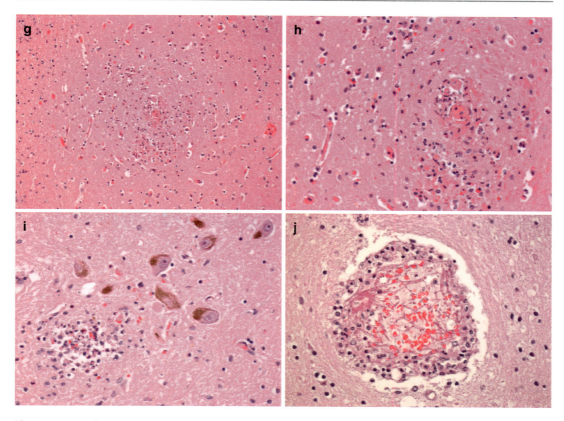

Fig. 25.14 (continued)

- Late cerebritis (day 4–9)
  - Pus surrounded by layer of inflammatory granulation tissue
  - Polymorphs
  - Lymphocytes
  - Macrophages
  - Perivascular spaces cuffed with polymorphs and lymphocytes
- Early abscess capsule (day 10–13)
  - Granulation tissue and lymphocytes
  - Plasma cells
  - Monocytes
  - Macrophages
  - Newly formed blood vessels
  - Fibroblasts
- Firm capsule (day 14–later)
  - Fibroblasts
  - Capsule consists of five layers:
    – Necrotic center invaded by macrophages
    – Granulation tissue with fibroblasts and capillaries
    – Zone of lymphocytes and plasma cells in granulation tissue
    – Dense fibrous tissue with astrocytes
    – Surrounding edematous area of gliosis
- Septic embolism (Fig. 25.14a–j)
  – Septic embolus implanted in a cerebral artery "mycotic aneurysm"

Tuberculosis (Fig. 25.16)
- Epidural or subdural abscess
  – Epidural abscess: complication of the spine (Pott disease)
- Meningitis (Fig. 25.16)
  – Most common form of CNS tuberculosis
  – Thick exudates involving the basal meninges

25.6 Neuropathology Findings

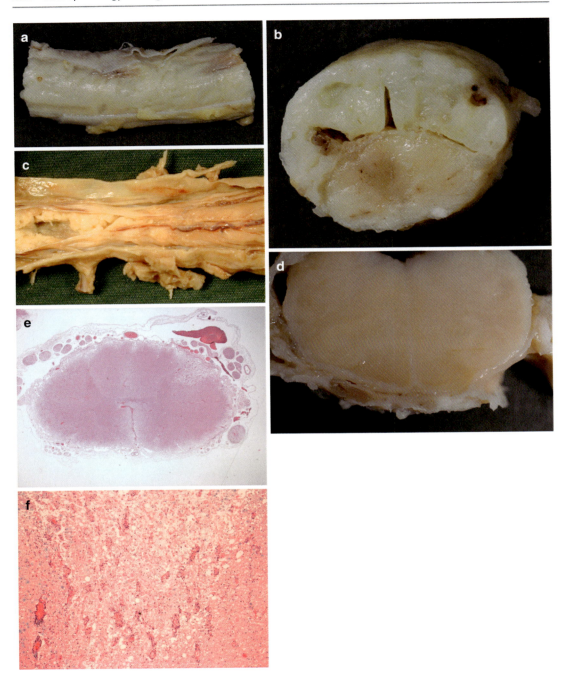

Fig. 25.15 Radiculomyelitis: The spinal cord is surrounded by masses of pus (**a–d**); focal areas of necrosis are evident (**e, f**: HE) (**g, h**: LFB), macrophages (**i, j**: CD68) and microglia (**k, l**: HLA-DRII) populate the necrotic areas. Reactive astrogliosis is pronounced at the border of the necrosis (**m, n**: GFAP); infiltration of a spinal ganglion by lymphocytes (**o, p**); infiltration of nerve roots and vessels by CD3-positive T-lymphocytes (**q, r**)

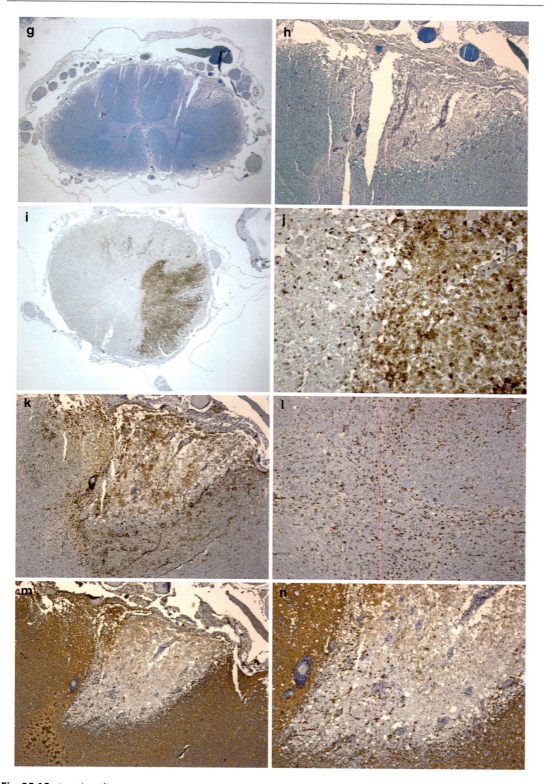

Fig. 25.15 (continued)

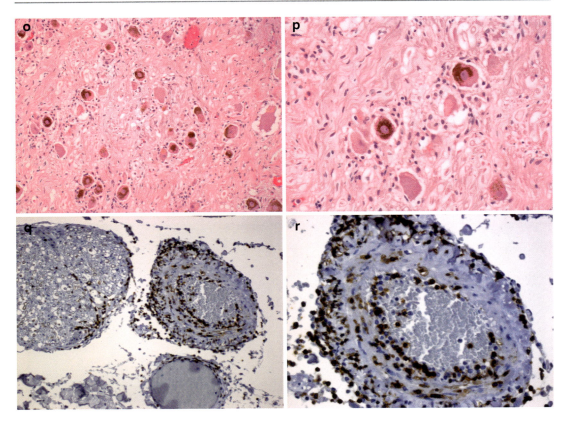

Fig. 25.15 (continued)

- Inflammatory infiltrates in the leptomeninges and subpial region
- Lymphocytes, mononuclear cells
- Epitheloid nodules with few giant cells
- Tubercles:
  ○ central area of caseous necrosis
  ○ surrounded by epitheloid macrophages
  ○ peripheral ring of lymphocytes
- Vascular changes leading to endarteritis obliterans causing ischemic parenchymal lesions
- Tuberculomas of the brain and spinal cord
  ○ Single or multiple
  ○ Spherical lesion with caseous center surrounded by granulomatous tissue including giant cells, lymphocytes, and fibrosis
- Tuberculous abscess

Immunophenotype
- Antibodies specific for various strains of bacteria
- GFAP
- Macrophage markers
- Microglia markers

Differential Diagnosis
- Necrosis of malignant brain tumor or metastasis

25.7 Molecular Neuropathology

- General mechanisms
  - Bacterial invasion and dissemination
  - Bacterial translocation into the CNS
  - Immune activation and inflammatory response in the brain
- Tissue destruction by release of
  - Degradative enzymes
  - Toxins to directly harm tissue
  - Endotoxins altering cell function (cytolytic, receptor-binding)

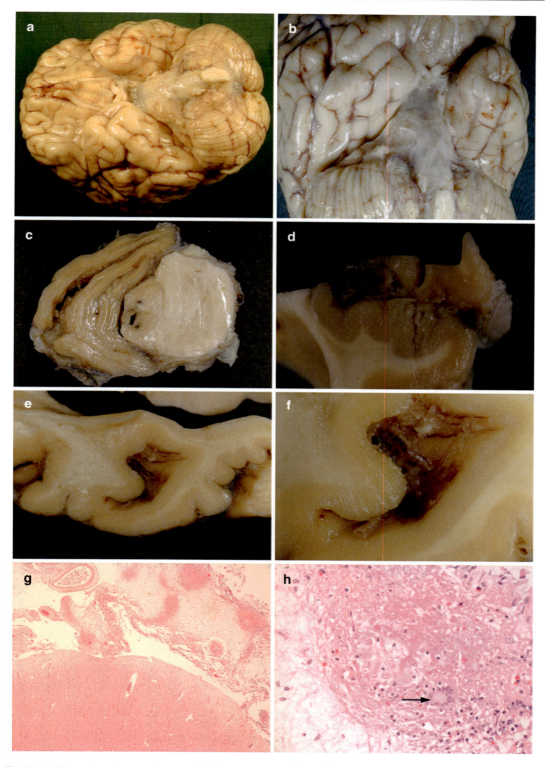

Fig. 25.16 Tuberculous leptomeningoencephalitis: Yellowish-white infiltrates predominantly in the basal leptomeninges (**a–c**) but also cortical leptomeninges (**d–f**). Widened leptomeningeal spaces containing inflammatory cells as well as multinucleated giant cells (arrow) (**g, h**) and demonstration of bacteria in Ziehl-Neelsen stain (**i, j**). CD3-positive T-lymphocytes are evident (**k, l**). Macrophages infiltrate the cerebral cortex from the leptomeninges (**m, n**)

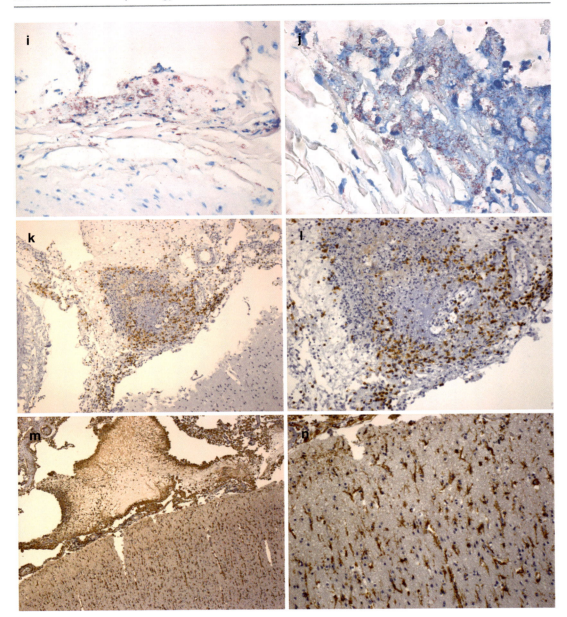

Fig. 25.16 (continued)

- Superantigens
- Inhibition of protein synthesis
- Host genetic factors are major determinants of susceptibility to infectious diseases.
- Differences in susceptibility are due to single base-pair variations (single nucleotide polymorphisms (SNPs)).
- Genes controlling the host response to microbes coding for:
  - Complement system
  - Toll-like receptor (TLR) pathways
  - Cytokines
  - Complement factor H
  - Cytokine and fibrinolysis genes (N. meningitides)
- Genetic polymorphisms associated with TBM
  - SPN—Surface glycoprotein (CD43) involved in Mycobacterium tuberculosis adhesion and pro-inflammatory cytokine induction

- MBL2—Lectin involved in recognition and uptake of M. tuberculosis
- TLR2—Innate pattern recognition receptor
- TLR9—Innate pattern recognition receptor
- TIRAP—Toll adaptor protein
- PKP3–SIGIRR–ANO9—gene region negative regulator of toll-like receptor/IL-1R signaling
- VDR—Vitamin D receptor
- LTA4H—Leucotriene A4 hydrolase
- CCL2—Chemokine
- Epidural abscess
  - Spread from osteomyelitis secondary to frontal or mastoid sinusitis, trauma, or surgery
- Subdural abscess or empyema
  - Extends from adjacent sinusitis, otitis, or osteomyelitis
- Purulent leptomeningitis
  - Hematogeneous dissemination of bacteria
- Brain abscess
  - Local or blood-borne
  - Posttraumatic
  - Hematogeneous origin

Brain Abscess
- Brain abscess development can be divided into four stages (Muzumdar et al. 2011):
  - Early cerebritis (1–4 days)
  - Late cerebritis (4–10 days)
  - Early capsule formation (11–14 days)
  - Late capsule formation (>14 days).
- The glial cell activation in brain abscesses is through parenchymal microglia and astrocytes.
- Activated microglia influence the type and extent of antibacterial adaptive immune response through
  - upregulation of MHC class II
  - costimulatory molecule expression
- The continued release of pro-inflammatory mediators could damage the surrounding brain parenchyma.
- Cytokines IL-1 and TNF-alpha individually dictate essential functions for establishment of an effective antibacterial response in the CNS parenchyma.
- Persistent immune activation associated with elevated levels of

- Interleukin-1β (IL-1β)
- Tumor necrosis factor-alpha (TNFα)
- Macrophage inflammatory protein-2 (MIP-2)

Tuberculous Meningitis (Wilkinson et al. 2017)
- Bacilli reach brain blood capillaries within cells or as extracellular bacilli; the precise mechanism is unknown.
- The endothelium itself can be infected, or infected cells can adhere and undergo diapedesis.
  - Both processes result in breakdown of tight endothelial junctions and the basement membrane.
- Microglial cells can become infected.
  - Together with infiltrating cells, they produce inflammatory chemoattractants that result in further breakdown of the blood–brain barrier and influx of uninfected cells, including innate and specific T- and B-lymphocytes.
- The nascent granuloma might rupture, leading to meningeal and intracerebral dissemination of infection.

25.8 Treatment and Prognosis

Treatment
- Antibiotic medication having the following mechanisms:
  - Inhibition of cell wall synthesis
    - Penicillin, cephalosporin
  - Inhibition of protein synthesis
    - Tetracyclines, macrolides
  - Inhibition of nucleic acid synthesis
    - Quinolones, metronidazole
  - Antimetabolite
    - Sulphonamides
- Surgery for brain abscess
  - Extirpation
  - Aspiration

Treatment of Patients with Abscess
- Operation: 87%
- Aspiration: 66%
- Excision: 26%
- Aspiration and excision: 14%
- Stereotactic operation: 22%

- Reoperation: 31%
- Medical treatment: 12%
- Steroids: 55%

Biologic Behavior–Prognosis–Prognostic Factors
- Abscess:
  - Raised intracranial pressure with cerebral herniation
  - Rupture of the abscess with ventricular empyema
  - Outcome
    - Mortality 20%
    - Mortality studies using only stereotactic aspiration 3%
    - Good outcome 57%

Selected References

Agarwal R, Sze G (2009) Neuro-lyme disease: MR imaging findings. Radiology 253(1):167–173. https://doi.org/10.1148/radiol.2531081103

Alper G, Knepper L, Kanal E (1996) MR findings in listerial rhombencephalitis. AJNR Am J Neuroradiol 17(3):593–596

Alvis Miranda H, Castellar-Leones SM, Elzain MA, Moscote-Salazar LR (2013) Brain abscess: current management. J Neurosci Rural Pract 4(suppl 1):S67–S81. https://doi.org/10.4103/0976-3147.116472

Barichello T, Generoso JS, Simoes LR, Goularte JA, Petronilho F, Saigal P, Badawy M, Quevedo J (2016) Role of microglial activation in the pathophysiology of bacterial meningitis. Mol Neurobiol 53(3):1770–1781. https://doi.org/10.1007/s12035-015-9107-4

Bernardini GL (2004) Diagnosis and management of brain abscess and subdural empyema. Curr Neurol Neurosci Rep 4(6):448–456

Bleck TP (2013) Bacterial meningitis and other nonviral infections of the nervous system. Crit Care Clin 29(4):975–987. https://doi.org/10.1016/j.ccc.2013.07.001

Boucher A, Herrmann JL, Morand P, Buzele R, Crabol Y, Stahl JP, Mailles A (2017) Epidemiology of infectious encephalitis causes in 2016. Med Mal Infect 47(3):221–235. https://doi.org/10.1016/j.medmal.2017.02.003

Bourgi K, Fiske C, Sterling TR (2017) Tuberculosis meningitis. Curr Infect Dis Rep 19(11):39. https://doi.org/10.1007/s11908-017-0595-4

Brook I (2017) Microbiology and treatment of brain abscess. J Clin Neurosci 38:8–12. https://doi.org/10.1016/j.jocn.2016.12.035

Brouwer MC, Coutinho JM, van de Beek D (2014a) Clinical characteristics and outcome of brain abscess: systematic review and meta-analysis. Neurology 82(9):806–813. https://doi.org/10.1212/wnl.0000000000000172

Brouwer MC, Tunkel AR, McKhann GM II, van de Beek D (2014b) Brain abscess. N Engl J Med 371(5):447–456. https://doi.org/10.1056/NEJMra1301635

Brouwer MC, Wijdicks EF, van de Beek D (2016) What's new in bacterial meningitis. Intensive Care Med 42(3):415–417. https://doi.org/10.1007/s00134-015-4057-x

Doran KS, Fulde M, Gratz N, Kim BJ, Nau R, Prasadarao N, Schubert-Unkmeir A, Tuomanen EI, Valentin-Weigand P (2016) Host-pathogen interactions in bacterial meningitis. Acta Neuropathol 131(2):185–209. https://doi.org/10.1007/s00401-015-1531-z

Erdogan E, Cansever T (2008) Pyogenic brain abscess. Neurosurg Focus 24(6):E2. https://doi.org/10.3171/foc/2008/24/6/e2

Esen N, Kielian T (2009) Toll-like receptors in brain abscess. Curr Top Microbiol Immunol 336:41–61. https://doi.org/10.1007/978-3-642-00549-7_3

Falcone S, Post MJ (2000) Encephalitis, cerebritis, and brain abscess: pathophysiology and imaging findings. Neuroimaging Clin N Am 10(2):333–353

Gaieski DF, Nathan BR, O'Brien NF (2015) Emergency neurologic life support: meningitis and encephalitis. Neurocrit Care 23(suppl 2):S110–S118. https://doi.org/10.1007/s12028-015-0165-2

Gordon SM, Srinivasan L, Harris MC (2017) Neonatal meningitis: overcoming challenges in diagnosis, prognosis, and treatment with omics. Front Pediatr 5:139. https://doi.org/10.3389/fped.2017.00139

Haimes AB, Zimmerman RD, Morgello S, Weingarten K, Becker RD, Jennis R, Deck MD (1989) MR imaging of brain abscesses. AJR Am J Roentgenol 152(5):1073–1085. https://doi.org/10.2214/ajr.152.5.1073

Hazany S, Go JL, Law M (2014) Magnetic resonance imaging of infectious meningitis and ventriculitis in adults. Top Magn Reson Imaging 23(5):315–325. https://doi.org/10.1097/rmr.0000000000000034

Heckenberg SG, Brouwer MC, van de Beek D (2014) Bacterial meningitis. Handb Clin Neurol 121:1361–1375. https://doi.org/10.1016/b978-0-7020-4088-7.00093-6

Hemmert AC, Gilbreath JJ (2016) The current state of diagnostics for meningitis and encephalitis. MLO Med Lab Obs 48(7):12–14. quiz 16

Honda H, Warren DK (2009) Central nervous system infections: meningitis and brain abscess. Infect Dis Clin N Am 23(3):609–623. https://doi.org/10.1016/j.idc.2009.04.009

Kumar R, Pandey CK, Bose N, Sahay S (2002) Tuberculous brain abscess: clinical presentation, pathophysiology and treatment (in children). Childs Nerv Syst 18(3-4):118–123. https://doi.org/10.1007/s00381-002-0575-2

Lucas MJ, Brouwer MC, van de Beek D (2016) Neurological sequelae of bacterial meningitis. J Infect 73(1):18–27. https://doi.org/10.1016/j.jinf.2016.04.009

Mailles A, Stahl JP, Bloch KC (2017) Update and new insights in encephalitis. Clin Microbiol Infect 23(9):607–613. https://doi.org/10.1016/j.cmi.2017.05.002

McGill F, Heyderman RS, Panagiotou S, Tunkel AR, Solomon T (2016) Acute bacterial meningitis in adults. Lancet 388(10063):3036–3047. https://doi.org/10.1016/s0140-6736(16)30654-7

Muzumdar D, Jhawar S, Goel A (2011) Brain abscess: an overview. Int J Surg (London, England) 9(2):136–144. https://doi.org/10.1016/j.ijsu.2010.11.005

Radetsky M (2014) Fulminant bacterial meningitis. Pediatr Infect Dis J 33(2):204–207. https://doi.org/10.1097/01.inf.0000435508.67490.f0

Rath TJ, Hughes M, Arabi M, Shah GV (2012) Imaging of cerebritis, encephalitis, and brain abscess. Neuroimaging Clin N Am 22(4):585–607. https://doi.org/10.1016/j.nic.2012.04.002

Richie MB, Josephson SA (2015) A practical approach to meningitis and encephalitis. Semin Neurol 35(6):611–620. https://doi.org/10.1055/s-0035-1564686

Rosenberg J, Galen BT (2017) Recurrent meningitis. Curr Pain Headache Rep 21(7):33. https://doi.org/10.1007/s11916-017-0635-7

Saez-Llorens X, Nieto-Guevara J (2013) Brain abscess. Handb Clin Neurol 112:1127–1134. https://doi.org/10.1016/b978-0-444-52910-7.00032-5

Sarrazin JL, Bonneville F, Martin-Blondel G (2012) Brain infections. Diagn Interv Imaging 93(6):473–490. https://doi.org/10.1016/j.diii.2012.04.020

Sheehan JP, Jane JA, Ray DK, Goodkin HP (2008) Brain abscess in children. Neurosurg Focus 24(6):E6. https://doi.org/10.3171/foc/2008/24/6/e6

Skoura E, Zumla A, Bomanji J (2015) Imaging in tuberculosis. Int J Infect Dis 32:87–93. https://doi.org/10.1016/j.ijid.2014.12.007

Sonneville R, Ruimy R, Benzonana N, Riffaud L, Carsin A, Tadie JM, Piau C, Revest M, Tattevin P (2017) An update on bacterial brain abscess in immunocompetent patients. Clin Microbiol Infect 23(9):614–620. https://doi.org/10.1016/j.cmi.2017.05.004

Stephanov S, Sidani AH (2002) Intracranial subdural empyema and its management. A review of the literature with comment. Swiss Surg 8(4):159–163

Sundaram C, Lakshmi V (2006) Pathogenesis and pathology of brain abscess. Indian J Pathol Microbiol 49(3):317–326

Swanson D (2015) Meningitis. Pediatr Rev 36(12):514–524.; quiz 525–526. https://doi.org/10.1542/pir.36-12-514

Thacker S, Cruce C, Rowlett JD (2015) Update on meningitis in adolescents and young adults. Adolesc Med State Art Rev 26(3):658–674

Viallon A, Botelho-Nevers E, Zeni F (2016) Clinical decision rules for acute bacterial meningitis: current insights. Open Access Emerg Med 8:7–16. https://doi.org/10.2147/oaem.s69975

Wilkinson RJ, Rohlwink U, Misra UK, van Crevel R, Mai NTH, Dooley KE, Caws M, Figaji A, Savic R, Solomons R, Thwaites GE (2017) Tuberculous meningitis. Nat Rev Neurol 13(10):581–598. https://doi.org/10.1038/nrneurol.2017.120

Wong AM, Zimmerman RA, Simon EM, Pollock AN, Bilaniuk LT (2004) Diffusion-weighted MR imaging of subdural empyemas in children. AJNR Am J Neuroradiol 25(6):1016–1021

Infections: Viruses

26.1 Clinical Signs and Symptoms

Signs and symptoms of (Table 26.1):

- Meningitis
- Encephalitis
  - Cerebral dysfunctions (delirium, lethargy, confusion, stupor, coma)
  - Seizures
  - Focal neurologic deficits

26.2 Classification of Viruses

Classification of viruses based on their nuclei acid into (Tables 26.2 and 26.3):

- DNA viruses
- RNA viruses

The diseases caused by viruses are listed in Table 26.4 while brain diseases caused by viruses are depicted in Tables 26.5 and 26.6.

26.3 Epidemiology

Incidence
- 1.5–7 cases/100,000 inhabitants/year, excluding epidemics
- True incidence of these infections is difficult to determine because

Table 26.1 Neurologic signs and syndromes related to affected regions

Localization	Syndrome	Neurologic signs
Meninges	• Meningitis	• Headache • Vomiting • Photophobia • Focal neurologic deficits • Alterations in consciousness
Brain parenchyma diffuse	• Encephalitis	• Alterations in consciousness • Seizures • Multifocal neurologic deficits
Brain parenchyma focal	• Encephalitis • Cerebritis	• Focal neurologic deficits • Seizures
Brain stem and posterior cranial fossa	• Brain stem encephalitis • Cerebellitis	• Opto- and pupillomotor disturbances • Nuclear cranial nerve lesions • Dysarthria • Bilateral pyramidal tract signs • Alterations in consciousness • Breathing insufficiency • Vegetative signs
Spinal cord	• Myelitis	• Paraplegia • Brown Séquard syndrome
Arteries	• Arteritis	• Sudden focal neurologic deficit
Veins	• Septic venous sinus thrombosis	• Headache • Seizures • Raised brain pressure • Focal neurologic deficits

Table 26.2 Subdivision of viruses

DNA viruses	Enveloped	• Pox • Herpes • Hepadna
	Naked capsid	• Polyoma, Papilloma, Adeno • Parvo
RNA viruses	+RNA	• Naked capsid: Picorna, Calici • Enveloped: Toga, Flavi, Corona
	−RNA	• Enveloped: Rhabdo, Filo, Orthomyxo, Paramyxo, Bunya, Arena
	±RNA	• Double capsid: Reo
	+RNA via DNA	• Enveloped: Retro

– Many cases are unreported.
– The diagnosis may not be considered.
– A specific viral etiology is never confirmed.

Age Incidence
– all ages possible
– CMV: congenital, adulthood
– HIV: adulthood

Sex Incidence
• dependent on virus
  – HIV: predominantly males
  – CMV: equal distribution

Table 26.3 A detailed subdivision of viruses

Viral genome		Family name of virus	Family members
DNA	Double-stranded	Herpesviridae	• HSV-1 • HSV-2 • Varicella-zoster virus • Cytomegalovirus • Epstein-Barr virus • Human herpesvirus 6 • Human herpesvirus 7 • Human herpesvirus 8 • Herpes simiae
		Adenoviridae	• Adenovirus
		Papovaviridae	• JC virus • Simian virus 40
	Single-stranded	Parvoviridae	• Parvovirus B19
RNA	Double-stranded	Reoviridae	• Coltivirus • Seadornavirus
	Single-stranded sense non-segmented	Retroviridae	• Deltaretrovirus • Lentivirus
		Coronaviridae	• Coronavirus
		Togaviridae	• Alphavirus
		Flaviviridae	• Flavivirus
		Picornaviridae	• Enterovirus
	Single-stranded antisense segmented	Bunyaviridae	• Orthobunyavirus • Phlebovirus
		Arenaviridae	• Arenavirus
	Single-stranded antisense non-segmented	Orthomyxoviridae	• Influenza viruses
		Paramyxoviridae	• Henipavirus • Morbilivirus • Rubulavirus
		Rhabdoviridae	• Rabies • Borna
		Filoviridae	• Ebola

Table 26.4 List of viruses and related diseases of viruses

	Viral family	Virus	Disease
DNA	Papillomavirus		• Warts • Condylomas • Cervical cancer
	Polyomaviridae	BK virus	• Renal disease
		JC virus	• Progressive multifocal leukoencephalopathy
	Adenoviridae		• Respiratory disease • Meningoencephalitis
	Alphaherpesvirinae	Herpesvirus 1	• Encephalitis
		Herpesvirus 2	• Encephalitis
		Varicella-zoster virus	• Encephalitis
	Gammaherpesvirinae	Epstein-Barr virus	• Encephalitis
	Betaherpesvirinae	Cytomegalovirus	• Encephalitis
	Poxviruses		• Smallpox
	Parvoviruses		• Erythema infectiosum
	Picornaviruses	Enterovirus	• Encephalitis • Meningitis • Poliovirus infections (polyomyelitis, paralytic polio)
		Hepatovirus	• Hepatitis
RNA	Picornaviridae	Poliovirus	• Poliomyelitis • Postpolio syndrome
		Enteroviruses	
		Cardiovirus genus	
		Encephalomyocarditis virus	
	Arboviruses	Togaviridae, alphavirus genus	• Eastern equine encephalitis • Western equine encephalitis • Venezuelan equine encephalitis
		Flaviviridae	• Japanese encephalitis • St. Louis Encephalitis • Russian spring-summer encephalitis • Central European encephalitis • Kyasanur forest disease • Murray valley encephalitis • Rocio
		Bunyaviridae	• La Crosse encephalitis • Snowshoe hare virus • California encephalitis • Jamestown canyon encephalitis
		Reoviridae	• Colorado tick fever
	Paramyxoviruses	Measles virus	• Measles
		Parainfluenza virus	• Limited respiratory tract infection
		Mumps virus	• Mumps
	Orthomyxoviruses	Influenza A and B viruses	• Influenza
	Rhabdoviruses	Rhabdovirus	• Rabies
	Retroviruses	Oncovirinae (HTLV)	• Tropical spastic paraparesis
		Lentivirinae (HIV)	• Acquired immune deficiency syndrome (AIDS)

Table 26.5 Viral infections of the brain and their causative viral agents

Encephalitis	• HSV-1 • Toga, Flavi, Bunya encephalitis viruses • Picornaviruses • Arboencephalitis virus • Varicella-zoster virus • Rabies virus • Polioviruses • Coxsackie A and B viruses

Meningitis	• HSV-2
	• Picornaviruses
	• Mumps virus
	• Enteroviruses
	  – Echoviruses
	  – Coxsackie virus
	  – Poliovirus
	• Adenoviruses

Paralysis	• Poliovirus • Enterovirus 70 and 71 • Coxsackie A7 virus
Postinfectious encephalitis (immune mediated)	• Measles virus • Mumps virus • Rubella virus • Varicella-zoster virus • Influenza virus
Other	• JC virus-progressive multifocal leukoencephalopathy (PML) • Human Immunodeficiency Virus (HIV) • Human T-cell lymphotropic virus 1 (HTLV-1) (tropical spastic paraparesis) • Measles variant (subacute sclerosing panencephalitis)

Table 26.6 Acute and chronic viral infection affecting the brain

Acute viral infection	• Aseptic meningitis
	• Polyomyelitis
	• Neonatal enteroviral encephalitis
	• Herpesvirus infections
	  – Herpes simplex virus infection
	  – Atypical herpes simplex encephalitis
	  – Chronic granulomatous herpes simplex encephalitis
	  – Necrotizing myelopathy
	  – Neonatal HSV encephalitis
	  – Varicella-zoster virus (ZVZ) infection
	  – Epstein-Barr virus (EBV) infection
	  – Cytomegalovirus (CMV) infection
	  – Human herpesviruses 6 and 7
	• Adenovirus
	• Paramyxoviruses
	  – Mumps virus
	  – Measles
	• Rubella encephalitis
	• Rabies
	• Arbovirus infections

Chromic and subacute viral infections	• Chronic enteroviral encephalomyelitis • Subacute measles encephalitis • Subacute sclerosing panencephalitis (SSPE) • Progressive rubella panencephalitis • Progressive multifocal leukoencephalopathy (PML) • Human T-cell leukemia/lymphotropic virus-1 (HTLV-1) • Human immunodeficiency virus (HIV) • Rasmussen encephalitis

Localization
- Brain, any region
- Temporal lobe for HSV

26.4 Neuroimaging Findings

General Imaging Findings
- Viral CNS infections can either lead to meningitis or (meningo-)encephalitis.
- Imaging of viral encephalitis often nonspecific—like focal or diffuse edema (acute infection) or focal atrophy (chronic infection)—except HSV encephalitis showing an almost pathognomonic involvement of limbic system.
- Location depends on causative agent.

CT Non-Contrast-Enhanced
- Meningitis: Normal
- Encephalitis: Hypodense edema, loss of gray-white matter differentiation, chronic infection may cause brain atrophy

CT Contrast-Enhanced
- Meningitis: Meningeal enhancement often missing
- Encephalitis: Enhancement possible

MRI-T2
- Encephalitis: Hyperintensity of involved brain areas

MRI-FLAIR
- Encephalitis: Hyperintensity of involved brain areas

MRI-T1
- Encephalitis: Hypointense edema with loss of gray-white matter differentiation

MRI-T1 Contrast-Enhanced
- Meningitis: Weak meningeal enhancement
- Encephalitis: Variable enhancement

MRI-T2*/SWI
- Encephalitis: Hemorrhages (HSV, VZV, Japanese encephalitis)

MR-Diffusion Imaging
- Encephalitis: Diffusion restriction common

Typical MR imaging patterns of specific viral encephalitides are listed in Table 26.7.

Nuclear Medicine Imaging Findings
- In HIV-infected patients
  - Reduced brain perfusion SPECT and reduced FDG-PET uptake of cortical structures (medial frontal, temporoparietal) are described.
  - FDG shows diffuse hypermetabolism in subcortical and deep white matter, basal ganglia, and thalami in some cases.
- In herpes simplex encephalitis
  - HMPAO showed increased uptake followed by a decrease in tracer uptake in the recovery phase and ECD decreased uptake of the affected temporal lobe (most likely due to disturbed membrane and intracellular metabolism).
  - FDG-PET shows hippocampal hypermetabolism in the acute phase of herpes simplex encephalitis followed by hypometabolism after 3–9 months, but it is reported, that hypometabolism can persist for years.
- Studies with various imaging agents are performed to assess different pathologic steps in neuroinflammation.

26.5 Neuropathology Findings

Macroscopic Features
- No discernible lesion
- Hemorrhagic lesion
- Necrotic lesion

Table 26.7 Typical MR imaging patterns of specific viral encephalitides

HSV	• Limbic system and temporal lobe • Often hemorrhages and enhancement
CMV	• Periventricular white matter, subependymal enhancement • Calcifications in perinatal CMV
EBV	• Symmetric involvement of basal ganglia, thalami, cortex, or brain stem • Rarely EBV-cerebellitis
VZV	• Multifocal cortical areas • Hemorrhagic infarctions possible
HIV	• Brain atrophy • Symmetric confluent white matter lesions (periventricular, basal ganglia, centrum semiovale, brain stem, cerebellum), • No enhancement
Rabies virus	• Diffuse involvement of basal ganglia, thalami, periventricular white matter, brain stem, and hippocampi
TBEV (Tick-borne encephalitis virus)	• MRI and CT often normal • Rarely lesions in thalamus, cerebellum, caudate nucleus, and brain stem
JC Virus (PML)	• Confluent subcortical white matter lesions, predominantly in parieto-occipital lobes • U-fibers involved
JEV (Japanese encephalitis virus)	• Bilateral symmetric lesions in thalami, basal ganglia, and midbrain
Enteroviruses	• Posterior medulla oblongata and pons, dentate nuclei, and midbrain

Microscopic Features
- See specific subchapters
- Perivascular lymphocytic cuffing
- Gliomesenchymal nodules
- Multinucleated giant cells
- Large cells with inclusion bodies
- Reactive astrogliosis
- Leukoencephalopathies

Immunohistochemical Staining Characteristics
- Antibodies directed against a specific virus or part of the virus
- HIV: p24, gp41

Differential Diagnosis
- Necrosis of malignant tumors or metastases
- Necrosis from other infectious agents

26.6 Molecular Neuropathology

Properties of viruses, i.e., DNA versus RNA viruses (Table 26.8)
- Entry into the body
  - Viral receptors (Table 26.9)
- Delivery of the virus to the target tissue
- Interaction of virus with target tissue
  - Stability of virus in the body
  - Ability to establish viremia
  - Ability to spread through the reticuloendothelial system
- Cytopathogenesis
  - Failed infection (abortive infection)
  - Cell death (lytic infection)
  - Replication without cell death (persistent infection)
  - Presence of virus without production but with potential for reactivation (latent-recurrent infection)
- Host responses
  - Antigen-nonspecific (innate) host defenses
  - Antigen-specific immune responses
  - Viral mechanisms of escape to immune responses
- Immunopathology
  - Interferon
  - T-cell responses: cell killing, inflammation

Table 26.8 Properties of DNA viruses and RNA viruses

DNA viruses	RNA viruses
• DNA is not transient or labile.	• RNA is labile and transient.
• Many DAN viruses establish persistent infections.	• Most RNA viruses replicate in the cytoplasm.
• DNA genomes reside in the nucleus.	• Cells cannot replicate RNA. RNA viruses must encode an RNA-dependent RNA polymerase.
• Viral DNA resembles host DNA for transcription and replication.	• The genome structure determines the mechanism of transcription and replication.
• Viral genes must interact with host transcriptional machinery.	• RNA viruses are prone to mutation.
• Viral gene transcription is temporally regulated.	• The genome structure and polarity determine how viral messenger RNA is generated and proteins are processed.
• Early genes encode DNA-binding proteins and enzymes.	
• Late genes encode structural and other proteins.	• RNA viruses, except (+) RNA genome, must carry polymerases
• DNA polymerases require a primer to replicate the viral genome.	• All (−) RNA viruses are enveloped.
• The larger DNA viruses encode means and promote efficient replication of their genome.	

Table 26.9 Viral receptors

Virus	Target cell	Receptor
Epstein-Barr virus	B-cell	C3d complement receptor CR2 (CD21)
Human immunodeficiency virus	Helper T-cell	CD4 molecule and chemokine co-receptor
Rhinovirus	Epithelial cells	ICAM-1 (immunoglobulin superfamily protein)
Poliovirus	Epithelial cells	Immunoglobulin superfamily protein
Herpes simplex virus	Many cells	Herpesvirus entry mediator (HVEM), nectin 1
Rabies virus	Neuron	Acetylcholine receptor, NCAM
Influenza A virus	Epithelial cells	Sialic acid
B19 parvovirus	Erythroid precursors	Erythrocyte P antigen (globoside)

- Antibody: complement, antibody-dependent cellular cytotoxicity, immune complexes
  - Other inflammatory responses
- Virus production in a tissue with release of the virus to other people (contagion)
- Transmission of viruses depends
  - On source of the virus (tissue site of viral replication and secretion)
  - Ability of the virus to endure hazards and barriers of the environment

26.7 Treatment and Prognosis

Treatment

Antiviral drugs aim at altering:

- Virion disruption
- Attachment
- Penetration and uncoating
- RNA synthesis
- Genome replication
- Protein synthesis
- Virion assembly and release

Antiviral drugs include:

- Nucleoside analogs
  - Acyclovir
  - Ganciclovir
- Nonnucleoside polymerase inhibitors
- Protease inhibitors
- Immunomudulators

Biologic Behavior–Prognosis–Prognostic Factors
- Age of infection
  - Congenital
- Nature of disease
  - Target tissue
  - Portal of entry of virus
  - Access of virus to target tissue
  - Tissue tropism of virus
  - Permissiveness of cells for viral replication
  - Pathogenic activity (strain)
- Severity of disease
  - Cytopathic ability of virus
  - Immune status
  - Competence of the immune system
  - Prior immunity to the virus
  - Immunopathology
- Progression of viral disease
  - Acquisition
  - Activation of innate protections
  - Incubation period
  - Target tissue
  - Host responses
  - Contagion
  - Resolution or persistent infection/chronic disease

26.8 Unspecified Nodular Encephalitis

The only histological finding in unspecified nodular encephalitis is the presence of gliomesenchymal nodules (GMN) (Fig. 26.1a–d). The finding is indicative of a viral infection.

GMN are:

- composed of microglia, macrophages, and reactive astrocytes
- found in the gray and white matter
- absence of multinucleated giant cells (MGC) or large cells containing inclusion bodies

The differential diagnosis for GMN includes

- HIV-1 encephalopathy/leukoencephalopathy
- Cytomegalovirus encephalitis
  - The nodules are very suspicious to contain CMV when further serial sectioning is performed.
- Toxoplasma gondii encephalitis

Complete clarification and identification of an infectious agent is sometimes not possible.

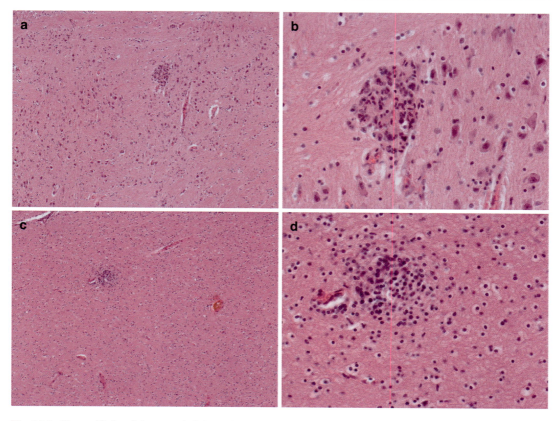

Fig. 26.1 Unspecified nodular encephalitis (**a–d**) (Stain: H&E)

26.9 RNA Viruses: Human Immunodeficiency Virus (HIV)-1

Human immunodeficiency virus (HIV)-1 infection is a serious health problem worldwide as 33 million adults and 2 million children are infected with HIV-1. Despite preventive efforts, the epidemic continues to spread rapidly and the socioeconomic consequences of the neurologic dysfunction caused by HIV-1 infection are of enormous proportions. Most of the affected patients live in developing countries, where antiretroviral medications are not available.

HIV-viruses (1, 2) are

- Retroviruses, lentivirinae subfamily
- Roughly spheric, enveloped, RNA viruses
- Diameter of 80–120 nm
- RNA-dependent DNA polymerase
- Encode accessory genes
  - *Gag*: group-specific antigen: core and capsid proteins
  - *Int*: integrase
  - *Pol*: polymerase: reverse transcriptase, protease, integrase
  - *Pro*: protease
  - *Env*: envelope: glycoproteins
  - *Tat*: transactivation of viral and cellular genes
  - *Rev*: regulation of RNA splicing and promotion of export to cytoplasm
  - *Nef*: decreases cell surface CD4, facilitates T-cell activation, progression to AIDS
  - *Vif*: virus infectivity, promotion of assembly, blocks a cellular antiviral protein

- *Vpu*: facilitates virion assembly and release, induces degradation of CD4
- *Vpr*: transport of complementary DNA to nucleus, arresting of cell growth, replication in macrophages
- LTR: promoter, enhancer elements

Following involvement of the lung (75–85%), the brain is the second most frequently affected organ (60–80%) in HIV-1 infection.

Neurological signs and symptoms are seen:

- In about 50% of HIV-1-infected patients.
- In approximately 10% of the cases, they are the first presentation of the disease.

The term "AIDS dementia complex (ADC)" was coined in 1986 (Navia et al. 1986a, b) to describe impaired memory and concentration, psychomotor slowing and behavioral disturbances in 65% of patients, and has been attributed mainly to subcortical damage of AIDS brains (subcortical dementia). The name ADC was later changed into HIV-1-associated cognitive and motor complex with HIV-1-associated dementia complex (motor)/(behavior) (HAD) and HIV-1-associated myelopathy as its severe manifestations and HIV-1-associated minor cognitive/motor disorder as its mild manifestation (Force 1991).

Classification of HIV-associated neurocognitive disorders (HAND) (Antinori et al. 2007)

- Asymptomatic neurocognitive impairment (ANI)
  - No evidence of pre-existing cause. Cognitive impairment must be attributable to HIV and no other etiology (e.g., dementia, delirium).
  - The cognitive impairment does not interfere with activities of daily living.
  - Involves at least two cognitive areas (memory, attention, language, processing speed, sensory perceptual, motor skills) documented by performance of >1 standard deviation below the mean of standardized neuropsychological testing.
  - 30% prevalence in combination antiretroviral therapies (CART)-treated HIV+ individuals.
- Mild neurocognitive disorder (MND)
  - No evidence of pre-existing cause. Cognitive impairment must be attributable to HIV and no.
  - Other etiology (e.g., dementia, delirium).
  - At least mild interference in >1 activities of daily living including mental acuity, inefficiency at work, homemaking or social functioning.
  - 20–30% prevalence in combination antiretroviral therapies (CART)-treated HIV+ individuals.
- HIV-associated dementia (HAD)
  - No evidence of another pre-existing cause for dementia (i.e., CNS infections, CNS neoplasm, cerebrovascular disease).
  - Marked interference in activities of daily living.
  - Marked cognitive impairment involving at least two cognitive domains by performance of >2 standard deviation below the mean of standardized neuropsychological tests, especially in learning of new information, slowed information processing and defective attention or concentration.
  - 2–8% prevalence in combination antiretroviral therapies (CART)-treated HIV+ individuals.

Despite the introduction of antiretroviral therapies with a greater life expectancy of HIV-1-infected individuals, epidemiologic data suggest that involvement of the brain in AIDS patients continues to be a frequent autopsy finding.

Neuropathological examinations show in up to 95% of the brains changes that may be due to:

- primary effect of HIV-1
- probable effect of HIV-1
- opportunistic agents
- neoplasias

The neuropathological changes seen in the brains (Table 26.10) and peripheral nerve and skeletal muscle (Table 26.11) of HIV-1-infected patients are manifold.

Table 26.10 The neuropathological changes seen in the brains of HIV-1-infected patients

Changes primarily due to HIV-1	• HIV-1 encephalitis (HIVE) • HIV-1 leukoencephalopathy (HIVL) • HIV-1 myelitis • Lymphocytic meningitis (LM) • Meningeal lymphocytic infiltration (MLI) • Perivascular lymphocytic infiltration (PLI)
Changes probably due to HIV-1	• Vacuolar myelopathy • Vacuolar leukoencephalopathy
Opportunistic infections—viruses	• Cytomegalovirus infection (CMV) • Progressive multifocal leukoencephalopathy (PML) • Herpes simplex virus 1 • Herpes simplex virus 2 • Herpes zoster • HTLV-1 • Varicella-zoster virus
Opportunistic infections—parasites	• Toxoplasma gondii • Acanthamoeba • Leptomyxid amoeba • Trypanosoma cruzi • Strongyloides
Opportunistic infections—fungi	• Aspergillus fumigatus • *Candida albicans* • *Cryptococcus neoformans* • Others including: Histoplasma, Phycomyces, Coccidioides, Blastomyces, Acremonium, Cladosporium
Opportunistic infections—bacteria	• Pyogenic: *Escherichia coli*, Listeria, Staphylococcus, Salmonella • Mycobacterial: *Mycobacterium tuberculosis*, *Mycobacterium avium* intracellulare • Spirochetal: Treponema pallidum • Filamentous: Nocardia • Miscellaneous: Whipple's disease
Neoplasias	• Lymphoma (primary and secondary) • Kaposi sarcoma

Table 26.11 The changes occurring in the peripheral nervous system and in skeletal muscles of HIV-1-infected patients

Peripheral nervous system	• Acute inflammatory demyelinating (poly) (radiculo) neuropathy • Chronic inflammatory demyelinating (poly) (radiculo) neuropathy • Axonal neuropathy • Ganglionitis, ganglioradiculitis, (poly) (radiculo) neuritis • necrotizing vasculitis, vasculitic neuropathy
Skeletal muscle	• (Poly) myositis • Necrotizing myopathy • Nemaline rod myopathy • Vesicular myopathy, mitochondrial myopathy • Necrotizing vasculitis

examination is required. If focal lesions are present, they are almost always due to opportunistic infections, cerebrovascular complications, or neoplasms.

26.9.1.1 Neuroimaging Findings

General Imaging Features
- Brain atrophy and symmetric confluent white matter lesions (periventricular, basal ganglia, centrum semiovale, brain stem, cerebellum), no enhancement

CT Non-Contrast-Enhanced
- Brain atrophy
- Symmetric confluent white matter hypodensities

CT Contrast-Enhanced
- No enhancement

MRI-T2/FLAIR (Fig. 26.2a–d)
- Focal white matter hyperintensities
- Diffuse white matter hyperintensities

MRI-T1 (Fig. 26.2e, f)
- Lesions usually not seen

MRI-T1 Contrast-Enhanced (Fig. 26.2g, h)
- No enhancement

26.9.1 HIV-1 Encephalitis (HIVE)

Since HIV-1 is rarely the cause of focal macroscopic lesions even in severely infected patients, systematic sampling of specimens for histological

MRI-DWI (Fig. 26.2i, j)
- No restricted diffusion.

26.9.1.2 Microscopical Findings

HIV-1 encephalitis is characterized by (Fig. 26.3a–j)

- Multiple disseminated foci composed of microglia, macrophages, and multinucleated giant cells (MGCs). The foci are predominantly located in the cortex, deep gray matter, and the white matter.
- The multinucleated giant cells (MGC) are the hallmark for HIV-1 encephalitis.
  - They contain up to 20 round or elongated and basophilic nuclei which are usually arranged at the periphery of the cell.
  - The cytoplasm is eosinophilic and appears densely stained in the center and vacuolated at the periphery.
  - The cells are of monocyte/histiocyte lineage which includes microglia and macrophages.
  - They are derived from HIV-1-mediated fusion of infected microglia and macrophages.
  - The nucleic acids of HIV proteins have been demonstrated to be located in their cytoplasm.
- In their absence, the presence of HIV-antigen or HIV nucleic acids has to be demonstrated either by immunohistochemistry, i.e., gp41 and p24 (Fig. 26.3j) or by in situ hybridization.
- HIVE usually occurs in the later stages of the AIDS infection.
- The electron microscopical analysis revealed retroviral particles either free in the cytoplasm or in cytoplasmic cisternae.
- Microglia/macrophages and MGC are capable of HIV synthesis and, thus, constitute the major reservoir and vehicle for the spread of the virus.
- Synonyms previously used: giant cell encephalitis, multifocal giant cell encephalitis, multinucleated cell encephalitis, subacute encephalitis

There is no strong correlation between HIVE and the clinical stages of the HAD.

Despite the introduction of HAART with a greater life expectancy of infected individuals, epidemiologic data suggest that the prevalence of HIVE is on the rise.

26.9.2 HIV-1 Leukoencephalopathy (HIVL)

HIV-1 leukoencephalopathy is chararcterized by (Fig. 26.4a–j)

- diffuse damage to the white matter including
  - myelin loss
  - reactive astrogliosis
  - macrophages
  - multinucleated giant cells
- Myelin pallor is usually found around the gliomesenchymal nodule containing the MGC.
- Little or no inflammatory infiltrates are seen.
- In the absence of multinucleated giant cells, the presence of HIV-antigen or HIV nucleic acids has to be demonstrated either by immunohistochemistry or by in situ hybridization.
- Axonal damage can be demonstrated with immunohistochemistry for β-amyloid precursor protein.
- HIVL usually occur in the later stages of the AIDS infection.
- Synonyms previously used: progressive diffuse leukoencephalopathy

26.9.3 Lymphocytic Meningitis (LM) and Perivascular Lymphocytic Infiltration (PLI)

Lymphocytic meningitis (LM) is characterized by (Fig. 26.5a–f)

- Significant lymphocytic infiltrates in the leptomeninges.
- No opportunistic pathogens are encountered in the meninges.

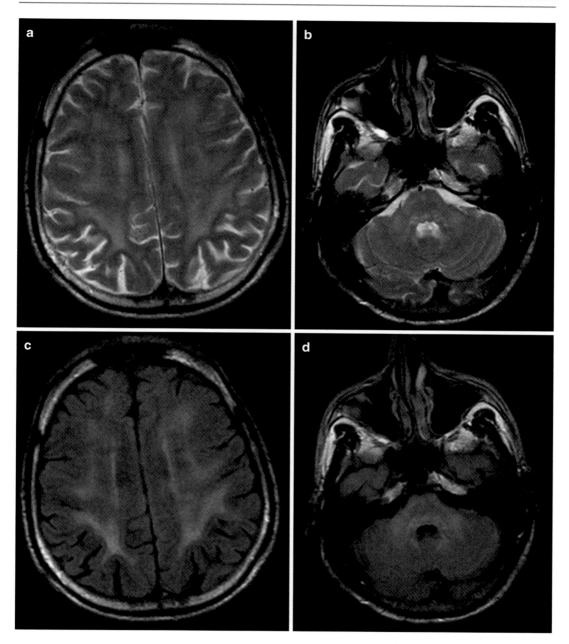

Fig. 26.2 HIV encephalopathy, T2 (**a**, **b**), FLAIR (**c**, **d**), T1 (**e**, **f**), T1 contrast (**g**, **h**), DWI (**i**, **j**)

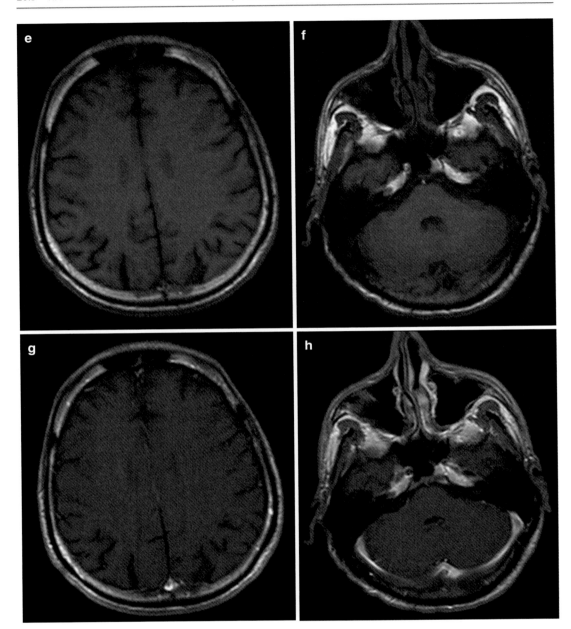

Fig. 26.2 (continued)

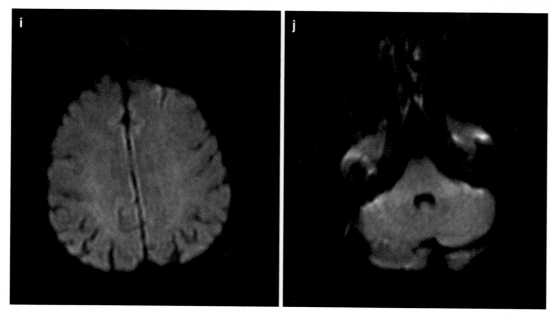

Fig. 26.2 (continued)

Perivascular lymphocytic infiltration (PLI) is characterized by (Fig. 26.5g–j)

- Significant lymphocytic infiltrates in the perivascular spaces of the brain tissue.
- No opportunistic pathogens are encountered in the perivascular brain tissue.

It seems that lymphocytic infiltrates in the leptomeninges and in the perivascular spaces of the brain tissue constitute changes occurring in the early stages of the HIV-1 infection.

26.9.4 Vacuolar Myelopathy (VM) and Vacuolar Leukoencephalopathy (VL)

Vacuolar myelopathy is characterized by (Fig. 26.6a–f)

- Numerous vacuolar myelin swellings.
- Macrophages in multiple areas of the spinal cord.
- Predominant involvement of the dorsolateral spinal tracts.

- Some macrophages may be found in the vacuoles.
- Might not be specific for HIV-1 since they can occur in the absence of HIV.
- The axon is at first unaffected, but it is damaged in the later stages of the disease.
- VM might not be specific for HIV-1

Vacuolar leukoencephalopathy is characterized by

- Numerous vacuolar myelin swellings in the central white matter.
- Some macrophages may be found in the vacuoles.
- VL is a rare condition.

26.9.5 Neuropathological Changes in Early Stages of HIV-1 Infection

Brain changes in HIV-1 seropositive, non-AIDS cases include:

- Cerebral vasculitis was significantly more frequent and marked in HIV seropositive cases and was often associated with lymphocytic

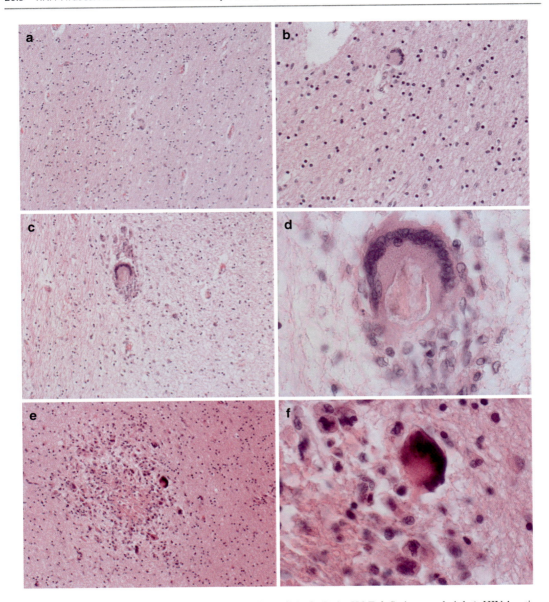

Fig. 26.3 HIV-1-encephalitis: multinucleated giant cells (**a–i**) (**a–h**: Stain: H&E; **i**: Stain: cresyl violet). HIV-1 antigen shown in a small gliomesenchymal nodule (**j**: stain: immunohistochemistry for p24)

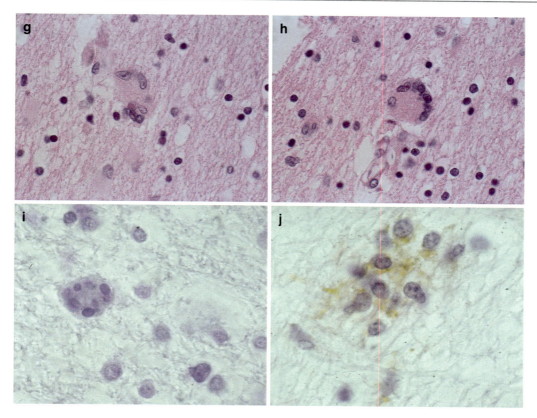

Fig. 26.3 (continued)

meningitis (Gray et al. 1992).
- Granular ependymitis, myelin pallor with reactive astrocytosis, and microglial proliferation were also more frequent and more severe in HIV seropositive cases. Immunohistochemistry was negative for HIV-antigens. Highly expressed cytokines (tumor necrosis factor-α, interleukin (IL)-1,4,6) (Gray et al. 1992).
- Perivascular lymphocytic infiltrates (PLI) as well as lymphocytic infiltrates in the meninges (MLI) were found in 62.8% of the cases. PLI alone was seen in 61% of the cases, MLI alone in 43% of the cases, and the combination of PLI and MLI in 34% of the cases (Weis et al., unpublished data).

26.9.6 Neuropathological Changes in HIV-1-Infected Children

Children born to HIV-1-infected mothers are in 10–40% of the cases also infected by the virus (Kozlowski et al. 1993). These children develop symptoms before the age of 2 years.

- About 30% of the HIV-1 children develop opportunistic infection or HIV-1 encephalopathy within the first year of life.
- Brain growth is impaired leading to intellectual deficiency.
- The gross-anatomical analysis shows brains which are too small for the age.
- Sometimes atrophic gyri may be noted.

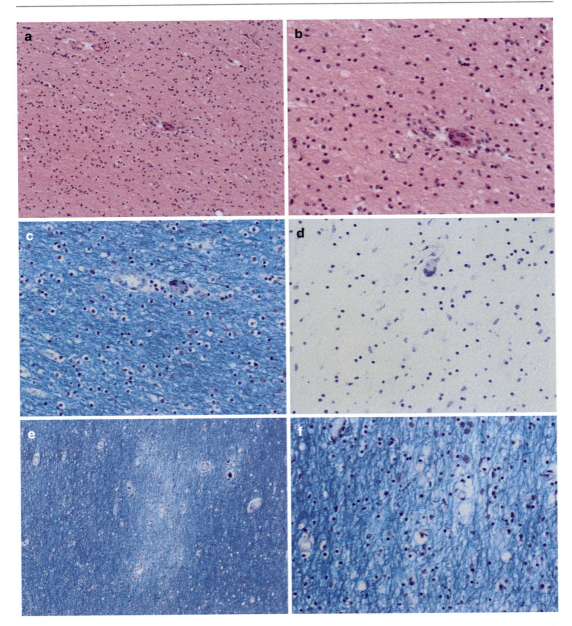

Fig. 26.4 HIV-leukoencephalopathy: presence of multinucleated giant cells in the white matter (**a**, **b**: H&E, **c**: LFB, **d**: cresyl violet) and myelin pallor loss (**e–j**)

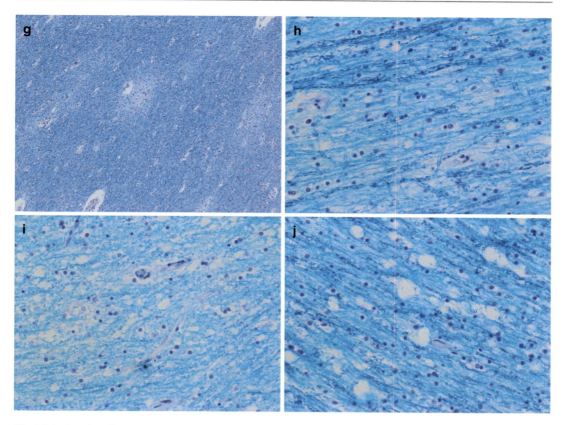

Fig. 26.4 (continued)

- Microcephaly and/or brain atrophy is present.
- The most common findings in brains of HIV-1-infected children are
  - Mineralization of predominantly small vessels found in 95% of the case.
  - Myelin pallor and gliosis are the noted changes of the white matter that occur in 78% of the cases.
  - MGC are seen in 62% of HIV-1-infected children.
- Opportunistic infections are comparatively uncommon.

26.9.7 Therapy: HAART Effects and Therapy-Induced Immune Restitution Inflammatory Syndrome (IRIS)

In 1995/1996, highly active antiretroviral therapies (HAART) were introduced which combine

- nucleoside reverse transcriptase inhibitors (NRTI)
  - specifically inhibit the viral reverse transcriptase enzyme necessary for DNA chain elongation of the virus
- protease inhibitors (PI)
  - prevent the production of active virus by interfering with the cleavage of proteins necessary for viral assembly

Effects of the therapy results in:

- The frequency of HIV-1-related CNS diseases has been reduced through
  - the reduction of both viral load in the blood
  - the reduced continuous penetration of virus into the brain (Tardieu 1999)
- HIV-positive patients live longer.
- The median survival

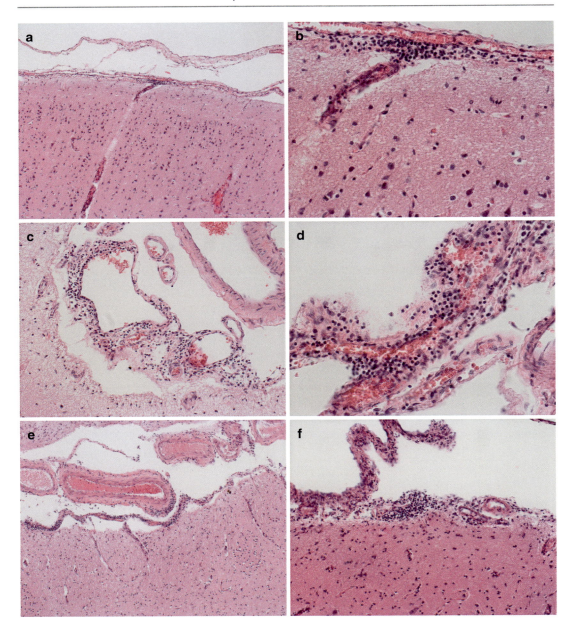

Fig. 26.5 Meningeal lymphocytic infiltrates (**a–f**: Stain: H&E). Perivascular lymphocytic infiltrates (**g–j**: Stain: H&E)

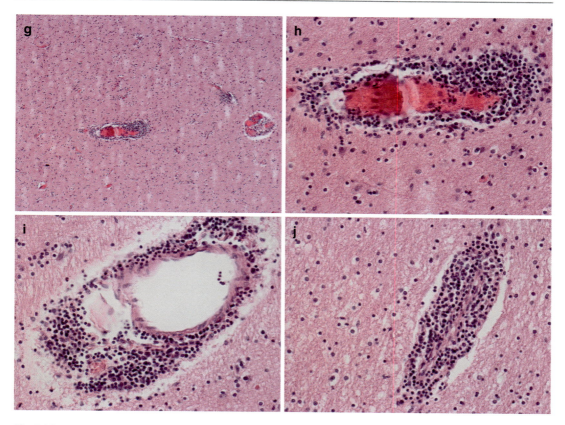

Fig. 26.5 (continued)

- following AIDS increased from 19.6 months in 1993–1995 to 39.6 months for those diagnosed in 1996–2000
- following ADC increased from 11.9 months in 1993–1995 to 48.2 in 1996–2000.
• The proportion of patients with AIDS dementia complex (ADC) increased from 5.2% in 1993–1995 to 6.8% in 1996–2000.

Larger cohort autopsy studies of HIV-infected patients over longer time periods suggest that, despite the beneficial effects of modern antiretroviral combination therapy, involvement of the brain in AIDS subjects continues to be a frequent autopsy finding (Gray et al. 1988, 2003; Jellinger et al. 2000; Langford et al. 2003) (Tables 26.12 and 26.13).

Immune reconstitution inflammatory syndrome (IRIS) is a syndrome that emerges when the immune system recovers after an immune deficiency state (Table 26.14) (Nelson et al. 2017; Chahroudi and Silvestri 2012; McCarthy and Nath 2010). IRIS is an adverse clinical manifestation that occurs in HIV-infected individuals treated successfully with ART and consists of a paradoxical deterioration of clinical status despite improved CD4-T-cell counts and immunologic conditions.

A new variant of HIVE has emerged in the era of HAART as a severe leukoencephalopathy with significant perivascular infiltration of macrophages and lymphocytes which is assumed to be the result of an exaggerated response from a newly reconstituted immune system (Persidsky and Gendelman 2003).

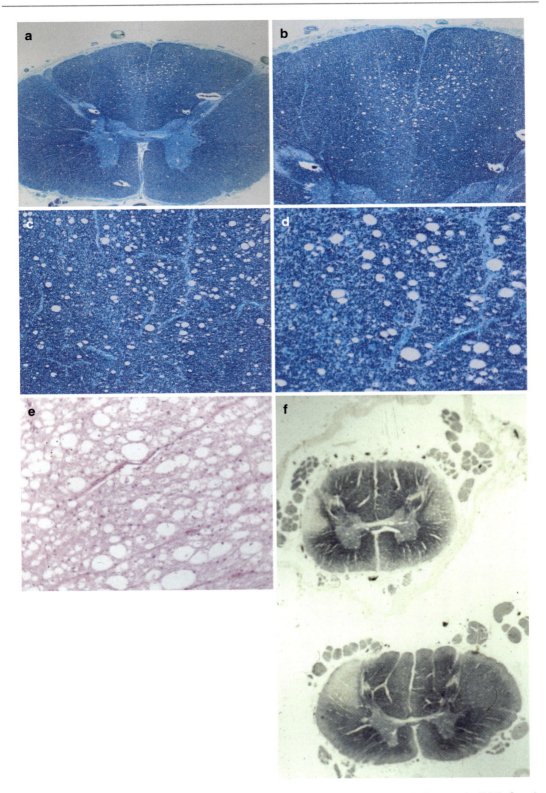

Fig. 26.6 Spinal cord showing vacuolar myelopathy of the dorsal tracts (**a–d**: stain LFB, **e**: stain H&E, **f**: stain: Woelcke's myelin stain)

Table 26.12 Review of 1597 consecutive autopsies of HIV-1-positive patients performed between 1984 and 2000, and division into four time periods on the basis of the therapeutic regimens available (Vago et al. (2002) reproduced with kind permission by Wolters Kluwer Health)

Year	Therapy	n	HIV-E/L	Opportunistic infections
1984–1987	No therapy	119	53.8	40.3
1988–1994	Monotherapy (zidovudine)	1116	32.2	46.8
1995–1996	Dual combination therapy with nucleoside reverse transcriptase inhibitors	256	17.9	42.6
1997–2000	Triple combination therapy including two NRTIs and at least one protease inhibitor or non-NRTI	106	15.1	42.5

Table 26.13 Frequencies for various neuropathological changes in pre-HAART era compared to HAART era

Author (year)		n	HIVE	HIVL	CMV	PML	TOXO	LYM
Gray et al. (1988)	Pre-HAART	40	37.5	Nip	20.0	5.0	47.5	2.5
Gray et al. (2003)[a]	HAART	23	17.4	Nip	8.7	17.4	13.0	13.0
Jellinger et al. (2000)	Pre-HAART	352	8.5	4.3	18.5	7.1	22.2	8.5
	HAART	98	8.0	5.0	11.0	5.0	8.0	6.0
Langford (2003)	Pre-HAART	62	25.8	Nip	16.1	6.4	6.4	19.3
	HAART	89	43.8	Nip	16.8	5.6	0.0	8.9

n sample size, *HIVE* HIV-1 encephalitis, *HIVL* HIV-1 leukoencephalopathy, *CMV* cytomegalovirus encephalitis, *PML* progressive multifocal leukoencephalopathy, *TOXO* toxoplasma gondii encephalitis, *LYM* primary non-Hodgkin lymphoma

[a]Frequencies for pre-HAART could not be calculated due to lack of original data in their paper

Table 26.14 Clinical manifestations of IRIS in patients with HIV-1 infection on cART modified after McCarthy and Nath (2010) reproduced with kind permission by Springer Nature

Infection	Typical clinical manifestations	Atypical clinical manifestations
HIV encephalitis	• Asymptomatic • Mild cognitive decline	• Fulminant decline in mental status over days with brain swelling and inflammation
PML with JCV	• Subacute focal neurologic deficits	• Focal areas of contrast enhancement and swelling
Varicella-zoster virus	• Shingles • CNS vasculitis	• Strokes without skin rash
Cytomegalovirus	• Retinitis • Cerebritis	• Vasculitis
Epstein-Barr virus	• CNS lymphoma	• Optic neuropathy
Tuberculosis	• Meningitis	• Cerebral infarcts • Subarachnoid hemorrhage
Cryptococcus	• Meningitis	• Enhancing mass lesions in posterior fossa
Candida	• Meningitis	• Vasculitis with strokes

Neuropathological examination revealed

- Severe inflammatory lesions.
- Demyelinating lesions with marked intraparenchymal and perivascular infiltration by macrophages and T-lymphocytes.
- In some cases, abundant viral proliferation was identified by immunocytochemistry or in situ hybridization, but in others the infectious agent could only be detected using PCR.
- T-lymphocytes were predominantly CD8(+).
- In those cases with the more favorable course, inflammation was less severe with marked macrophage activation and a number of CD4(+) lymphocytes.
- In the lethal cases, inflammation was severe and mostly composed of CD8(+) cytotoxic lymphocytes.

26.9.8 The Sequalae of HIV-1 Infection of the Nervous System

In summary, the following changes of the brain have been described to be due to the HIV-1 infection:

- Brain weight (Weis, unpublished data)
  - no changes
- Brain edema (Weis, unpublished data)
  - no significant difference
- Gross-anatomy (Gelman and Guinto 1992)
  - No apparent macroscopical signs of atrophy are seen by bare visual inspection.
  - Cerebrospinal fluid (CSF) space greater than two standard deviations above the mean of the age-matched control subjects.
  - CSF spaces expanded most in the frontal and temporal lobe.
- Ventricular system (Weis, unpublished data) (Gelman and Guinto 1992)
  - Widening of the lateral ventricles.
  - Ventricular spaces expanded more than the sulcal spaces.
- Volume of brain regions (Oster et al. 1993; Subbiah et al. 1996; Weis et al. 1993c)
  - No significant changes in volume, surface area, mean cortical thickness.
  - Reduction of the mean volume of the neocortex.
  - Reduction in volume of the central brain nuclei.
  - Reduction in volume of the internal capsule.
  - Mean neocortical thickness was reduced by 12%.
  - There were no differences in white matter volumes between groups.
  - The mean volume of the white matter was reduced by 13%.
  - Mean ventricular volume was increased by 55%.
  - There were no significant differences between the AIDS groups with and without HIV-associated dementia.
- Neuronal number
  - Cerebral cortex (Ketzler et al. 1990; Weis et al. 1993b)
    - Loss of neurons in different cortical regions.
    - Neuronal loss is not be correlated with development of dementing symptoms and of HIV-specific neuropathology.
  - Basal ganglia
    - decrease in neuronal density (21%) in the putamen especially in those cases with HIV-1 encephalitis (Everall et al. 1993).

- Cerebellum
  - significant reduction of the volume density, the numerical density of neurons as well as neuronal size was apparent in the cerebellar dentate nucleus and in both inferior olivary nuclei (Abe et al. 1996)
- Substantia nigra
  - The total number of neuronal cell bodies was 25% lower in AIDS than in age-matched controls although the volume density of neuronal melanin did not differ from that of controls because the percentage of pigmented cell bodies was higher and the cell bodies were more fully packed with melanin in AIDS (Reyes et al. 1991).
  - The size of total neurons (pigmented and non-pigmented neurons) and of pigmented neurons was significantly reduced in all investigated nuclei (anteromedial, antero-intermediolateral, posterolateral, and posteromedial nuclei) of HIV-1-infected brains.
  - Furthermore, the nigral neuronal loss showed no relationship with immunohistochemical detection of HIV-1 antigens (gp41, p24).
  - The numerical density of non-pigmented large neurons (type II neurons) was significantly increased in HIV-1-infected brains suggesting that (1) non-pigmented, dopaminergic neurons or non-pigmented, non-dopaminergic neurons might be relatively preserved in the SN of HIV-1 infection, or (2) that pigmented dopaminergic neurons loose their melanin pigments during the early stages of degeneration, which also might be responsible for functional deterioration (Itoh et al. 2000).
- Neuronal size (Weis et al. 1993b)
  - no changes in perikaryal size
- Synapses (Wiley et al. 1991)
  - Loss of synapses as shown by a decrease in the immunoreactivity against synaptophysin
- Dendrites (Masliah et al. 1992a, b)
  - Apical dendrites
    - dilated, vacuolated, and tortuous
    - decreased length and branching
  - Basal and oblique dendrites
    - show the same alterations, but to a lesser extent
  - Some dendrites present lacunae and filopodia consistent with remodeling.
  - 40–60% decrease in spine density throughout the entire length of dendrites.
  - Fewer spines on neurons; 55% fewer on the first segment, 40% fewer on the second, 45% fewer on the third, 60% fewer on the fourth, and 65% fewer in the fifth segment.
  - Aberrant spines in regions of abnormal second-order dendritic branches.
- Nerve fibers
  - White matter
    - Loss of nerve fibers in the white matter
  - Corpus callosum (Wohlschlaeger et al. 2009)
    - Reduced thickness of the myelin sheath of nerve fibers in the corpus callosum.
    - Calculation of the g-ratio revealed a relative increase in size of the axon and a relative decrease in the myelin sheath thickness.
    - The data indicated a reduction in the size of nerve fibers and axons as well as thinner myelin sheaths, whereas in other callosal regions axons and myelin sheaths were swollen and enlarged.
    - These changes were observed in regions which are unaffected, as revealed by light-microscopic analysis of sections stained for myelin.
  - Optic nerve (Tenhula et al. 1992)
    - Degeneration was often severe and was scattered throughout all of the AIDS-affected optic nerves.
    - Despite the approximate 40% loss of axons in the AIDS-affected optic nerves, the mean axonal population was markedly lower than the mean obtained from normal optic nerves (880,000 vs. 1,507,000).
    - The mean axonal diameters were not markedly different, that the changes may not only be secondary to damage at the

retina, but may reflect an AIDS-associated primary optic neuropathy.
- Astroglia (Weis et al. 1993a; Ciardi et al. 1990)
  – no change in the number of all astrocytes (i.e., GFAP-positive and GFAP-negative astrocytes)
  – reduction of the number of GFAP-negative cells
  – increase of reactive GFAP-positive astrocytes
  – not correlated with loss of nerve cells
  – increase in nuclear size of GFAP-negative and GFAP-positive astrocytes
  – increase of the size of the cytoplasm of GFAP-positive astroglia
  – no correlation between the neuronal loss and the pattern of reactive astrocytosis
- Oligodendroglia (Esiri et al. 1991)
  – significant increase in the number of oligodendrocytes associated with mild degree of myelin damage
  – decrease of oligodendrocytes in severely affected areas
  – slight increase in immunoreactivity for the enzymes carbonic anhydrase II and 2′,3′-cyclic nucleotide 3′-phosphodiesterase
  – significant increase in the numerical density of transferrin-immunopositive cells of the white matter
  – an initial reactive hyperplasia which may represent an attempt to repair myelin damage taking place already early during the HIV-1 infection
- Microglia/macrophages (Weis et al. 1994)
  – Activated in gray and white matter of all brain regions.
  – Activation pattern is not correlated with the presence of HIV-antigen gp41 and p24 in the brain tissue.
- Vessels (Buttner et al. 1996; Weis et al. 1996)
  – Significant increase in the diameter of cortical vessels
  – Increase of the volume fraction, surface area of vessels
  – No changes in length density indicating no changes in the number of vessels
  – Increase of the numerical density of vessels in the gray matter
  – No changes in the numerical density of vessels in the white matter
  – Thinning of the basal lamina as seen by electron microscopy
  – Reduced immunoreactivity for collagen IV and laminin (thinning of the basal lamina)
- Vascular endothelial cell (Buttner et al. 1996; Weis et al. 1996)
  – loss of glycoproteins SBA, UEA-I, and WGA of the endothelial cell membrane
  – decrease of immunoreactivity for von Willebrand factor (Factor VIII)
  – no significant differences RCA-I
  – No changes in size at the electron microscopic level
- Capillaries (Weis and Haug 1989)
  – region-specific changes
  – increased capillary profile area
  – increased capillary diameter
  – decreased basal lamina thickness
  – increased endothelial cell size
  – unchanged pericyte size

26.9.9 Pathogenetic Mechanisms

26.9.9.1 Mode of Entrance of HIV-1 to the Brain

HIV-1 enters the CNS by

- HIV-1 is passively carried by T-lymphocytes and monocytes—the "Trojan Horse" hypothesis.
- Cell-free HIV-1 particles may also penetrate brain microvascular endothelial cells.
- After crossing the BBB into the CNS, macrophages spread productive HIV-1 infection to neighboring microglia.
- Microglia serve as
  – a reservoir for persistent viral infection and replication
  – a vehicle for viral dissemination throughout the brain
  – a major source of neurotoxic products that affect glial function, the blood–brain

barrier and neuronal function, and finally lead to cell death
- Microglia and monocyte-derived macrophages express both the CD4 and chemokine coreceptors (CCR5, CXCR4), the prerequisite for HIV-1 to enter a cell.
- The potential role of the cerebrospinal fluid or the choroid plexus as a means for HIV-1 entry in the brain is still unclear.
- At the time of primary HIV-1 infection, an acute aseptic meningitis or encephalitis indicates central nervous system invasion.
- The point in time when the migration of HIV-1-infected lymphocytes into the brain takes place is not known. It has been shown that, at the time of seroconversion, HIV-1 can be detected in the CSF; this is the time when, clinically, a subacute meningitis develops, thus, suggesting that HIV-1 enters the CNS at a very early stage of the disease.
- Opportunistic infectious agents or drugs of abuse disturbing the BBB may further attract more HIV-1-infected T-lymphocytes and macrophages into the brain.

26.9.9.2 Target Cells of HIV-1 Infection

The cells in the brain identified to contain HIV-1 are:

- Microglia
- Macrophages
- Multinucleated giant cells
- Astrocytes (possibly)
- Endothelial cells (possibly)
- Oligodendrocytes (possibly)

Mechanisms of Brain Lesions
- The development of brain lesions due to opportunistic infections and lymphomas might be explained by the lack of a competent immunologic defense system.
- One might assume that the changes described in Sect. 26.5.8 might result by direct infection with HIV-1.
  - However, it has been shown that neither neurons, nor astrocytes nor endothelial cells are infected with HIV-1.
  - Thus, these changes more probably result from indirect toxic factors that are produced either by infected multinucleated giant cells or by activated microglia.
- Neuronal dropout occurs in brain regions
  - That are free from any neuropathological changes.
  - Neuronal damage in AIDS was, at least, partly due to apoptosis.
  - No correlation was found between the presence and severity of neuronal loss or of neuronal apoptosis and a history of cognitive disorders.
  - No correlation between the presence of HIV-1 proteins and neuronal loss.
- The reactive astrogliosis was not correlated with the loss of nerve cells, indicating that this reaction pattern is rather a response to toxic factors secreted into the brain tissue.
- The number of activated microglia/macrophages is significantly increased in all brain regions. This activation of microglia is not correlated with the presence of HIV-1 antigen in the brain tissue. Activated microglia/macrophages, rather than MGCs, most probably secrete toxic factors.
- The neurotoxicity associated with HIV-1 infection is mediated, in part, through
  - cytokines
  - arachidonic acid metabolites
  - produced during cell-to-cell interactions between HIV-1-infected brain macrophages and astrocytes
- Pathobiological events underlying the neurodegenerative processes in HIV-1-associated dementia are believed to begin with productive infection of monocytes/macrophages by HIV-1.
  - Peripheral activation causes the differentiation of macrophages to produce a variety of immune products that lead to the upregulation of adhesion molecules on brain microvascular endothelial cells and the expression of adhesins on the monocyte-macrophage cell surface.
  - After penetration of the BBB, the differentiated brain macrophages and microglia can be vehicles for viral dissemination

- throughout the brain and focal reservoirs for productive HIV-1 replication.
- The neurotoxic events in the brain are caused by neurotoxins produced by these cells which are primed by HIV-1 and secondarily activated by factors such as immune stimuli or by T-cells trafficking through the nervous system.
- The primed and immune-activated brain macrophages/microglia secrete a variety of factors which affect neural and glial function and eventually lead to CNS inflammation.
- A pro-inflammatory cytokine response from blood-derived monocytes/macrophages, microglia, and astrocytes is amplified and leads finally to neurodegeneration.
- Immune neurotoxic factors may contribute to the breakdown of the BBB and affect the generation of chemokines, leading to transendothelial migration of monocytes into the brain perpetuating the inflammatory cascade.
- As a result of the neurotoxic activities of activated macrophages/microglia, astrocytes may suppress or increase-macrophages/microglia secretory functions and toxicity, depending on the astrocytic functional status.
- Cytolytic T-lymphocytes serve to eliminate infected cells, but are lost in late-stage HIV-1 disease, allowing the virus-induced, neurodegenerative response to continue unabated.
- Other factors include:
  - viral proteins
  - CA^{2+} channels
  - NMDA receptors
  - chemokines and cytokines
- Expression of developmental proteins (Malik and Eugenin 2016):
  - Dickkopf homolog 1 (DKK1): upregulated
  - Rho-associated, coiled-coil containing protein kinase 2 (ROCK2)—upregulated
  - Low density lipoprotein receptor-related protein-associated protein 1 (LRPAP1)—upregulated
  - Low density lipoprotein receptor-related protein 5-like (LRP5L)—downregulated
  - Low density lipoprotein-related protein 12 (LRP12)—upregulated
  - Low density lipoprotein receptor-related protein 8, apolipoprotein e receptor (LRP8)—downregulated
  - Catenin (cadherin-associated protein), alpha-like 1 (CTNNAL1)—upregulated
  - Catenin, beta-like 1 (CTNNBL1)—downregulated
  - Catenin (cadherin-associated protein), delta 1 (CTNND1)—downregulated
  - Catenin (cadherin-associated protein), alpha-like 1 (CTNNAL1)—upregulated
  - Glycogen synthase kinase 3 beta (GSK3B)—downregulated
  - Wingless-type MMTV integration site family, member 10A (WNT10A)—downregulated
- For more details, see (Zayyad and Spudich 2015; Singh 2016; Ru and Tang 2017; Rao et al. 2014; Malik and Eugenin 2016; Lamers et al. 2016; Joseph et al. 2016; Chen et al. 2014; Carroll and Brew 2017).

Interactions between the blood–brain barrier (BBB) and HIV (Hong and Banks 2015)

Mechanisms involving the BBB in HIV-infection

- Passage of HIV cell-free virus across the BBB
  - Transcytotic (mannose 6 phosphate receptor dependent)
  - Paracellular (tight junction dissolution)
- Passage of HIV-1 proteins (gp120, Tat) across the BBB
- Increased immune Ccll trafficking across the BBB
  - Activated and infected T cells
  - Activated and infected monocytes
- Transport of cytokines across the BBB
- Induction of cytokine release from barrier cells
- Increased BBB leakiness
- Brain-to-blood efflux of antivirals
  - Protease inhibitors by P-glycoprotein
  - AZT by organic ion transporter
- Altered BBB transporter expression and function (e.g., P-glycoprotein)
- Neurovascular unit effects

Table 26.15 Therapy and effects on involved pathways (Sanchez and Kaul 2017) reproduced with kind permission from MDPI open access

	HIV or methamphetamine or HIV + Meth	HIV + cART	HIV + METH + cART
Microglia activation	↑	↑	↑
Astrocytosis	↑	↑	↑
Alteration of neurotransmission	↑		↑
HAND/HAD	↑	↓	
Oxidative stress	↑	↑	↑
Mitochondrial impairment	↑		
ER stress		↑	
Autophagy			↓
Neuronal dendrites	↓		↓
Synapses	↓		↓
Neuronal ATP	↓	↓	↓
Viral load		↓	

Therapeutic effects on involved pathways are illustrated in Table 26.15.

26.10 DNA-Virus: Cytomegalovirus Infection (CMV)

Cytomegalovirus
- Herpesviruses, subfamily Betaherpesvirinae
- Large, enveloped viruses containing double-stranded DNA
- 150 nm in diameter

26.10.1 Neuroradiology Findings

General Imaging Features
- Periventricular white matter lesions, subependymal enhancement
- Calcifications in perinatal CMV

CT Non-Contrast-Enhanced (Fig. 26.7a)
- Periventricular hypodense lesions
- Periventricular hyperdense calcifications in perinatal CMV

CT Contrast-Enhanced
- Subependymal enhancement possible

MRI-T2/FLAIR (Fig. 26.7b, c)
- Periventricular hyperintensities

MRI-T1 (Fig. 26.7e)
- Subependymal enhancement

MRI-T1 Contrast-Enhanced (Fig. 26.7e)
- Subependymal enhancement

MRI-T2∗/SWI (Fig. 26.7f)
- Periventricular hypointense calcifications in perinatal CMV

26.10.2 Neuropathology Findings

Macroscopic Features
- In general, there are no gross-anatomical changes.
- Rarely, some small areas of necrosis are seen lining the ventricles, i.e., necrotizing ependymitis.

Microscopic Features (Fig. 26.8a–j)
- Microglial nodules are seen scattered throughout the nervous system.
- Large cells containing inclusion bodies are found within the microglial nodules.
- The microglial nodules located in the gray and white matter are usually not surrounded by a necrotic area.
- Along the periventricular spaces CMV-containing cells are found within the necrotic areas.

26.6 DNA-Virus: Cytomegalovirus Infection (CMV)

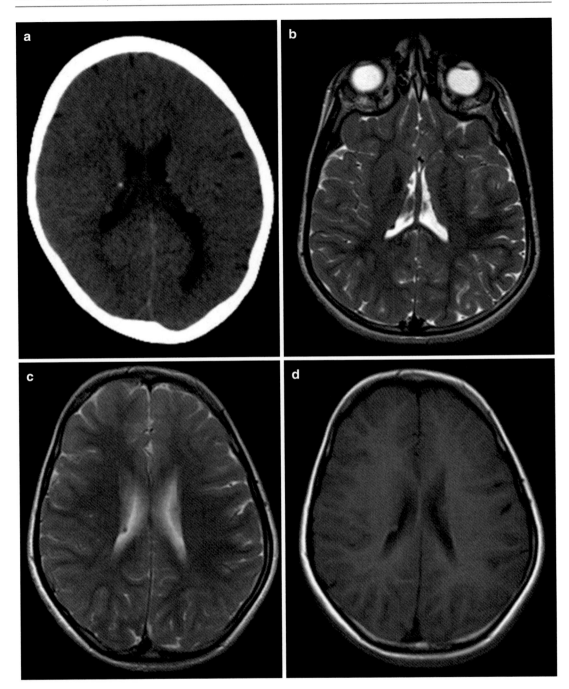

Fig. 26.7 Cytomegalovirus (CMV) infection: periventricular calcifications after perinatal CMV. CT non-contrast (**a**), T2 (**b**, **c**), T1 (**d**), T1 contrast (**e**), T2∗ (**f**)

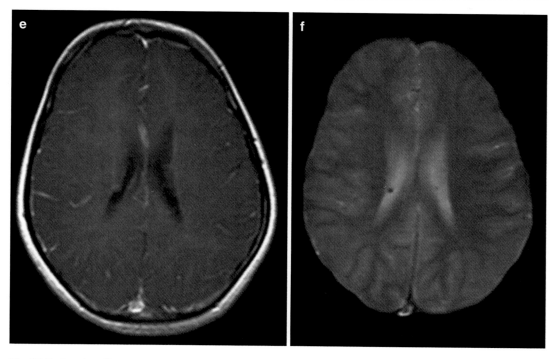

Fig. 26.7 (continued)

26.11 Progressive Multifocal Leukoencephalopathy (PML)

John Cunningham Virus (JCV) is a member of the Polyomaviridae family
Polyomaviruses BK and JC are ubiquitous.

- Are 45 nm in diameter.
- Contain less than 5000 base pairs.
- Genomes of BK and JC are closely related.
  - divided in early, late, and non-coding regions

- JC virus etiological agent of the progressive multifocal leukoencephalopathy (PML)
- JC is an ubiquitous, neurotropic virus:
  - 50–90% of adult healthy individuals have been exposed to this virus.
  - 19–27% of those people shedding JCV in their urine.
- The seroprevalence increases with age but acquisition of this virus is not associated with a clinical syndrome.
- JC binds to sialylated carbohydrates and serotonin receptors to enter glial cells by endocytosis.

- DNA genome is uncoated and delivered to the nucleus.

26.11.1 Clinical Signs and Symptoms

- The pre-AIDS era
  - Impaired vision
    - homonymous hemianopsia
  - Motor weakness
    - hemiparesis or hemiplegia
  - Changes in mentation:
    - personality change
    - difficulty with memory
    - emotional lability
    - dementia
- AIDS-related PML
  - weakness (42%)
  - speech abnormalities (40%)
  - cognitive abnormalities (36%)
  - gait abnormalities (29%)
  - sensory loss (19%)
  - visual impairment (19%)
  - seizures

26.7 Progressive Multifocal Leukoencephalopathy (PML)

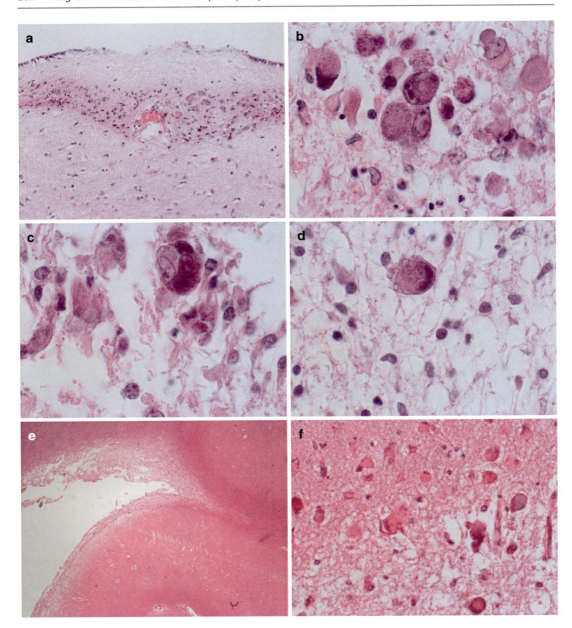

Fig. 26.8 Cytomegalovirus (CMV) infection (**a–n**). Cells with inclusion bodies (**a–j**) (stain: H&E); cytomegalic cell with inclusion body (**k–n**) (stain: immunohistochemistry for CMV)

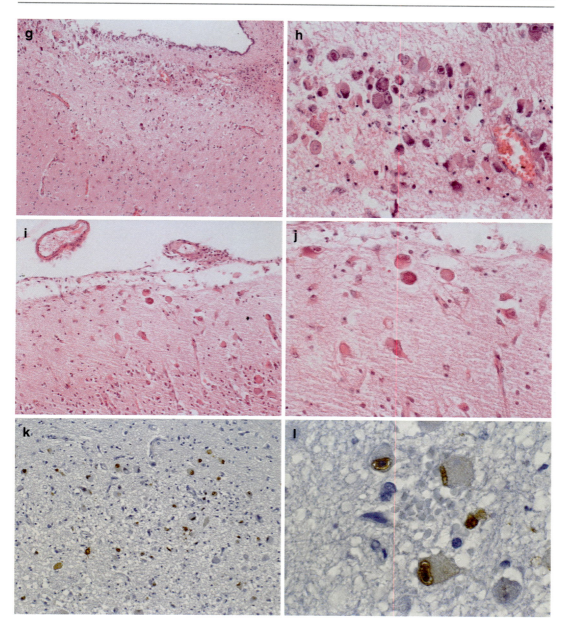

Fig. 26.8 (continued)

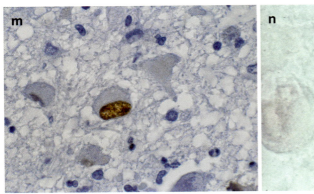
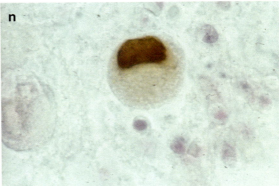

Fig. 26.8 (continued)

- diplopia
- limb incoordination
- PML associated with monoclonal antibody therapy
  - cognitive disorders (48%)
  - motor abnormalities (37%)
  - language disturbances (31%)
  - visual defects (26%)
- PML–IRIS immune reconstitution inflammatory syndrome
  - Paradoxical worsening of clinical or radiographic finding with recovery of the immune system
  - New or increased neurologic deficits
  - Increase in the number or size of lesions on neuroimaging
  - Contrast enhancement of brain lesions
  - Brain edema
  - Concurrent with diagnosis of PML

26.11.2 Neuroimaging Findings

General Imaging Features
- Confluent subcortical white matter lesions, predominantly in parieto-occipital or frontal lobes, U-fibers involved

CT Non-Contrast-Enhanced (Fig. 26.9a)
- Multiple hypodensities in white matter
- No mass effect
- If bilateral often asymmetric
- Natalizumab-associated PML often monofocal

CT Contrast-Enhanced (Fig. 26.9b)
- Usually no enhancement
- Enhancement possible in HIV-associated PML and natalizumab-associated PML

MRI-T2 (Fig. 26.9c)
- Hyperintense

MRI-FLAIR (Fig. 26.9d)
- Hyperintense

MRI-T1 (Fig. 26.9e)
- Hypointense

MRI-T1 Contrast-Enhanced (Fig. 26.9f)
- Usually no enhancement
- Enhancement possible in HIV-associated PML and natalizumab-associated PML

MRI-DWI (Fig. 26.9g)
- Acute lesions hyperintense

MRI-ADC (Fig. 26.9h)
- Acute lesions hypointense

26.11.3 Neuropathology Findings

Macroscopic Features (Fig. 26.10a–d)
- Multiple areas of discoloration of the white matter.
- Sometimes, the white matter may appear softened and mottled.

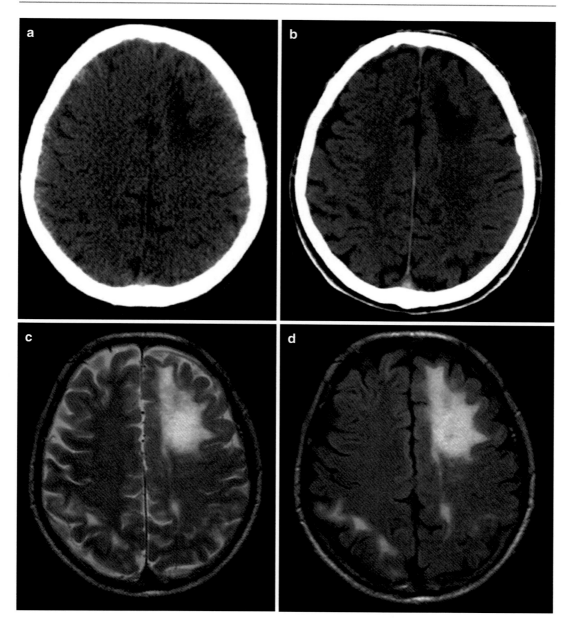

Fig. 26.9 Progressive multifocal leukoencephalopathy (PML). CT non-contrast (**a**), CT contrast (**b**), T2 (**c**), FLAIR (**d**), T1 (**e**), T1 contrast (**f**), DWI (**g**), ADC (**h**)

26.7 Progressive Multifocal Leukoencephalopathy (PML)

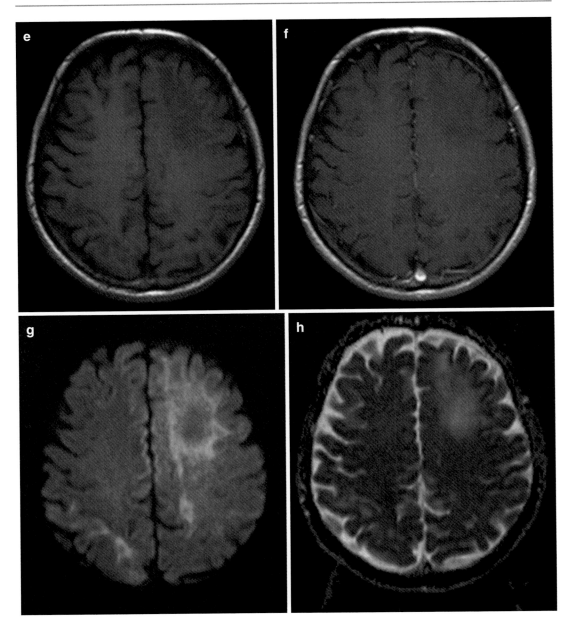

Fig. 26.9 (continued)

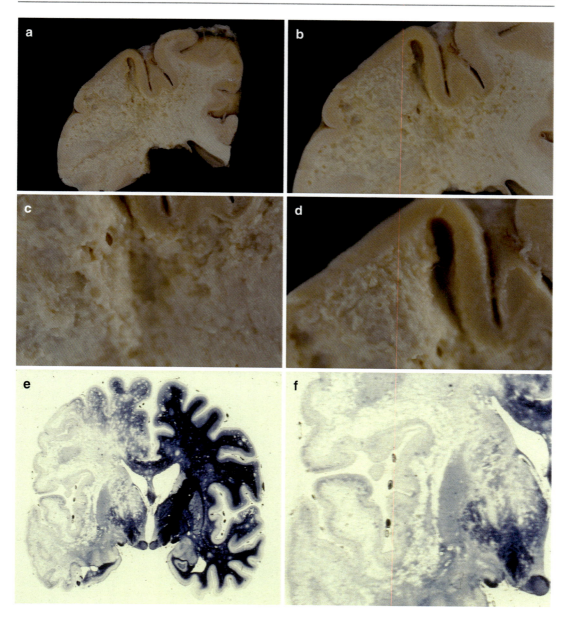

Fig. 26.10 Progressive multifocal leukoencephalopathy: macroscopically, the white matter shows a moth-eaten appearance (**a–d**). The myelin of the left hemisphere is completely lost (stain: Woelcke's myelin stain) (**e, f**). Histology shows degeneration of myelin accompanied by the presence of reactive astrocytes, bizarre astrocytes/oligodendrocytes with large eccentric cytoplasm and lymphocytic infiltrates (**g–j**). Reactive astrogliosis (stain: GFAP) (**k, l**) and reactive microgliosis (stain: HLA-DRII) (**m, n**). Lymphocytes (stain: CD45) (**o, p**) are found in the perivascular spaces and within the brain tissue

26.7 Progressive Multifocal Leukoencephalopathy (PML)

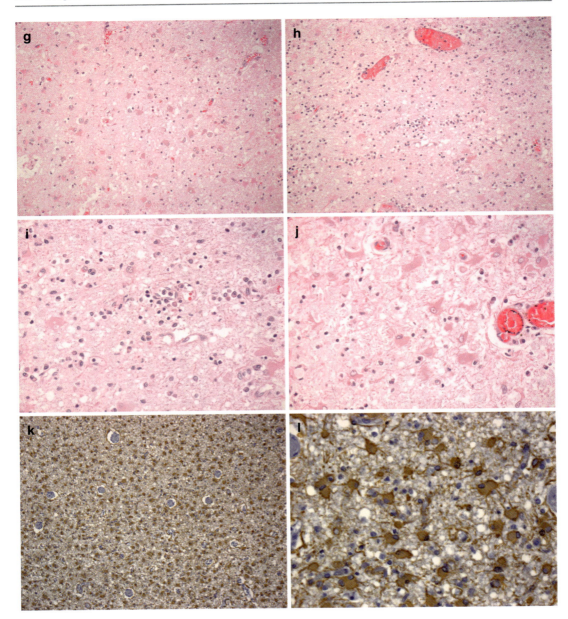

Fig. 26.10 (continued)

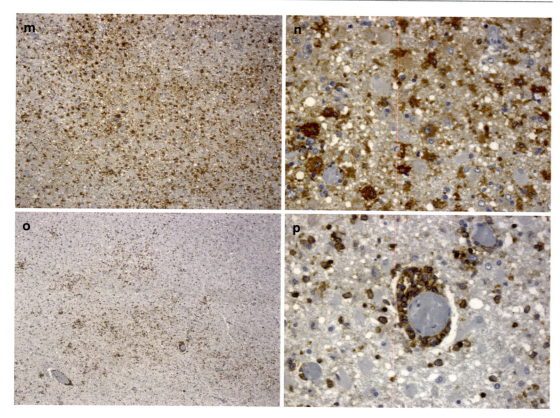

Fig. 26.10 (continued)

Microscopic Features (Fig. 26.10e–p)
- Multiple foci of demyelination in the white matter consisting of loss of myelin sheaths.
- The oligodendrocytes are enlarged, amphophilic, and contain intranuclear inclusions.
- Enlarged, bizarre astrocytes.

26.11.4 Molecular Nauropathology

Development of PML (Berger and Khalili 2011)

- infection with JC virus
- establishment of latent and/or persistent JC virus infection
- rearrangement of JC virus into a neurotropic strain if initial infection has been with the archetype strain
- reactivation of the neurotropic JC virus strain from sites of viral persistence/latency
- entry into the brain
- establishment of productive infection of oligodendrocytes
- ineffective immune system that prevents immunosurveillance from eliminating the infection

Drugs which cause PML are listed in Table 26.16.

The differences between progressive multifocal leukoencephalopathy (PML), progressive multifocal leukoencephalopathy—immune reconstitution inflammatory syndrome (PML–IRIS) and multiple sclerosis (MS) with regard to anatomical, neuropathological, and MRI features are shown in Table 26.17.

Prognostic factors of the evolution of progressive multifocal leukoencephalopathy have been described (Gheuens et al. 2013) and include:

- Favorable factors:
  - Detectable JCV-specific cellular immune response in blood or CSF

26.8 Herpes Simplex Virus (HSV) Encephalitis

Table 26.16 Drug-induced cases of PML (Bauer et al. 2015) reproduced with kind permission by Springer Nature

Medication	Treatment
Azathioprine	Transplantation/autoimmune disease
Cyclosporine	Transplantation
Cyclophosphamide	Cancer/transplantation/autoimmune disease
Dimethylfumarate	Autoimmune disease
Efalizumab	Autoimmune disease (psoriasis)
Fingolimod	Autoimmune disease
Infliximab	Autoimmune disease
Leflunomid	Autoimmune disease
Methotrexate	Cancer/autoimmune disease
Mycophenolate	Transplantation/autoimmune disease
Natalizumab	Autoimmune disease
Rituximab	Cancer/autoimmune disease
Tacrolimus	Transplantation

- Rapid clearance of JCV from CSF
- CD4 count >200 μL − 1 at onset
- Unfavorable factors:
  - Undetectable JCV-specific cellular immune response in blood or CSF
  - Mass effect on MRI
  - Posterior fossa lesions
  - High JC viral load in CSF
  - CD4 count <200 μL − 1 at onset

26.12 Herpes Simplex Virus (HSV) Encephalitis

Herpesviruses are
Large, enveloped viruses.
- Contain double-stranded DNA.
- 150 nm in diameter.
- DNA core surrounded by an icosadeltahedral capsid containing 162 capsomeres.
- Capsid is enclosed by a glycoprotein-containing envelope.
- Encode proteins that manipulate the host cell and immune response.
- DNA replication and capsid assembly occurs in the nucleus.
- Virus is released by
  - Exocytosis
  - Cell lysis
  - Through cell-to-cell bridges
- Cause lytic, persistent, latent, and immortalizing infections

26.12.1 Clinical Signs and Symptoms

- Headache
- Neck stiffness
- Drowsiness
- Coma
- Dysphagia
- Hemiparesis
- Focal seizures

26.12.2 Neuroimaging Findings

General Imaging Features
- Involvement of limbic system and temporal lobe
- Often hemorrhages and enhancement
- Often bilateral, but asymmetric

CT Non-Contrast-Enhanced (Fig. 26.11a)
- Normal (early) to mild hypodense, swollen temporal lobes and insula

CT Contrast-Enhanced
- Patchy enhancement possible

MRI-T2/FLAIR (Fig. 26.11b–d)
- Hyperintense, swollen white matter and cortex of affected areas.
- Hemorrhages may be hypointense.

Table 26.17 Comparative anatomical, neuropathological, and MRI features of progressive multifocal leukoencephalopathy (PML), progressive multifocal leukoencephalopathy—immune reconstitution inflammatory syndrome (PML–IRIS) and multiple sclerosis (MS) (Bauer et al. 2015) reproduced with kind permission by Springer Nature

PML	PML–IRIS	MS
Anatomical features		
• Lesions mostly reside in cerebral hemispheres but periventricular lesions are rare. • Lesions predominantly affect the deep and subcortical white matter and can expand into the cortical gray matter. • Intracortical lesions are present. • Spinal cord and optic nerves are spared.	• Lesion distribution is similar to PML.	• Lesions can be found in white and gray matter, but are often found in a periventricular position. • Unlike in PML, lesions can be found in spinal cord and optic nerves.
Neuropathological features		
• Demyelinating lesions reveal oligodendrocytes with enlarged nucleus and cytoplasm. The nucleus may show inclusion bodies. • Oligodendrocytes are mostly found on the border of the lesion. • Subpial lesions are absent. • Remyelination is absent. • Within the demyelinated lesions, large (the so-called bizarre) astrocytes are found. • Lesions contain low to moderate numbers of T-cells. • few B-cells • few plasma cells • Activated microglial cells and macrophages are present in high numbers.	• Like PML, lesions contain infected cells, especially on the border. • In small samples (biopsies) however, infected cells may be low in numbers or may be absent. • Subpial lesions are absent. • Remyelination is absent. • Like in PML, lesions contain bizarre astrocytes. • Lesions contain extremely high numbers of T-cells and B-cells. • Numbers of microglia and macrophages do not differ with PML.	• Unlike in PML, lesions are perivenous and show finger-like extensions (i.e., Dawson fingers). • Subpial lesions are present and are specific for MS. • Lesions can show variable remyelination. • Lesions can show activated astrocytes and/or astrogliosis. • Extremely large bizarre astrocytes are absent. • Lesions contain moderate to high numbers of T-cells. • Low numbers of B-cell • Low numbers of plasma cells • Numbers of (foamy) macrophages do not differ from PML or PML–IRIS.
MRI features		
• Usually larger than 3 cm • Lesions always start in subcortical regions, probably related to a high blood flow. • Borders are sharp towards the GM and ill-defined towards the WM. • In first scans of 28% of patients, lesions extend in deep GM. • 23–57% of (HIV-associated) cases have contrast-enhancing lesions. • T1 lesions are mostly hypointense. • Diffusion-weighted images are always hyperintense. • Punctate T2-hyperintense lesions can be found in the immediate vicinity of the main lesion.	• Usually larger than 3 cm • Lesions always start in subcortical regions, probably related to a high blood flow. • Borders are sharp towards the GM and ill-defined towards the WM. • In first scans of 71% of patients, lesions extend in deep GM. • 86% of PML–IRIS cases have contrast-enhancing lesions. • T1 lesions may have hyperintense rims. • Diffusion-weighted images are always hyperintense. • Punctate T2-hyperintense lesions can be found in the immediate vicinity of the main lesion.	• All MRI features seen in PML and/or PML–IRIS also can be seen in MS. • However, MS lesions usually are and stay smaller in size than in PML or PML–IRIS. • Homogeneous or open-ring enhancing lesions are present in MS but not observed in PML.

26.8 Herpes Simplex Virus (HSV) Encephalitis

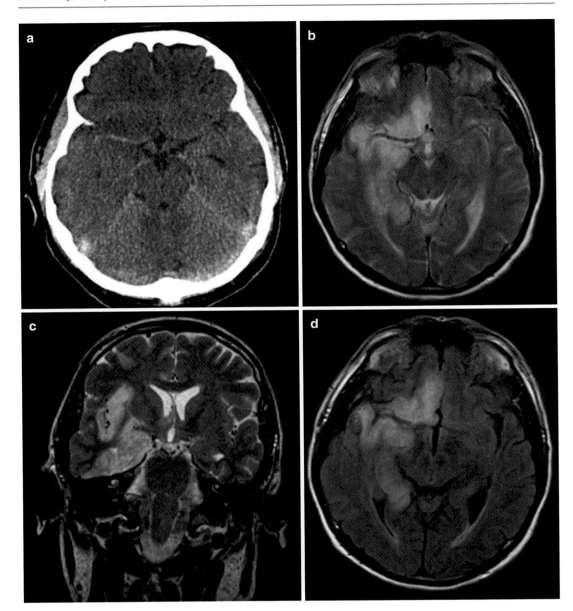

Fig. 26.11 Herpes encephalitis with characteristic involvement of right limbic system, temporal and basal frontal lobe, restricted diffusion and weak enhancement; CT non-contrast (**a**), T2 ax/cor (**b**, **c**), FLAIR (**d**), T1 (**e**), T1 contrast (**f**), DWI (**g**), ADC (**h**)

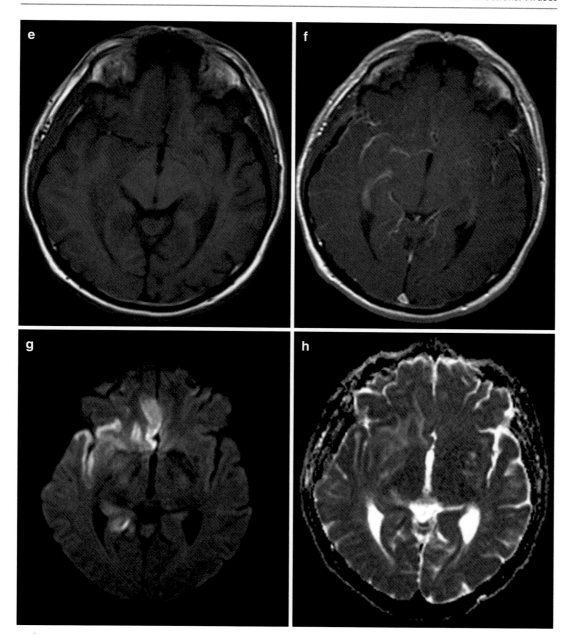

Fig. 26.11 (continued)

MRI-T1 (Fig. 26.11e)
- Hypointense edema
- Loss of gray-white matter differentiation

MRI-T1 Contrast-Enhanced (Fig. 26.11f)
- Diffuse enhancement

MRI-T2∗/SWI
- Hemorrhages hypointense

MR-Diffusion Imaging (Fig 26.11g)
- Often restricted diffusion

MRI-ADC (Fig. 26.11h)
- Often restricted diffusion

Nuclear Medicine Findings (Fig. 26.12)
- Decreased FDG uptake
- After recovery FDG uptake appears regular

26.8 Herpes Simplex Virus (HSV) Encephalitis

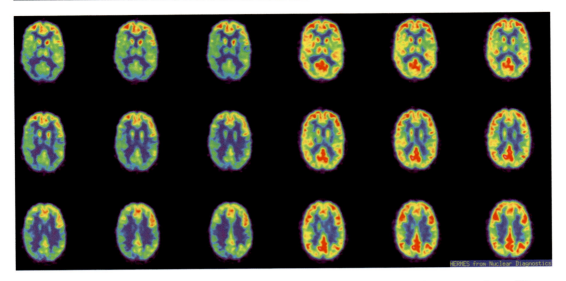

Fig. 26.12 Herpes encephalitis: decreased FDG uptake (left 3 rows) in a patient during the recovery phase of Herpes simplex encephalitis and regular FDG uptake after recovery (right 3 rows)

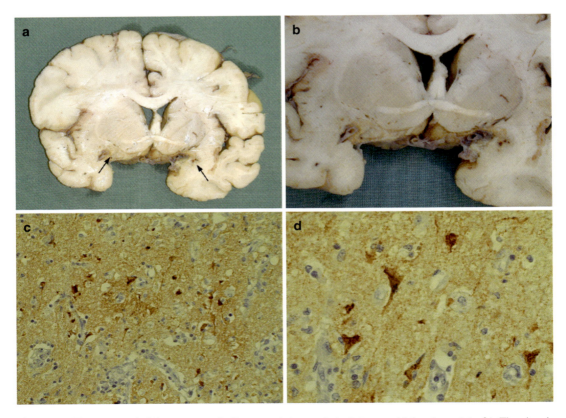

Fig. 26.13 Herpes encephalitis: macroscopically, necrosis is seen in both temporal lobes (arrow) (**a**, **b**). The virus is demonstrated by immunohistochemistry mainly in neurons (**c**, **d**)

26.12.3 Neuropathology Findings

Macroscopic Features (Fig. 26.13a, b)
- Congestion
- Hemorrhagic necrosis of the
  - Temporal lobe
  - Insula
  - Cingulate gyrus
  - Posterior orbitofrontal cortex

Microscopic Features (Fig. 26.13c, d)
- Acute phase
  - parenchymal inflammation
  - lymphocytes and macrophages in the leptomeninges
  - necrotic cells
  - foci of hemorrhages
  - perivascular and interstitial infiltrate of lymphocytes
  - microglial nodules
  - neuronophagia
- Chronic phase
  - glial scar tissue
  - clusters of lymphocytes

26.12.4 Molecular Neuropathology

Pathogenesis
- Primary mucocutaneous infection
  - mucocutaneous border of lips or oropharyngeal mucosa
- Latency in trigeminal ganglion
  - by retrograde axonal transport along sensory fibers to the trigeminal ganglion
  - further replication
  - latent infection (latency-associated transcripts)
- Reactivation of virus
  - anterograde transport to the skin or mucose
  - development of cold sores
  - reactivation
    - spontaneously
    - mucocutaneous trauma
    - ultraviolet irradiation
    - emotional stress
    - pyrexia
    - fluctuations in estrogen and progesterone concentrations
    - immunosuppression

26.12.5 Treatment and Prognosis

Outcome
- Fatal outcome within a few days when untreated
- Treatment

26.13 Tick-Borne Encephalitis

Tick-borne encephalitis (TBE) is an infection of the central nervous system (CNS) caused by tick-borne encephalitis virus (TBEV) and transmitted by ticks, with a variety of clinical manifestations (Table 26.18). The incidence of TBE in Europe is increasing due to an extended season of the infection and the enlargement of endemic areas.

Causative agents:

- Togaviridae
- Flaviviridae
- Reoviridae
- Bunyaviridae

TBE is a caused by flavivirus

- Western Europe subtype, tick vector: *Ixodes ricinus*
- Siberian subtype, tick vector: *Ixodes persulcatus*
- Far eastern subtype, tick vector: *Ixodes persulcatus*

26.13.1 Clinical Signs and Symptoms

- Meningitis typically manifests with
  - High fever
  - Headache
  - Nausea
  - Vomiting
- Encephalitis can be manifested by
  - Impaired consciousness
  - Somnolence
  - Stupor
  - Coma
- Myelitis
- Other manifestations comprise
  - Personality changes
  - Behavioral disorders

26.9 Tick-Borne Encephalitis

Table 26.18 Viruses causing tick-borne encephalitis

Virus	Brain region affected	Mortality	Morbidity	Geographic distribution
Eastern equine encephalitis		50–75%	90% of survivors have persistent neurologic disability.	• Eastern and Gulf coast states of the USA. • Caribbean • South America
Western equine encephalitis	• Basal ganglia • Thalamus • Brain stem	<5%		• Western and Midwestern USA
St. Louis encephalitis	• Midbrain • Thalamus	<5%	25% of survivors have persistent neurologic disability.	• The USA • Central America • South America
Japanese encephalitis	• Thalamus • Substantia nigra • Brain stem • Spinal cord	Up to 50%	High percentage of survivors have persistent neurologic disability.	• Southeast Asia • Bangladesh • Pakistan
West Nile virus	• Thalamus • Cerebellum • Substantia nigra • Pons • Medulla oblongata • Spinal cord	3–15%	50–75% of survivors have residual neurologic disability.	• Africa • Eastern Europe • West Asia • Middle East • North America
Tick-borne encephalitis		1–10%	Small percentage develop chronic encephalitis with intractable epilepsy and progressive paralysis (Russian spring-summer encephalitis).	

- Concentration and cognitive function disturbances
- Tongue fasciculations and tremor of extremities
- Focal or generalized seizures
- Delirium
- Psychosis

26.13.2 Epidemiology

Incidence
- Highly endemic areas (≥5 cases/100 000/year)

26.13.3 Neuroimaging Findings

General Imaging Features
- MRI and CT often normal, rarely lesions in thalamus, cerebellum, or basal ganglia

CT Non-Contrast-Enhanced
- Usually normal

MRI-T2/FLAIR (Fig. 26.14a, b)
- Lesions hyperintense

MRI-T1 (Fig. 26.14c)
- Lesions hypointense

MRI-T1 Contrast-Enhanced (Fig. 26.14d)
- Meningeal or parenchymal enhancement possible

MR-Diffusion Imaging (Fig. 26.14e)
- Restricted diffusion possible

MRI-ADC (Fig. 26.14f)
- Restricted diffusion possible

Nuclear Medicine Imaging Findings (Fig. 26.15)
- decreased FDG uptake

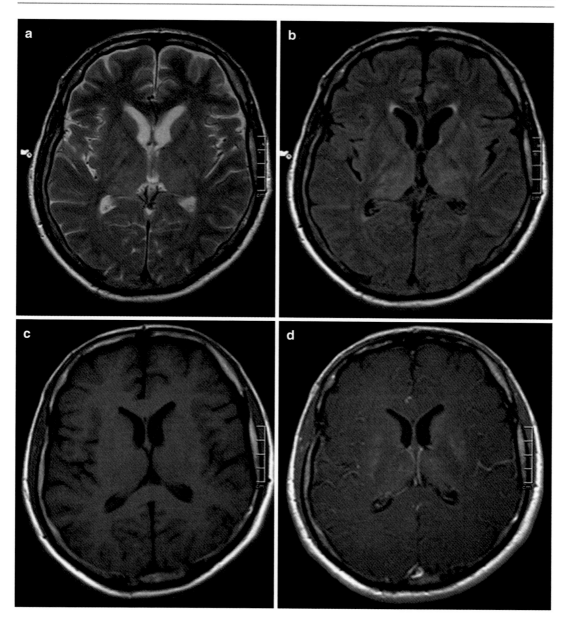

Fig. 26.14 Tick-borne encephalitis with T2-hyperintensity and mild enhancement of thalami and basal ganglia. T2 (**a**), FLAIR (**b**), T1 (**c**), T1 contrast (**d**), DWI (**e**), ADC (**f**)

26.9 Tick-Borne Encephalitis

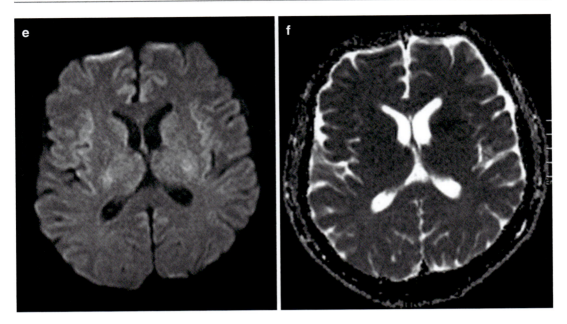

Fig. 26.14 (continued)

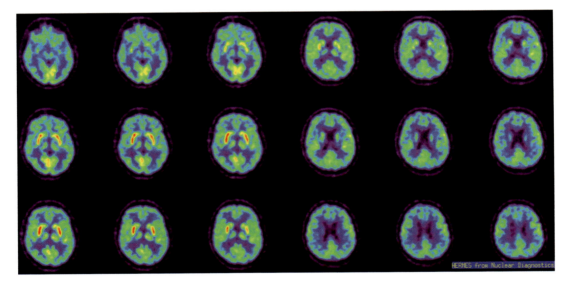

Fig. 26.15 Tick-borne encephalitis: totally decreased FDG uptake in cerebral cortex

26.13.4 Neuropathology Findings

Macroscopic Features
- moderate to sever congestion (Fig. 26.15)
- petechial hemorrhages

Microscopic Features (Fig. 26.16a–l)
- lymphocytic infiltrates
  – leptomeningeal
  – perivascular
  – parenchymal
- microglial nodules and macrophages
- focal necrosis of white matter myelinated fibers
- thrombosed small vessels

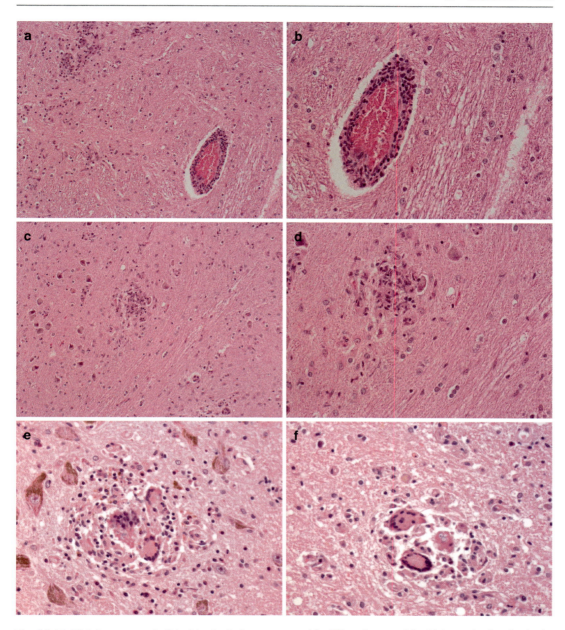

Fig. 26.16 Tick-borne encephalitis: histological examination reveals perivascular lymphocytic infiltrates (**a**, **b**) and the presence of gliomesenchymal nodules (**c**, **d**) which may contain multinucleated giant cells (**e**, **f**). The perivascular infiltrates are mainly made up of CD3-positive T-lymphocytes (**g**) which are also homing in the surrounding brain tissue (**h**). Reactive astrogliosis (stain: GFAP) (**i**, **j**) and reactive microgliosis (stain: HLA-DRII) (**k**, **l**) might be moderate

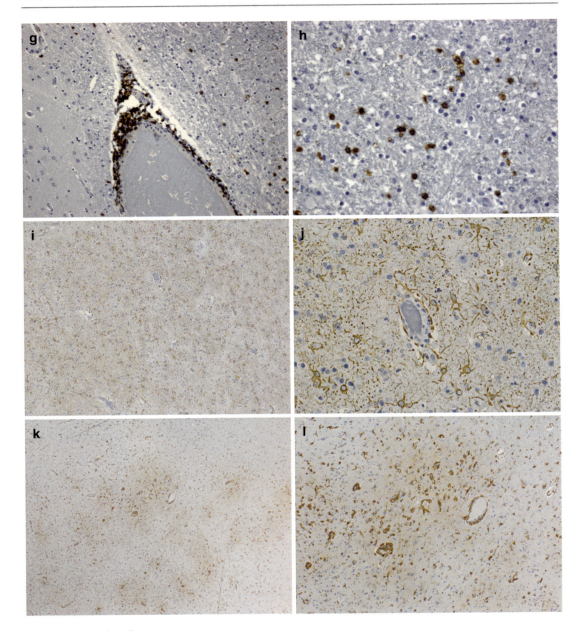

Fig. 26.16 (continued)

26.13.5 Molecular Neuropathology

- Virus enters the vector (mosquito or tick) while it is feeding on the blood of an infected host.
- Is transmitted to other hosts in the salivary secretions of the vector.
- Natural hosts are birds or small mammals (rodents).
- Humans are dead-end hosts.
- Virus replicates at the site of host inoculation.
- Spreads to regional lymph nodes and other lymphoreticular tissues.
- Disseminates hematogenously to systemic tissues (CNS).

26.13.6 Treatment and Prognosis

Treatment

- No specific drug therapy
- Corticosteroids
- Tracheal intubation and respiratory support

Outcome

- Complete restitution to fatal
- Prevention:
  - vaccination

Selected References

Abe H, Mehraein P, Weis S (1996) Degeneration of the cerebellar dentate nucleus and the inferior olivary nuclei in HIV-1-infected brains: a morphometric analysis. Acta Neuropathol 92(2):150–155

Adang L, Berger J (2015) Progressive multifocal leukoencephalopathy. F1000Res:4. https://doi.org/10.12688/f1000research.7071.1

Aksamit AJ Jr (2012) Progressive multifocal leukoencephalopathy. Continuum (Minneapolis, Minn) 18(6 Infectious Disease):1374–1391. https://doi.org/10.1212/01.CON.0000423852.70641.de

Amicizia D, Domnich A, Panatto D, Lai PL, Cristina ML, Avio U, Gasparini R (2013) Epidemiology of tick-borne encephalitis (TBE) in Europe and its prevention by available vaccines. Hum Vaccin Immunother 9(5):1163–1171. https://doi.org/10.4161/hv.23802

Ances BM, Hammoud DA (2014) Neuroimaging of HIV-associated neurocognitive disorders (HAND). Curr Opin HIV AIDS 9(6):545–551. https://doi.org/10.1097/coh.0000000000000112

Andreula C (2004) Cranial viral infections in the adult. Eur Radiol 14(Suppl 3):E132–E144. https://doi.org/10.1007/s00330-003-2040-3

Antinori A, Arendt G, Becker JT, Brew BJ, Byrd DA, Cherner M, Clifford DB, Cinque P, Epstein LG, Goodkin K, Gisslen M, Grant I, Heaton RK, Joseph J, Marder K, Marra CM, McArthur JC, Nunn M, Price RW, Pulliam L, Robertson KR, Sacktor N, Valcour V, Wojna VE (2007) Updated research nosology for HIV-associated neurocognitive disorders. Neurology 69(18):1789–1799. https://doi.org/10.1212/01.WNL.0000287431.88658.8b

Aurelian L (2005) HSV-induced apoptosis in herpes encephalitis. Curr Top Microbiol Immunol 289:79–111

Bale JF Jr (2014) Congenital cytomegalovirus infection. Handb Clin Neurol 123:319–326. https://doi.org/10.1016/b978-0-444-53488-0.00015-8

Baringer JR (2008) Herpes simplex infections of the nervous system. Neurol Clin 26(3):657–674, viii. https://doi.org/10.1016/j.ncl.2008.03.005

Baskin HJ, Hedlund G (2007) Neuroimaging of herpesvirus infections in children. Pediatr Radiol 37(10):949–963. https://doi.org/10.1007/s00247-007-0506-1

Bauer J, Gold R, Adams O, Lassmann H (2015) Progressive multifocal leukoencephalopathy and immune reconstitution inflammatory syndrome (IRIS). Acta Neuropathol 130(6):751–764. https://doi.org/10.1007/s00401-015-1471-7

Bellizzi A, Anzivino E, Rodio DM, Palamara AT, Nencioni L, Pietropaolo V (2013) New insights on human polyomavirus JC and pathogenesis of progressive multifocal leukoencephalopathy. Clin Dev Immunol 2013:839719. https://doi.org/10.1155/2013/839719

Beltrami S, Gordon J (2014) Immune surveillance and response to JC virus infection and PML. J Neurovirol 20(2):137–149. https://doi.org/10.1007/s13365-013-0222-6

Berger JR (2011) The clinical features of PML. Cleve Clin J Med 78(Suppl 2):S8–S12. https://doi.org/10.3949/ccjm.78.s2.03

Berger JR (2014) Progressive multifocal leukoencephalopathy. Handb Clin Neurol 123:357–376. https://doi.org/10.1016/b978-0-444-53488-0.00017-1

Berger JR (2017) Classifying PML risk with disease modifying therapies. Mult Scler Relat Disord 12:59–63. https://doi.org/10.1016/j.msard.2017.01.006

Berger JR, Khalili K (2011) The pathogenesis of progressive multifocal leukoencephalopathy. Discov Med 12(67):495–503

Berger JR, Aksamit AJ, Clifford DB, Davis L, Koralnik IJ, Sejvar JJ, Bartt R, Major EO, Nath A (2013) PML diagnostic criteria: consensus statement from the AAN Neuroinfectious Disease Section. Neurology 80(15):1430–1438. https://doi.org/10.1212/WNL.0b013e31828c2fa1

Birkmann A, Zimmermann H (2016) HSV antivirals—current and future treatment options. Curr Opin Virol 18:9–13. https://doi.org/10.1016/j.coviro.2016.01.013

Bloom DC (2004) HSV LAT and neuronal survival. Int Rev Immunol 23(1–2):187–198

Bradshaw MJ, Venkatesan A (2016) Herpes simplex virus-1 encephalitis in adults: pathophysiology, diagnosis, and management. Neurotherapeutics 13(3):493–508. https://doi.org/10.1007/s13311-016-0433-7

Brown JC (2017) Herpes simplex virus latency: the DNA repair-centered pathway. Adv Virol 2017:7028194. https://doi.org/10.1155/2017/7028194

Buttner A, Mehraein P, Weis S (1996) Vascular changes in the cerebral cortex in HIV-1 infection. II An immunohistochemical and lectinhistochemical investigation. Acta Neuropathol 92(1):35–41

Cantey JB, Sanchez PJ (2013) Neonatal herpes simplex virus infections: past progress and future challenges. Pediatr Infect Dis J 32(11):1205–1207. https://doi.org/10.1097/INF.0b013e3182a1915e

Carletti T, Zakaria MK, Marcello A (2017) The host cell response to tick-borne encephalitis virus. Biochem Biophys Res Commun 492(4):533–540. https://doi.org/10.1016/j.bbrc.2017.02.006

Carroll A, Brew B (2017) HIV-associated neurocognitive disorders: recent advances in pathogenesis, biomarkers, and treatment. F1000Res 6:312. https://doi.org/10.12688/f1000research.10651.1

Chahroudi A, Silvestri G (2012) IRIS: the unfortunate rainbow of HIV. Blood 119(13):2971–2972. https://doi.org/10.1182/blood-2012-01-403683

Chen MF, Gill AJ, Kolson DL (2014) Neuropathogenesis of HIV-associated neurocognitive disorders: roles for immune activation, HIV blipping and viral tropism. Curr Opin HIV AIDS 9(6):559–564. https://doi.org/10.1097/coh.0000000000000105

Ciardi A, Sinclair E, Scaravilli F, Harcourt-Webster NJ, Lucas S (1990) The involvement of the cerebral cortex in human immunodeficiency virus encephalopathy: a morphological and immunohistochemical study. Acta Neuropathol 81(1):51–59

Cinque P, Koralnik IJ, Gerevini S, Miro JM, Price RW (2009) Progressive multifocal leukoencephalopathy in HIV-1 infection. Lancet Infect Dis 9(10):625–636. https://doi.org/10.1016/s1473-3099(09)70226-9

Clifford DB, Ances BM (2013) HIV-associated neurocognitive disorder. Lancet Infect Dis 13(11):976–986. https://doi.org/10.1016/s1473-3099(13)70269-x

Corey L, Wald A (2009) Maternal and neonatal herpes simplex virus infections. N Engl J Med 361(14):1376–1385. https://doi.org/10.1056/NEJMra0807633

Del Valle L, Pina-Oviedo S (2006) HIV disorders of the brain: pathology and pathogenesis. Front Biosci 11:718–732

Desai DV, Kulkarni SS (2015) Herpes simplex virus: the interplay between HSV, host, and HIV-1. Viral Immunol 28(10):546–555. https://doi.org/10.1089/vim.2015.0012

Descamps M, Hyare H, Stebbing J, Winston A (2008) Magnetic resonance imaging and spectroscopy of the brain in HIV disease. J HIV Ther 13(3):55–58

Dorrbecker B, Dobler G, Spiegel M, Hufert FT (2010) Tick-borne encephalitis virus and the immune response of the mammalian host. Travel Med Infect Dis 8(4):213–222. https://doi.org/10.1016/j.tmaid.2010.05.010

Eggers C, Arendt G, Hahn K, Husstedt IW, Maschke M, Neuen-Jacob E, Obermann M, Rosenkranz T, Schielke E, Straube E (2017) HIV-1-associated neurocognitive disorder: epidemiology, pathogenesis, diagnosis, and treatment. J Neurol 264(8):1715–1727. https://doi.org/10.1007/s00415-017-8503-2

Ellis R, Langford D, Masliah E (2007) HIV and antiretroviral therapy in the brain: neuronal injury and repair. Nat Rev Neurosci 8(1):33–44. https://doi.org/10.1038/nrn2040

Esiri MM, Morris CS, Millard PR (1991) Fate of oligodendrocytes in HIV-1 infection. AIDS (London, England) 5(9):1081–1088

Everall I, Luthert P, Lantos P (1993) A review of neuronal damage in human immunodeficiency virus infection: its assessment, possible mechanism and relationship to dementia. J Neuropathol Exp Neurol 52(6):561–566

Ferenczy MW, Marshall LJ, Nelson CD, Atwood WJ, Nath A, Khalili K, Major EO (2012) Molecular biology, epidemiology, and pathogenesis of progressive multifocal leukoencephalopathy, the JC virus-induced demyelinating disease of the human brain. Clin Microbiol Rev 25(3):471–506. https://doi.org/10.1128/cmr.05031-11

Force WGotAAoNAT (1991) Nomenclature and research case definitions for neurologic manifestations of human immunodeficiency virus-type 1 (HIV-1) infection. Report of a Working Group of the American Academy of Neurology AIDS Task Force. Neurology 41(6):778–785

Fournier A, Martin-Blondel G, Lechapt-Zalcman E, Dina J, Kazemi A, Verdon R, Mortier E, de La Blanchardiere A (2017) Immune reconstitution inflammatory syndrome unmasking or worsening AIDS-related progressive multifocal leukoencephalopathy: a literature review. Front Immunol 8:577. https://doi.org/10.3389/fimmu.2017.00577

Garden GA (2002) Microglia in human immunodeficiency virus-associated neurodegeneration. Glia 40(2):240–251. https://doi.org/10.1002/glia.10155

Gartner S (2000) HIV infection and dementia. Science (New York, NY) 287(5453):602–604

Gelman BB, Guinto FC Jr (1992) Morphometry, histopathology, and tomography of cerebral atrophy in the acquired immunodeficiency syndrome. Ann Neurol 32(1):31–40. https://doi.org/10.1002/ana.410320107

Gendelman HE, Lipton SA, Tardieu M, Bukrinsky MI, Nottet HS (1994) The neuropathogenesis of HIV-1 infection. J Leukoc Biol 56(3):389–398

Gheuens S, Wuthrich C, Koralnik IJ (2013) Progressive multifocal leukoencephalopathy: why gray and white matter. Annu Rev Pathol 8:189–215. https://doi.org/10.1146/annurev-pathol-020712-164018

Gilden DH (2008) Brain imaging abnormalities in CNS virus infections. Neurology 70(1):84. https://doi.org/10.1212/01.wnl.0000286937.09760.e4

Gnann JW Jr, Whitley RJ (2017) Herpes simplex encephalitis: an update. Curr Infect Dis Rep 19(3):13. https://doi.org/10.1007/s11908-017-0568-7

Gougeon ML (2017) Alarmins and central nervous system inflammation in HIV-associated neurological disorders. J Intern Med 281(5):433–447. https://doi.org/10.1111/joim.12570

Gray F, Gherardi R, Scaravilli F (1988) The neuropathology of the acquired immune deficiency syndrome (AIDS). A review. Brain J Neurol 111(Pt 2):245–266

Gray F, Lescs MC, Keohane C, Paraire F, Marc B, Durigon M, Gherardi R (1992) Early brain changes in HIV infection: neuropathological study of 11 HIV seropositive, non-AIDS cases. J Neuropathol Exp Neurol 51(2):177–185

Gray F, Chretien F, Vallat-Decouvelaere AV, Scaravilli F (2003) The changing pattern of HIV neuropathology in the HAART era. J Neuropathol Exp Neurol 62(5):429–440

Grosche L, Kummer M, Steinkasserer A (2017) What goes around, comes around—HSV-1 replication in monocyte-derived dendritic cells. Front Microbiol 8:2149. https://doi.org/10.3389/fmicb.2017.02149

Hartman EA, Huang D (2008) Update on PML: lessons from the HIV uninfected and new insights in pathogenesis and treatment. Curr HIV/AIDS Rep 5(3):112–119

Holt JL, Kraft-Terry SD, Chang L (2012) Neuroimaging studies of the aging HIV-1-infected brain. J Neurovirol 18(4):291–302. https://doi.org/10.1007/s13365-012-0114-1

Honce JM, Nagae L, Nyberg E (2015) Neuroimaging of natalizumab complications in multiple sclerosis: PML and other associated entities. Mult Scler Int 2015:809252. https://doi.org/10.1155/2015/809252

Hong S, Banks WA (2015) Role of the immune system in HIV-associated neuroinflammation and neurocognitive implications. Brain Behav Immun 45:1–12. https://doi.org/10.1016/j.bbi.2014.10.008

Horger M, Beck R, Fenchel M, Ernemann U, Nagele T, Brodoefel H, Heckl S (2012a) Imaging findings in tick-borne encephalitis with differential diagnostic considerations. AJR Am J Roentgenol 199(2):420–427. https://doi.org/10.2214/ajr.11.7911

Horger M, Beschorner R, Beck R, Nagele T, Schulze M, Ernemann U, Heckl S (2012b) Common and uncommon imaging findings in progressive multifocal leukoencephalopathy (PML) with differential diagnostic considerations. Clin Neurol Neurosurg 114(8):1123–1130. https://doi.org/10.1016/j.clineuro.2012.06.018

Hu XT (2016) HIV-1 tat-mediated calcium dysregulation and neuronal dysfunction in vulnerable brain regions. Curr Drug Targets 17(1):4–14

Itoh K, Mehraein P, Weis S (2000) Neuronal damage of the substantia nigra in HIV-1 infected brains. Acta Neuropathol 99(4):376–384

Jelcic I, Jelcic I, Faigle W, Sospedra M, Martin R (2015) Immunology of progressive multifocal leukoencephalopathy. J Neurovirol 21(6):614–622. https://doi.org/10.1007/s13365-014-0294-y

Jellinger KA, Setinek U, Drlicek M, Bohm G, Steurer A, Lintner F (2000) Neuropathology and general autopsy findings in AIDS during the last 15 years. Acta Neuropathol 100(2):213–220

Jiang YC, Feng H, Lin YC, Guo XR (2016) New strategies against drug resistance to herpes simplex virus. Int J Oral Sci 8(1):1–6. https://doi.org/10.1038/ijos.2016.3

Joseph J, Colosi DA, Rao VR (2016) HIV-1 induced CNS dysfunction: current overview and research priorities. Curr HIV Res 14(5):389–399

Kaiser R (2008) Tick-borne encephalitis. Infect Dis Clin N Am 22(3):561–575, x. https://doi.org/10.1016/j.idc.2008.03.013

Kastrup O, Wanke I, Maschke M (2005) Neuroimaging of infections. NeuroRx 2(2):324–332. https://doi.org/10.1602/neurorx.2.2.324

Kastrup O, Wanke I, Maschke M (2008) Neuroimaging of infections of the central nervous system. Semin Neurol 28(4):511–522. https://doi.org/10.1055/s-0028-1083688

Kaul M, Garden GA, Lipton SA (2001) Pathways to neuronal injury and apoptosis in HIV-associated dementia. Nature 410(6831):988–994. https://doi.org/10.1038/35073667

Ketzler S, Weis S, Haug H, Budka H (1990) Loss of neurons in the frontal cortex in AIDS brains. Acta Neuropathol 80(1):92–94

Kolson DL (2002) Neuropathogenesis of central nervous system HIV-1 infection. Clin Lab Med 22(3):703–717

Kolson D (2017) Neurologic complications in persons with HIV infection in the era of antiretroviral therapy. Top Antivir Med 25(3):97–101

Kozlowski PB, Sher JH, Rao C, Anzil PA, Wrzolek MA, Sharer L, Cho ES, Dickson DW, Weidenheim KM, Llena JF et al (1993) Central nervous system in pediatric AIDS. Results from Neuropathologic Pediatric AIDS Registry. Ann N Y Acad Sci 693:295–296

Lamers SL, Rose R, Ndhlovu LC, Nolan DJ, Salemi M, Maidji E, Stoddart CA, McGrath MS (2016) The meningeal lymphatic system: a route for HIV brain migration? J Neurovirol 22(3):275–281. https://doi.org/10.1007/s13365-015-0399-y

Langford TD, Letendre SL, Larrea GJ, Masliah E (2003) Changing patterns in the neuropathogenesis of HIV during the HAART era. Brain Pathol (Zurich, Switzerland) 13(2):195–210

Laothamatas J, Hemachudha T, Mitrabhakdi E, Wannakrairot P, Tulayadaechanont S (2003) MR imaging in human rabies. AJNR Am J Neuroradiol 24(6):1102–1109

Laothamatas J, Sungkarat W, Hemachudha T (2011) Neuroimaging in rabies. Adv Virus Res 79:309–327. https://doi.org/10.1016/b978-0-12-387040-7.00014-7

Le LT, Spudich SS (2016) HIV-associated neurologic disorders and central nervous system opportunistic infections in HIV. Semin Neurol 36(4):373–381. https://doi.org/10.1055/s-0036-1585454

Levine AJ, Panos SE, Horvath S (2014) Genetic, transcriptomic, and epigenetic studies of HIV-associated neurocognitive disorder. J Acquir Immune Defic Syndr 65(4):481–503. https://doi.org/10.1097/qai.0000000000000069

Lindquist L (2014) Tick-borne encephalitis. Handb Clin Neurol 123:531–559. https://doi.org/10.1016/b978-0-444-53488-0.00025-0

Liner KJ 2nd, Ro MJ, Robertson KR (2010) HIV, antiretroviral therapies, and the brain. Curr HIV/AIDS Rep 7(2):85–91. https://doi.org/10.1007/s11904-010-0042-8

Lipton SA (1991) HIV-related neurotoxicity. Brain Pathol (Zurich, Switzerland) 1(3):193–199

Liu H, Xu E, Liu J, Xiong H (2016) Oligodendrocyte injury and pathogenesis of HIV-1-associated neurocognitive disorders. Brain Sci 6(3):E23. https://doi.org/10.3390/brainsci6030023

Lopez-Labrador FX, Berenguer M, Navarro D (2015) Overcoming drug resistance in HSV, CMV, HBV and HCV infection. Future Microbiol 10(11):1759–1766. https://doi.org/10.2217/fmb.15.74

Louboutin JP, Strayer DS (2012) Blood-brain barrier abnormalities caused by HIV-1 gp120: mechanistic and therapeutic implications. Sci J 2012:482575. https://doi.org/10.1100/2012/482575

Malik S, Eugenin EA (2016) Mechanisms of HIV neuropathogenesis: role of cellular communication systems. Curr HIV Res 14(5):400–411

Marban C, Forouzanfar F, Ait-Ammar A, Fahmi F, El Mekdad H, Daouad F, Rohr O, Schwartz C (2016) Targeting the brain reservoirs: toward an HIV cure. Front Immunol 7:397. https://doi.org/10.3389/fimmu.2016.00397

Maschke M, Kastrup O, Forsting M, Diener HC (2004) Update on neuroimaging in infectious central nervous system disease. Curr Opin Neurol 17(4):475–480

Masliah E, Achim CL, Ge N, DeTeresa R, Terry RD, Wiley CA (1992a) Spectrum of human immunodeficiency virus-associated neocortical damage. Ann Neurol 32(3):321–329. https://doi.org/10.1002/ana.410320304

Masliah E, Ge N, Morey M, DeTeresa R, Terry RD, Wiley CA (1992b) Cortical dendritic pathology in human immunodeficiency virus encephalitis. Lab Invest 66(3):285–291

McCarthy M, Nath A (2010) Neurologic consequences of the immune reconstitution inflammatory syndrome (IRIS). Curr Neurol Neurosci Rep 10(6):467–475. https://doi.org/10.1007/s11910-010-0138-y

McRae M (2016) HIV and viral protein effects on the blood brain barrier. Tissue Barriers 4(1):e1143543. https://doi.org/10.1080/21688370.2016.1143543

Meeker RB, Asahchop E, Power C (2014) The brain and HAART: collaborative and combative connections. Curr Opin HIV AIDS 9(6):579–584. https://doi.org/10.1097/coh.0000000000000110

Menendez CM, Carr DJJ (2017) Defining nervous system susceptibility during acute and latent herpes simplex virus-1 infection. J Neuroimmunol 308:43–49. https://doi.org/10.1016/j.jneuroim.2017.02.020

Molloy ES, Calabrese CM, Calabrese LH (2017) The risk of progressive multifocal leukoencephalopathy in the biologic era: prevention and management. Rheum Dis Clin N Am 43(1):95–109. https://doi.org/10.1016/j.rdc.2016.09.009

Monaco MC, Major EO (2015) Immune system involvement in the pathogenesis of JC virus induced PML: what is learned from studies of patients with underlying diseases and therapies as risk factors. Front Immunol 6:159. https://doi.org/10.3389/fimmu.2015.00159

Navia BA, Cho ES, Petito CK, Price RW (1986a) The AIDS dementia complex: II. Neuropathology. Ann Neurol 19(6):525–535. https://doi.org/10.1002/ana.410190603

Navia BA, Jordan BD, Price RW (1986b) The AIDS dementia complex: I. Clinical features. Ann Neurol 19(6):517–524. https://doi.org/10.1002/ana.410190602

Nelson AM, Manabe YC, Lucas SB (2017) Immune reconstitution inflammatory syndrome (IRIS): what pathologists should know. Semin Diagn Pathol 34(4):340–351. https://doi.org/10.1053/j.semdp.2017.04.010

Netravathi M, Mahadevan A, Satishchandra P, Shobha N, Mailankody P, Kandavel T, Jitender S, Anantaram G, Nagarathna S, Govekar S, Ravikumar BV, Ravi V, Shankar SK (2013) Progressive multifocal leukoencephalopathy (PML) associated with HIV Clade C–is not uncommon. J Neurovirol 19(3):198–208. https://doi.org/10.1007/s13365-013-0168-8

Nicoll MP, Proenca JT, Efstathiou S (2012) The molecular basis of herpes simplex virus latency. FEMS Microbiol Rev 36(3):684–705. https://doi.org/10.1111/j.1574-6976.2011.00320.x

Nightingale S, Winston A, Letendre S, Michael BD, McArthur JC, Khoo S, Solomon T (2014) Controversies in HIV-associated neurocognitive disorders. Lancet Neurol 13(11):1139–1151. https://doi.org/10.1016/s1474-4422(14)70137-1

Oster S, Christoffersen P, Gundersen HJ, Nielsen JO, Pakkenberg B, Pedersen C (1993) Cerebral atrophy in AIDS: a stereological study. Acta Neuropathol 85(6):617–622

Pavlovic D, Patera AC, Nyberg F, Gerber M, Liu M (2015) Progressive multifocal leukoencephalopathy: current treatment options and future perspectives. Ther Adv Neurol Disord 8(6):255–273. https://doi.org/10.1177/1756285615602832

Persidsky Y, Gendelman HE (2003) Mononuclear phagocyte immunity and the neuropathogenesis of HIV-1 infection. J Leukoc Biol 74(5):691–701. https://doi.org/10.1189/jlb.0503205

Pires de Mello CP, Bloom DC, Paixao IC (2016) Herpes simplex virus type-1: replication, latency, reactivation and its antiviral targets. Antivir Ther 21(4):277–286. https://doi.org/10.3851/imp3018

Rao VR, Ruiz AP, Prasad VR (2014) Viral and cellular factors underlying neuropathogenesis in HIV associated neurocognitive disorders (HAND). AIDS Res Ther 11:13. https://doi.org/10.1186/1742-6405-11-13

Reyes MG, Faraldi F, Senseng CS, Flowers C, Fariello R (1991) Nigral degeneration in acquired immune deficiency syndrome (AIDS). Acta Neuropathol 82(1):39–44

Rocha AJ, Littig IA, Nunes RH, Tilbery CP (2013) Central nervous system infectious diseases mimicking multiple sclerosis: recognizing distinguishable features using MRI. Arq Neuropsiquiatr 71(9b):738–746. https://doi.org/10.1590/0004-282x20130162

Roizman B, Whitley RJ (2013) An inquiry into the molecular basis of HSV latency and reactivation. Annu Rev Microbiol 67:355–374. https://doi.org/10.1146/annurev-micro-092412-155654

Rozenberg F, Deback C, Agut H (2011) Herpes simplex encephalitis: from virus to therapy. Infect Disord Drug Targets 11(3):235–250

Ru W, Tang SJ (2017) HIV-associated synaptic degeneration. Mol Brain 10(1):40. https://doi.org/10.1186/s13041-017-0321-z

Rumboldt Z (2008) Imaging of topographic viral CNS infections. Neuroimaging Clin N Am 18(1):85–92; viii. https://doi.org/10.1016/j.nic.2007.12.006

Ruzek D, Dobler G, Donoso Mantke O (2010) Tick-borne encephalitis: pathogenesis and clinical implications. Travel Med Infect Dis 8(4):223–232. https://doi.org/10.1016/j.tmaid.2010.06.004

Ryan LA, Cotter RL, Zink WE 2nd, Gendelman HE, Zheng J (2002) Macrophages, chemokines and neuronal injury in HIV-1-associated dementia. Cell Mol Biol (Noisy-le-Grand) 48(2):137–150

Sabri F, Titanji K, De Milito A, Chiodi F (2003) Astrocyte activation and apoptosis: their roles in the neuropathology of HIV infection. Brain Pathol (Zurich, Switzerland) 13(1):84–94

Sahraian MA, Radue EW, Eshaghi A, Besliu S, Minagar A (2012) Progressive multifocal leukoencephalopathy: a review of the neuroimaging features and differential diagnosis. Eur J Neurol 19(8):1060–1069. https://doi.org/10.1111/j.1468-1331.2011.03597.x

Sanchez AB, Kaul M (2017) Neuronal stress and injury caused by HIV-1, cART and drug abuse: converging contributions to HAND. Brain Sci 7(3):E25. https://doi.org/10.3390/brainsci7030025

Saylor D, Dickens AM, Sacktor N, Haughey N, Slusher B, Pletnikov M, Mankowski JL, Brown A, Volsky DJ, McArthur JC (2016) HIV-associated neurocognitive disorder—pathogenesis and prospects for treatment. Nat Rev Neurol 12(4):234–248. https://doi.org/10.1038/nrneurol.2016.27

Schwab N, Schneider-Hohendorf T, Melzer N, Cutter G, Wiendl H (2017) Natalizumab-associated PML: challenges with incidence, resulting risk, and risk stratification. Neurology 88(12):1197–1205. https://doi.org/10.1212/wnl.0000000000003739

Senocak E, Oguz KK, Ozgen B, Kurne A, Ozkaya G, Unal S, Cila A (2010) Imaging features of CNS involvement in AIDS. Diagn Interv Radiol (Ankara, Turkey) 16(3):193–200. https://doi.org/10.4261/1305-3825.dir.2182-08.1

Shah R, Bag AK, Chapman PR, Cure JK (2010) Imaging manifestations of progressive multifocal leukoencephalopathy. Clin Radiol 65(6):431–439. https://doi.org/10.1016/j.crad.2010.03.001

Singh SK (2016) Overview on the tricks of HIV tat to hit the blood brain barrier. Curr HIV Res 14(5):382–388

Smit R, Postma MJ (2015) Review of tick-borne encephalitis and vaccines: clinical and economical aspects. Expert Rev Vaccines 14(5):737–747. https://doi.org/10.1586/14760584.2015.985661

Sotrel A, Dal Canto MC (2000) HIV-1 and its causal relationship to immunosuppression and nervous system disease in AIDS: a review. Hum Pathol 31(10):1274–1298. https://doi.org/10.1053/hupa.2000.19293

Steiner I, Berger JR (2012) Update on progressive multifocal leukoencephalopathy. Curr Neurol Neurosci Rep 12(6):680–686. https://doi.org/10.1007/s11910-012-0313-4

Subbiah P, Mouton P, Fedor H, McArthur JC, Glass JD (1996) Stereological analysis of cerebral atrophy in human immunodeficiency virus-associated dementia. J Neuropathol Exp Neurol 55(10):1032–1037

Taba P, Schmutzhard E, Forsberg P, Lutsar I, Ljostad U, Mygland A, Levchenko I, Strle F, Steiner I (2017) EAN consensus review on prevention, diagnosis and management of tick-borne encephalitis. Eur J Neurol 24(10):1214–e1261. https://doi.org/10.1111/ene.13356

Tan CS, Koralnik IJ (2010) Progressive multifocal leukoencephalopathy and other disorders caused by JC virus: clinical features and pathogenesis. Lancet Neurol 9(4):425–437. https://doi.org/10.1016/s1474-4422(10)70040-5

Tardieu M (1999) HIV-1-related central nervous system diseases. Curr Opin Neurol 4:377–81

Tenhula WN, Xu SZ, Madigan MC, Heller K, Freeman WR, Sadun AA (1992) Morphometric comparisons of optic nerve axon loss in acquired immunodeficiency syndrome. Am J Ophthalmol 113(1):14–20

Thellman NM, Triezenberg SJ (2017) Herpes simplex virus establishment, maintenance, and reactivation: in vitro modeling of latency. Pathogens (Basel, Switzerland) 6(3). https://doi.org/10.3390/pathogens6030028

Thompson PM, Jahanshad N (2015) Novel neuroimaging methods to understand how HIV affects the brain. Curr HIV/AIDS Rep 12(2):289–298. https://doi.org/10.1007/s11904-015-0268-6

Tselis AC (2014) Cytomegalovirus infections of the adult human nervous system. Handb Clin Neurol 123:307–318. https://doi.org/10.1016/b978-0-444-53488-0.00014-6

Uzasci L, Nath A, Cotter R (2013) Oxidative stress and the HIV-infected brain proteome. J Neuroimmune Pharmacol 8(5):1167–1180. https://doi.org/10.1007/s11481-013-9444-x

Vago L, Bonetto S, Nebuloni M, Duca P, Carsana L, Zerbi P, D'Arminio-Monforte A (2002) Pathological findings in the central nervous system of AIDS patients on assumed antiretroviral therapeutic regimens: retrospective study of 1597 autopsies. AIDS (London, England) 16(14):1925–1928

Vartak-Sharma N, Nooka S, Ghorpade A (2017) Astrocyte elevated gene-1 (AEG-1) and the A(E)Ging HIV/AIDS-HAND. Prog Neurobiol 157:133–157. https://doi.org/10.1016/j.pneurobio.2016.03.006

Vera JH, Ridha B, Gilleece Y, Amlani A, Thorburn P, Dizdarevic S (2017) PET brain imaging in HIV-associated neurocognitive disorders (HAND) in the era of combination antiretroviral therapy. Eur J Nucl Med Mol Imaging 44(5):895–902. https://doi.org/10.1007/s00259-016-3602-3

Verma R (2012) MRI features of Japanese encephalitis. BMJ Case Rep 2012:bcr0320126088. https://doi.org/10.1136/bcr.03.2012.6088

von Stulpnagel C, Winkler P, Koch J, Zeches-Kansy C, Schottler-Glas A, Wolf G, Niller HH, Staudt M, Kluger G, Rostasy K (2016) MRI-imaging and clinical findings of eleven children with tick-borne encephalitis and review of the literature. Eur J Paediatr Neurol 20(1):45–52. https://doi.org/10.1016/j.ejpn.2015.10.008

Wattjes MP, Richert ND, Killestein J, de Vos M, Sanchez E, Snaebjornsson P, Cadavid D, Barkhof F (2013) The chameleon of neuroinflammation: magnetic resonance imaging characteristics of natalizumab-associated progressive multifocal leukoencephalopathy. Mult Scler (Houndmills,

Basingstoke, England) 19(14):1826–1840. https://doi.org/10.1177/1352458513510224

Weis S, Haug H (1989) Capillaries in the human cerebral cortex: a quantitative electronmicroscopical study. Acta Stereologica 8:139–144

Weis S, Haug H, Budka H (1993a) Astroglial changes in the cerebral cortex of AIDS brains: a morphometric and immunohistochemical investigation. Neuropathol Appl Neurobiol 19(4):329–335

Weis S, Haug H, Budka H (1993b) Neuronal damage in the cerebral cortex of AIDS brains: a morphometric study. Acta Neuropathol 85(2):185–189

Weis S, Llenos IC, Büttner A, Rebhan A, Soreth D, Mehraein P (1993c) Macroscopic morphometry of human brains in neurodegeneration. Acta Stereologica 12:299–304

Weis S, Neuhaus B, Mehraein P (1994) Activation of microglia in HIV-1 infected brains is not dependent on the presence of HIV-1 antigens. Neuroreport 5(12):1514–1516

Weis S, Haug H, Budka H (1996) Vascular changes in the cerebral cortex in HIV-1 infection: I. A morphometric investigation by light and electron microscopy. Clin Neuropathol 15(6):361–366

Weller SK, Coen DM (2012) Herpes simplex viruses: mechanisms of DNA replication. Cold Spring Harb Perspect Biol 4(9):a013011. https://doi.org/10.1101/cshperspect.a013011

White MK, Khalili K (2011) Pathogenesis of progressive multifocal leukoencephalopathy—revisited. J Infect Dis 203(5):578–586. https://doi.org/10.1093/infdis/jiq097

White MK, Sariyer IK, Gordon J, Delbue S, Pietropaolo V, Berger JR, Khalili K (2016) Diagnostic assays for polyomavirus JC and progressive multifocal leukoencephalopathy. Rev Med Virol 26(2):102–114. https://doi.org/10.1002/rmv.1866

Wiley CA, Masliah E, Morey M, Lemere C, DeTeresa R, Grafe M, Hansen L, Terry R (1991) Neocortical damage during HIV infection. Ann Neurol 29(6):651–657. https://doi.org/10.1002/ana.410290613

Williams KC, Hickey WF (2002) Central nervous system damage, monocytes and macrophages, and neurological disorders in AIDS. Annu Rev Neurosci 25:537–562. https://doi.org/10.1146/annurev.neuro.25.112701.142822

Wilson AC, Mohr I (2012) A cultured affair: HSV latency and reactivation in neurons. Trends Microbiol 20(12):604–611. https://doi.org/10.1016/j.tim.2012.08.005

Wohlschlaeger J, Wenger E, Mehraein P, Weis S (2009) White matter changes in HIV-1 infected brains: a combined gross anatomical and ultrastructural morphometric investigation of the corpus callosum. Clin Neurol Neurosurg 111(5):422–429. Epub 2009 Jan 2029

Zambito Marsala S, Pistacchi M, Gioulis M, Mel R, Marchini C, Francavilla E (2014) Neurological complications of tick borne encephalitis: the experience of 89 patients studied and literature review. Neurol Sci 35(1):15–21. https://doi.org/10.1007/s10072-013-1565-8

Zayyad Z, Spudich S (2015) Neuropathogenesis of HIV: from initial neuroinvasion to HIV-associated neurocognitive disorder (HAND). Curr HIV/AIDS Rep 12(1):16–24. https://doi.org/10.1007/s11904-014-0255-3

Infections: Parasites

27.1 Classification of Parasitic Agents

Parasites are classified into (Table 27.1):

- Protozoa
- Animalia (metazoa)
- Fungi (see Chap. 28)
- Stramenopila (formerly chromista)

The main protozoa and helminthes responsible for human infections are listed in Tables 27.2 and 27.3, respectively.

27.2 Clinical Signs and Symptoms

Clinical signs include (Table 27.4):

- Fever
- Headache
- Nausea and vomiting
- Meningism
- Seizures
- Neck pain
- Sensitivity to light
- Confusion or changes in behavior

Parasites associated with diseases of the central nervous system are listed in Table 27.5.

27.3 *Toxoplasma gondii*

Basically, the following two forms of cerebral toxoplasmosis are distinguished:

- Congenital toxoplasmosis
- Acquired toxoplasmosis

Toxoplasmosis restricted to the CNS can be pathogenetically classified as reactivation of a latent infection, whereas acute, systemic toxoplasmosis involving other organs is seen in patients who probably acquired the infection during HIV-induced immunosuppression.

27.3.1 Clinical Signs and Symptoms

- Acute disease
  - Flu-like illness
    - Chills
    - Fever
    - Headaches
  - Myalgia
  - Lymphadenitis, cervical lymphadenopathy
  - Fatigue
- Congenital
  - acute primary infection acquired by the mother during pregnancy
    - devastating effect

Table 27.1 Examples of parasitic pathogens

Protozoan infections	• Toxoplasmosis • Amoebic meningoencephalitis or cerebral amebic abscess • Cerebral malaria • Trypanosomiasis • Babesiosis • Microsporidiosis • Leishmaniasis • Sarcocystosis	
Metazoan infections	• Cestodes	• Cysticercosis • Coenurosis • Hydatid disease • Sparganosis
	• Trematode	• Schistosomiasis • Paragonimiasis • Other trematode infections
	• Nematodes	• Eosinophilic meningoencephalitis • Toxocariasis • Trichinosis
	• Filariasis	• Onchocerciasis • Loiasis

Table 27.2 Main protozoa responsible for human infections

Amebiasis	Cerebral amebic abscess	• *Entamoeba histolytica*
	Primary amebic meningoencephalitis	• *Naegleria fowleri*
	Primary granulomatous amebic encephalitis	• *Acanthamoeba* spp. • *Leptomyxid*
	Keratitis	• *Acanthamoeba*
Cerebral malaria		• *Plasmodium falciparum*
Toxoplasmosis		• *Toxoplasma gondii*
Trypanosomiasis	African trypanosomiasis	• *Trypanosoma brucei*
	South American trypanosomiasis	• *Trypanosoma cruzi*

Table 27.3 Major helminthic infections

Cestodes	Neurocysticercosis	• *Taenia solium*
	Hydatid cyst	• *Echinococcus granulosus*
	Coenurosis	• *Taenia multiceps*
	Sparganosis	• *Spirometra*
Trematodes	Paragonimiasis	• *Paragonimus westermani*
	Schistosomiasis	• *Schistosoma mansoni, japonicum, haematobium, mekongi*
	Other trematode infections	
Nematodes	Eosinophilic meningoencephalitis	• *Angiostrongylus cantonensis* • *Gnathostoma spinigerum*
	Toxocariasis	• *Trichinella spiralis* • Other forms of larva migrans
	Human filariasis, Loa-loa	• *Dracunculus medinensis* • *Onchocerca volvulus*
	Nematodes and immunosuppression	• *Strongyloides stercoralis*

27.3 Toxoplasma gondii

Table 27.4 Neurologic signs and syndromes related to affected regions

Localization	Syndrome	Neurologic signs
Meninges	• Meningitis • Sub- or epidural empyema	• Headache • Vomiting • Photophobia • Focal neurologic deficits • Alterations in consciousness
Brain parenchyma diffuse	• Encephalitis	• Alterations in consciousness • Seizures • Multifocal neurologic deficits
Brain parenchyma focal	• Encephalitis • Cerebritis • Abscess	• Focal neurologic deficits • Seizures
Brain stem and posterior cranial fossa	• Brain stem encephalitis • Cerebellitis	• Opto- and pupillomotor disturbances • Nuclear cranial nerve lesions • Dysarthria • Bilateral pyramidal tract signs • Alterations in consciousness • Breathing insufficiency • Vegetative signs
Spinal cord	• Myelitis • Paraspinal empyema/abscess	• Paraplegia • Brown Séquard syndrome
Arteries	• Arteritis	• Sudden focal neurologic deficit
Veins	• Septic venous sinus thrombosis	• Headache • Seizures • Raised brain pressure • Focal neurologic deficits

Table 27.5 Parasites associated with diseases of the central nervous system

Disease entity	Pathogen
Meningoencephalitis	• *Naegleria fowleri* • *Trypanosoma brucei gambiense* • *Trypanosoma brucei rhodesiense* • *Trypanosoma cruzi* • *Toxoplasma gondii* • Microsporidia
Granulomatous encephalitis	• *Acanthamoeba* spp. • *Balamuthia mandrillaris*
Mass lesion—brain abscess	• *Toxoplasma gondii* • *Taenia solium* • *Schistosoma japonicum* • *Acanthamoeba* spp. • *Balamuthia mandrillaris*
Eosinophilic meningitis	• *Angiostrongylus cantonensis* • *Toxocara* spp. • *Baylisascaris*
Cerebral malaria	• *Plasmodium falciparum*
Cerebral paragonimiasis	• *Paragonimus westermani*

- Immunocompromised old patient
  - Diffuse encephalopathy
  - Meningoencephalitis
  - Signs of cerebral mass lesion
  - Hemiparesis
  - Seizures
  - Visual impairment, retinochoroiditis
  - Confusion
  - Lethargy

  - first trimester:
    o spontaneous abortion
    o stillbirth
    o severe disease
  - after first trimester
    o epilepsy
    o encephalitis
    o microcephaly
    o hydrocephalus
    o intracerebral calcifications
    o psychomotor or mental retardation
    o chorioretinitis

27.3.2 Epidemiology

Incidence
- Human infection with *Toxoplasma gondii* is ubiquitous.

Age Incidence
- Any age

Sex Incidence
- Any sex

Localization
- Any part of the brain

27.3.3 Neuroimaging Findings

General Imaging Findings
- Supratentorial, often cystic mass with enhancement

CT Non-Contrast-Enhanced (Fig. 27.1a)
- Often multiple iso- or hypodense lesions with perifocal edema.
- Predominantly located in basal ganglia, thalamus, and juxtacortical.
- Hyperdense calcifications and hemorrhages may be seen after medical treatment.

CT Contrast-Enhanced
- Ring or nodular enhancement

MRI-T2 (Fig. 27.1b)
- Hyperintense lesions

MRI-FLAIR (Fig. 27.1c, d)
- Iso- or hyperintense lesions
- Hyperintense perifocal edema

MRI-T1 (Fig. 27.1e)
- Hypointense lesions

MRI-T1 Contrast-Enhanced (Fig. 27.1f, g)
- Ring or nodular enhancement

MRI-T2∗/SWI
- Hemorrhages or calcifications may occur.

MR-Diffusion Imaging (Fig. 27.1h)
- Elevated diffusivity if center of lesion is necrotic.

MR-Spectroscopy
- Lipid and lactate peaks

27.3.4 Neuropathology Findings

Macroscopic Features (Fig. 27.2a–d)
- Focal and space-occupying lesions.
- Lesions appear as zones of necrosis with an area of hyperemia and/or small hemorrhages surrounded by a poorly defined area of edema.
- Cerebral hemispheres, basal ganglia.

Microscopic Features (Figs. 27.3a, b, 27.4a–n, 27.5a–j, 27.6a–h, and 27.7a–d)
- Large zones of necrosis are found in brain tissue.
- Chronic inflammatory cell response may be seen in the area of necrosis which might be intense and gives sometimes the appearance of a lymphoma.
- The infiltrates contain lymphocytes, plasma cells, and histiocytes.
- The necrotic lesion is surrounded by reactive astrocytes, activated microglia and inflammatory cells.
- Hemorrhages are frequent.
- Toxoplasma may be found in two forms:
  - Bradyzoites: organisms in pseudocysts
  - Tachyzoites: free forms found in small or larger collections diffusely distributed near the junction area of necrosis and brain tissue
- After treatment or during the course of the illness, the lesions appear:
  - Necrotizing
  - Organizing abscesses
  - Chronic treated lesions with central cystic space

Differential Diagnosis
- Macroscopic level
  - Hemorrhagic ischemic necroses
- Microscopic level
  - Swollen dying neurons
  - Debris-filled macrophages

27.3.5 Molecular Neuropathology

- Congenital toxoplasmosis
  - Secondary to transplacental infection

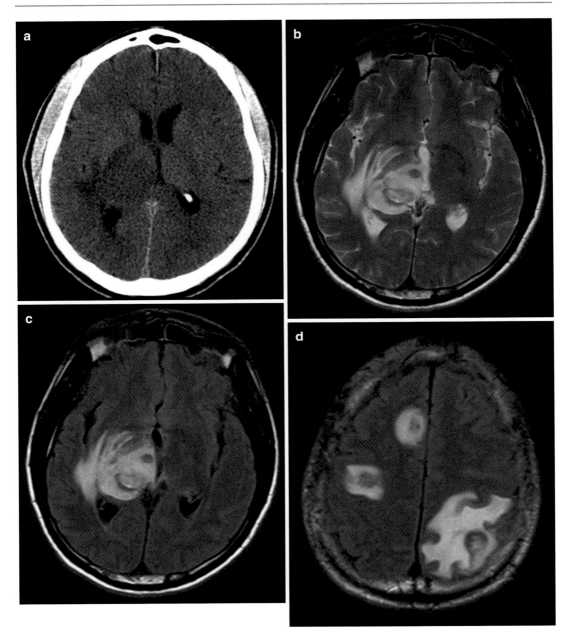

Fig. 27.1 Toxoplasmosis in an HIV-infected patient—multiple lesions juxtacortical and right thalamus CT (**a**), T2 (**b**), FLAIR (**c, d**), T1 (**e**), T1 contrast (**f, g**), DWI (**h**), ADC (**i**)

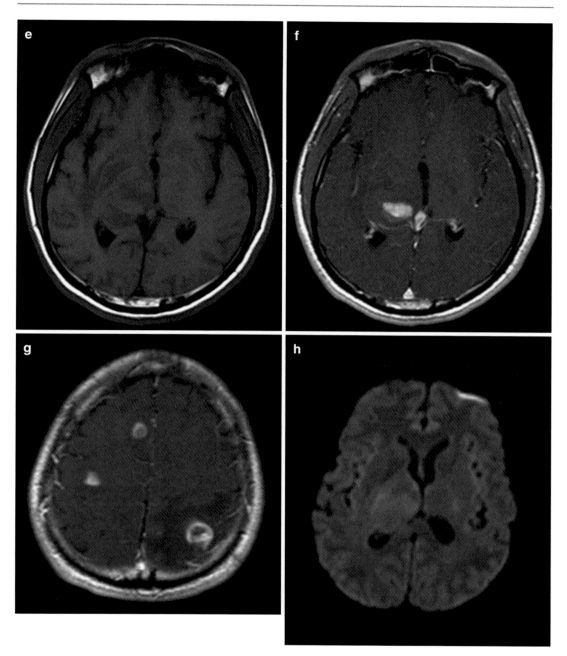

Fig. 27.1 (continued)

27.3 Toxoplasma gondii

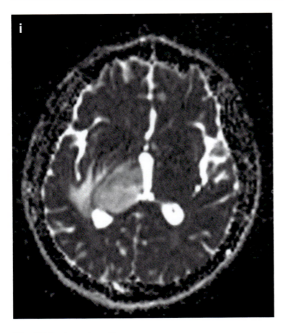

Fig. 27.1 (continued)

- Acquired toxoplasmosis
  - Immunocompromised patients
    o HIV
    o Post-transplantation
    o Congenital immunodeficiencies
- Can also occur in immunocompetent individuals
- Essential reservoir host:
  - members of family Felidae (domestic cats and their relatives)
- Unsporulated oocysts are shed in the cat's feces.
  - Although oocysts are usually only shed for 1–2 weeks, large numbers may be shed.
- Oocysts take 1–5 days to sporulate in the environment and become infective.
  - Intermediate hosts in nature (including birds and rodents) become infected after ingesting soil, water, or plant material contaminated with oocysts.
- Oocysts transform into tachyzoites shortly after ingestion.

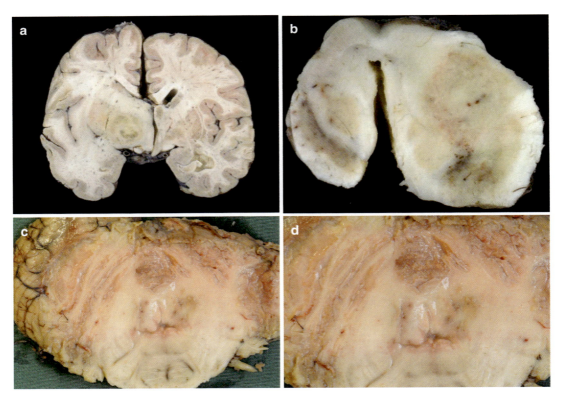

Fig. 27.2 *Toxoplasma gondii* infection. Yellowish abscess-like destruction of the left basal ganglia (**a**) and right substantia nigra (**b**) is evident, putrid formation in the brain stem around the cerebral aqueduct, extending into the cerebellum (**c**, **d**)

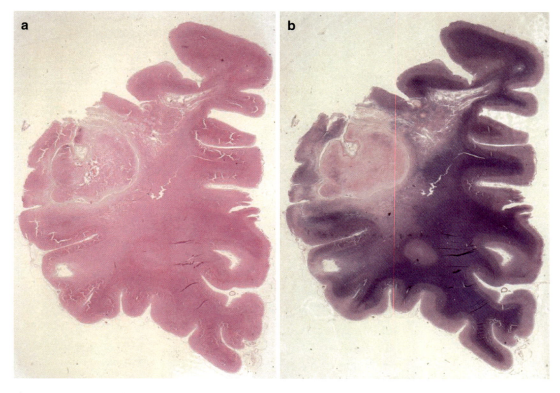

Fig. 27.3 Large area of necrosis in the frontal lobe (**a**, stain: H&E; **b**: stain: PAS)

- These tachyzoites localize in neural and muscle tissue and develop into tissue cyst bradyzoites.
- Cats become infected after consuming intermediate hosts harboring tissue cysts.
- Cats may also become infected directly by ingestion of sporulated oocysts.
- Animals bred for human consumption and wild game may also become infected with tissue cysts after ingestion of sporulated oocysts in the environment.
- Humans can become infected by any of several routes:
  - eating undercooked meat of animals harboring tissue cysts
  - consuming food or water contaminated with cat feces or by contaminated environmental samples (such as fecal-contaminated soil or changing the litter box of a pet cat)
  - blood transfusion or organ transplantation
  - transplacentally from mother to fetus
- In the human host, the parasites form tissue cysts, most commonly in skeletal muscle, myocardium, brain, and eyes.
- These cysts may remain throughout the life of the host.

27.3.6 Treatment and Prognosis

Treatment
- Mononucleosis-like infection
  - no specific therapy
- Immunocompromised patients
  - Initial high dose of pyrimethamine + sulfadiazine (4–6 weeks)
  - Indefinite continuation of lower doses of pyrimethamine + sulfadiazine

27.3 Toxoplasma gondii

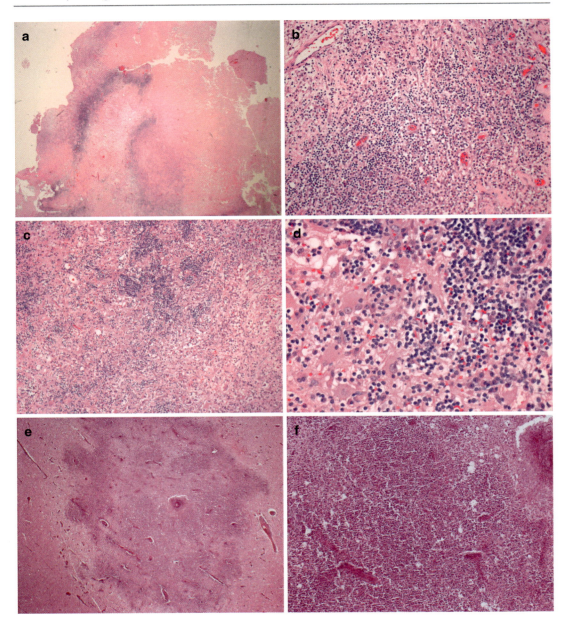

Fig. 27.4 Areas of necrotic tissue destruction surrounded by a rim of lymphocytes (**a–d**), abscess formation (**e, f**). Brain tissue is diffusely infiltrated by lymphocytes (**g, h**) forming perivascular cuffs (**i, j**) and gliomesenchymal nodules (**k, l**). Reactive astrocytes might also be encountered (**m, n**) (**a–n**: stain: H&E)

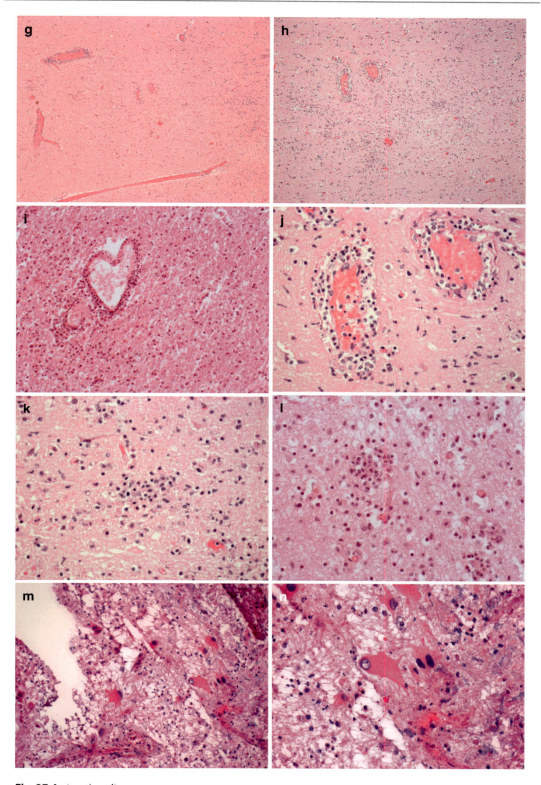

Fig. 27.4 (continued)

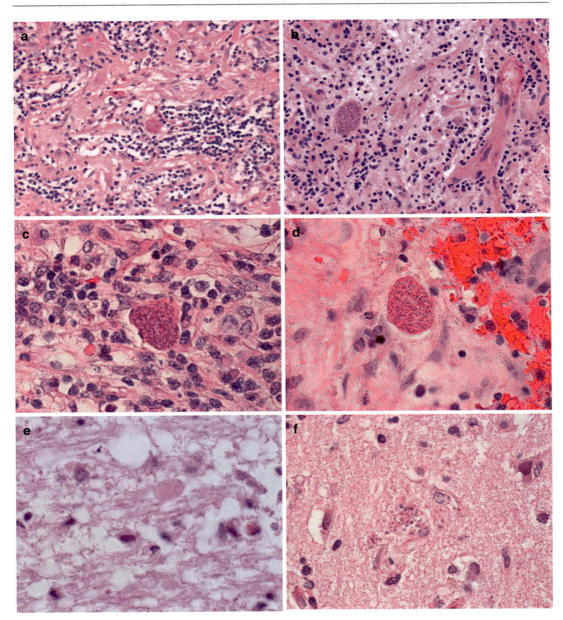

Fig. 27.5 The parasite is found in form of bradyzoites (**a–e**), ruptured cyst with free tachyzoites (**f**) Encysted organisms found in a gliomesenchymal nodule (**g, h**) in the near proximity of a neuron (**g**) or in the tissue (**i, j**) (**a–f**, stain: H&E; **g–j**, stain: cresyl violet)

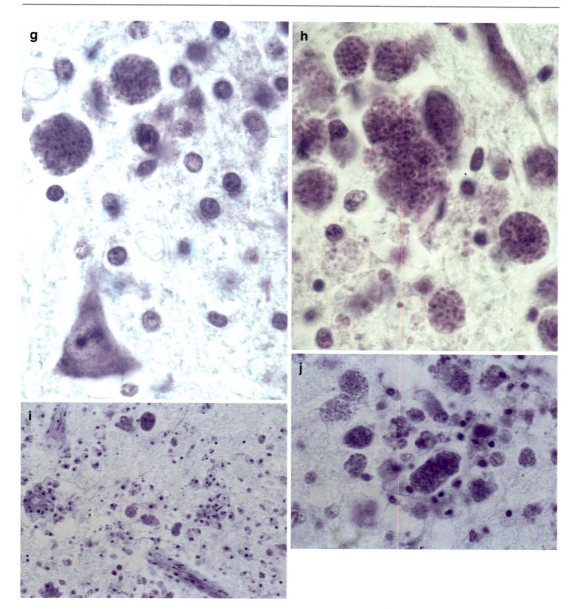

Fig. 27.5 (continued)

- Management of maternal and fetal infection
  - **Spiramycin** is recommended (for the first and early second trimesters)
  - **Pyrimethamine/sulfadiazine** and leucovorin (for late second and third trimesters)

Biologic Behavior–Prognosis–Prognostic Factors
- Underlying cause of immunodeficiency

- Congenital:
  - devastating effect
  - first trimester: spontaneous abortion, stillbirth, or severe disease
  - after first trimester: epilepsy, encephalitis, microcephaly, hydrocephalus, intracerebral calcifications psychomotor or mental retardation, chorioretinitis

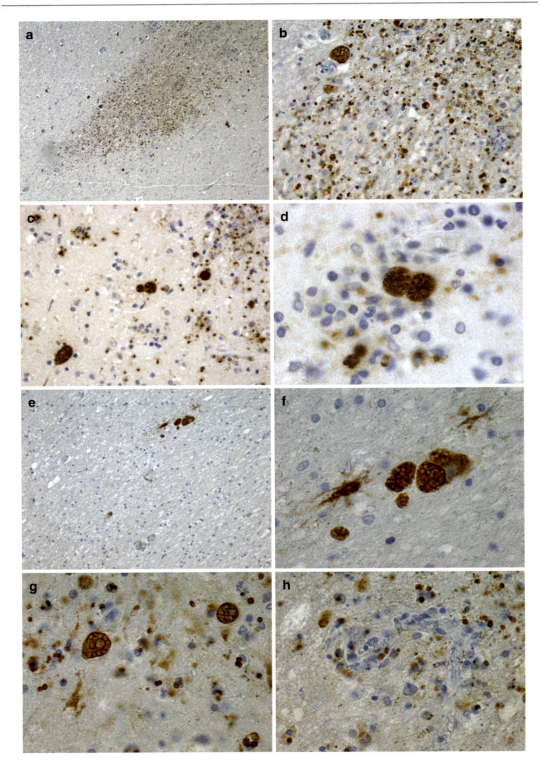

Fig. 27.6 Immunohistochemical demonstration of *Toxoplasma gondii* as free tachyzoites and as bradyzoites (**a–h**, stain: IHC against *Toxoplasma gondii*)

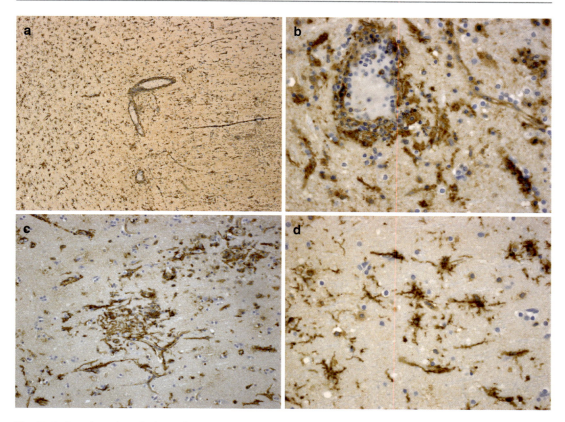

Fig. 27.7 Reactive microgliosis (**a–d**, stain: IHC HLA-DRII)

27.4 Taeniasis: Coenurosis/Cysticercosis

27.4.1 Cysticercosis: Clinical Signs and Symptoms

Neurocysticercosis
- Defined as the infection of the central nervous system and its covering by the larval stage of the tapeworm *Taenia solium*.
- The disease complex of taeniasis/cysticercosis is closely linked to poverty and ignorance, disproportionately affecting underserved populations.
- The most common cause of acquired epilepsy in the world.

The symptoms of cysticercosis are caused by the development of cysticerci in various sites.

- Cerebral cysticercosis (or neurocysticercosis)
  - Seizures.
  - Mental disturbances.
  - Focal neurologic deficits.
  - Signs of space-occupying intracerebral lesions.
  - Death can occur suddenly.
- Extracerebral cysticercosis can cause ocular, cardiac, or spinal lesions with associated symptoms.
- Asymptomatic subcutaneous nodules and calcified intramuscular nodules can be encountered.

27.4.2 Coenurosis: Clinical Signs and Symptoms

- Coenuri in the skin or subcutaneous tissue
  - Usually present as painless nodules.
  - Are often fluctuant and tender lesions.

- Most subcutaneous nodules manifest on the trunk, sclera, subconjuctiva, neck, shoulders, head, and limbs.
- Coenuri in the neck may affect neck movement and swallowing.
- Clinically, coenuri may mimic lymphomas, lipomas, pseudotumors, or neurofibromas.
• Coenuri in the eye
  - Cause both intraocular and orbital infections.
  - Patients may present with varying degrees of visual impairment.
  - May cause painful inflammation, glaucoma, and eventually blindness.
• Coenuri in the central nervous system
  - Headache
  - Fever
  - Vomiting
  - Meningitis
  - Hydrocephalus
  - Cranial nerve damage
  - Seizures
  - Hyperactive reflexes
  - Nerve palsies
  - Jacksonian epilepsy
  - Pachymeningitis
  - Obstructive or communicating hydrocephalus
  - Intracranial arteritis with transient hemiparesis

27.4.3 Epidemiology

Incidence
• Found in areas where *Taenia solium* is prevalent and is directly correlated with human fecal contamination

Age Incidence
• Any age

Sex Incidence
• Equally distributed

Localization
• Any part of the brain

27.4.4 Neuroimaging Findings

CT Non-Contrast-Enhanced (Figs. 27.8a and 27.9a)
• Vesicular stage:
  - CSF-isodense cyst with hyperdense scolex
• Colloidal vesicular stage:
  - Cyst fluid becomes more hyperdense, perifocal edema
• Granular nodular stage:
  - Decreased edema
• Nodular calcified stage:
  - Residual hyperdense calcified lesion

CT Contrast-Enhanced (Fig. 27.8b)
• Vesicular stage:
  - No or faint enhancement
• Colloidal vesicular stage:
  - Rim enhancement
• Granular nodular stage:
  - Ring or nodular enhancement
• Nodular calcified stage:
  - Calcified lesion hyperdense

MRI-T2 (Figs. 27.8c and 27.9b)
• Vesicular stage:
  - Cyst fluid isointense to CSF
• Colloidal vesicular stage:
  - Cyst fluid hyperintense to CSF, perifocal hyperintense edema
• Granular nodular stage:
  - Retracted cyst, decreased edema
• Nodular calcified stage:
  - Signal dropout due to calcifications

MRI-FLAIR (Figs. 27.8d and 27.9c)
• Intraventricular cysts:
  - hyperintense
• Vesicular stage:
  - cyst fluid isointense to CSF
  - scolex hyperintense
• Colloidal vesicular stage:
  - cyst fluid hyperintense to CSF
  - hyperintense perifocal edema
• Granular nodular stage:
  - less extensive perifocal edema
• Nodular calcified stage:
  - calcified lesions

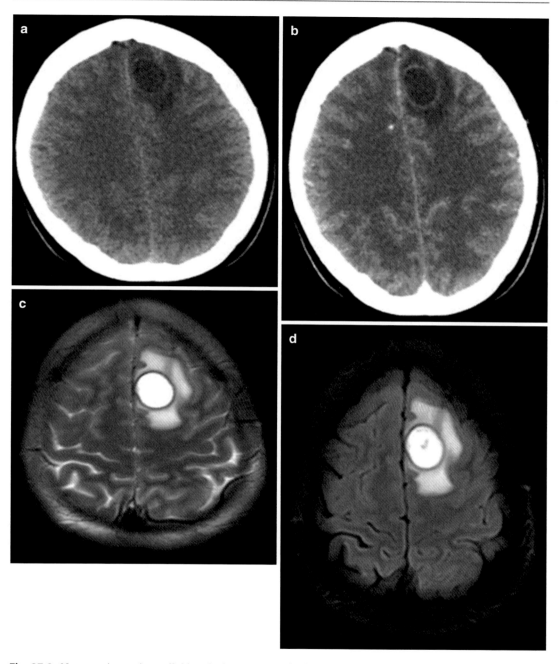

Fig. 27.8 Neurocysticercosis—colloid vesicular stage cyst in the left frontal lobe CT (**a**), CT contrast (**b**), T2 (**c**), FLAIR (**d**), T1 (**e**), T1 contrast (**f**), T2∗ (**g**)

MRI-T1 (Figs. 27.8e and 27.9d)
- Vesicular stage:
  – Cyst fluid isointense to CSF
  – Scolex hyperintense
- Colloidal vesicular stage:
  – Cyst fluid hyperintense to CSF
- Granular nodular stage:
  – Retraction of cyst

27.4 Taeniasis: Coenurosis/Cysticercosis

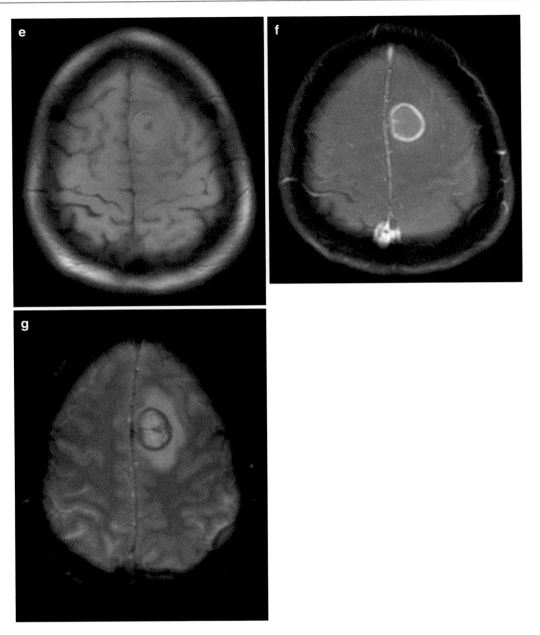

Fig. 27.8 (continued)

- Nodular calcified stage:
  - Calcified lesions

MRI-T1 Contrast-Enhanced (Figs. 27.8f and 27.9e)
- Vesicular stage:
  - No or faint enhancement
- Colloidal vesicular stage:
  - Enhancement of cyst wall and scolex
- Granular nodular stage:
  - Decreased enhancement of retracted cyst wall
- Nodular calcified stage:
  - Persisting enhancement possible

MRI-T2∗/SWI (Fig. 27.8g)
- Calcified scolex
- Calcified lesions in nodular calcified stage

MR-Diffusion Imaging (Fig. 27.9f)
- Cyst fluid isointense to CSF

MR-Spectroscopy
- Elevated lactate, alanine, and choline values
- Decreased NAA values

Nuclear Medicine Imaging Findings
- Parasites detection is no indication for nuclear medicine diagnostic.

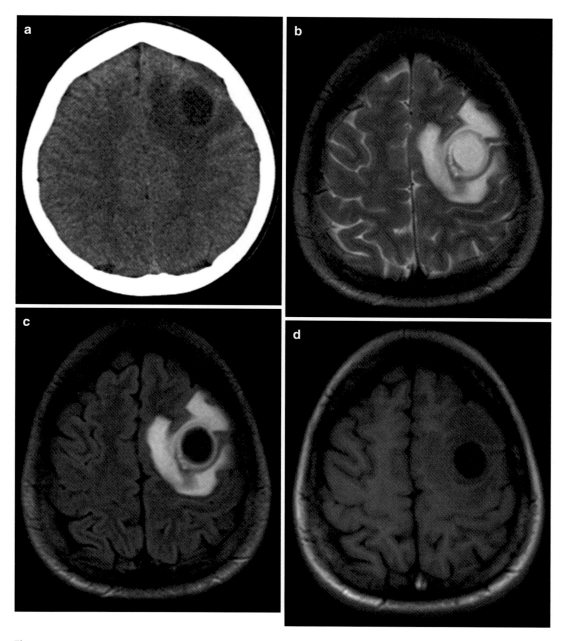

Fig. 27.9 Human coenurosis (Taenia serialis): CT (**a**), T2 (**b**), FLAIR (**c**), T1 (**d**), T1 contrast (**e**), DWI (**f**), ADC (**g**)

27.4 Taeniasis: Coenurosis/Cysticercosis

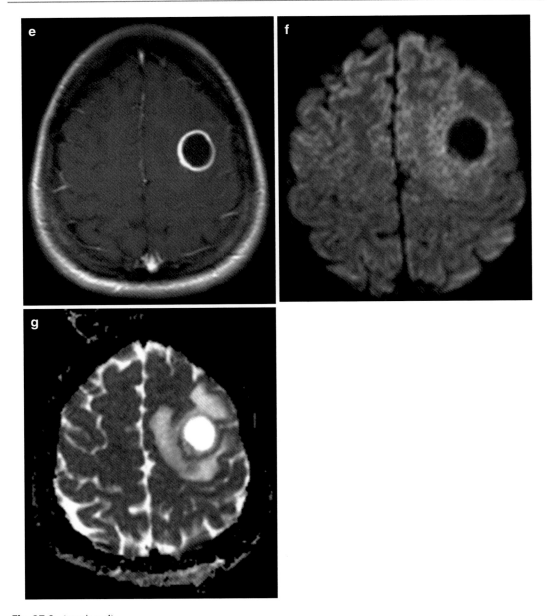

Fig. 27.9 (continued)

- Reports state that especially in HIV patients distinguishing lymphoma (high FDG uptake) from toxoplasmosis (low FDG uptake) is possible with FDG-PET.

27.4.5 Neuropathology Findings

Macroscopic Features (Fig. 27.10a–d)
- Cyst formations of various sizes.
- Number of cysts varies from one to several hundreds.

Microscopic Features (Fig. 27.10e–p)
- Cysts contain
  - Single scolex with four suckers
  - Double row of hooklets
- Cysts consists of three layers:
  - Outer or cuticular layer

- Middle cellular layer with pseudoepithelial appearance
- Inner reticular or fibrillary layer
• After death of the organism
  - Granulomatous reaction
  - Fibrosis
  - Calcifications

Differential Diagnosis
• Granulomatous process

27.4.6 Molecular Neuropathology

Pathogenesis: Cysticercosis
• Endemic in all countries, particularly Latin America.
• Cysticercus, the larval stage of *Taenia solium*, infects pigs.
• Human ingestion of water or vegetables contaminated with *T. solium* eggs from human feces initiates the infection.
• After ingestion, the eggs hatch in the stomach of the intermediate host, releasing the hexacanth embryo or oncosphere.
• The oncosphere penetrates the intestinal wall and migrates in the circulation to striated muscles, as well as the brain, liver, and other tissues.
• In the tissues, the oncosphere develops into cysticercus over 3–4 months.
• Cysticerci may develop in muscle, connective tissue, brain, lungs, and eyes.

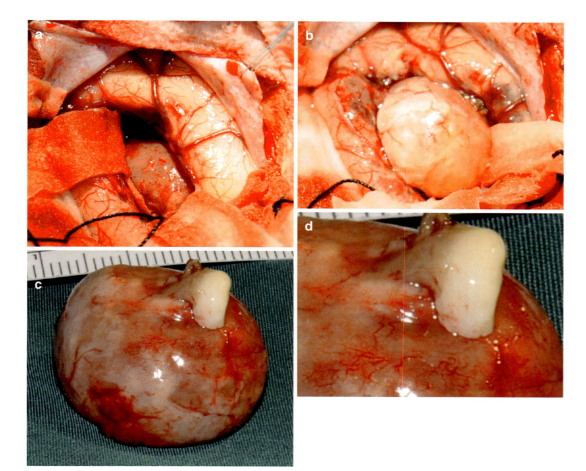

Fig. 27.10 *Taenia serialis*. Intraoperative (**a**, **b**), gross-anatomical appearance of the cystic formation after surgical removal (**c**, **d**), soft-tissue structures containing collagen fibers and small thin-walled vessels interspersed with lymphocytes, granulocytes, and plasmocytes (**e**) adjacent to parts of the worm (**f**). The scolex with suckers is shown in (**g–l**) (alternating H&E and PAS stains). Calcareous corpuscles (**m**, **n**; stain: H&E). Parts of the parasite intestinal tract (**o**, **p**; stain: PAS). Classification as *Taenia serialis* was based on molecular biologic analysis

27.4 Taeniasis: Coenurosis/Cysticercosis

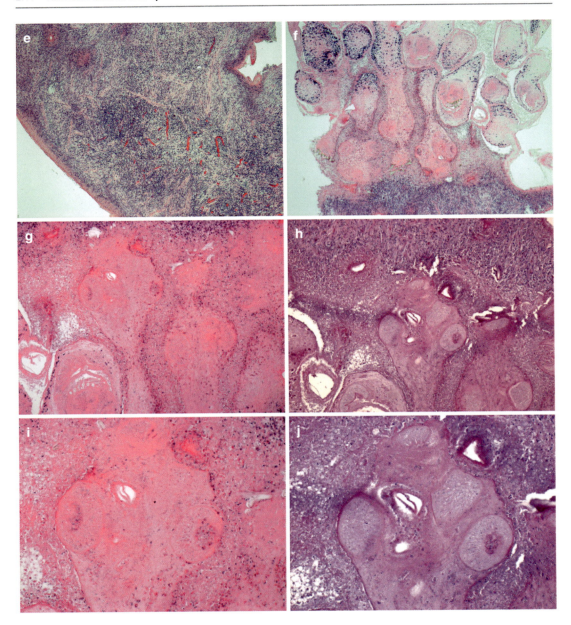

Fig. 27.10 (continued)

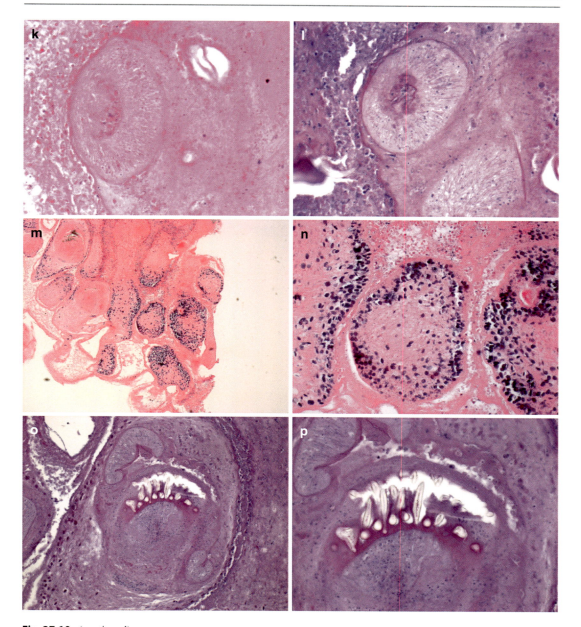

Fig. 27.10 (continued)

- Cysticerci remain viable for as long as 5 years.
- Cysts evaginate and attach to the small intestine by their scolex.
- Adult tapeworms develop (up to 2–7 m in length) and produce less than 1000 proglottids, each with approximately 50,000 eggs, and reside in the small intestine for years.
- *Taenia solium* is found worldwide.

Pathogenesis: Coenurosis
- The definitive hosts for *Taenia multiceps* and *T. serialis:* members of the family Canidae.
  - Dogs and foxes can serve as hosts for *T. serialis.*
- Eggs and gravid proglottids are shed in feces into the environment.
- They are ingested by an intermediate host.
  - rodents, rabbits, horses, cattle, sheep, and goats

- Eggs hatch in the intestine, and oncospheres are released.
- The oncospheres circulate in blood until they lodge in suitable organs (including skeletal muscle, eyes, brain, and subcutaneous tissue),
- After about 3 months, oncospheres develop into coenuri.
- The definitive host becomes infected by ingesting the tissue of an infected intermediate host containing a coenurus.
- The adult cestodes reside in the small intestine of the definitive host.
- Humans become infected after the accidental ingestion of eggs on fomites or in food and water contaminated with dog feces.
  - Eggs hatch in the intestine, and oncospheres are released.
  - The oncospheres circulate in blood until they lodge in suitable organs.
  - After about 3 months, they develop into coenuri.
  - Coenuri of *T. multiceps* are usually found in the eyes and brain; those of *T. serialis* are usually found in subcutaneous tissue.

27.4.7 Treatment and Prognosis

Treatment
- Before surgical treatment: praziquantel or albendazole
- Concomitant steroid medication for minimizing the inflammatory response to dying larvae

Biologic Behavior–Prognosis–Prognostic Factors
- Depends on the brain regions involved
- Worse prognosis when cyst ruptures during surgical removal

Selected References

Alday PH, Doggett JS (2017) Drugs in development for toxoplasmosis: advances, challenges, and current status. Drug Des Devel Ther 11:273–293. https://doi.org/10.2147/dddt.s60973

Ambekar S, Prasad C, Dwarakanath S, Mahadevan A (2013) MRS findings in cerebral coenurosis due to Taenia multiceps. J Neuroimaging 23(1):149–151. https://doi.org/10.1111/j.1552-6569.2011.00616.x

Chang L, Cornford ME, Chiang FL, Ernst TM, Sun NC, Miller BL (1995) Radiologic-pathologic correlation. Cerebral toxoplasmosis and lymphoma in AIDS. AJNR Am J Neuroradiol 16(8):1653–1663

Chong-Han CH, Cortez SC, Tung GA (2003) Diffusion-weighted MRI of cerebral toxoplasma abscess. AJR Am J Roentgenol 181(6):1711–1714. https://doi.org/10.2214/ajr.181.6.1811711

Christodoulopoulos G, Dinkel A, Romig T, Ebi D, Mackenstedt U, Loos-Frank B (2016) Cerebral and non-cerebral coenurosis: on the genotypic and phenotypic diversity of Taenia multiceps. Parasitol Res 115(12):4543–4558. https://doi.org/10.1007/s00436-016-5246-4

Del Brutto OH, Garcia HH (2013) Neurocysticercosis. Handb Clin Neurol 114:313–325. https://doi.org/10.1016/b978-0-444-53490-3.00025-x

Del Brutto OH, Garcia HH (2015) Taenia solium cysticercosis—the lessons of history. J Neurol Sci 359(1–2):392–395. https://doi.org/10.1016/j.jns.2015.08.011

Garcia HH, Gonzalez AE, Gilman RH (2011) Cysticercosis of the central nervous system: how should it be managed? Curr Opin Infect Dis 24(5):423–427. https://doi.org/10.1097/QCO.0b013e32834a1b20

Garcia HH, Rodriguez S, Friedland JS (2014) Immunology of Taenia solium taeniasis and human cysticercosis. Parasite Immunol 36(8):388–396. https://doi.org/10.1111/pim.12126

Gonzales I, Rivera JT, Garcia HH (2016) Pathogenesis of Taenia solium taeniasis and cysticercosis. Parasite Immunol 38(3):136–146. https://doi.org/10.1111/pim.12307

Haitchi G, Buchroithner J, Sonnberger M, Weis S, Fellner FA (2012) AIRP best cases in radiologic-pathologic correlation: human coenurosis (Taenia Larva). Radiographics 32(2):517–521. https://doi.org/10.1148/rg.322105230

Hampton MM (2015) Congenital toxoplasmosis: a review. Neonatal Netw 34(5):274–278. https://doi.org/10.1891/0730-0832.34.5.274

Hermos JA, Healy GR, Schultz MG, Barlow J, Church WG (1970) Fatal human cerebral coenurosis. JAMA 213(9):1461–1464

Ing MB, Schantz PM, Turner JA (1998) Human coenurosis in North America: case reports and review. Clin Infect Dis 27(3):519–523

Ito A, Yanagida T, Nakao M (2016) Recent advances and perspectives in molecular epidemiology of Taenia solium cysticercosis. Infect Genet Evol 40:357–367. https://doi.org/10.1016/j.meegid.2015.06.022

Jayakumar PN, Chandrashekar HS, Ellika S (2013) Imaging of parasitic infections of the central nervous system. Handb Clin Neurol 114:37–64. https://doi.org/10.1016/b978-0-444-53490-3.00004-2

Kieffer F, Wallon M (2013) Congenital toxoplasmosis. Handb Clin Neurol 112:1099–1101. https://doi.org/10.1016/b978-0-444-52910-7.00028-3

Kimura-Hayama ET, Higuera JA, Corona-Cedillo R, Chavez-Macias L, Perochena A, Quiroz-Rojas LY, Rodriguez-Carbajal J, Criales JL (2010) Neurocysticercosis: radiologic-pathologic correlation. Radiographics 30(6):1705–1719. https://doi.org/10.1148/rg.306105522

Kravetz J (2013) Congenital toxoplasmosis. BMJ Clin Evid 2013. pii: 0906.

Kristensson K, Masocha W, Bentivoglio M (2013) Mechanisms of CNS invasion and damage by parasites. Handb Clin Neurol 114:11–22. https://doi.org/10.1016/b978-0-444-53490-3.00002-9

Lee GT, Antelo F, Mlikotic AA (2009) Best cases from the AFIP: cerebral toxoplasmosis. Radiographics 29(4):1200–1205. https://doi.org/10.1148/rg.294085205

Lescano AG, Zunt J (2013) Other cestodes: sparganosis, coenurosis and Taenia crassiceps cysticercosis. Handb Clin Neurol 114:335–345. https://doi.org/10.1016/b978-0-444-53490-3.00027-3

Lightowlers MW (2013) Cysticercosis and echinococcosis. Curr Top Microbiol Immunol 365:315–335. https://doi.org/10.1007/82_2012_234

Liu Q, Wang ZD, Huang SY, Zhu XQ (2015) Diagnosis of toxoplasmosis and typing of Toxoplasma gondii. Parasit Vectors 8:292. https://doi.org/10.1186/s13071-015-0902-6

Lucato LT, Guedes MS, Sato JR, Bacheschi LA, Machado LR, Leite CC (2007) The role of conventional MR imaging sequences in the evaluation of neurocysticercosis: impact on characterization of the scolex and lesion burden. AJNR Am J Neuroradiol 28(8):1501–1504. https://doi.org/10.3174/ajnr.A0623

Pereira-Chioccola VL, Vidal JE, Su C (2009) Toxoplasma gondii infection and cerebral toxoplasmosis in HIV-infected patients. Future Microbiol 4(10):1363–1379. https://doi.org/10.2217/fmb.09.89

Pittella JE (2013) Pathology of CNS parasitic infections. Handb Clin Neurol 114:65–88. https://doi.org/10.1016/b978-0-444-53490-3.00005-4

Pleyer U, Schluter D, Manz M (2014) Ocular toxoplasmosis: recent aspects of pathophysiology and clinical implications. Ophthalmic Res 52(3):116–123. https://doi.org/10.1159/000363141

Pomares C, Montoya JG (2016) Laboratory diagnosis of congenital toxoplasmosis. J Clin Microbiol 54(10):2448–2454. https://doi.org/10.1128/jcm.00487-16

Randall LM, Hunter CA (2011) Parasite dissemination and the pathogenesis of toxoplasmosis. Eur J Microbiol Immunol 1(1):3–9. https://doi.org/10.1556/EuJMI.1.2011.1.3

Rodriguez S, Wilkins P, Dorny P (2012) Immunological and molecular diagnosis of cysticercosis. Pathog Glob Health 106(5):286–298. https://doi.org/10.1179/2047773212y.0000000048

Saadatnia G, Golkar M (2012) A review on human toxoplasmosis. Scand J Infect Dis 44(11):805–814. https://doi.org/10.3109/00365548.2012.693197

Sheth TN, Pillon L, Keystone J, Kucharczyk W (1998) Persistent MR contrast enhancement of calcified neurocysticercosis lesions. AJNR Am J Neuroradiol 19(1):79–82

Teitelbaum GP, Otto RJ, Lin M, Watanabe AT, Stull MA, Manz HJ, Bradley WG Jr (1989) MR imaging of neurocysticercosis. AJR Am J Roentgenol 153(4):857–866. https://doi.org/10.2214/ajr.153.4.857

Venkat B, Aggarwal N, Makhaik S, Sood R (2016) A comprehensive review of imaging findings in human cysticercosis. Jpn J Radiol 34(4):241–257. https://doi.org/10.1007/s11604-016-0528-4

Wilkins PP (2013) Immunodiagnosis of CNS parasitic infections. Handb Clin Neurol 114:23–36. https://doi.org/10.1016/b978-0-444-53490-3.00003-0

Infections: Fungi

28.1 General Aspects

28.1.1 Clinical Signs and Symptoms

Clinical signs and symptoms include (Table 28.1):

- Fever
- Headache
- Nausea and vomiting
- Meningism
- Seizures
- Neck pain
- Sensitivity to light
- Confusion or changes in behavior

28.1.2 Epidemiology

Incidence
- among immunocompromised individuals (transplant patients, HIV-infected patients, cancer patients undergoing chemotherapy)
- hospitalized people with serious underlying diseases

Age Incidence
- any age group

Sex Incidence
- Male:Female: 1:1

Localization
- Leptomeninges
- Cerebral hemispheres
- Brain stem

Fungi causing meningitis and brain abscess are listed in Table 28.2.

28.1.3 Classification of Fungi

Major disease-causing fungal classes in humans include:

- Mucormycetes
- Basidiomycetes
- Pneumocystidiomycetes
- Hemiascomycetes
- Euascomycetes

Based on morphology and mode of spore production (Table 28.3):

- yeast
- molds

Yeasts
- unicellular
- produce round, pasty, or mucoid colonies on agar

Table 28.1 Neurologic signs and syndromes related to affected regions

Localization	Syndrome	Neurologic signs
Meninges	• Meningitis • Sub- or epidural empyema	• Headache • Vomiting • Photophobia • Focal neurologic deficits • Alterations in consciousness
Brain parenchyma diffuse	• Encephalitis	• Alterations in consciousness • Seizures • Multifocal neurologic deficits
Brain parenchyma focal	• Encephalitis • Cerebritis • Abscess	• Focal neurologic deficits • Seizures
Brain stem and posterior cranial fossa	• Brain stem encephalitis • Cerebellitis	• Opto- and pupillomotor disturbances • Nuclear cranial nerve lesions • Dysarthria • Bilateral pyramidal tract signs • Alterations in consciousness • Breathing insufficiency • Vegetative signs
Spinal cord	• Myelitis • Paraspinal empyema/abscess	• Paraplegia • Brown Séquard syndrome
Arteries	• Arteritis	• Sudden focal neurologic deficit
Veins	• Septic venous sinus thrombosis	• Headache • Seizures • Raised brain pressure • Focal neurologic deficits

Table 28.2 Fungi causing meningitis and brain abscess

	Pathogens
Meningitis	• *Candida* spp. • *Cryptococcus neoformans/gattii* • *Aspergillus* spp. • Mucormycetes • *Coccidioides immitis/posadasii* • *Histoplasma capsulatum* • *Blastomyces dermatitidis* • *Rhodotorula* spp. • *Blastoschizomyces capitatus* • *Penicillium marneffei*
Brain abscess	• *Candida* spp. • *Cryptococcus neoformans/gattii* • *Aspergillus* spp. • Mucormycetes • *Scedosporium apiospernum* • *Trichosporon* spp. • *Trichoderma* spp.

Table 28.3 Morphological features for fungal identification in tissue

Organism	Size (width in μm)	Defining morphology
Aspergillus spp.	3–5	• Acute-angle branching • Septate • Conidial head
Cryptococcus neoformans	5–20	• Narrow-neck bud
Histoplasma capsulatum	2–5	• Narrow-neck bud
Blastomyces dermatitidis	15–30	• Broad-based bud
Candida glabrata	3–5	• Budding • No pseudohyphae
Candida ssp.	2–3	• Yeast • Pseudohyphae • Hyphae
Zygomycetes spp.	5–8	• Right-angle branching • Ribbons • Pauciseptate
Pseudallescheria spp.	3–4	• Acute-angle branching • Septate • Terminal chlamydospore • Pigmented conidia
Fusarium spp.	4–5	• Acute and right-angle branching • Septate • Narrowed branch points
Coccidioides immitis	20–200	• Endosporulation

- a cell reproducing by budding or by fission
- progenitor cell pinches off a portion of itself forming "pseudohyphae"

Molds

- multicellular organisms
- consist of hyphae (threadlike tubular structures)
  - septate hyphae (divided by partitions or cross-walls)
  - coenocytic hyphae (hollow or multinucleate)
- produce hyphae on agar

28.1 General Aspects

Table 28.4 List of mycoses caused by various fungi

	Etiologic agents
Opportunistic mycoses	• *Candida* spp. • *Cryptococcus neoformans* • *Aspergillus* spp. • *Mucormycetes* • Other hyaline molds • Dematiaceous molds
Superficial and cutaneous mycoses	• Dermatophytic • Nondermatophytic
Subcutaneous mycoses	• Various etiologic agents
Systemic mycoses	• *Blastomyces dermatitidis* • *Coccidioides immitis* • *Histoplasma capsulatum* • *Paracoccidioides brasiliensis* • *Penicillium marneffei*

Heterotrophic existence as:

- saprobes (live of dead or decaying matter)
- symbionts (live together and in which the association is of mutual advantage)
- commensals (live in close relationship in which one profits from the relationship and the other neither benefits nor is harmed)
- parasites (live on or within host from which they derive benefits without making any useful contribution in turn)

Function:

- degrade organic matter

A list of mycoses caused by various fungi is given in Table 28.4.

28.1.4 Neuroimaging Findings

General Imaging Findings
- Variable imaging features depending on causative organism
- In general, multiple parenchymal lesions with variable parenchymal and leptomeningeal enhancement

CT Non-Contrast-Enhanced
- Unspecific imaging features
  - multiple hypointense lesions
  - hydrocephalus
  - hemorrhages

CT Contrast-Enhanced
- Multifocal enhancement
- Ring enhancement possible

MRI-T2
- Multiple hyperintense parenchymal lesions
- *Aspergillosis*:
  - multiple abscesses with hypointense rim and hyperintense surrounding edema
- *Cryptococcosis*:
  - enlarged perivascular spaces

MRI-FLAIR
- Multiple hyperintense parenchymal lesions
- *Aspergillosis*:
  - hyperintense perifocal edema, subarachnoid hemorrhages possible (caused by mycotic aneurysms)
- *Cryptococcosis*:
  - multiple hyperintense pseudocysts in basal ganglia

MRI-T1
- Lesions hypo- or hyperintense (subacute hemorrhage)

MRI-T1 Contrast-Enhanced
- Leptomeningeal enhancement, solid or ring enhancement
- *Cryptococcosis*:
  - nodular leptomeningeal and parenchymal enhancement

MRI-T2*/SWI
- *Aspergillosis*:
  - Subarachnoid hemorrhages, hemorrhagic infarctions

MR-Diffusion Imaging
- Restricted diffusion in abscesses and hemorrhagic infarctions

Nuclear Medecine Imaging Findings
- Most nuclear medicine studies are dealing with cutaneous or pulmonary mycosis.
- There have been some trials for imaging fungal infections by labeling fluconazole and differentiate them from bacterial infections or sterile inflammation but not in the brain.
- A case report states uptake of 201Tl-chloride in a mixed fungal/bacterial brain abscess.
- Another case report states increased HMPAO-uptake in the parasitic infectious region of the cerebrum with reduced contralateral cerebellar uptake due to diaschisis.
- Some efforts are made by labeling antibiotics.

28.1.5 Neuropathology Stains

Special Stains Include:
- Gomori methenamine silver (GMS)
  - Stains fungi in histological sections
  - Detects all fungi
  - Stains hyphae and yeasts
- Grocott
  - Stains fungi in histological sections
  - Detects all fungi
  - Stains hyphae and yeasts
- Periodic acid-Schiff (PAS)
  - Stain for fungi
  - Stains yeasts and hyphae
  - CAVE: PAS-positive artifacts might resemble yeast cells
- Mucicarmine
  - Stain for mucin
  - Stains capsular material of *Cryptococcus neoformans*
- Gram stain
  - Stains bacteria and fungi
  - Stains most yeasts and hyphae
  - Most fungi stain Gram-positive
- Giemsa stain
  - Used for peripheral blood smears
  - Detects intracellular *Histoplasma capsulatum*
  - Detects intracystic and trophic forms of *Pneumocystis jirovecii*

Neuropathological changes seen in various mycoses and fungal morphology summarized in Table 28.5.

Immunophenotype
- Specific antibodies might be available

Differential Diagnosis
- Bacterial infections
- Necroses of malignant brain tumors or metastases
- Intravascular lymphoma

28.1.6 Molecular Neuropathology

Pathogenesis
- among immunocompromised individuals (transplant patients, HIV-infected patients, cancer patients undergoing chemotherapy)
- hospitalized people with serious underlying diseases
- modulation of yeast and host immune system interactions
- presentation of surface antigens modulating the T-helper pathway
- stimulation of an ineffective TH2 immune response
- urease production
- extracellular proteinases
- modulation of the pH of the phagolysosome

28.1.7 Treatment

Antifungal agents include:
- Allylamines
- Antimetabolite
- Imiazoles
- Triazoles
- Echinocandins
- Polyenes
- Chitin synthesis inhibitors

28.2 Aspergillus Fumigatus

Table 28.5 Neuropathological changes seen in various mycosis and fungal morphology

Mycosis	Neuropathologic changes	Fungal morphology
Aspergillosis	• Abscess • Granuloma • Extensive hemorrhage	• Branching hyphae • Septate hyphae
Blastomycosis	• Epiduritis • Pachymeningitis • Purulent or granulomatous meningitis	• Central, basophilic body with wall • Single bud
Candidiasis	• Abscess or granuloma • Meningitis (rare)	• Chains of elongated cylindrical pseudohyphae
Chromomycosis	• Meningitis • Abscess • Diffuse encephalitis	• Hyphae • Rarely spores
Cledosporiosis	• Abscess • Meningitis	• Hyphae
Coccidioidomycosis	• Basal meningitis • Vasculitis	• Hyphae
Cryptococcosis	• Meningitis	• Spores with capsule
Histoplasmosis	• Meningitis with vasculitis • Granuloma (rare)	• Small ovoid budding bodies • intracellular
Paracoccidioidomycosis	• Meningitis • Space-occupying lesions	• Multiple budding
Pseudoallescheriosis	• Meningitis • Abscess • Vasculitis	• Septated hyphae • Clamidospores
Zygomycosis	• Necrosis • Polymorphs with giant cells • Vasculitis with hemorrhage	• Broad branching, non-septated hyphae

Biologic Behavior–Prognosis–Prognostic Factors
- Sanitation of the primary focus
- State of immunodeficiency or immunocompetence

28.2 Aspergillus Fumigatus

28.2.1 Neuroimaging Findings

MRI-T2 (Fig. 28.1a)
- Multiple hyperintense parenchymal lesions
- Multiple abscesses with hypointense rim and hyperintense surrounding edema

MRI-FLAIR (Fig. 28.1b)
- Multiple hyperintense parenchymal lesions
- Hyperintense perifocal edema, subarachnoid hemorrhages possible (caused by mycotic aneurysms)

MRI-T1 (Fig. 28.1c)
- Lesions hypo- or hyperintense (subacute hemorrhage)

MRI-T1 Contrast-Enhanced (Fig. 28.1d)
- Leptomeningeal enhancement, solid or ring enhancement

MRI-T2∗/SWI
- Subarachnoid hemorrhages, hemorrhagic infarctions

MR-Diffusion Imaging (Fig. 28.1e, f)
- Restricted diffusion in abscesses and hemorrhagic infarctions

28.2.2 Neuropathology Findings

Fungal Morphology
- Hyphae
  - Septate
  - Dichotomous, acute-45° branches
  - Uniform width 3–6 μm

Macroscopic Features (Fig. 28.2a–l)
- A wide spectrum of changes of the brain might be seen.
- Abscess formation.
- Granuloma formation.
- Aspergillus is located in large vessels, thus the lesions are associated with hemorrhage and hemorrhagic infarctions in large areas of the brain.

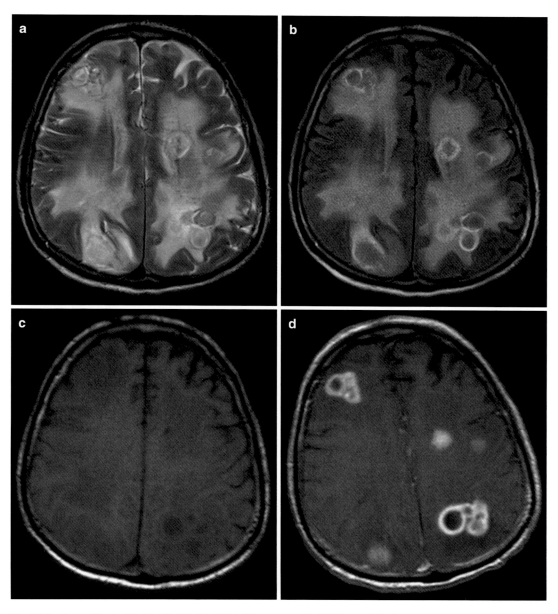

Fig. 28.1 Aspergillosis; T2 (**a**), FLAIR (**b**), T1(**c**), T1 contrast (**d**), DWI (**e**), ADC (**f**)

28.2 Aspergillus Fumigatus

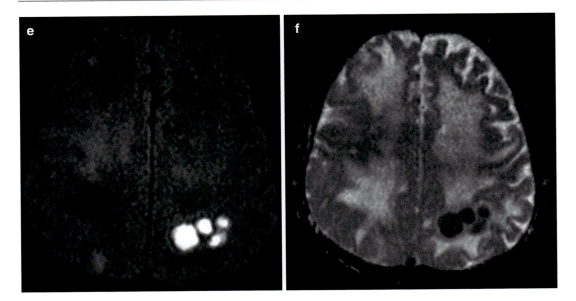

Fig. 28.1 (continued)

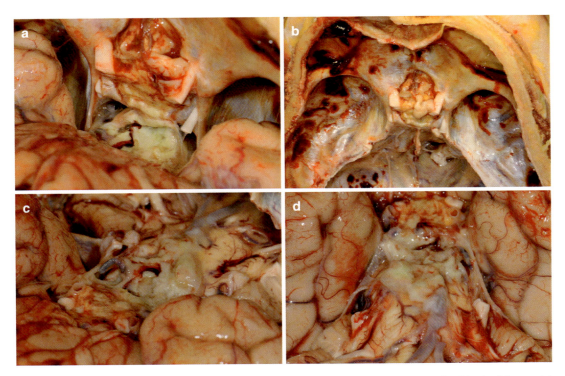

Fig. 28.2 Macroscopic appearance of leptomeningoencephalitis due to *Aspergillus fumigatus*. Yellowish pus in the tuberculum sellae (**a**, **b**), pus covering the base of the brain extending from the optic chiasm until the medulla oblongata (**c**, **d**) in the unfixed brain, pus covering the base of the brain extending from the optic chiasm until the medulla oblongata (**e**, **f**) in the fixed brain. Discrete (**g**) and severe (**h**) signs of leptomeningitis with destruction of the underlying tissue (**h**), cystic necroses in the cerebellum (**i**, **j**), yellowish-reddishly colored softened tissue undergoing necrosis and abscess formation (**k**, **l**)

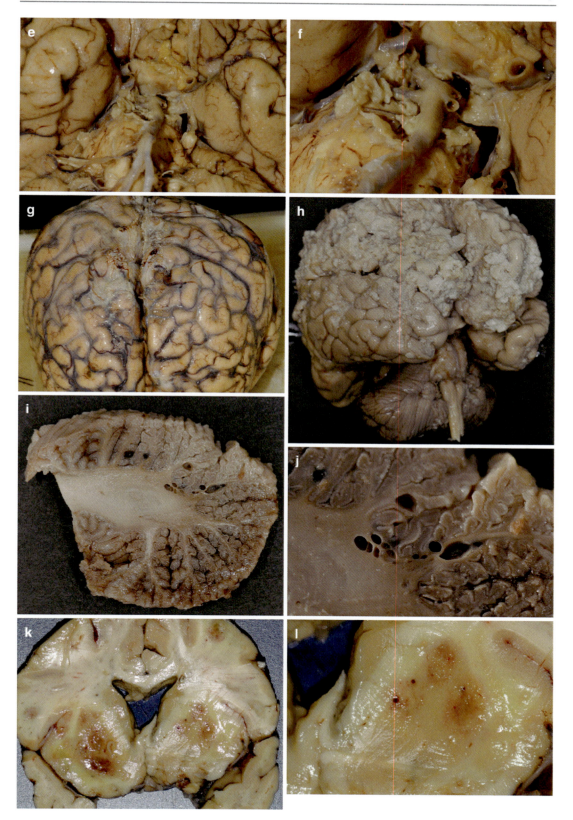

Fig. 28.2 (continued)

28.2 Aspergillus Fumigatus

Microscopic Features (Fig. 28.3a–l)
- The vessel walls are invaded by septated and branching hyphae.
- Thrombosis of the vessels and invasion of the tissue by the organisms is associated with necrosis.

28.2.3 Molecular Neuropathology

Pathogenesis
- *Aspergillus* is very common both indoors and outdoors.
- Most people breathe in fungal spores every day.

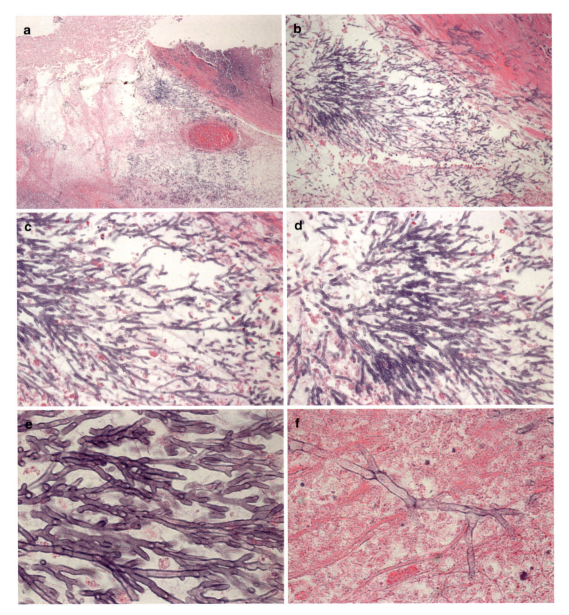

Fig. 28.3 Microscopic appearance of leptomeningoencephalitis due to *Aspergillus fumigatus*. Tissue destruction with the presence of bluish septated and branched hyphae (**a–f**, stain: H&E), Special staining of hyphae by Grocott (**g–j**, stain Grocott) and budding (**j**). Hyphae within a vessel wall (**k**, **l**, stain: PAS)

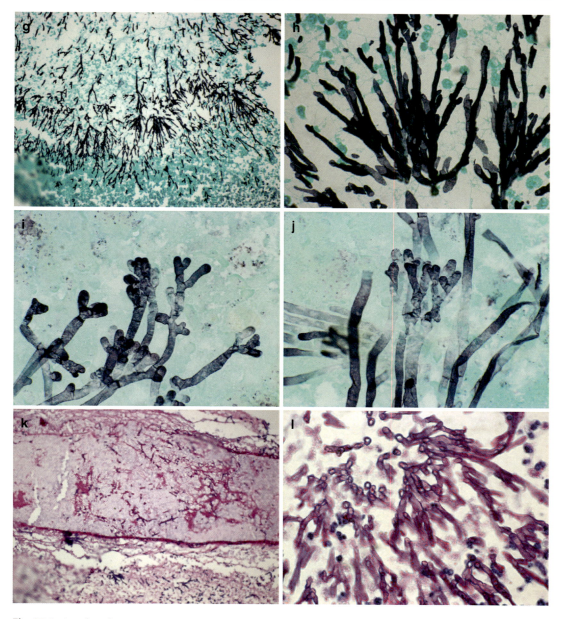

Fig. 28.3 (continued)

- Immunocompromised people (weakened immune system after a stem cell transplant or organ transplant, chemotherapy for cancer, or high doses of corticosteroids develop invasive aspergillosis).
- Foci in the lungs and gastrointestinal tract.

28.3 *Cryptococcus Neoformans*

28.3.1 Neuroimaging Findings

MRI-T2 (Fig. 28.4a)
- multiple hyperintense parenchymal lesions
- enlarged perivascular spaces

28.3 Cryptococcus Neoformans

MRI-FLAIR (Fig. 28.4b)
- multiple hyperintense parenchymal lesions
- multiple hyperintense pseudocysts in basal ganglia

MRI-T1 (Fig. 28.4c)
- Lesions hypointense

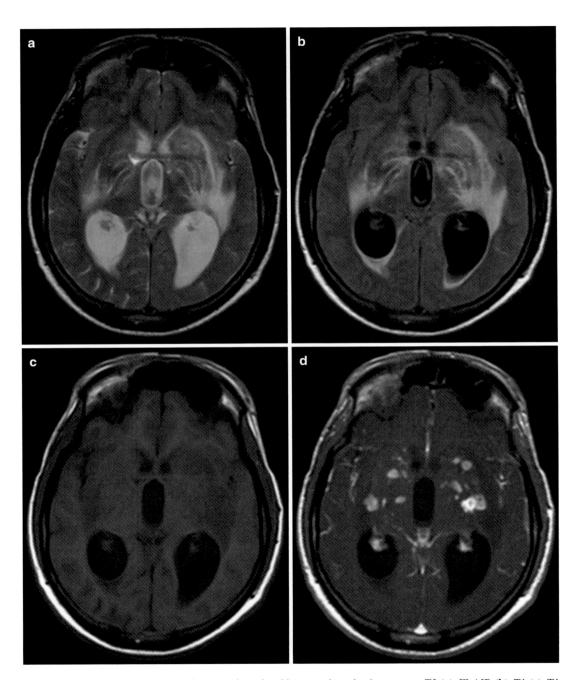

Fig. 28.4 Cryptococcosis with nodular parenchymal and leptomeningeal enhancement; T2 (**a**), FLAIR (**b**), T1 (**c**), T1 contrast (**d, e**), DWI (**f**), ADC (**g**)

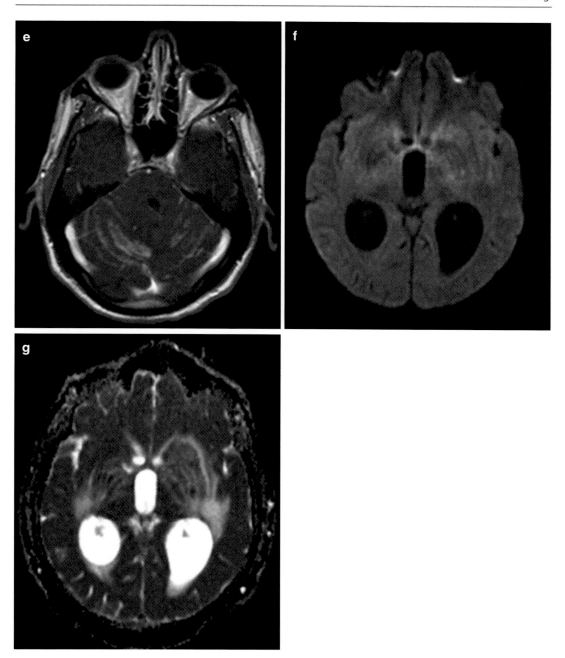

Fig. 28.4 (continued)

28.3 Cryptococcus Neoformans

MRI-T1 Contrast-Enhanced (Fig. 28.4d, e)
- Leptomeningeal enhancement, solid or ring enhancement
- Nodular leptomeningeal and parenchymal enhancement

MR-Diffusion Imaging (Fig. 28.4g, f)
- Restricted diffusion in abscesses

28.3.2 Neuropathology Findings

Fungal Morphology
- Yeast
  - spherical budding
  - variable size 2–15 μm

Macroscopic Features (Fig. 28.5a–l)
- The appearance of the brain lesions due to cryptococcus is diverse.
  - Sometimes no changes can be discerned.
  - Small or large foci of gelatinous material may be seen either in the leptomeninges or within the brain parenchyma.

Microscopic Features (Figs. 28.6a–r and 28.7a–d)
- The gelatinous areas are composed of thick mucin-positive capsules that contain the cryptococcus spores.
- There may be minimal inflammatory response in the neighborhood of the capsules.

28.3.3 Molecular Neuropathology

Pathogenesis
- People can become infected with *C. neoformans* after inhalation of the microscopic fungus followed by a state of latency in the lungs.
- Most people who are exposed to the fungus never get sick from it.
- Cryptococcosis occurs predominantly in immunocompromised patients, most commonly those with HIV/AIDS as well as in solid organ transplant recipients, and in people with no apparent immune defects.
- Cryptococcosis occurs during latency breakdown in the setting of immune deficiency.
- HIV-associated cryptococcosis is heralded by CD4 T-cell counts less than 100 cells/μL and detectable serum cryptococcal antigen (CrAg).
- Cryptococcal virulence
  - The central virulence factor of C. neoformans is its polysaccharide capsule.
  - Other virulence determinants include capacity to grow at mammalian temperatures as well as intracellular replication.
- Host response to C. neoformans
  - Innate and acquired immune mechanisms contribute to resistance to cryptococcosis.
  - CD4 T-cells and cytokines enhance phagocytosis and cryptococcal containment.
  - CD8 T-cells enhance cryptococcal killing.
  - Macrophage phagocytosis promotes cryptococcal containment, but C. neoformans can replicate in macrophages.
  - B-cells enhance resistance to C. neoformans in experimental models.
  - Natural IgM promotes containment of C. neoformans in murine lungs, preventing dissemination to brain.
  - HIV-associated cryptococcosis was linked to reduced levels of IgM memory B-cells and lower levels of IgM.
- Genetic susceptibility to cryptococcosis
  - MBL and Fc-γ receptor polymorphisms have been associated with cryptococcosis.
  - Genetic factors influence susceptibility and resistance to C. neoformans.

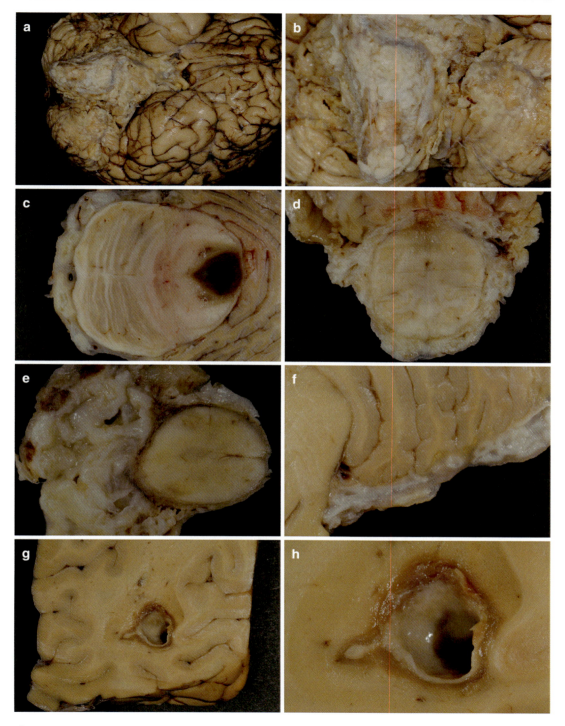

Fig. 28.5 Macroscopic appearance of leptomeningoencephalitis due to *Cryptococcus neoformans*. The leptomeninges of the brain stem and cerebellum (**a–f**) are engorged by a whitish material [brain stem (**a**, **b**), pons (**c**), medulla oblongata (**d**), upper cervical spinal segment (**e**), cerebellum (**f**), Abscess formation (**g**, **h**), and ventriculitis (**i**, **j**)]. Leptomeningeal involvement (**k**, **l**)

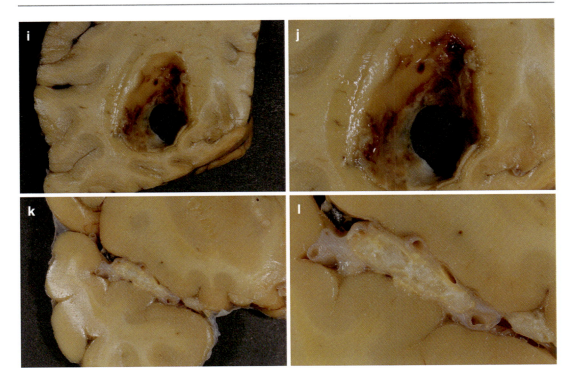

Fig. 28.5 (continued)

28.4 Candida Albicans

28.4.1 Neuropathology Findings

Fungal Morphology
- Yeast
  - Oval
  - Budding
  - Diameter 2–6 μm

Macroscopic Features
- Nonspecific changes are found in the brain.
- Occasionally, a mild to moderate edema with yellow softening of the brain tissue is noted.
- Abscess formation.
- Granuloma formation.
- Meningitis.

Microscopic Features (Fig. 28.8a–l)
- Chains of elongated cylindrical pseudohyphae
- Multifocal microabscesses might be found containing
  - Polymorphonuclear cells
  - Monocytic cells
  - Microglia
  - Sometimes surrounded by tissue necrosis

28.4.2 Molecular Pathology

Pathogenesis
- *Candida* normally lives in the gastrointestinal tract and on skin without causing any problems.

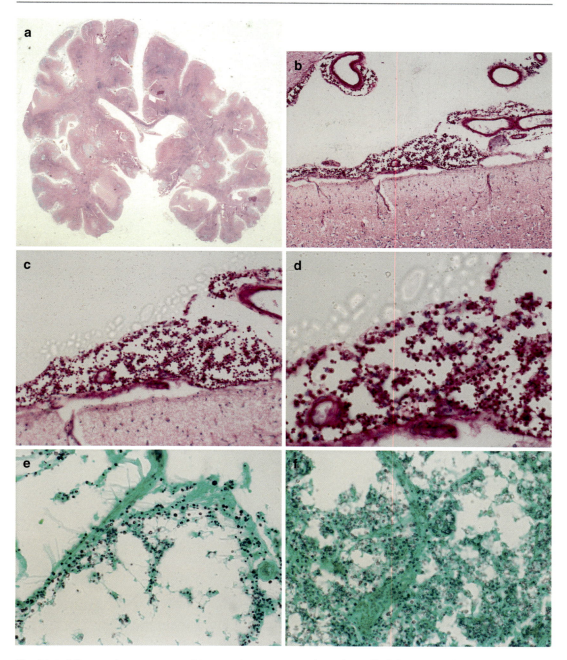

Fig. 28.6 Microscopic appearance of leptomeningoencephalitis due to *Cryptococcus neoformans*. Whole hemispheric section showing the lesions in blue affecting the leptomeninges as well as the brain tissue in the form of gelatinous cystic formations (**a**, stain H&E). Thickened leptomeninges harboring encapsulated organisms (**b–d**, stain PAS) and appearing like black round structures (**e, f**, stain: Grocott). Ventriculitis with accumulation of mono- morphonuclear cells lining the ventricular wall (**g**) and the presence of multinucleated macrophages phagocytosing the parasite (**h–j**, stain **h–i**: H&E, **j**: stain: Grocott). Gelatinous cyst containing parasites (**k, l**, stain: H&E), cyst containing the parasites and macrophages (**m, n**, stain: H&E). Cryptococcus can be well demonstrated with the PAS stain (**o, p**) and even with the cresyl violet (Nissl) stain (**q, r**)

28.4 Candida Albicans

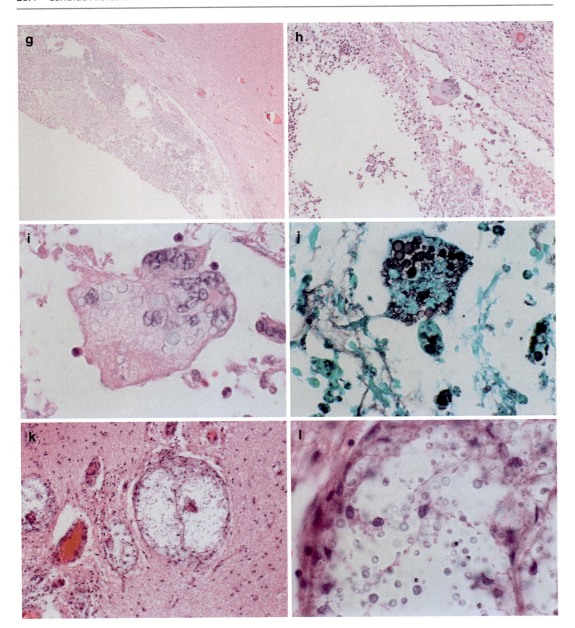

Fig. 28.6 (continued)

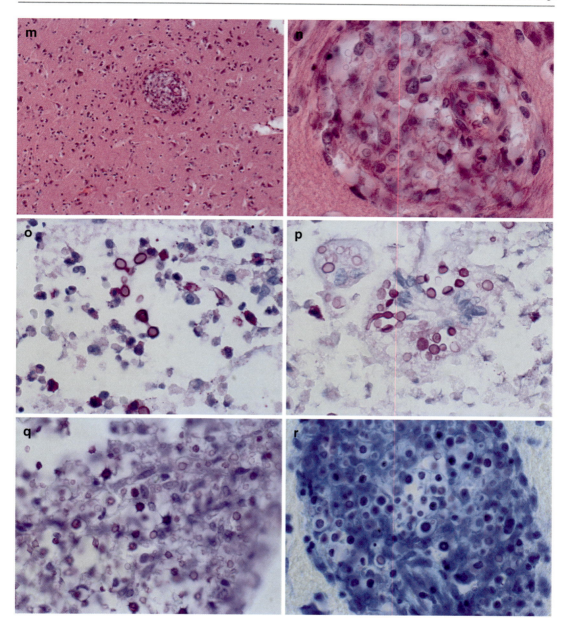

Fig. 28.6 (continued)

28.4 Candida Albicans

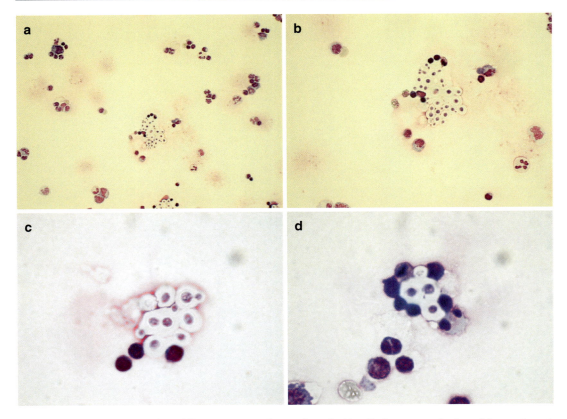

Fig. 28.7 Encapsulated organisms (*Cryptococcus neoformans*) can be identified upon examination of the cerebrospinal fluid (**a–d**)

- Saprophyte in digestive and genital mucosa.
- In the following patients, *Candida* can enter the bloodstream and cause an infection.
  - who have a central venous catheter
  - who are in the intensive care unit (ICU)
  - who have weakened immune systems (organ transplant, HIV/AIDS, or are on cancer chemotherapy)
  - who have taken broad-spectrum antibiotics
  - who have a very low neutrophil (a type of white blood cell) count (neutropenia)
  - who have kidney failure or are on hemodialysis
  - who have had surgery, especially gastrointestinal surgery
  - who have diabetes
- Invasive candidiasis is a serious infection that can affect the blood, heart, brain, eyes, bones, or other parts of the body.

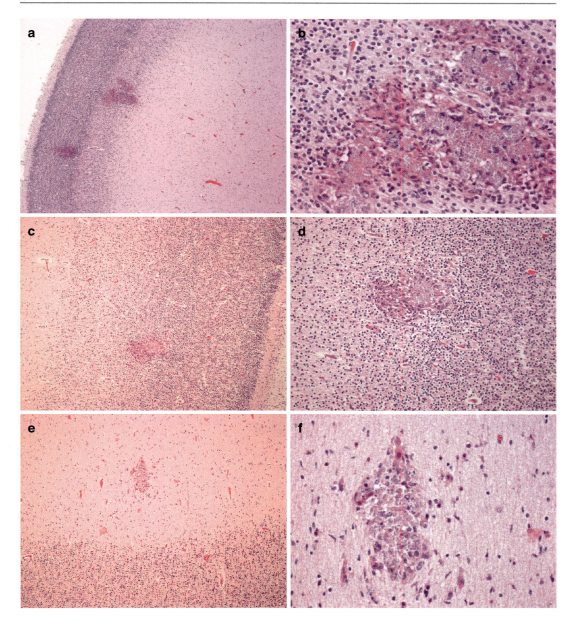

Fig. 28.8 *Candida albicans* encephalitis in a fetal brain. Foci of necroses with the presence of the parasite in the cerebral cortex (**a–d**, stain (H&E)) and white matter (**e, f**, stain H&E), demonstration of the parasite with special stains (**g, h**, stain Grocott; **i–j**, stain: PAS), scant reactive astrogliosis mostly encountered around the lesion (**k–l**, stain: IHC-GFAP)

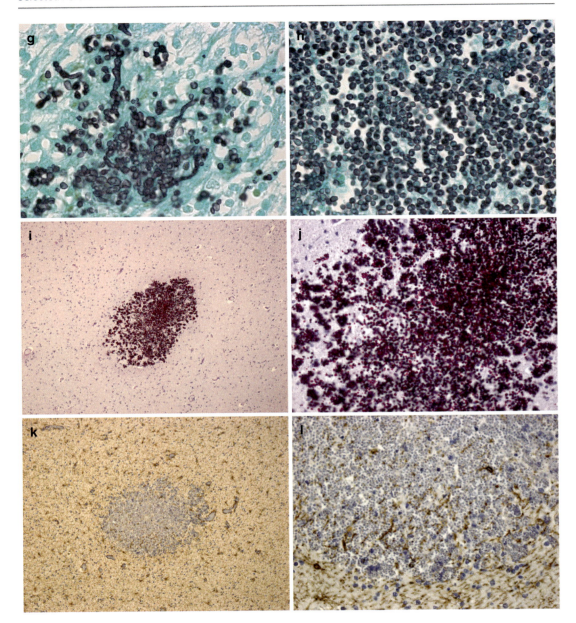

Fig. 28.8 (continued)

Selected References

Almeida F, Wolf JM, Casadevall A (2015) Virulence-associated enzymes of cryptococcus neoformans. Eukaryot Cell 14(12):1173–1185. https://doi.org/10.1128/ec.00103-15

Ashdown BC, Tien RD, Felsberg GJ (1994) Aspergillosis of the brain and paranasal sinuses in immunocompromised patients: CT and MR imaging findings. AJR Am J Roentgenol 162(1):155–159. https://doi.org/10.2214/ajr.162.1.8273655

Brown SM, Campbell LT, Lodge JK (2007) Cryptococcus neoformans, a fungus under stress. Curr Opin Microbiol 10(4):320–325. https://doi.org/10.1016/j.mib.2007.05.014

Chai LY, Vonk AG, Kullberg BJ, Netea MG (2011) Immune response to Aspergillus fumigatus in compromised hosts: from bedside to bench. Future Microbiol 6(1):73–83. https://doi.org/10.2217/fmb.10.158

Cheng YC, Ling JF, Chang FC, Wang SJ, Fuh JL, Chen SS, Teng MM, Chang CY (2003) Radiological manifestations of cryptococcal infection in central nervous system. J Chin Med Assoc 66(1):19–26

Coelho C, Bocca AL, Casadevall A (2014a) The intracellular life of Cryptococcus neoformans. Annu Rev Pathol 9:219–238. https://doi.org/10.1146/annurev-pathol-012513-104653.

Coelho C, Bocca AL, Casadevall A (2014b) The tools for virulence of Cryptococcus neoformans. Adv Appl Microbiol 87:1–41. https://doi.org/10.1016/b978-0-12-800261-2.00001-3. 10.2217/fmb.14.132

da Silva Dantas A, Lee KK, Raziunaite I, Schaefer K, Wagener J, Yadav B, Gow NA (2016) Cell biology of Candida albicans-host interactions. Curr Opin Microbiol 34:111–118. https://doi.org/10.1016/j.mib.2016.08.006

Dagenais TR, Keller NP (2009) Pathogenesis of Aspergillus fumigatus in Invasive Aspergillosis. Clin Microbiol Rev 22(3):447–465. https://doi.org/10.1128/cmr.00055-08

DeLeon-Rodriguez CM, Casadevall A (2016) Cryptococcus neoformans: tripping on Acid in the Phagolysosome. Front Microbiol 7:164. https://doi.org/10.3389/fmicb.2016.00164

Ghazaei C (2017) Molecular insights into pathogenesis and infection with aspergillus fumigatus. Malays J Med Sci 24(1):10–20. https://doi.org/10.21315/mjms2017.24.1.2

Gibbons JG, Rokas A (2013) The function and evolution of the Aspergillus genome. Trends Microbiol 21(1):14–22. https://doi.org/10.1016/j.tim.2012.09.005

Goncalves SS, Souza AC, Chowdhary A, Meis JF, Colombo AL (2016) Epidemiology and molecular mechanisms of antifungal resistance in Candida and Aspergillus. Mycoses 59(4):198–219. https://doi.org/10.1111/myc.12469

Hall RA, Cottier F, Muhlschlegel FA (2009) Molecular networks in the fungal pathogen Candida albicans. Adv Appl Microbiol 67:191–212. https://doi.org/10.1016/s0065-2164(08)01006-x

Harrison TS (2000) Cryptococcus neoformans and cryptococcosis. J Infect 41(1):12–17. https://doi.org/10.1053/jinf.2000.0695

Hohl TM, Feldmesser M (2007) Aspergillus fumigatus: principles of pathogenesis and host defense. Eukaryot Cell 6(11):1953–1963. https://doi.org/10.1128/ec.00274-07

Hole C, Wormley FL Jr (2016) Innate host defenses against Cryptococcus neoformans. J Microbiol (Seoul, Korea) 54(3):202–211. https://doi.org/10.1007/s12275-016-5625-7

Jabra-Rizk MA, Kong EF, Tsui C, Nguyen MH, Clancy CJ, Fidel PL Jr, Noverr M (2016) Candida albicans pathogenesis: fitting within the host-microbe damage response framework. Infect Immun 84(10):2724–2739. https://doi.org/10.1128/iai.00469-16

Karkowska-Kuleta J, Rapala-Kozik M, Kozik A (2009) Fungi pathogenic to humans: molecular bases of virulence of Candida albicans, Cryptococcus neoformans and Aspergillus fumigatus. Acta Biochim Pol 56(2):211–224

Kim J, Sudbery P (2011) Candida albicans, a major human fungal pathogen. J Microbiol (Seoul, Korea) 49(2):171–177. https://doi.org/10.1007/s12275-011-1064-7

Lamoth F (2016) Aspergillus fumigatus-related species in clinical practice. Front Microbiol 7:683. https://doi.org/10.3389/fmicb.2016.00683

Lin X (2009) Cryptococcus neoformans: morphogenesis, infection, and evolution. Infect Genet Evol 9(4):401–416. https://doi.org/10.1016/j.meegid.2009.01.013

Lin X, Heitman J (2006) The biology of the Cryptococcus neoformans species complex. Annu Rev Microbiol 60:69–105. https://doi.org/10.1146/annurev.micro.60.080805.142102

Mayer FL, Wilson D, Hube B (2013) Candida albicans pathogenicity mechanisms. Virulence 4(2):119–128. https://doi.org/10.4161/viru.22913

Naglik JR, Richardson JP, Moyes DL (2014) Candida albicans pathogenicity and epithelial immunity. PLoS Pathog 10(8):e1004257. https://doi.org/10.1371/journal.ppat.1004257

Nobile CJ, Johnson AD (2015) Candida albicans biofilms and human disease. Annu Rev Microbiol 69:71–92. https://doi.org/10.1146/annurev-micro-091014-104330

Noble SM, Gianetti BA, Witchley JN (2017) Candida albicans cell-type switching and functional plasticity in the mammalian host. Nat Rev Microbiol 15(2):96–108. https://doi.org/10.1038/nrmicro.2016.157

O'Meara TR, Alspaugh JA (2012) The Cryptococcus neoformans capsule: a sword and a shield. Clin Microbiol Rev 25(3):387–408. https://doi.org/10.1128/cmr.00001-12

Perfect JR (2006) Cryptococcus neoformans: the yeast that likes it hot. FEMS Yeast Res 6(4):463–468. https://doi.org/10.1111/j.1567-1364.2006.00051.x

Poulain D (2015) Candida albicans, plasticity and pathogenesis. Crit Rev Microbiol 41(2):208–217. https://doi.org/10.3109/1040841x.2013.813904

Powers-Fletcher MV, Hanson KE (2016) Molecular diagnostic testing for Aspergillus. J Clin Microbiol 54(11):2655–2660. https://doi.org/10.1128/jcm.00818-16

Rohatgi S, Pirofski LA (2015) Host immunity to Cryptococcus neoformans. Future Microbiol 10(4):565–581. https://doi.org/10.2217/fmb.14.132.

Sabiiti W, May RC (2012) Mechanisms of infection by the human fungal pathogen Cryptococcus neoformans. Future Microbiol 7(11):1297–1313. https://doi.org/10.2217/fmb.12.102

Sellam A, Whiteway M (2016) Recent advances on Candida albicans biology and virulence. F1000Res 5:2582. https://doi.org/10.12688/f1000research.9617.1

Starkey J, Moritani T, Kirby P (2014) MRI of CNS fungal infections: review of aspergillosis to histoplasmosis and everything in between. Clin Neuroradiol 24(3):217–230. https://doi.org/10.1007/s00062-014-0305-7

Sugui JA, Kwon-Chung KJ, Juvvadi PR, Latge JP, Steinbach WJ (2014) Aspergillus fumigatus and related species. Cold Spring Harb Perspect Med 5(2):a019786. https://doi.org/10.1101/cshperspect.a019786

Tam JM, Mansour MK, Acharya M, Sokolovska A, Timmons AK, Lacy-Hulbert A, Vyas JM (2016) The role of autophagy-related proteins in Candida albicans infections. Pathogens (Basel, Switzerland) 5(2):E34. https://doi.org/10.3390/pathogens5020034

Zhang M, Sun D, Shi M (2015) Dancing cheek to cheek: Cryptococcus neoformans and phagocytes. Mycoses 4:410. https://doi.org/10.1186/s40064-015-1192-3. 10.1111/myc.12415

Prion Encephalopathies

29.1 General Aspects

Human prion encephalopathies include (Table 29.1):
- Creutzfeldt–Jakob disease (CJD)
- Sporadic Creutzfeldt–Jakob disease (sCJD)
- Familial (genetic) Creutzfeldt–Jakob disease (fCJD)
- New variant Creutzfeldt–Jakob disease (vCJD)
- Iatrogenic Creutzfeldt–Jakob disease
- Variable proteinase-sensitive prionopathy (VPSPr)
- Gerstmann–Sträussler–Scheinker syndrome (GSSS)
- Fatal familial insomnia (FFI)
- Kuru
- PrP cerebral amyloid angiopathy

Prion encephalopathies of animals include (Table 29.1):
- Scrapie (among flocks of sheep in the field)
  - Typical forms
  - Atypical or Nor98 scrapie
- Bovine spongiform encephalopathy (BSE)
  - Classical BSE
  - Atypical BSE (H- and L-type)
  - BSE in goats
- Transmissible mink encephalopathy (TME)
- Chronic wasting disease of mule, elk, and deer (CWD)
- Feline spongiform encephalopathy (FSE)
- Lemurs (NHP)
- Exotic ruminant spongiform encephalopathy
- Laboratory transmission of scrapie

Prion diseases are also named "transmissible spongiform encephalopathies" (TSE) as they are characterized by:

- Vacuolization of neurons and neuropil (spongiform changes) (severe form: status spongiosus)
- Transmissibility to other humans and/or animals

Prion diseases are:
- Transmissible
- Infectious
- Neurodegenerative
- Fatal

Prion diseases are microscopically characterized by:
- Spongiform changes in the gray matter
- Neuronal loss
- Reactive astrogliosis
- Reactive microgliosis
- Accumulation of an abnormal form of prion protein in the brain

Table 29.1 List of prion diseases, modified after Aguzzi et al. (2013) reproduced with kind permission by Springer Nature

Disease	Natural host species	Route of transmission or disease-induction mechanism	Other susceptible species
Sporadic CJD	Humans	Unknown	Primates, hamsters, guinea pigs, bank voles, humanized and chimeric human–mouse transgenic mice, and wild-type mice
Iatrogenic CJD	Humans	Accidental medical exposure to CJD-contaminated tissues (dura mater grafts, cornea grafts), hormones, or blood derivatives	Primates, humanized and chimeric human–mouse transgenic mice, and wild-type mice
Familial CJD	Humans	Genetic (germline PRNP mutations)	Primates, bank voles, chimeric human–mouse transgenic mice and wild-type mice
Variant CJD	Humans	Genetic (germline PRNP mutations)	Primates, guinea pigs, humanized transgenic mice, and wild-type mice
Kuru	Humans	Ritualistic cannibalism	Primates and humanized transgenic mice
Fatal familial insomnia	Humans	Genetic (germline PRNP mutations)	Humanized and chimeric human–mouse transgenic mice, and wild-type mice
Sporadic fatal insomnia	Humans	Unknown	Chimeric human–mouse transgenic mice
Gerstmann–Sträussler–Scheinker syndrome	Humans	Genetic (germline PRNP mutations)	Primates, guinea pigs, mutated Prnp transgenic mice, and wild-type mice
Scrapie sheep, goat, and mouflon		Horizontal and possibly vertical	Primates, elk, hamsters, raccoons, bank voles, ovinized transgenic mice (which express sheep PrP^C), and wild-type mice
Atypical scrapie	Sheep and goat	Unknown	Ovinized transgenic mice and porcinized transgenic mice (which express pig PrP^C)
Chronic wasting disease	Mule deer, white-tailed deer, Rocky Mountain elk, and moose	Horizontal and possibly vertical	Primates, ferrets, cattle, sheep, cats, hamsters, bank voles, cervidized transgenic mice (which express deer PrP^C), or murine Prnp-overexpressing transgenic mice
Bovine spongiform encephalopathy BSE	Cattle	Ingestion of BSE-contaminated food	Primates, guinea pigs, humanized and bovinized transgenic mice, and wild-type mice
Atypical bovine spongiform encephalopathy BSE	Cattle	Unknown	Primates, humanized and bovinized transgenic mice, and wild-type mice
Feline spongiform encephalopathy	Zoological and domestic felids	Ingestion of BSE-contaminated food	Wild-type mice
Transmissible mink encephalopathy	Farmed mink	Ingestion of BSE-contaminated food	Primates, cattle, hamsters, and raccoons
Spongiform encephalopathy of zoo animals	Zoological ungulates and bovids	Ingestion of BSE-contaminated food	Wild-type mice

29.1 General Aspects

The causing agent is the:
- Prion = *pro*teinaceous and *in*fectious
- An infectious misfolded amyloidogenic protein

29.1.1 Clinical Signs and Symptoms

- Rapid progressive dementia leading to death within several months to up to 2 years
- Extrapyramidal and/or cerebellar signs
- Myocloni
- Characteristic EEG changes

The criteria for probable, possible, and definite CJD are listed in Table 29.2.

29.1.2 Neuroimaging Findings

General Imaging Findings
- Progressive hyperintensities (T2, FLAIR, DWI) in basal ganglia (putamen and caudate), thalami, and cortex

Table 29.2 List of the criteria for probable, possible, and definite CJD

Possible CJD	• Progressive dementia
	• No or atypical EEG
	• At least 2 of:
	  – Myoclonus
	  – Visual or cerebellar disturbance
	  – Pyramidal/extrapyramidal dysfunction
	  – Akinetic mutism
	• Duration of less than 2 years

Probable CJD	• Progressive dementia
	• Typical EEG
	• At least 2 of:
	  – Myoclonus
	  – Visual or cerebellar disturbance
	  – Pyramidal/extrapyramidal dysfunction
	  – Akinetic mutism

Definite CJD	• Neuropathologic confirmation:
	  – Immunohistochemistry or Western blot
	  – Electron microscopy: scrapie-associated fibril

CT Non-Contrast-Enhanced
- Normal
- Demonstrates progressive atrophy

CT Contrast-Enhanced
- No enhancement

MRI-T2/FLAIR (Figs. 29.1a and 29.2a, b)
- Hyperintensities in basal ganglia, thalami, and cerebral cortex (frontal, temporal, parietal)
- Heidenhain variant predominantly occipital cortex
- Variant CJD:
  – hyperintense posterior thalami (pulvinar sign) or dorsomedial thalami (hockey stick sign), also in sporadic CJD

MRI-T1 (Figs. 29.1c and 29.2c)
- Often normal
- In sporadic CJD hyperintensities in globus pallidus are described.

MRI-T1 contrast-enhanced (Figs. 29.1d and 29.2d)
- No enhancement

MR-Diffusion Imaging (Figs. 29.1b, 29.2e, f and 29.3a–d)
- Most sensitive
- Restricted diffusion in basal ganglia, thalami, and cortex

MR - Spectroscopy
- Reduced NAA:creatine ratio

The UCSF 2011 MRI criteria for sCJD read as follows (Vitali et al. 2011):

MRI definitely CJD
DWI > FLAIR hyperintensities in:
- Classic pathognomonic: cingulate, striatum, and >1 neocortical gyrus (often precuneus angular, superior, or middle frontal gyrus)
- Supportive for subcortical involvement:
  – Striatum with anterior-posterior gradient
  – Subcortical ADC hypointensity

- Supportive for cortical involvement:
  - Asymmetric involvement of midline neocortex or cingulate
  - Sparing of the precentral gyrus
  - ADC cortical ribboning hypointensity
- Cortex only (>3 gyri); see supportive for cortex (above)

MRI probably CJD
- Unilateral striatum or cortex ≤3 gyri; see supportive for subcortical (above); see supportive for cortex (above).
- Bilateral striatum or postero-mesial thalamus; see supportive for subcortical (above).

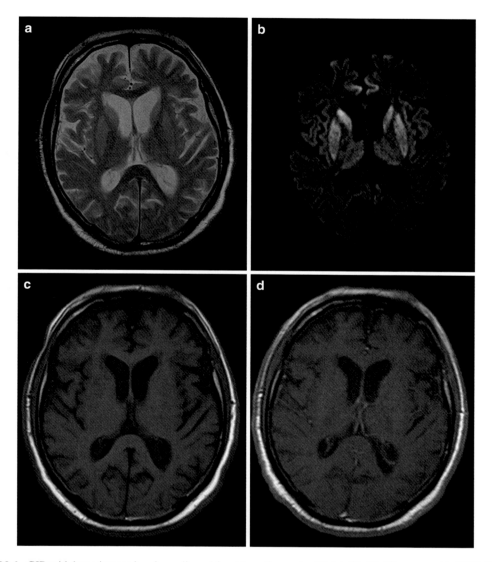

Fig. 29.1 CJD with hyperintense basal ganglia and frontal median cortex T2 (**a**), T1 (**b**), T1 contrast (**c**), DWI (**d**)

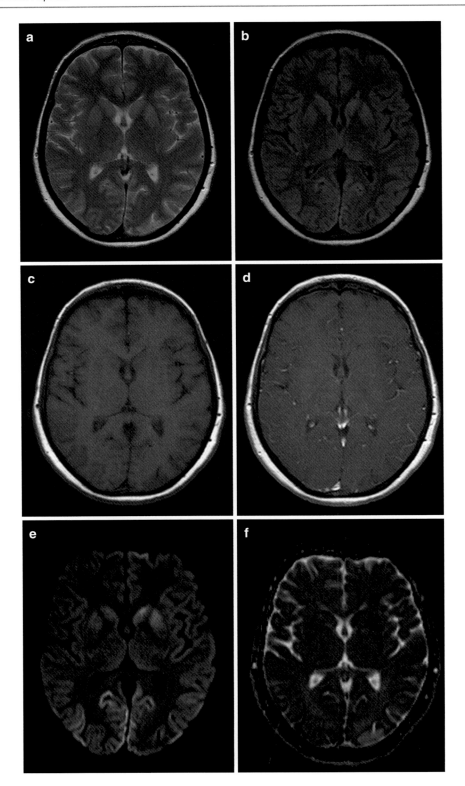

Fig. 29.2 Heidenhain variant with hyperintense lesions primary occipital T2 (**a**), FLAIR (**b**), T1 (**c**), T1 contrast (**d**), DWI (**e**), ADC (f)

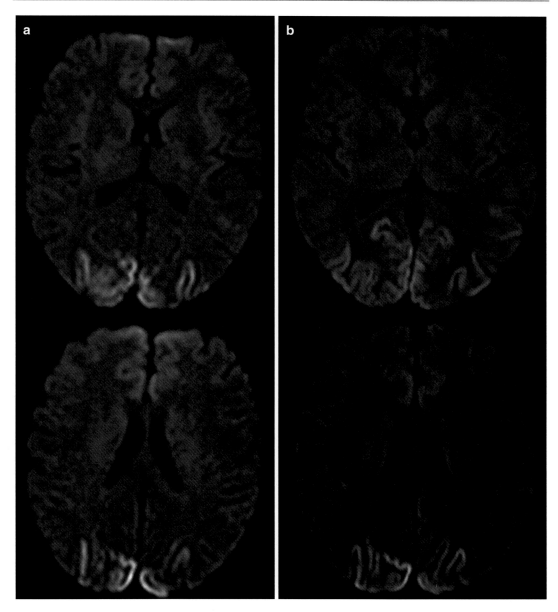

Fig. 29.3 Progression of hyperintense changes in DWI at day 1 (**a**), 1 month (**b**), 2 month (**c**), and 3 month (**d**)

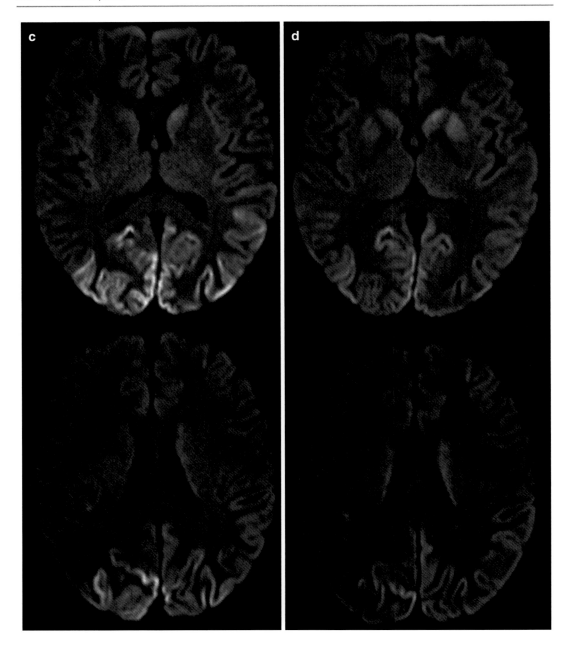

Fig. 29.3 (continued)

Table 29.3 Frequency of gray matter fluid-attenuated inversion recovery (FLAIR) or diffusion-weighted imaging (DWI) hyperintensities in different disease cohorts modified after (Vitali et al. 2011) reproduced with kind permission of Springer Nature

	Neocortical	Limbic	Subcortical
sCJD	85	90	64
fCJD	84	65	65
GSS	13	42	13
Non-prion rapidly progressive dementias	0	22	5

MRI probably not CJD
- Only FLAIR/DWI abnormalities in limbic areas, where hyperintensity can be normal (e.g., insula, anterior cingulate, hippocampi) and ADC map does not show restricted diffusion in these areas.
- DWI hyperintensities due to artifact (signal distortion); see other MRI issues (below).
- FLAIR > DWI hyperintensities; see other MRI issues (below).

MRI definitely not CJD
- No change from prior criteria
- Abnormalities not consistent with CJD

Other MRI Issues
- In prolonged courses of sCJD (>1 year), brain MRI might show significant atrophy with loss of DWI hyperintensity, particularly in areas previously with restricted diffusion.
- To help distinguish abnormality from artifact, obtain sequences in multiple directions (e.g., axial and coronal).

Hyperintensities differ in gray matter fluid-attenuated inversion recovery (FLAIR) or diffusion-weighted imaging (DWI) among sporadic CJD, familial CJD, Gerstmann–Sträussler–Scheinker disease and non-prion progressive dementias (Table 29.3).

Nuclear Medicine Imaging Findings (Figs. 29.4 and 29.5)
- In Creutzfeldt–Jakob disease, FDG-PET shows widespread hypometabolism which is correlated with histopathologic findings like astrocytosis, neuronal death and spongiform change. Studies showed hypometabolism to be more pronounced in the cerebellum, basal ganglia, occipital and temporoparietal lobes.
- In two thirds of the patients, the pattern is asymmetric. There is not one universal pattern of hypometabolism.
- FDG-PET is particular useful in demonstrating hypometabolism of the occipital lobe in patients with visual symptoms (i.e., the Heidenhain variant).
- The pattern of hypometabolism is different from other types of dementia (especially by including cerebellum and basal ganglia).
- Some studies are dealing with changes in cerebral blood flow (using ^{15}O labeled water) and astrocytosis (using a monoamine oxidase B inhibitor).
- PET tracers dealing with prion plaques are investigated.
- CBF-SPECT with HMPAO, ECD, and ^{123}Iodine HIPDM showed hypoperfusion similar to FDG-PET results.

29.1.3 Neuropathology Findings

Macroscopic Features (Fig. 29.6)
- No changes
- Atrophy
- Reduced brain weight

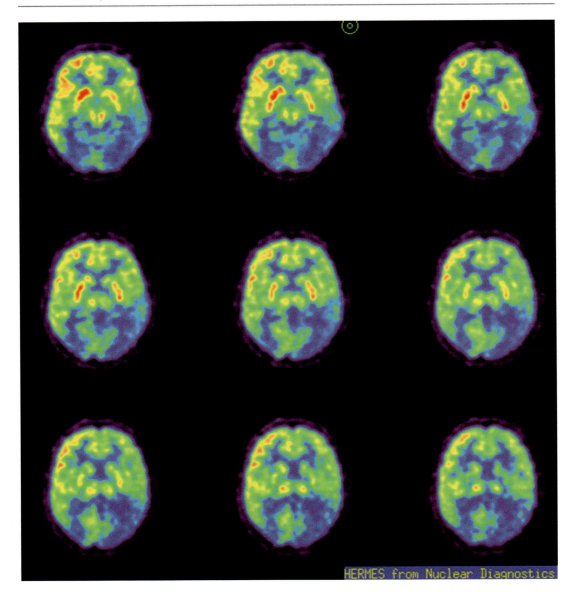

Fig. 29.4 FDG-PET (slices) of a patient with Creutzfeldt–Jakob disease (Heidenhain variant) with asymmetrical hypometabolism in the occipital, temporal, and parietal lobes

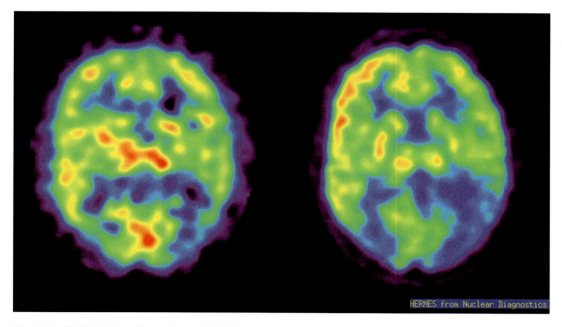

Fig. 29.5 CBF-SPECT and correlating FDG-PET of the same patient as in Fig. 29.4

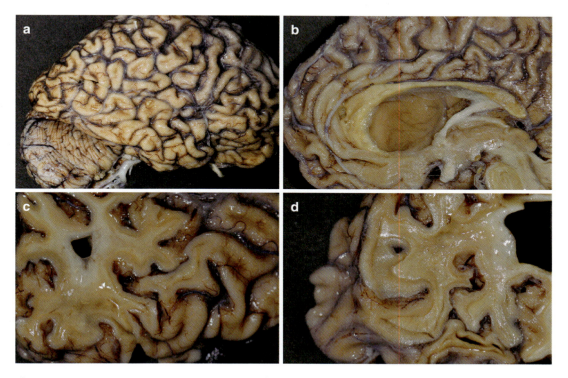

Fig. 29.6 Autopsy brain showing signs of atrophy (**a**, **b**) which are more evident on frontal sections (**c**, **d**)

29.1 General Aspects

Microscopic Features (Figs. 29.7, 29.8, 29.9, 29.10 and 29.11)
- Prion diseases are microscopically characterized by:
- Spongiform changes in the gray matter (Fig. 29.7a–p).
- Accumulation of an abnormal form of prion protein in the brain (Fig. 29.8a–m).
- Neuronal loss.
- Reactive astrogliosis (Fig. 29.9a–h).
- Reactive microgliosis (Fig. 29.10a–h).
- Associated pathology includes the presence of neurofibrillary tangles, amyloid plaques, Lewy bodies (Fig. 29.11a–f).

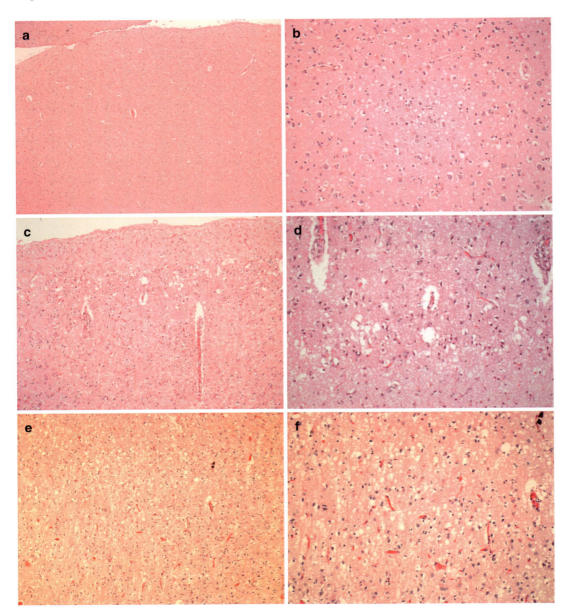

Fig. 29.7 Spongiform changes (**a–n**) in the cerebral cortex (**a–h**), basal ganglia (**i, j**), cerebellum (**k, l**) at various degrees: mild (**a–d**), moderate (**e, f**), severe (**g, h**). Intracytoplasmatic intraneuronal spongiform change (→) (**m, n**). Reactive astrogliosis (→) (**o, p**)

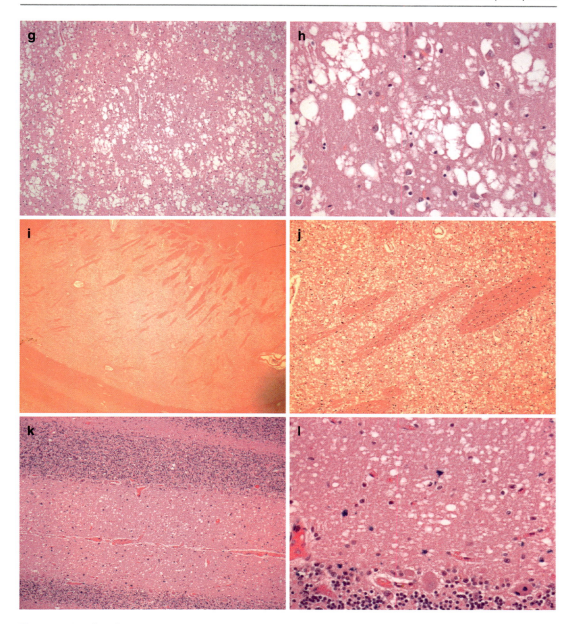

Fig. 29.7 (continued)

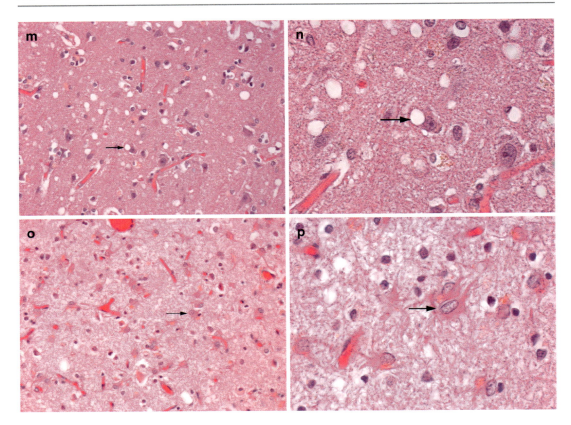

Fig. 29.7 (continued)

Spongiform changes
- Microvacuolar spongiform change
  - Multiple rounded vacuoles within the neuropil of the gray matter
  - Diameter: 2–20 µm
- Confluent spongiform change
  - Larger rounded overlapping vacuoles
- EM: vacuoles consist of membranous and amorphous fragments within distended neuritis

Immunophenotype of PrP deposits (Fig. 29.8a–n.)**:**
- Synaptic
- Perineuronal
- Perivacuolar
- Granular
- Plaque-like

Immunohistochemistry should be performed using various antibodies as each antibody recognizes different epitopes in the prion protein. Paraffin-embedded tissue (PET) blot has higher sensitivity and specificity then immunohistochemistry.

Western blot analysis for the detection of protease-resistant prion protein (PrP^{res}) types:

- Type 1: the non-glycosylated band is ≈ 21 kDa.
- Type 2: the non-glycosylated band is ≈ 19 kDa.
- Type 1 + 2: both bands are found.

Amyloid plaques
- Found in 5–10% of CJD cases
- Immunopositive for PrP-Antibodies
- Immunonegative for ß-Amyloid
- Composed of eosinophilic, PAS-positive round masses with radiating amyloid fibrils in the periphery

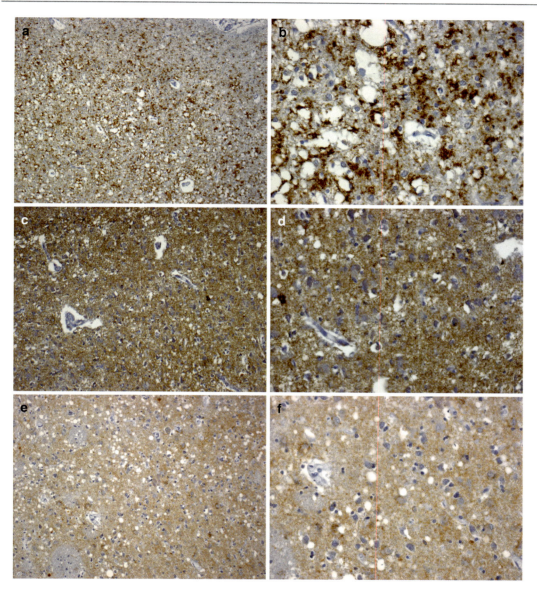

Fig. 29.8 Immunohistochemical staining patterns for prion protein (**a–m**): diffuse synaptic (**a–d**), perineuronal (**a, b**), perivacuolar (**g–j**), plaque-like (**k–n**)

29.1 General Aspects

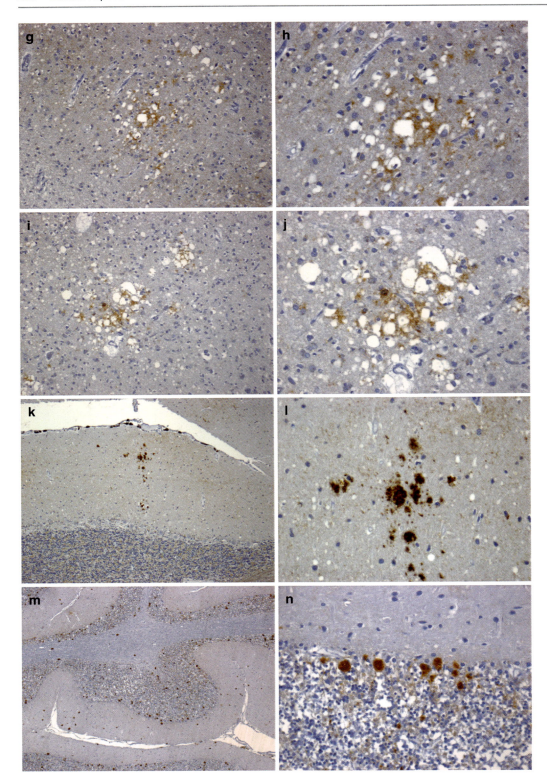

Fig. 29.8 (continued)

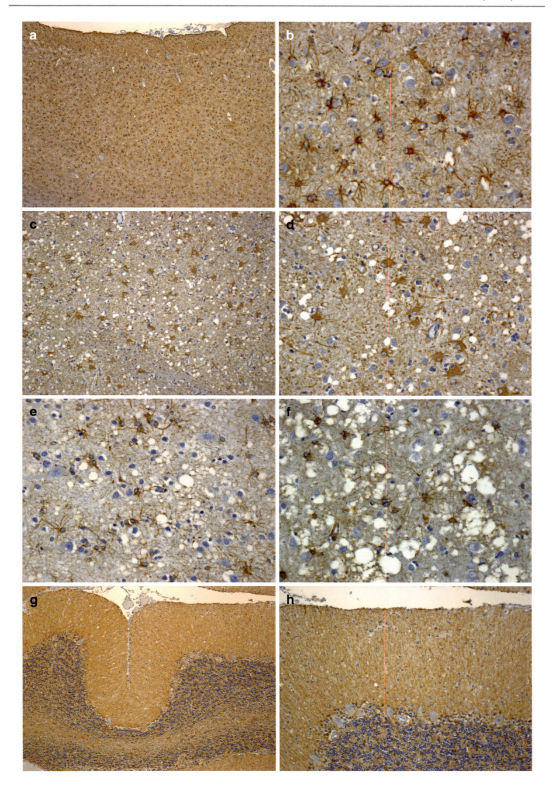

Fig. 29.9 Immunophenotype: reactive astrogliosis (GFAP) (**a–h**), cerebral cortex (**a–f**), cerebellum (**g, h**)

29.1 General Aspects

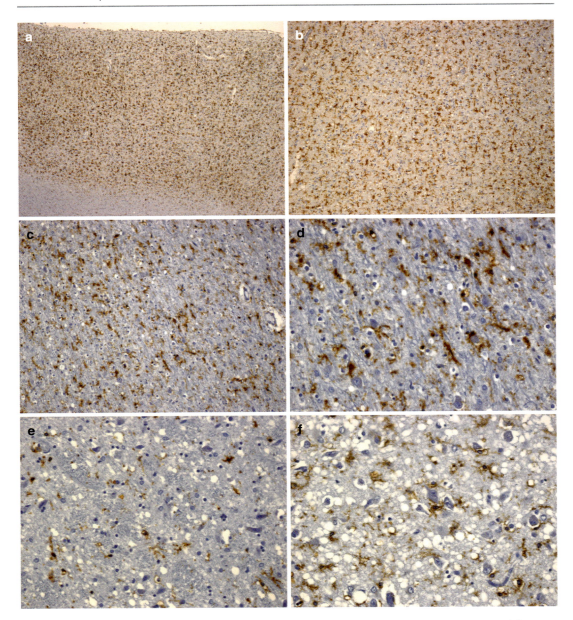

Fig. 29.10 Immunophenotype: reactive microgliosis (HLA-DRII) (**a–j**), cerebral cortex (**a–h**), cerebellum (**i, j**), severe (**a, b**), moderate (**c, d**), mild (**e–h**)

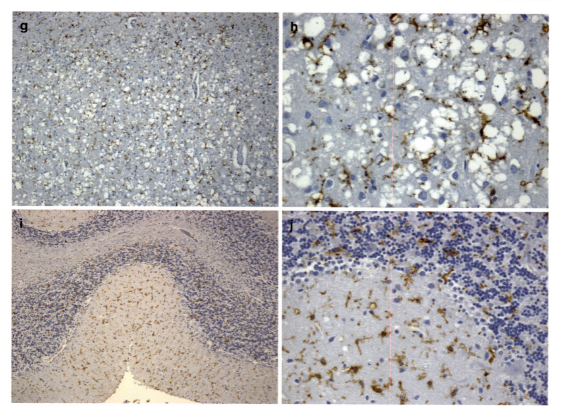

Fig. 29.10 (continued)

Amyloid plaques composed of abnormal PrP:
- Kuru-type plaques
  - Solid core
  - Radiating fibrils
  - Seen in sCJD (MV2 subtype), iCJD
- Multicentric plaques
  - Large irregular plaques
  - Variable multicentric structure
  - Seen in GSS
- Florid plaques
  - composed of a central eosinophilic amyloid core with radiating linear amyloid fibrils surrounded by a corona of spongiform change
  - Seen in vCJD
- Microplaques
  - Small plaques
  - Seen in VPSPr

Differential diagnosis
- Edema
  - vacuoles also in white matter
- Gray matter vacuolization
  - metabolic encephalopathies toxic disorders
- Temporal cortex
  - Pick disease
  - Lewy body dementia

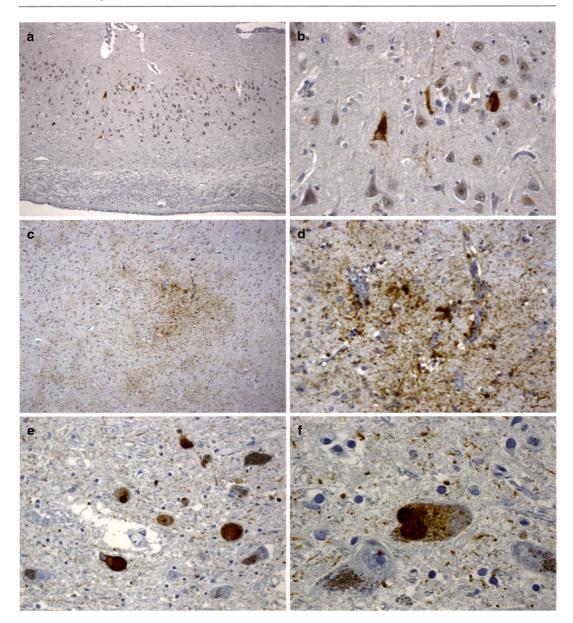

Fig. 29.11 Associated pathology: neurofibrillary tangles in the hippocampal formation (phosphorylated tau) (**a**, **b**), astrocytic plaque (phosphorylated tau) (**c**, **d**), Lewy bodies in the substantia nigra (**e**, **f**)

29.1.4 Treatment and Prognosis

Treatment
- No curative treatment
- Symptomatic
- Antiepileptic drugs

Biologic Behavior-Prognosis-Prognostic Factors
- Rapid progressive decline
- Death over 2–12 months
- GSS might last over several years

29.1.5 Molecular Neuropathology

Cellular Prion Protein (PrP^C)
- Glycosylphosphatidylinositol-anchored, extrinsic cell surface, copper-binding sialoglycoprotein
- Expressed by neurons and astrocytes
- PRNP (gene)
  - Chromosome 20p
  - Polymorphic at codon 129 Valine or Methionine
- Possible physiological role in:
  - Membranes of neurons and glial cells
  - Lymphoreticular system
  - Heart
  - Skeletal muscle
- Possible functional roles:
  - Copper-binding protein in brain membrane fractions.
  - Protects against oxidative stress.
  - Promotes neuroprotection.
  - Is a laminin receptor; laminin/PrP^C interaction plays a role in the learning/memory pathway.
  - Mediates neuronal survival and differentiation, involved in modulation of apoptosis.
  - Involved in signal transduction (cAMP, PKA, ERK).
  - Synaptic transmission and plasticity.
    o Reduced long-term potentiation
    o Reduced excitatory and inhibitory synaptic transmission
  - Memory formation.
    o Reduced spatial learning and memory
    o Reduced avoidance learning and memory
  - Stabilization of sleep and circadian rhythm.
    o Altered circadian rhythm, increased sleep fragmentation, increased SWA after sleep deprivation
  - Neuronal excitability.
    o Reduced Kv4.2 currents
    o Reduced sAHP and calcium-activated potassium currents
    o Increased susceptibility to Kainate-induced seizures
  - Calcium homeostasis.
    o Reduced VGCC currents
    o Increased calcium buffering
  - Glutamate receptor function.
    o Increased NMDA currents, nociception and depressive-like behavior
    o Upregulation of Kainate receptor subunits
  - Neurite outgrowth.
    o Delayed development of cerebellar circuitry
    o Reduced neurite outgrowth in vitro
  - Toxicity elicited by oligomeric species.
    o Protected from LTP reduction induced by toxic Aβ species
  - Neuroprotection.
    o Larger lesions in model of acute cerebral ischemia
    o Decreased SOD activity
  - Copper, zinc, iron, and lactate metabolism.
    o Reduced zinc content in primary neurons
    o Increased lactate-uptake in cultured astrocytes
    o Altered iron and copper metabolism
  - Peripheral myelin maintenance.
    o Age-dependent demyelinating neuropathy
  - PrP^C as a receptor for amyloid-β oligomers.
    o Binding of oligomeric amyloid-β to PrP^C results in a poorly understood signaling pathway, which possibly includes the phosphorylation of FYN, microtubule-associated protein tau (MAPT), and the N-methyl-D-aspartate receptor subunit 2B, ultimately leading to amyloid-β-mediated neurotoxicity.
  - Interactions with various partners (Table 29.4).

29.1 General Aspects

Table 29.4 Reported interacting partners of PrP^C modified after Castle and Gill (2017) reproduced with kind permission by Frontiers Journals, open access

Protein/protein complex	Subcellular localization and function
14-3-3 protein	Cytoplasmic adaptor protein involved in multiple signaling pathways
37/67 kDa laminin receptor	Cell surface receptor for laminin
60 kDa heat shock protein	Mitochondrial chaperone
Annexin A2	Calcium-regulated cell membrane protein with a poorly defined function
Desmoplakin	Organization of cell junctions
Dipeptidyl aminopeptidase-like protein 6	Cell membrane protein that binds to and modulates activity of potassium channels
Doppel	Cell membrane protein of unknown function
Junction plakoglobin (a.k.a. g-catenin)	Organization of cell junctions
Laminin	Extracellular matrix protein with multiple functions (cell migration, adhesion, differentiation, etc.)
Lactate dehydrogenase	Cytoplasmic enzyme that converts lactate to pyruvate and *vice versa*
Metabotropic glutamate receptor	Cell surface receptor for the neurotransmitter glutamate
Neural cell adhesion molecule 1	Cell membrane protein with multiple functions (adhesion, neurite outgrowth, etc)
Nicotinic acetylcholine receptor	Cell surface receptor for the neurotransmitter acetylcholine
Stress-induced phosphoprotein 1	Cytoplasmic co-chaperone; may also be secreted to function as a PrP^C ligand
Tubulin	Cytoskeletal protein (microtubules)
Vimentin	Cytoskeletal protein (intermediate filaments)

Pathological Prion protein PrP^{Sc}
- Abnormal, disease-associated form
- Increased ß-pleated sheet content
- Consists solely of proteins
- Lacks nucleic acid
- Decreased solubility
- Increased protease resistance
- Resists conventional sterilization
- No inflammatory or immune reaction
- Does not form neuronal inclusions
- Conversion from PrP^C to PrP^{Sc} proceeds by a seeded aggregation process
  - Location: cell surface, endocytotic pathway
  - Co-factors: polyanions (RNA, glycosaminoglycans), lipids
- Toxic by-product or intermediate in the PrP^C to PrP^{Sc} conversion
- *PRNP* codon 129 polymorphisms (Table 29.5)

Prion Strains
- Distinct versions of prion disease, which differ at the symptomatic and biochemical level, can occur in the same mammalian species, even though the PrP gene is identical in these animals.
- Strain-specific properties encoded by a nucleic acid genome?
- PrP^{Sc} must exist in various distinct pathological conformations, each of which can impart its own conformation onto PrP^C.
- Defined by
  - their biological properties on transmission to wild-type mice
  - characteristic incubation period
  - pattern of vacuolar pathology (lesion profile)

Table 29.5 *PRNP* codon 129 polymorphisms given in percent in prion diseases and normal population

	M/M	V/V	M/V
Sporadic CJD	72	17	12
Iatrogenic CJD (human growth hormone)	31	50	19
vCJD	100	0	0
Normal population	44	11	45
Control Caucasians	37	12	51
Control Japanese	92	0	8

Factors influencing phenotypic variability in human prion disease
- Etiology: sporadic, acquired, or inherited
- Route of infection in acquired disease
- Location of first propagation in inherited and sporadic disease
- Transmission barrier effect (kinetics of prion propagation)
- Infecting prion strain type
- Prion strain mutation or adaptation in host
- Multiple strain infection and strain competition within host
- PrP genotype of source of infecting prion
- Host PRNP genotype: 30 pathogenic mutations; coding polymorphisms; interaction mutations/polymorphisms; codon 129 zygosity; B haplotype; other non-coding changes
- Host genome type—other loci: known major effects on incubation, period, and strain selection
- Differential recruitment of wild-type PrP in inherited prion disease
- Subclinical (carrier) state
- Coexistent non-prion pathology (chronic inflammation)

Cytokines and chemokines involved in prion pathogenesis in the central nervous system
- Chemokine ligand
- Chemokine receptor
- Chemokine receptor (CXC)
- Extracellular signal-regulated kinase (ERK)
- Interleukin 1
- IL-1 receptor 1
- Transforming growth factor-β1
- Tumor necrosis factor
- TNF receptor

Peripheral prion replication and the involvement of follicular dendritic cells (FDCs):
- Peripherally acquired prions replicate in lymphoid follicles of secondary lymphoid organs (SLOs; such as tonsils, spleen, Peyer's patches in the intestines and lymph nodes) and are mainly associated with follicular dendritic cells (FDCs).
- Mature FDCs express high levels of cellular prion protein (PrP^C) and are involved in peripheral prion replication and accumulation.

Prion-induced neurodegeneration
- Prion infection elicits neuronal damage and glial activation.
- Astrocyte-released milk fat globule epidermal growth factor 8 (MFGE8) facilitates phagocytosis of apoptotic neurons by microglia.
- Microglia function as scavengers and have neuroprotective roles in prion pathogenesis.
- Microglia-mediated clearance might become overwhelmed by the progressive accumulation of scrapie prion protein (PrP^{Sc}).
- It is possible that excess prion accumulation in the brain could reprogram microglia into a pro-inflammatory phenotype, which might facilitate the spread of prions within the central nervous system, ultimately leading to worsening of the disease and neurodegeneration.

29.2 Creutzfeldt–Jakob Disease (CJD)

29.2.1 Clinical Signs

- Annual age-adjusted mortality 1–2:1.000.000
- Mean age at death: 67 years
- Rapidly progressing mental deterioration with dementia, myoclonus, motor disturbances
- EEG: period short-wave activity
- Diversity of clinical features (Table 29.7)
- Diverse distribution of neuropathological changes

A list of the criteria for probable, possible, and definite CJD is given in Table 29.6.

Symptoms and signs in pathologically confirmed sporadic Creutzfeldt–Jakob disease (sCJD) display a large variation-based codon 129 genotype, i.e., MM, MV, and VV (Will and Ironside2017).

29.2 Creutzfeldt–Jakob Disease (CJD)

Table 29.6 List of the criteria for probable, possible, and definite CJD

Possible CJD	• Progressive dementia
	• No or atypical EEG
	• At least 2 of:
	  – Myoclonus
	  – Visual or cerebellar disturbance
	  – Pyramidal/extrapyramidal dysfunction
	  – Akinetic mutism
	• Duration of less than 2 years

Probable CJD	• Progressive dementia
	• Typical EEG
	• At least 2 of:
	  – Myoclonus
	  – Visual or cerebellar disturbance
	  – Pyramidal/extrapyramidal dysfunction
	  – Akinetic mutism

Definite CJD	• Neuropathologic confirmation:
	  – Immunohistochemistry or Western blot
	  – Electron microscopy: scrapie-associated fibril

- Forgetfulness
  – MM: 98; MV: 100; VV: 100
- Gait disorder
  – MM: 98; MV: 93; VV: 100
- Language disturbance
  – MM: 61; MV: 49; VV: 44
- Behavioral symptoms
  – MM: 54; MV: 36; VV: 22
- Visual impairment
  – MM: 50; MV: 31; VV: 56
- Cognitive impairment
  – MM: 99; MV: 100; VV: 100
- Myoclonus
  – MM: 95; MV: 93; VV: 91
- Ataxia
  – MM: 64; MV: 76; VV: 94
- Spasticity
  – MM: 62; MV: 38; VV: 44
- Akinetic mutism
  – MM: 59; MV: 27; VV: 22

29.2.2 Macroscopic Features

- No obvious change
- Atrophy of the brain, basal ganglia, or cerebellum

29.2.3 Microscopic Features

- Spongiform degeneration of neurons and their ramifications
- Neuronal loss
- Reactive astrogliosis
- Reactive microgliosis
- Rarely presence of amyloid plaques
- Heterogeneity in the expression of the various changes
- Heterogeneous topographical involvement
  – Cerebral cortex
  – Subiculum of the hippocampal formation
  – Putamen, caudate nucleus
  – Thalamus
  – Molecular layer of the cerebellum
- Rare involvement of the following brain regions.
  – Hippocampus
  – Globus pallidus
  – Brain stem
  – Spinal cord

CJD types based on involved brain regions
- Cortical
- Cortico-striatal with visual loss
- Cortico-striatal without visual loss
- Cortico-striato-cerebellar
- Corticospinal
- Corticonigral

Sporadic CJD can be subtyped based on the *PRNP* codon 129 polymorphism and the PrP^{Sc} isoform (Table 29.7).

Ultrastructural Features
- focal swelling of neurites, i.e., axons and dendrites as well as synapses
- loss of internal organelles
- accumulation of abnormal membranes

Differential Diagnosis
- Alzheimer disease
- Lewy body disease
- Parkinsonism
- Pick disease
- Huntington disease
- Cerebellar disorders
- Amyotrophic lateral sclerosis

Table 29.7 Subclassification of sporadic CJD based on the *PRNP* codon 129 polymorphism and the PrP^{Sc} isoform

Codon 129 genotype PRP type	Previous terminology	Frequency (%)	Onset (years)	Duration (months)	Spongiform change	PrP deposits
MM1 MV1	Myoclonic or Heidenhain	72	63	3.9	Microvacuolar • Cerebral cortex • (Frontal and occipital lobes) • Thalamus • Cerebellum	• Synaptic • Granular
MM2 cortical	Long duration	2–7	52–65	17	Confluent spongiform change: • Cerebral cortex • Entorhinal cortex	• Perivacuolar
MM2 thalamic (sFI)		<1	53	16	Limited changes Patchy spongiform change: • Cerebral cortex • Entorhinal cortex • Cerebellum; marked • Anterior and medial • Thalamic gliosis • Neuronal loss	• Synaptic • Granular
MV2	Cerebellar or ataxic	8–14	59–65	11–18	Microvacuolar Microvacuolar/confluent spongiform change: • Cerebral cortex • Entorhinal cortex • Hippocampus • Basal ganglia • Thalamus kuru-type plaques in • Cerebellar cortex	• Kuru-plaques • Synaptic • Plaque-like deposits
VV1		1–2	39–53	10–15.3	Microvacuolar • Cerebral cortex (frontal lobe) • Entorhinal cortex • Basal ganglia	• Synaptic
VV2	Cerebellar or ataxic	15	60	6.6	Microvacuolar/Confluent spongiform change: • Cerebral cortex layer 3 • Hippocampus • Basal ganglia • Thalamus • Cerebellum severely involved, with neuronal loss, gliosis, and atrophy	• Synaptic • Perineuronal • Plaque-like

- Brain tumors
- Multi-infarct dementia
- Vascular malformations

29.3 Variant CJD

Variant CJD affects younger age groups than sCJD, with a mean age at death of 30 years.

29.3.1 Clinical Signs and Symptoms

- The initial symptoms of vCJD are predominantly psychiatric for a mean of 6 months.
- Progression to a neurological disorder typified by
  - progressive ataxia
  - cognitive impairment
  - involuntary movements
    o dystonia

- chorea
- myoclonus
- Terminal stages are similar to sCJD, with
  - Accumulating neurological deficits leading to helplessness.
  - Death often results from intercurrent infection.
- The median duration of illness is 14 months.

29.3.2 Microscopic Features

- The presence of large numbers of florid plaques.
- in the cerebral cortex and cerebellar cortex
- composed of a central eosinophilic amyloid core with radiating linear amyloid fibrils surrounded by a corona of spongiform change
- Spongiform change is present to a variable extent.
  - in the cerebral cortex, cerebellum, and thalamus
  - is most marked in the caudate nucleus and putamen
- The thalamus also shows severe neuronal loss and gliosis in the posterior nuclei, particularly the pulvinar (correlates with changes in MRI).

Immunophenotype
- intense labeling of the florid plaques
  - in the cerebral and cerebellar cortex
- numerous smaller cluster plaques
- small amorphous "feathery" deposits of PrP around small capillaries and neurons
- accumulation of PrP^{res} in lymphoid tissues outside the CNS
  - in follicular dendritic cells within lymphoid follicles
  - in peripheral autonomic ganglia

29.3.3 Molecular Neuropathology

- The incubation period in vCJD is unknown in individual cases.
  - most probably a mean of 15 years
- Approximately 250 cases of vCJD have been identified worldwide, with 177 occurring in the United Kingdom.
- The likely large exposure of the UK population to the BSE agent via the food chain in the 1980s and 1990s.
- Prevalence of asymptomatic vCJD infection in the UK population of 237–493 per million (assessed by immunohistochemical analyses of abnormal PrP accumulation in lymphoid tissues in appendix and tonsil specimens).
- All three PRNP codon 129 genotypes are susceptible to vCJD infection.

29.4 Gerstmann–Sträussler–Scheinker Disease (GSS)

29.4.1 Clinical signs

- Ataxia
- Tremor
- Extrapyramidal symptoms
- Dysarthria
- Cognitive impairment
- Duration of disease:
  - Median: 5 years
  - Range: 3–8 years
- Autosomal dominant disorder

29.4.2 Microscopic Features

- Multicentric PrP-amyloid plaques (GSS-plaques)
  - mainly found in the molecular layer of the cerebellum
  - also encountered in the cerebral cortex
  - consist of large central masses of amyloid
  - surrounded by small satellite deposits
- Amorphic or primitive plaques
  - molecular layer of the cerebellum
  - diameter 150–200 μm
- Degeneration of the white matter
- Neuronal loss in brain stem and spinal cord
- Rarely neurofibrillary tangles, mainly found in the cerebral cortex

The following two subtypes are described:
- Telencephalic GSS
- GSS with neurofibrillary tangles

Telencephalic GSS
- Abundant amyloid plaques in the cerebral cortex
- Multicentric GSS-plaques, diameter 150–500 μm
- Kuru-plaques, diameter 20–70 μm, mainly white matter

GSS with neurofibrillary tangles
- Abundant multicentric and unicentric plaques
  - Cerebral and cerebellar cortex

29.5 Fatal Familial Insomnia (FFI)

29.5.1 Clinical signs

- Disturbed sleep/wake rhythm
- Progressive insomnia
- Complex hallucinations
- Stupor
- Coma
- Autonomic signs:
  - Hyperhydrosis
  - Pyrexia
  - Tachycardia
  - Hypertension
  - Irregular breathing
- Additional signs:
  - Ataxia
  - Spontaneous and evoked myoclonus
  - Dysarthria
  - Pyramidal signs

29.5.2 Microscopic Features

- Neuronal loss (up to 50%) in the anterior ventral and mediodorsal thalamus
- Cerebral cortex only slightly involved with mild spongiosis in layers II-III
- Reactive astrogliosis
- Absence of amyloid plaques

29.6 Kuru

Neurodegenerative disease exclusively found in Papua and New Guinea among the Fore population.
Endemic in this region: incidence 1% of the total population
Disease transmission through ritual cannibalism

29.6.1 Clinical signs

- In the first (ambulant) stage
  - unsteady stance and gait
  - decreased muscle control
  - tremors
  - difficulty pronouncing words (dysarthria)
  - titubation
- In the second (sedentary) stage
  - Incapable of walking without support.
  - Suffers ataxia and severe tremors.
  - Signs of emotional instability and depression.
  - Uncontrolled and sporadic laughter.
  - Tendon reflexes are still intact.
- In the third and final (terminal) stage
  - Ataxia
  - No longer capable of sitting without support.
  - Dysphagia, or difficulty swallowing.
  - Develop incontinence.
  - Lose the ability to speak.
  - Unresponsive to their surroundings.
- Death occurs within 3 months to 2 years after the first terminal stage symptoms, often because of pneumonia or infection.

29.6.2 Macroscopical Features

- marked atrophy of the cerebellum

29.6.3 Microscopical Features

- Cerebellum:
  - Loss of Purkinje cells
  - Severe proliferation of Bergmann glia

- Mild to moderate vacuolization
- *Kuru-plaques:* plaques with central deposits of amyloid surrounded by a brighter granular or fibrillary ring
• Neuronal loss:
- Brain stem and diencephalon > basal ganglia and cerebral cortex
• No inflammatory reaction

Selected References

Aguzzi A, Nuvolone M, Zhu C (2013) The immunobiology of prion diseases. Nat Rev Immunol 13(12):888–902. https://doi.org/10.1038/nri3553

Annus A, Csati A, Vecsei L (2016) Prion diseases: new considerations. Clin Neurol Neurosurg 150:125–132. https://doi.org/10.1016/j.clineuro.2016.09.006

Atkinson CJ, Zhang K, Munn AL, Wiegmans A, Wei MQ (2016) Prion protein scrapie and the normal cellular prion protein. Prion 10(1):63–82. https://doi.org/10.1080/19336896.2015.1110293

Castle AR, Gill AC (2017) Physiological functions of the cellular prion protein. Front Mol Biosci 4:19. https://doi.org/10.3389/fmolb.2017.00019

Ciric D, Rezaei H (2015) Biochemical insight into the prion protein family. Front Cell Dev Biol 3:5. https://doi.org/10.3389/fcell.2015.00005

Fraser PE (2014) Prions and prion-like proteins. J Biol Chem 289(29):19839–19840. https://doi.org/10.1074/jbc.R114.583492

Galanaud D, Haik S, Linguraru MG, Ranjeva JP, Faucheux B, Kaphan E, Ayache N, Chiras J, Cozzone P, Dormont D, Brandel JP (2010) Combined diffusion imaging and MR spectroscopy in the diagnosis of human prion diseases. Am J Neuroradiol 31(7):1311–1318. https://doi.org/10.3174/ajnr.A2069

Gaudino S, Gangemi E, Colantonio R, Botto A, Ruberto E, Calandrelli R, Martucci M, Vita MG, Masullo C, Cerase A, Colosimo C (2017) Neuroradiology of human prion diseases, diagnosis and differential diagnosis. Radiol Med 122(5):369–385. https://doi.org/10.1007/s11547-017-0725-y

Geschwind MD (2015) Prion diseases. Continuum 21(6 Neuroinfectious Disease):1612–1638. https://doi.org/10.1212/con.0000000000000251

Hartmann A, Muth C, Dabrowski O, Krasemann S, Glatzel M (2017) Exosomes and the prion protein: more than one truth. Front Neurosci 11:194. https://doi.org/10.3389/fnins.2017.00194

Jackson WS, Krost C (2014) Peculiarities of prion diseases. PLoS Pathog 10(11):e1004451. https://doi.org/10.1371/journal.ppat.1004451

Kallenberg K, Schulz-Schaeffer WJ, Jastrow U, Poser S, Meissner B, Tschampa HJ, Zerr I, Knauth M (2006) Creutzfeldt-Jakob disease: comparative analysis of MR imaging sequences. Am J Neuroradiol 27(7):1459–1462

Kang HE, Mo Y, Abd Rahim R, Lee HM, Ryou C (2017) Prion diagnosis: application of real-time quaking-induced conversion. Biomed Res Int 2017:5413936. https://doi.org/10.1155/2017/5413936

Linsenmeier L, Altmeppen HC, Wetzel S, Mohammadi B, Saftig P, Glatzel M (2017) Diverse functions of the prion protein - Does proteolytic processing hold the key? Biochim Biophys Acta Mol Cell Res 1864(11 Pt B):2128–2137. https://doi.org/10.1016/j.bbamcr.2017.06.022

Lodi R, Parchi P, Tonon C, Manners D, Capellari S, Strammiello R, Rinaldi R, Testa C, Malucelli E, Mostacci B, Rizzo G, Pierangeli G, Cortelli P, Montagna P, Barbiroli B (2009) Magnetic resonance diagnostic markers in clinically sporadic prion disease: a combined brain magnetic resonance imaging and spectroscopy study. Brain 132(Pt 10):2669–2679. https://doi.org/10.1093/brain/awp210

Macedo B, Cordeiro Y (2017) Unraveling prion protein interactions with aptamers and other PrP-binding nucleic acids. Biomed Res Int 18(5):E1023. https://doi.org/10.3390/ijms18051023

Obst J, Simon E, Mancuso R, Gomez-Nicola D (2017) The role of microglia in prion diseases: a paradigm of functional diversity. Front Aging Neurosci 9:207. https://doi.org/10.3389/fnagi.2017.00207

Pandya HG, Coley SC, Wilkinson ID, Griffiths PD (2003) Magnetic resonance spectroscopic abnormalities in sporadic and variant Creutzfeldt-Jakob disease. Clin Radiol 58(2):148–153

Senatore A, Restelli E, Chiesa R (2013) Synaptic dysfunction in prion diseases: a trafficking problem? Int J Cell Biol 2013:543803. https://doi.org/10.1155/2013/543803

Takada LT, Geschwind MD (2013) Prion diseases. Semin Neurol 33(4):348–356. https://doi.org/10.1055/s-0033-1359314

Thompson A, MacKay A, Rudge P, Lukic A, Porter MC, Lowe J, Collinge J, Mead S (2014) Behavioral and psychiatric symptoms in prion disease. Am J Psychiatry 171(3):265–274. https://doi.org/10.1176/appi.ajp.2013.12111460

Tschampa HJ, Zerr I, Urbach H (2007) Radiological assessment of Creutzfeldt-Jakob disease. Eur Radiol 17(5):1200–1211. https://doi.org/10.1007/s00330-006-0456-2

Ukisu R, Kushihashi T, Tanaka E, Baba M, Usui N, Fujisawa H, Takenaka H (2006) Diffusion-weighted MR imaging of early-stage Creutzfeldt-Jakob disease: typical and atypical manifestations. Radiographics 26(Suppl 1):S191–S204. https://doi.org/10.1148/rg.26si065503

Vitali P, Maccagnano E, Caverzasi E, Henry RG, Haman A, Torres-Chae C, Johnson DY, Miller BL, Geschwind MD (2011) Diffusion-weighted MRI hyperintensity patterns differentiate CJD from other rapid dementias. Neurology 76(20):1711–1719. https://doi.org/10.1212/WNL.0b013e31821a4439

Will RG, Ironside JW (2017) Sporadic and infectious human prion diseases. Cold Spring Harb Perspect Med 7(1). https://doi.org/10.1101/cshperspect.a024364

Wulf MA, Senatore A, Aguzzi A (2017) The biological function of the cellular prion protein: an update. BMC Biol 15(1):34. https://doi.org/10.1186/s12915-017-0375-5